D1608403

Introduction to Radiation Therapy

Principles and Practice of Radiation Therapy

VOLUME I

Introduction to Radiation Therapy

Edited by

Charles M. Washington, BS, RT(T)

Director, Radiation Therapy Program
M.D. Anderson Cancer Center
The University of Texas
Houston, Texas

Dennis T. Leaver, MS, RT(R)(T)

Director, Radiation Therapy Program
Southern Maine Technical College
South Portland, Maine

with 211 illustrations

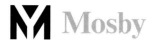 Mosby

St. Louis Baltimore Boston Carlsbad Chicago Naples New York Philadelphia Portland
London Madrid Mexico City Singapore Sydney Tokyo Toronto Wiesbaden

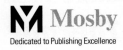

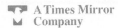

Vice President and Publisher: Don Ladig
Editor: Jeanne Rowland
Developmental Editor: Lisa Potts
Editorial Assistant: Carole Glauser
Project Manager: Linda McKinley
Associate Production Editor: Paul Stoecklein
Designer: Elizabeth Fett
Electronic Production Coordinator: Joan Herron
Manufacturing Supervisor: Karen Lewis

Printed in the United States of America

Composition by Mosby Electronic Production—St. Louis
Lithography by Top Graphics
Printing/binding by Maple Vail Book Manufacturing Group

Mosby–Year Book, Inc.
11830 Westline Industrial Drive
St. Louis, Missouri 63146

Library of Congress Cataloging in Publication Data
Principles and practice of radiation therapy / edited by Charles M.
    Washington, Dennis T. Leaver.
                    p.   cm.
        Includes bibliographical references and index.
        Contents: v. 1. Introduction to radiation therapy.
        ISBN 0-8151-9145-6 (hardback)
        1. Cancer--Radiotherapy.   I. Washington, Charles M. II. Leaver,
    Dennis T.
        [DNLM: 1. Radiation Oncology--methods.   WN 250 P957 1996]
    RC271.R3P734 1996
    616.99' 442--dc20
    DNLM/DLC
    for Library of Congress   96–4954
                                                         CIP

98 99 00 / 9 8 7 6 5 4 3 2

Contributors

Linda Alfred, BS, MEd, RT(T)
Applications Manager,
Varian Oncology Systems,
Palo Alto, California

Edward Aribisala, MS, RT(T)
Administrative Director,
Radiation Oncology Department,
Hurley Medical Center,
Flint, Michigan

Lana Havron Bass, BS, RT(R)(T)
Director,
Texas Oncology School of Radiation Therapy,
Sammons Cancer Center,
Baylor University Medical Center,
Dallas, Texas

Judith Bastin, MS, RT(R)(T)
Director, Radiation Therapy Program,
National-Louis University,
Evanston, Illinois

Diana Browning, MBA, RT(T)
Division Administrator,
Division of Radiotherapy,
M.D. Anderson Cancer Center,
The University of Texas,
Houston, Texas

Annette Coleman, BS, MA, RT(T)
Educational Coordinator/Technology,
Joint Center for Radiation Therapy,
Massachusetts College of Pharmacy and Allied Health Sciences,
Boston, Massachusetts

Stephanie Eatmon, EdD, RT(T)
Program Director,
Radiation Therapy Program,
Health Science Department,
California State University–Long Beach,
Long Beach, California

Wesley English, MD
Attending Surgeon,
Northeast Surgery, PA
Bangor, Maine

J.H. Hannemann, MD
Radiation Oncologist,
Department of Radiation Oncology,
Southern Maine Radiation Therapy Institute,
Portland, Maine

Dennis T. Leaver, MS, RT(R)(T)
Director, Radiation Therapy Program,
Southern Maine Technical College,
South Portland, Maine

Shirlee E. Maihoff, MEd, RT(T)
Associate Professor and Director,
Radiation Therapy Program,
The University of Alabama at Birmingham,
Birmingham, Alabama

Alan C. Miller, MEd, RT(R)
Radiography Program Director,
Moultrie Area Technical Institute,
Moultrie, Georgia

Shirley E. Otto, MSN, CRNI, AOCN
Clinical Nurse Specialist,
Via Christi Regional Medical Center,
Wichita, Kansas

Cathy Quane-Smyth, BA, RT(T)
Director, Radiation Therapy Program,
Nassau Community College,
Garden City, New York

Lynda N. Reynolds, BS, RT(R)(N)(T), FASRT
Associate Professor, Program Director,
Department of Radiologic Technology,
University of Oklahoma Health Sciences Center,
Oklahoma City, Oklahoma

Pamela J. Ross, RT(T)
Coordinator of Technology,
Clinical Coordinator,
School of Radiation Therapy,
New York Methodist Hospital,
Brooklyn, New York

Janet M. Salzmann, RT(R)(T)
Staff Radiation Therapist,
Houston Northwest Radiation Therapy,
Houston, Texas

Wanda Teasley, BS, MHSA, RT(R)(T), FASRT
Chairperson, Associate Professor,
Clinical Services Department,
College of Health Professions,
Medical University of South Carolina,
Charleston, South Carolina

Phyllis Thompson, MHPE, RT(T)
Director, Health Arts Program,
College of St. Francis,
Joliet, Illinois

Stephen M. Waldow, PhD
Associate Professor,
Department of Radiation Oncology,
Temple University School of Medicine,
Philadelphia, Pennsylvania

Charles M. Washington, BS, RT(T)
Director, Radiation Therapy Program,
M.D. Anderson Cancer Center,
The University of Texas,
Houston, Texas

Linda S. Wingfield, MEd, RT(R)(T)
Vice President, Clinical Services,
Central Arkansas Radiation Therapy Institute,
Little Rock, Arkansas

Reviewers

Eric Anderson, PhD
Assistant Professor of Physics,
Avila College,
Kansas City, Missouri

Sucha Asbell, MD
Chairman, Radiation Oncology,
Albert Einstein Medical Center,
Philadelphia, Pennsylvania

Joseph Baranowsky, BS
Field Service Engineer,
Dornier Medical Systems,
Kennesaw, Georgia

Cecelia Bouchard, MS, RT(R)(T)
Clinical Coordinator, Radiation Therapy Technology,
Southern Maine Technical College,
South Portland, Maine

Andrew P. Brown, MD
Radiation Oncologist,
Elliott Regional Cancer Center,
Manchester, New Hampshire

Cynthia P. Burns, AS, RT(R)(T)
Radiation Therapist,
Cynthia A. Rydholm Cancer Treatment Center,
Central Maine Medical Center,
Lewiston, Maine

Shaun T. Caldwell, BS, RT(R)(T)
Educational Director, Radiation Therapy,
College of Health Professions,
Weber State University,
Ogden, Utah

Anne T. Campbell, BHS, RT(R)(T)
Program Director, Radiation Therapy Technology Program,
Chandler Medical Center,
University of Kentucky,
Lexington, Kentucky

Sandra Bouquet Carslick, RT(R)(T)
Senior Radiation Therapist,
Costal Cancer Treatment Center,
Maine Medical Center,
Bath, Maine

Peter Y. Chen, MD
Associate Director of Education,
Department of Radiation Oncology,
William Beaumont Hospital,
Royal Oak, Michigan

Melvin C. Cheney, MS, RT(T)
Director of Patient Services,
Northwest Arkansas Radiation Therapy Institute;
Program Director, Radiation Therapist Program,
Northwest Arkansas Community College,
Springdale, Arkansas

Annette Coleman, BS, MA, RT(T)
Educational Coordinator/Technology,
Joint Center for Radiation Therapy,
Massachusetts College of Pharmacy and Allied Health Sciences,
Boston, Massachusetts

Joseph Digel, RT(R)(T)
Chief Therapist, Radiation Oncology,
Program Director, Radiation Therapy Program,
The Johns Hopkins Hospital,
Baltimore, Maryland

Barbara Flexner, BS, RT(T)
Educational Coordinator, Program Director,
Allied Health and Radiation Therapy Technology,
Vanderbilt University Medical Center,
Nashville, Tennessee

Diana Freeman, BS, RT(T)
Program Director, Certified Medical Dosimetrist,
Parkland College,
Decatur Memorial Hospital,
Decatur, Illinois

Tilly Gibbs, BA, RT(T)
Chief Therapist, Program Director,
Radiation Therapy Program,
University of Utah Hospital,
Salt Lake City, Utah

Patricia Giordano, MS, RT(T)
Program Director, Assistant Professor,
Gwynedd-Mercy College,
Gwynedd Valley, Pennsylvania

Charleen Gombert, BS, RT(T)
Professor, Program Director,
Radiation Therapy Technology Program,
Community College of Allegheny County,
Pittsburgh, Pennsylvania

Mark Graniero, BS, RT(T)
Chief Radiation Therapist,
Four County Radiation Medicine,
Utica, New York

Roslyn Ham, AS, RT(T)
Radiation Therapist,
Florida East Coast Cancer Center,
Ft. Pierce, Florida

Robert Holihan, BS, RT(R)
Instructor, Radiography Program,
Ferris State University,
Big Rapids, Michigan

Edna Holmes, MPA, RT(R)
Director, Radiography Program,
Lake Michigan College,
Benton Harbor, Michigan

Kathleen Kienstra, BS, RT(R)(T)
Program Director,
Barnes Hospital School of Radiation Therapy,
St. Louis, Missouri

Julianne Kinsman, MEd, RT(T)
Department Chairperson, Radiation Therapy Technology,
Springfield Technical Community College,
Springfield, Massachusetts

Druellen Kolker, BS, RT(T)
Program Director, Radiation Therapy Technology,
University of Chicago Hospitals,
Roosevelt University,
Chicago, Illinois

Sue M. Merkel, BS, RT(R)(T)
Program Director, Radiation Oncology,
University of Michigan Medical Center,
Ann Arbor, Michigan

Carmen Mesina, MS, RT(R)(T)
Clinical Radiation Therapy Physicist,
Harper Hospital,
Wayne State University,
Detroit, Michigan

Roy A. Miller, BS, RT(T)
Coordinator, Radiation Therapy Program,
Owens Community College,
Toledo, Ohio

Sharon J. Morretti, RT(T)
Supervisor, Radiation Therapy Program,
North Shore Cancer Center,
Peabody, Massachusetts

Cindy Mueller, BS, RT(R)(T)
Program Director, School of Radiation Therapy,
St. Joseph's Hospital,
Milwaukee, Wisconsin

Diane Mulkhey, AS, RT(T)
Manager, Radiation Therapy Department,
Central Maine Medical Center,
Lewiston, Maine

Joann M. Murray, BS, RT(R)(T)
Program Director, School of Radiation Therapy,
Welborn Cancer Center,
Evansville, Indiana

Larry Oliver, RT(T)
Program Director, Radiation Therapy Technology,
University of Kansas Medical Center,
Kansas City, Kansas

Brad Owen, RT(T)
Radiation Therapist,
Southern Maine Technical College,
Lisbon Falls, Maine

Christina M. Paugh, BA, RT(R)(T)
Program Director, Educational Coordinator,
Radiation Oncology,
West Virginia University Hospital,
Morgantown, West Virginia

Joan Pierson, RT(R)(T)
Program Coordinator,
School of Radiation Therapy,
Henry Ford Hospital,
Detroit, Michigan

Nancy Quinn-Fagan, MEd, RT(R)(T)
Director of Education,
M.D. Anderson-Moncrief Cancer Center,
Ft. Worth, Texas

Marie L.A. Racine, BS, RT(R)(T)
Program Director, Radiation Therapy Technology,
Galveston College/University of Texas School of Allied
   Health Sciences,
Galveston, Texas

Mary Jo Repasky, MHSA, RT(R)(T)
Program Director, Radiation Therapy Technology,
College of Health Professions,
Medical University of South Carolina,
Charleston, South Carolina

Pamela J. Ross, RT(T)
Coordinator of Technology,
Clinical Coordinator,
School of Radiation Therapy,
New York Methodist Hospital,
Brooklyn, New York

David Schatanoff, MD
Radiation Oncologist,
Radiation Oncology Department,
Mercy Regional Health System,
Altoona, Pennsylvania

Deborah Semanchik, RT(R)(T)
Radiation Therapist,
Radiation Oncology Department,
Mercy Regional Health System,
Altoona, Pennsylvania

Diane Skog, BS, RT(T)
Senior Radiation Therapist,
Maine Medical Center,
Portland, Maine

Shirley N. Smith, MPA, RT(R)(T)
Program Director, Radiation Therapy Technology,
Lansing Community College,
Lansing, Michigan

Carole A. Sullivan, PhD, RT(R)(T), FASRT
Dean, College of Allied Health,
Health Sciences Center,
University of Oklahoma,
Oklahoma City, Oklahoma

Larry Swafford, BS, RT(T)
Program Director, Radiation Therapy Technology,
Virginia Commonwealth University/Medical College of Virginia,
Richmond, Virginia

Wanda Teasley, BS, MHSA, RT(R)(T), FASRT
Chairperson, Associate Professor,
Clinical Services Department,
College of Health Professions,
Medical University of South Carolina,
Charleston, South Carolina

Giles Toole, MS, RT(R)(T)
Program Director, Radiation Therapy Technology,
Thomas Technical Institute,
Thomasville, Georgia

George M. Ushold, EdD, RT(T)
Director of Education, School of Radiation Therapy,
University of Rochester Cancer Center,
Rochester, New York

Ann Marie Vann, MEd, RT(R)(T)
Program Director, Radiation Therapy,
Medical College of Georgia,
Augusta, Georgia

David G. Ward, BS, Ed, RT(R)(T)
Program Director, Radiation Therapy Technology,
University Hospital of Cleveland,
Cleveland, Ohio

To those who have run and continue to run the race against cancer.
We sincerely hope those who read this work will grow in the knowledge
and understanding necessary to provide direction and compassion to their patients.
Let us not grow tired in running our own race,
but instead encourage those around us.

Preface

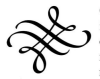 Cancer is the second leading cause of death in the United States. According to estimates of the American Cancer Society, over 1.2 million new cases of cancer were diagnosed in 1995. The problem of controlling the disease and the important role of those involved in clinical and research activities is evident by the vast amount of money spent on cancer research each year and the immeasurable cost in compromised quality and loss of human life. Radiation therapy, a vital resource involved in cancer management, is used in well over half the diagnosed cases.

Introduction to Radiation Therapy is one of three texts in the *Principles and Practice of Radiation Therapy* series designed to contribute to a comprehensive understanding of cancer management, improve techniques involved in delivering a prescribed dose of radiation therapy, and apply knowledge and complex concepts associated with radiation therapy treatment. Each text is designed to stand on its own and at the same time provide a continuum of information in the series to the student, therapist, dosimetrist, oncologist, nurse, and others involved in radiation oncology.

This first-ever text offers a comprehensive overview of radiation therapy with pertinent introductory chapters on cancer management, etiology, epidemiology, detection and diagnoses, and historical and state-of-the-art information. Additional chapters focus on the principles of surgical, medical, and radiation oncology; incorporate an in-depth approach to high-energy equipment used in radiation therapy; and emphasize the importance of patient care with specific chapters on patient assessment, education, and pharmacology.

Pedagogical features designed to enhance comprehension and high-level learning are incorporated into each chapter. Elements include chapter outlines, key terms, and a complete glossary. Other notable features are the review questions and questions to ponder at the end of each chapter. The review questions reiterate the cognitive information presented in the chapter to help the reader incorporate the information into the basic understanding of radiation therapy concepts. The questions to ponder are open-ended, divergent questions intended to stimulate critical thinking and analytical judgment during information processing. Each chapter offers a reference list, thus providing the reader with additional sources. Again, the focus on each chapter is the comprehensive needs of the radiation therapy management team.

Creating a series of this magnitude has been a collaborative effort by numerous individuals. Although the idea for such a work began several years ago as one comprehensive text, the impossibility of the task was soon realized, considering the complexity and vast amount of information. Instead, three texts were proposed: *Introduction to Radiation Therapy; Radiation Therapy Physics, Simulation, and Treatment Planning;* and *Practical Applications in Radiation Therapy.* A survey of nearly all radiation therapy, dosimetry, and radiation oncology resident program directors and a smaller number of oncology nurses revealed a strong need for such a work with a notable percentage of the respondents recommending a multivolume approach. Survey results not only were encouraging, but also provided us with various individuals interested in lending their expertise as contributing authors, consultants, and reviewers. The result is a truly collaborative effort from the oncology community. This has been especially helpful because a great deal of individuality exists among treatment centers, hospitals, and universities in the techniques of irradiation.

Our hope is that the *Principles and Practice of Radiation Therapy* series will add to the body of knowledge specific to the profession. In addition, we sincerely hope the expanded knowledge and progress gained in administering a prescribed dose of radiation will ultimately enrich the quality of life of the patient and reduce suffering from cancer.

Charles M. Washington
Dennis T. Leaver

Acknowledgments

This book is the result of a tremendous team effort involving 61 contributing authors, over 50 reviewers, our illustrators, and the dedicated professionals at Mosby–Year Book, Inc. All of us have had individuals who believed in and encouraged us when we encountered obstacles. We would like to acknowledge and thank those professionals who were instrumental in helping us build our professional foundation: Diane Chadwell and Adam Kempa from Wayne State University in Detroit, Michigan, and Dr. Banice Webber and Beverly Raymond from Radiation Oncology Associates in Providence, Rhode Island. Without their guidance and support, we could not have addressed the need for this work.

We would like to give special thanks to our students and reviewers who provided suggestions and comments that improved the manuscript. The continued support and encouragement of our colleagues at The University of Texas M.D. Anderson Cancer Center and Southern Maine Technical College are greatly appreciated. We are also grateful to Deborah Nickson and Jeanne Leaver for their dedicated service, secretarial assistance, and help with the glossary.

Above all, we gratefully acknowledge our families because they are the silent force behind this book. The idea for this project began at a conference in 1992. The idea was developed by many colleagues, friends, and the challenge to add to the body of knowledge in radiation oncology. We are grateful for the love, support, and encouragement from our wives, Connie Washington and Jeanne Leaver. They are also extremely important to this project. Finally, a special thanks goes to our heavenly Father, who sustains us and makes things grow.

Contents

Introduction

Cancer: An Overview

Stephanie Eatmon

Outline

Key terms

Cellular differentiation
Epidemiology
Etiology
Metastasize

Palliative
Prognosis
Tumoricidal Dose

HISTORICAL OVERVIEW

 Throughout recorded history, cancer has been the subject of investigation. Lacking current surgical techniques and diagnostic and laboratory equipment, early investigators relied on their senses to determine characteristics of the disease. Investigators were unable to examine cells, so infections and other benign conditions were present in these early observations. Knowledge about early observations, including examinations, diagnosis, and treatment comes in part from Egyptian papyri dating back to 1600 BC.[4,5]

Initially investigators believed that an excess of black bile caused cancer. This belief defined cancer as a systemic disease for which local treatment (such as surgery) only made the patient worse.[4,5] In light of this, cancer was considered to be fatal with little possibility of a cure. When investigators could not prove the existence of black bile, the theory of cancer as an initially localized disease emerged. With this theory came the possibility of treatment and a cure.

The cause of this deadly disease remained a mystery, and for some time, people thought cancer was contagious. This theory brought isolation and shame to cancer victims, and although this belief has long since vanished, patients not long ago expressed concern about spreading the disease to loved ones and losing their jobs as a consequence of the diagnosis.

Hippocrates began the classification of tumors by observation, but the discovery of the microscope enabled early investigators to classify tumors on the basis of cellular characteristics.[5] Classification of tumors and their stages of growth continues and will continue as technology advances.

BIOLOGICAL PERSPECTIVE

Building on the work of early investigators and aided by technological advances, researchers today are able to diagnose tumors in extremely early stages and examine tumor cell deoxyribonucleic acid (DNA) to determine mechanisms causing uncontrolled growth. Although knowledge about cancer has increased tremendously since early investigators began examining patients, much remains to be learned.

Theory of cancer initiation

Tumors are the result of abnormal cellular proliferation. This can occur because the process by which **cellular differentiation** takes place is abnormal or a normally nondividing, mature cell begins to proliferate. Cellular differentiation occurs when a stem cell undergoes mitosis and divides into daughter cells. These cells continue to divide and differentiate until a mature cell with a specific function results. When this process is disrupted, the daughter cells may continue to divide with no resulting mature cell, thus causing abnormal cellular proliferation.

The cause of this cellular dysfunction has been the subject of research for many years. Researchers now believe that "cancer is a disease of the genes."[3] Normal somatic cells contain genes that promote growth and genes that suppress growth, both of which are important to control the growth of a cell. In a tumor cell, this counterbalanced regulation is missing. Mutations occurring in genes that promote or suppress growth are implicated in the deregulation of cellular growth. Mutations in genes that promote growth force the growth of cells, whereas mutations to the genes that suppress growth allow unrestrained cellular growth. For many tumors, both mutations may be required for progression to full malignancy.[2,3,6-8]

The terms for the genes involved in the cancer process are *protooncogenes, oncogenes,* and *antioncogenes.* Protooncogenes are the normal genes that play a part in controlling normal growth and differentiation. These genes are the precursors of oncogenes, or cancer genes. The conversion of protooncogenes to oncogenes can occur through point mutations, translocations, and gene amplification, all of which are DNA mutations. Oncogenes are implicated in the abnormal proliferation of cells. Antioncogenes are also called *cancer-suppressor genes.* Inactivation of antioncogenes allows the malignant process to flourish.

What causes these mutations to occur? For somatic cells, exposure to carcinogens such as sunlight, radiation, and cigarette smoke is implicated. In some situations, such as the familial form of retinoblastoma, gene mutations are passed down through generations. Random mutations that occur during normal cellular replication can also lead to unregulated cellular growth.

Researchers have identified several gene mutations, including recently the gene implicated in the familial form of breast cancer. With the use of gene mapping and advanced technology, study in this area will continue.

Tumor classification

Tumors are classified by their anatomical site, cell of origin, and biological behavior. Tumors can originate from any cell. This accounts for the large variety of tumors. Well-differentiated tumors (those that closely resemble the cell of origin) can be easily classified according to their histology. Undifferentiated cells, however, do not resemble normal cells, so classification is more difficult. These tumors are called *undifferentiated* or *anaplastic.*

Tumors are divided into two categories: benign or malignant (Table 1-1). Benign tumors are generally well differentiated and do not metastasize or invade surrounding normal tissue. Often benign tumors are encapsulated and slow growing. Although the majority of benign tumors do little harm to the host, benign tumors of the brain (because of their location) are considered behaviorally malignant because of the adverse effect on the host. Benign tumors are noted by the suffix *oma,* which is connected to the term indicating the cell of origin. For example, a chondroma is a benign tumor of the cartilage.

Malignant tumors range from well differentiated to undifferentiated. They have the ability to **metastasize,** or spread to a site in the body distant from the primary site. Malignant tumors often invade and destroy normal surrounding tissue and, if left untreated, can cause the death of the host.

Tumors arising from mesenchymal cells are termed *sarcomas.* These cells include connective tissue such as cartilage and bone. An example is a chondrosarcoma or a sarcoma of the cartilage. Although blood and lymphatics are mesenchymal tissues, they are classified separately as *leukemias* and *lymphomas.*

Carcinomas are tumors that originate from the epithelium. These include all the tissues that cover a surface or line a cavity. For example, the aerodigestive tract is lined with squamous cell epithelium. Tumors originating from the lin-

Table 1-1	General characteristics of benign and malignant disease	
Characteristics	**Benign**	**Malignant**
Local spread	Expanding, pushing	Infiltrative and invasive
Distant spread	Rare	Metastasize early or late by lymphatics, blood, or seeding
Differentiation	Well differentiated	Well differentiated to undifferentiated
Mitotic activity	Normal	Normal to increased mitotic rate
Morphology	Normal	Normal to pleomorphic
Effect on host	Little (depending on treatment and location of tumor)	Life treating
Doubling time	Normal	Normal to accelerated

ing are called *squamous cell carcinoma of the primary site.* An example is squamous cell carcinoma of the lung. Epithelial cells that are glandular are called *adenocarcinoma.* An example is the tissue lining the stomach. A tumor originating in the cells of this lining is called *adenocarcinoma of the stomach.* (Table 1-2 lists examples of nomenclature used in neoplastic classification.)

As in any classification system, some situations do not follow the rules. Examples include Hodgkin's disease, Wilms' tumor, and Ewing's sarcoma. This system of classification continues to change as more knowledge of the origin and behavior of tumors becomes available. (Table 1-3 lists histologies associated with common anatomical cancer sites.)

Cancer outlook

The American Cancer Society[1] has estimated that "about one in three" people or "85 million Americans . . . will eventually have cancer." After taking into account normal life expectancy, 52% of these people will be alive 5 years after the diagnosis. In addition, 50% of individuals who have cancer will receive radiation therapy.

Excluding carcinoma of the skin, the most common types of cancer include prostate, lung, and colorectal in men and breast, colorectal, and lung in women.[1] These statistics are

Table 1-2	Classifications of neoplasms	
Tissue of Origin	**Benign**	**Malignant**
Glandular epithelium	Adenoma	Adenocarcinoma
Squamous epithelium	Papilloma	Squamous cell carcinoma
Connective tissue smooth muscle	Leiomyoma	Leiomyosarcoma
Hematopoietic	—	Leukemia
Lymphoreticular	—	Lymphoma
Neural	Neuroma	Blastoma

Table 1-3	Histologies associated with common anatomical cancer sites
Site	**Most common histology**
Oral cavity	Squamous cell carcinoma
Pharynx	Squamous cell carcinoma
Lung	Squamous cell carcinoma
Breast	Infiltrating ductal carcinoma
Colon and rectum	Adenocarcinoma
Anus	Squamous cell carcinoma
Cervix	Squamous cell carcinoma
Endometrium	Adenocarcinoma
Prostate	Adenocarcinoma
Brain	Astrocytoma

not static and change with environmental, lifestyle, technological, and other influences in society. Lung cancer in the 1930s was much less prevalent than it is today because of the increase in the number of cigarette smokers and improved diagnostic abilities. Invasive carcinoma of the cervix decreased over the past 10 years as a result of the Papanicolaou (Pap) smear. Currently, more carcinoma in situ, or preinvasive, cancers of the cervix are found than invasive tumors.

Depending on the geographical location, the incidence of tumor sites also varies. For example, the incidence of stomach cancer is much greater in Japan than in the United States, and skin cancer is found more frequently in New Zealand than in Iceland.

PATIENT PERSPECTIVE

Although cancer is a curable disease, the diagnosis is a life-changing event. In studying the various aspects of neoplasia, care providers can easily lose sight of the person suffering from the disease. The patient should be the focal point of all the radiation therapist's actions. Quality care is, however, derived from knowledge of the disease process, psychosocial issues, patient care, and principles and practices of cancer management, including an in-depth knowledge of radiation therapy as a treatment option. This knowledge provides the radiation therapist with the tools necessary for optimal treatment, care, and education of the cancer patient. Providing care that does not consider the whole person is unacceptable.

The person behind the diagnosis

When reviewing the large number of people who develop cancer, care providers can easily forget that the patient has a life outside of treatment with concerns and worries continuing and adding to the emotional, social, psychological, physical, and financial burdens that come with the diagnosis. In addition, other medical concerns unrelated to cancer may complicate treatment and further burden the patient.

Factors such as age, culture, support systems, education, and family background play important roles in medical-treatment compliance, attitudes toward treatment, and responses to treatment. By knowing as much as possible about the patient and factors that influence the treatment outcome, the radiation therapist can provide quality patient care. Remembering that the cancer and the whole person are receiving treatment is essential to providing the type of care every cancer patient deserves. A knowledge of available patient resources is essential to ensure that all patients receive the care and help they need to deal with the disease and resulting life issues.

Cancer-patient resources

In each medical facility is generally a myriad of cancer-support services. These services can include general education, cancer-site-specific education, financial aid, travel to and from treatment, and activity programs. Social work departments are available to assist with the financial, emotional, and logistic issues that arise, and community services through churches and other organizations are available to support individuals and their families. National organizations such as the American Cancer Society have also been established. Radiation therapists must become familiar with the services offered in their communities to better serve the patients they treat. Educating patients about programs or referring patients to specific services to address individual needs is an important part of quality care.

ETIOLOGY AND EPIDEMIOLOGY OVERVIEW

Today a tremendous amount of knowledge exists about factors that influence the development of cancer and the incidence at which it occurs. **Etiology** and **epidemiology** are the two areas of study that have contributed to the growing knowledge in these areas.

Etiology

Etiology is the study of disease causes. Although the cause of cancer is unknown, many carcinogenic agents have been identified. Experts use this information, as they have done with tobacco use, to establish prevention programs.

Etiological and epidemiological information is helpful in determining screening tests for early detection, producing patient-education programs, and identifying target populations. An example is the set of guidelines of the American Cancer Society for screening mammograms to detect breast cancer in its early stages.

Epidemiology

Epidemiology is the study of disease incidence. National databases provide statistical information about patterns of cancer occurrence and death rates. With this information, researchers can determine the incidence of cancer occurrence in a population for factors such as age, gender, race, and geographical location. Researchers can also determine which specific type of cancer affects which specific group of people. An example is the high incidence of stomach cancer in Japan compared with that in the United States. Epidemiological studies also help determine trends in disease such as the increase of lung cancer and the decline of stomach cancer in the United States.

DETECTION AND DIAGNOSIS

Early detection and diagnosis are keys to the successful treatment of cancer. The earlier a tumor is discovered, the less chance remains that it has spread to other parts of the body. For some tumors such as carcinoma of the larynx, early symptoms cause the patient to seek medical care early in the course of the disease. As a result, the cure rate for glottic tumors is extremely high. Cancer of the ovary, however, is associated with vague symptoms that could be the result of a number of medical problems. Therefore a diagnosis is often made late in the course of the disease. Cure rates for ovarian cancer reflect the results of late diagnosis.

Screening examinations

To identify cancer in its earliest stages (before symptoms appear and while the chance of cure is greatest), screening tests are performed. Examples include the Pap smear for cervical cancer, fecal occult blood testing for colorectal cancer, and mammograms for breast cancer. For many cancer sites, screening examinations are not readily available because of the inaccessibility of the tumor and the high cost associated with the tests.

To be useful, screening examinations must be sensitive and specific for the tumors they identify. If an examination is sensitive, it can identify a tumor in its extremely early stages. For example, a Pap smear is sensitive because it can help detect carcinoma of the cervix before the problem becomes invasive. If a test is specific, it can identify a particular type of cancer. Carcinoembryonic antigen (CEA) may be elevated because of a number of benign and malignant conditions. For this reason the test is not specific but is useful in determining recurrences.

Screening tests may also yield false-positive or false-negative readings. A false-positive reading indicates disease when in reality none is present. A false-negative reading is the reverse; the test indicates no disease when in fact the disease is present.

For a screening test to be highly useful, it should be sensitive, specific, cost effective, and accurate. The cost of the screening examination often limits its use to all but extremely high-risk populations.

Work-up components

After a tumor is suspected, a work-up, or series of diagnostic examinations, begins. The purpose of the work-up is to determine the general health status of the patient and collect as much information about the tumor as possible. To treat the patient effectively, the physician needs to know the type, location, and size of the tumor; the distance the tumor has invaded normal tissue; the presence of spread to distant sites; and lymph-node involvement if any. These questions are answered in the work-up.

The work-up depends on the type of cancer suspected and the symptoms experienced by the patient. The work-up for a suspected lung tumor is different than that for a suspected prostate tumor. The same questions are answered, but because the two tumors are extremely different, the tests are based on the specific tumor characteristics.

With advancing technology, more information is available to the physician than ever before. As new technologies emerge and prove useful in the information-gathering process, treatment becomes more effective. Before computed tomography (CT) became available, small tumor extension into normal lung tissues was not readily visible on chest radiographs. The physician had to make an educated guess about the extent of the tumor invasion and treat the patient based on the suspected condition. As a result, treatment fields had to be larger to encompass all the suspected disease. With CT, much of the guesswork is eliminated and treatment volumes can include areas of known disease while limiting even more the areas of normal tissue, therefore producing a more effective treatment.

Staging

Tumor staging is a means of defining the tumor size and extension at the time of diagnosis and is important for many reasons. Tumor staging provides a means of communication about tumors, helps in determining the best treatment, aids in predicting prognosis, and provides a means for continuing research. Staging systems have changed with advancing technologies and increased knowledge and will continue to progress as more information becomes known. For this reason, tumors that occur frequently have detailed staging classifications, whereas those that are rare have primitive or no working stages.

A common staging system adopted by the International Union Against Cancer (UICC) and the American Joint Committee on Cancer (AJCC), is the TNM system. The T category defines the size or extent of the primary tumor and is assigned numbers 1 through 4. A T_1 tumor is small and/or confined to a small area, whereas a T_4 tumor is extremely large and/or extends into other tissues. N designates the status of lymph nodes and the extent of lymph node involvement. A 0-through-4 designation exists depending on the extent of involvement with N_0 indicating that no positive nodes are present. N_1 indicates positive nodes close to the site of the primary tumor, whereas N_4 indicates positive nodes at more distant nodal sites. M is the category that defines the presence and extent of metastasis. Again, the M category is divided into a 0-through-4 designation depending on the extent of metastatic disease. The designation M_0 indicates no evidence of metastatic disease found, whereas M_4 indicates metastasis in multiple organs distant from the primary tumor.

In the TNM staging are additional subcategories for commonly occurring tumors. Notations are often used to determine whether the staging was accomplished through clinical, surgical, or pathological methods. Although the TNM system is widely used, numerous staging systems exist that more accurately detail important tumor characteristics for prognostic and treatment information. For example, the International Federation of Gynecology and Obstetrics (FIGO) system is used in the staging of gynecologic tumors. (A detailed explanation for staging is available in Chapter 6.)

Grade

The grade of a tumor provides information about its aggressiveness and is based on the degree of differentiation. For some tumors, such as a high-grade astrocytoma, grade is the most important prognostic indicator.

The stage and grade offer an accurate picture of the tumor and its behavior. When physicians know the exact types of tumors with which they are dealing, treatment decisions can be made that effectively eradicate the tumors. (A detailed description of cancer detection and diagnosis is provided in Chapter 6.)

TREATMENT OPTIONS

Cancer treatment demands a multidisciplinary approach. Tumor boards were established to have cancer specialists work together to review information about newly diagnosed tumors and devise effective treatment plans. Participants of a tumor board can include surgeons, radiation oncologists, medical oncologists, social workers, plastic surgeons, and other medical personnel. All these individuals play key roles in developing a treatment plan that effectively treats the tumor while helping the patient maintain a high quality of life.

Surgery

As a local treatment modality, surgery plays a role in diagnosis, staging, treatment, **palliation**, and identification of treatment response. As a tool for diagnosis, surgery is used to perform a biopsy of a suspected mass to determine whether the mass is malignant and, if so, the cellular origin. Many biopsy methods exist, and the characteristics of the suspected mass determine the use of a particular method. The information obtained from the biopsy is essential for accurate treatment.

Surgery provides a means for accurate staging. For example, with ovarian cancer the surgeon performs an exploratory laparotomy to identify the extent of tumor spread. Without this information, treatment is a hit-and-miss proposition because the true extent of the disease is unknown. Physicians also use surgery as a treatment modality alone or with radiation therapy and/or chemotherapy. Surgical intervention may be the only treatment necessary if it can completely remove the tumor. If, however, the surgical margins are positive for cancer cells, an incomplete resection was done, or the tumor has a high recurrence rate, further treatment is necessary.

The purpose of surgical palliation is to relieve symptoms the patient may be experiencing as a result of the disease. An example is an obstruction of the bowel. The surgery does not have a curative effect on the disease but provides the patient with symptom relief for an improved quality of life.

Second-look surgeries are performed to determine treatment outcome. With an ovarian tumor, a second-look surgery provides information about tumor response to the previous treatment. If the surgeon finds malignant cells during the second-look surgery, more treatment is indicated.

Surgery is limited by the tumor's accessibility, the patient's medical condition, and the tumor's extent. If a tumor is located in an area that is inaccessible or close to critical structures, surgery may not be possible. Critical structures are organs or structures that, if damaged, are incompatible with life or leave the patient in worse condition than before treatment. A cancer of the nasopharynx is located in an area in which accessibility is difficult because the cancer is close to the base of the brain and the cranial nerves. For these reasons, cancers of the nasopharynx are not good candidates for surgical intervention. Extremely large tumors involving many organs are not candidates for surgery because the amount of tissue that would need to be removed is too great. Surgery is further limited by the medical condition of the patient. If the patient's pulmonary function is compromised, general anesthesia may be contraindicated and surgical procedures impossible. (Detailed information about the use of surgery in the treatment of cancer is contained in Chapter 7.)

Radiation therapy

Radiation therapy is a local treatment that can be used alone or with other treatment modalities. Benefits of radiation therapy include preservation of function and better cosmetic results. An early stage laryngeal tumor can be effectively treated by surgery or radiation. Surgery may require removal of the vocal cords, thus leaving the patient without a voice. Radiation therapy, however, can obtain the same results while preserving the patient's voice. In the past, surgery for patients with prostate cancer always left the patient impotent with a high chance for incontinence. Radiation therapy can preserve function while providing an effective treatment.

Surgery and radiation therapy combined can also obtain an optimal cosmetic result. In the past, breast cancer was treated with a radical mastectomy, leaving the patient disfigured. Currently the treatment consisting of a lumpectomy followed by radiation therapy leaves the patient with minimal disfigurement and an equal chance of cure.

Radiation therapy plays a major role in palliation. An example is the treatment of bone metastasis. If the condition is left untreated, the patient experiences a great deal of pain and is at risk for broken bones. Radiation therapy to these sites usually eliminates the pain and prevents fractures. If a tumor is pressing on nerves, radiation therapy may be given to reduce the size of the tumor, thus eliminating pressure on the nerves and providing pain relief.

Radiation therapy is limited to a local area of treatment. Tumors that are diffuse throughout the body are not candidates for radiation therapy. Radiation therapy is further limited to areas in which a **tumoricidal dose** may be delivered without harming critical structures.

As with surgery, the patient's medical condition must be such that the patient can tolerate the treatment. If a patient is suffering from lung cancer and has little pulmonary function, radiation therapy may not be a suitable treatment option because it may further compromise the patient's ability to breathe.

Chemotherapy

Chemotherapy is a relatively young field. Over the past 30 years, however, great strides have been made in the treatment of cancer using chemotherapy. Chemotherapeutic drugs or agents are administered orally, through injection, through perfusion, and topically. Chemotherapy is given with surgery and/or radiation therapy or used alone in the treatment of specific cancers. Usually combinations of chemotherapeutic agents rather than a single agent are used. The agents act on the cell during the cell cycle. With the selection of a combination of agents that each affect the cell during a different phase of the cell cycle, a maximum number of cells are destroyed. Unfortunately, these agents also affect actively dividing normal cells. Cells such as bone marrow, hair follicles, and the epithelium in the gastrointestinal tract become dose-limiting factors. (More information on chemotherapy and specific chemotherapeutic agents is available in Chapter 8.)

Immunotherapy

Still in its infancy, immunotherapy carries great hope for the future. The goal of immunotherapy is to amplify the body's own disease-fighting system to destroy the cancer.

Cells at the forefront of the immune system are B, T, and natural killer cell lymphocytes. B cells produce the protein molecules or antibodies that circulate throughout the body, attacking and destroying foreign substances such as cancer. T cells, in response to contact with antigens found on the surface of a foreign substance, mature into killer cells that directly attack and destroy the foreign substance. Natural killer cells have the ability to spontaneously attack and destroy foreign substances.

Immunotherapy uses this knowledge to boost the naturally occurring defense mechanisms of the body. Monoclonal antibodies, for example, are produced to react to a specific antigen. The patient is given the monoclonal antibodies, which seek out and destroy the specific antigen found on the surface of the tumor cells. Studies are also being conducted in which a cytotoxic agent is tagged to the antibody, so when the antibody attacks the antigen, additional cell kill occurs. Similarly, vaccines are available for specific tumors that boost the body's own immune response toward a specific tumor antigen.

Interferons are naturally occurring body proteins capable of killing or slowing the growth of cancer cells. Interferons administered to a patient can enhance the cytotoxic activity of the immune system and provide a means to make tumor cell antigens more easily identified by the immune system. Interleukin-2 is a growth factor that stimulates an increase in the number of lymphocytes, especially killer cells.

While these three forms of immunotherapy are being used and researched, many other areas are currently under investigation.

PROGNOSIS

A **prognosis** is an estimation of the life expectancy of a cancer patient based on all the information obtained about the tumor and from clinical trials. A prognosis is, however, only an estimate. The duration of a person's life is a mystery, and thousands of cancer patients have outlived or underlived their estimated life expectancies.

Prognosis plays a role in the treatment plan. If a patient has a prognosis of 2 months, treatment is given in a manner such that the patient has the maximum time allowable to spend with family and friends. A treatment lasting 7 weeks would likely be more intrusive than helpful. Because the goal of treatment is to eradicate the tumor or provide palliation while preserving quality of life for the patient, the prognosis provides the information to ensure that this goal is accomplished.

For patients and their families, this information provides a time line to accomplish tasks or goals in preparation for impending death. This may include making a will, taking a long-awaited trip, and gathering family members from across the country. A patient's mental attitude plays an important role in the prognosis but is not a factor usually considered.

Factors specific to each tumor determine the prognosis. The natural history (the normal progression of a tumor without treatment) provides information about the tumor behavior. For example, some tumors grow slowly and cause the host few problems until late in the disease process, whereas other tumors grow rapidly and spread to distant sites at an early stage of tumor development. Generally, slow-growing tumors have better prognoses than those that have already metastasized at the time of presentation. Natural history information is also valuable in determining the most effective treatment for the patient (as it is with Hodgkin's disease), thus affecting the prognosis. For example, Hodgkin's disease has a systematic pattern of spread through the lymphatics. Therefore treatment of early stage Hodgkin's disease includes the known area of involvement plus the next level of lymph nodes. With this information the patient has a better chance for cure and a more favorable prognosis.

The method of treatment also determines the prognosis based on information obtained through clinical trials. As more effective treatment is delivered, the prognosis improves. As stated earlier, cancer demands a multidisciplinary approach to treatment. Finding the most effective combination of treatments has a profound effect on the prognosis.

Patterns of spread

Growth characteristics and spread patterns of a tumor have important prognostic implications. Tumors that tend to stay localized are more easily treated and thus generally have a better prognosis than those that are diffuse or spread to distant sites early in the development of the malignancy.

Tumors that are exophytic, or grow outward, have better prognoses than those that invade and ulcerate underlying tissues because of the communication with blood vessels and lymphatics, which are the highways of cancer cell transport to distant sites. Multicentric tumors, or tumors that have more than one focus of disease, can be more difficult to treat because the volume of tissue required for treatment is larger to encompass the entire organ or region. In addition, detecting all the tumor foci that may be at different stages in the development process is difficult.

Tumor dissemination, or spread, can be accomplished through the blood, lymphatics, and seeding. Tumor cells invading blood or lymph vessels can be transported to distant sites in the body. The mechanisms responsible for these cells taking root and growing in one area and not another is unknown. However, many tumors have a propensity to spread to specific sites. Prostate cancer commonly metastasizes to the bones. For this reason a bone scan is included in the work-up if evidence exists that metastasis has already occurred at the time of diagnosis. In addition, when the primary tumor is unknown and the patient has a metastatic disease, looking at the sites of the metastasis gives a clue about the primary tumor's location. Table 1-4 lists metastatic sites associated with common primary sites.

Tumor cells may also disseminate through seeding. Cells break off from the primary tumor and spread to new sites, where they grow. Ovarian cancer cells often spread to the abdominal cavity by this method, which is the reason that the staging laparotomy is an important diagnostic and staging tool. Cells from a medulloblastoma of the brain often seed into the spinal canal by means of the cerebrospinal fluid, thus necessitating the treatment of the spinal cord and brain.

Prognostic factors

For each tumor, specific prognostic factors are based on the cellular and behavioral characteristics, tumor site, and patient-related factors. Determination of prognostic factors is made through clinical trials in which factors related to the disease and patient are statistically analyzed for a group of patients. With this method, factors that have the greatest influence on prognosis are determined.

Table 1-4	Common metastatic sites of primary tumors	
Primary site	**Common metastatic sites**
Lung	Liver, adrenal glands, bone, and brain
Breast	Lungs, bone, and brain
Stomach	Liver
Anus	Liver and lungs
Bladder	Lungs, bone, and liver
Prostate	Bone, liver, and lungs
Uterine cervix	Lungs, bone, and liver

Tumor-related factors that are often of prognostic significance include grade, stage, tumor size, status of lymph nodes, depth of invasion, and histology. Patient-related prognostic factors include age, gender, race, and medical condition. Each factor displays a different level of importance in specific tumors. For example, the main prognostic indicator for breast cancer is the status of the axillary lymph nodes, whereas for a soft tissue sarcoma, it is histological grade.

CLINICAL TRIALS

Much of the progress made in the management of cancer is the result of carefully planned clinical trials. This type of research can be conducted at a single clinical site or in collaboration with many institutions. The advantage of collaboration is that a greater number of patients can participate in the study, thus increasing the significance of the results. Because cancer management is multidisciplinary, clinical trials are often a collaborative effort among disciplines.

Retrospective studies

Studies that review information from a group of patients treated in the past are retrospective. The treatment has already been delivered, and the information is collected (often on a national basis) and analyzed. Retrospective studies have an advantage in that the information can be obtained rather quickly; the investigator does not have to wait years to see the results of a particular treatment. However, a number of drawbacks are apparent with retrospective studies and can lead to errors. Complete information about a treatment is not always easy to obtain and is often incomplete. Outside factors that may have influenced the treatment and results are not controlled and may not be accurately documented.

Prospective studies

A clinical trial that is planned before treatment with eligibility criteria for patient selection is a prospective study. Investigators have the advantage of knowing the information that is essential to the study, thus leading to more complete and accurate documentation. In addition, better control of external factors that might influence the results of the study is possible. A disadvantage of prospective studies is the length of time needed to observe the results of a particular treatment. Depending on the length of the follow-up necessary to accurately assess the results, prospective trials can last 5 years or longer.

Randomized studies

Clinical studies often include several methods of treatment to determine which method results in the best outcome. After meeting all eligibility requirements for the study, patients are randomly selected for one of the treatment arms. The purpose of randomization is to eliminate any unintentional "stacking of the deck" and increase the accuracy of results and conclusions. Although patients may have the same type, grade, stage, and extent of cancer, each person responds individually to the disease and treatment. Care providers cannot control these factors, but randomization helps minimize their effects on the end result. With randomization, each arm of the study has approximately equal numbers of individuals with varying reactions.

Survival reporting

In the planning stages of a clinical trial an end point must be established. Otherwise the study can continue indefinitely with no data analysis. Rates of survival at a set end point are one type of information used to determine the benefit of one treatment over another. Survival reporting, however, can be accomplished with many methods. With absolute survival reporting, patients alive at the end point and those who have died are counted. Patients lost to follow-up are included, but the fact that patients may have died from other causes is not considered. Adjusted survival reporting includes patients who died from other causes and had no evidence of disease (NED) at the times of their deaths. Relative survival reporting involves the normal mortality rate of a similar group of people based on factors such as age, gender, and race.

In addition, survival reporting at the end point includes information about the status of the disease. At the end point the patient may be alive with NED, disease free, or alive with disease. Of equal importance is the information about treatment failures. Treatment failures are classified as local, locoregional, or distant and are based on tumor recurrences at the primary or nearby lymph node sites or metatastatic disease. This information is valuable for ongoing clinical trials and for determining types of treatment techniques to prevent future failures.

SUMMARY

Cancer has been a focus of scientific attention for decades. As technology improves and knowledge about the disease increases, detection, diagnosis, and treatment improve. The future of cancer management looks bright, with improved surgical techniques, more precise and advanced radiation therapy techniques, and improved chemotherapeutic agents.

Review Questions

Fill in the Blank

1. _____ _____ occurs when a stem cell undergoes mitosis and divides with daughter cells.

2. _____ are also called cancer-suppressor genes.

3. Tumors arising from mesenchymal cells are termed _____.

4. _____ are tumors that originate from the epithelium.

5. _____ _____ is a means of defining tumor size, extent, and extension at the time of diagnosis.

Listing

6. List three classifications of tumors.
   a. _____
   b. _____
   c. _____

7. List five factors that play important roles in the medical compliance with, attitude toward, and response to the treatment of cancer.
   a. _____
   b. _____
   c. _____
   d. _____
   e. _____

8. Name four cancer-treatment options.
   a. _____
   b. _____
   c. _____
   d. _____

Questions to Ponder

1. What cancer patient resources are available in the hospital in which you work? What resources are available in your community?

2. Mr. Jones has a T_2 tumor of the larynx, and Mrs. Smith has a T_4 tumor of the larynx. What differences would you expect to see in the tumors and in the treatment plans for each of these patients?

3. What effects have etiology and epidemiology had on cigarette smoking?

4. How does a prognosis help or hinder a physician, care provider, or patient?

5. Analyze a clinical trial taking place in the hospital in which you work. What type of research is being done?

6. Discuss the process of carcinogenesis.

7. Discuss differences between benign and malignant neoplasms.

REFERENCES

1. American Cancer Society: *Cancer facts and figures,* New York, 1994, The Society.
2. Cotran RS, Kumar V, Robbins SL: *Robbins pathologic basis of disease,* Philadelphia, 1989, WB Saunders.
3. Henshaw EC: The biology of cancer. In Rubin P, editor: *Clinical oncology: a multidisciplinary approach for physicians and students,* ed 7, Philadelphia, 1993, WB Saunders.
4. Kardinal CG, Strnad BN: Confrontation with cancer: historical and existential aspects. In Gross SC, Garb S, editors: *Cancer treatment and research in humanistic perspective,* New York, 1985, Springer Publishing .
5. Raven RW: The development and practice of oncology. In Gross SC, Garb S, editors: *Cancer treatment and research in humanistic perspective,* New York, 1985, Springer Publishing.
6. Solomon E, Borrow J, Goddard, AD: Chromosome aberrations and cancer, *Science* 254:1153-1159, 1991.
7. Weinberg RA: Tumor suppressor genes, *Science* 254:1138-1145, 1991.
8. Yunis JJ: The chromosomal basis of human neoplasia, *Science* 221:227-235, 1983.

BIBLIOGRAPHY

Aaronson SA: Growth factors and cancer, *Science* 254:1146-1152, 1991.
McCune CS, Chang AY: Basic concepts of tumor immunology and principles of immunotherapy. In Rubin P, editor: *Clinical oncology: a multidisciplinary approach for physicians and students,* ed 7, Philadelphia, 1993, WB Saunders.
Pajak T: Methodology of clinical trials. In Perez C, Brady L, editors: *Principles and practice of radiation oncology,* ed 2, Philadelphia, 1992, JB Lippincott.
Perez C, Brady L: Overview. In Perez C, Brady L, editors: *Principles and practice of radiation oncology,* ed 2, Philadelphia, 1992, JB Lippincott.
Ruben P, McDonald S, Keller J: Staging and classification of cancer: a unified approach. In Perez C, Brady L, editors: *Principles and practice of radiation oncology,* ed 2, Philadelphia, 1992, JB Lippincott.
Weiss DW: Immunological intervention in neoplasia. In Beers RF, Tilghman RC, Bassett EG, editors: *The role of immunological factors in viral and oncogenic processes.* Seventh International Symposium, Baltimore, 1974, Johns Hopkins University Press.

Epidemiology and Etiology

Wanda Teasley

Outline

Key terms

For the radiation therapist to fully understand the treatment delivered in the attempt to control cancer, a thorough understanding of cancer and its causes is essential. When patients seek health care, they expect to receive total care from health professionals. To do this, the radiation therapist must go beyond treatment and provide the patient with steps to prevent the disease. A general understanding of the disease process, treatment, and causes and trends of development begins with a discussion of the **etiology** and **epidemiology** of cancer.

Etiology is defined as the cause of a disease or the study of the cause.[8] For many diseases, this is a relatively simple process. The factors affecting the diseased group are compared with those that affect the normal group. By the process of elimination a person can determine the most likely cause. Further study on this theory usually yields the cause of the disease. For cancer the answer is not a simple one. Although numerous theories exist about the development of cancer, no single cause has been identified.

Epidemiology, like etiology, is the study of the cause of disease. However, epidemiology carries the study one step further. After a cause is identified, the information is used to relate the incidence and relationships of the disease to the population.[8] The application of this knowledge toward treatment and prevention is then used to help control the disease. For example, after experts determined that smoking was the major cause of lung cancer, the next step was to identify smokers and begin programs to reduce the number of lung cancer patients. For tobacco companies a program was initiated to lower the amount of tar and nicotine in tobacco products to reduce the dangers of smoking.

SOURCES OF INFORMATION

Information concerning cancer has been collected for years. A vast bank of knowledge is available concerning the development of cancer, its victims, its causes, and the reasons some persons get the disease and others do not. No national tumor registry or place to report actual cancer incidence exists. For the past 80 years the American Cancer Society (ACS) has been instrumental in collecting information about cancer and encouraging others to do so on local and national levels. In the 1930s, the ACS began a project with the American College of Surgeons to collect cancer information from various facilities across the country. This project eventually became the American College of Surgeons Commission on Cancer. Through this effort a database on cancer was established with cooperation from hospitals throughout the country. By 1988 over 67% of those involved in the project were using a computerized system to obtain data with endless possibilities of matching information across the country.[7]

Another source of information about cancer is the Surveillance, Epidemiology, and End Results (**SEER**) program. In 1973 the National Cancer Institute began the SEER program, which collects and compiles data from cancer registries across the country. A total of 11 population-based cancer registries now participate in the program, which samples about 10% of the population of the United States.[2,3] The SEER program represents enough of the population in the United States that this information can be used to project numbers for the entire population. Much of the information available today concerning incidence was collected as a result of SEER.

For years the ACS collected information and combined it with the data from SEER to help project deaths resulting from cancer. Because no sure way to determine these numbers existed, the ACS used mortality figures provided by the National Center for Health Statistics and the 1970 U.S. census.[2] This information and the reported incidence of cancers led to the estimation of the number of cancers and expected deaths during the coming year. This method provided a good estimate. However, in 1990 the ACS acquired access to the information provided by the World Health Organization (WHO),[2] which allowed more complete information and a mechanism to compare the data with information from around the world and not just in the United States. The 1992 edition of *CA Cancer Journal for Clinicians,* published by the ACS, was the first to use this expanded data bank of information. The 1996 issue of the journal projects cancer incidence and mortality by site for men and women based on collection of these data (Figs. 2-1 and 2-2).

Most medium-to-large treatment centers participate in **tumor registries**. All cancers are registered according to the same characteristics and treatment information. A tumor registry collects data on a local level and may be expanded to include the community, state, or nation. If these tumor registries are part of the SEER program, the institution can use these data to compare its method of treatment with others. The information supplied in the 1994 *CA Cancer Journal for Clinicians* had the benefit of collection from 937 hospitals during 1991 to make predictions.[7]

Purposes of data collection

Predictions are only as good as the information used to make them. The ACS tested its predictions and found that the projections were extremely close to the actual number of cancer cases and deaths for that year.[3] Incidence rates can even be categorized in such a way to determine the exact group, age,

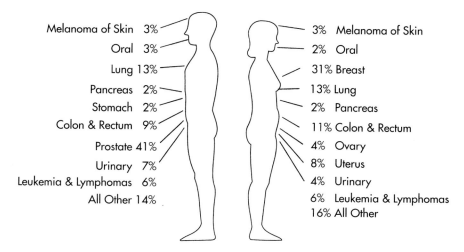

Melanoma of Skin 3%
Oral 3%
Lung 13%
Pancreas 2%
Stomach 2%
Colon & Rectum 9%
Prostate 41%
Urinary 7%
Leukemia & Lymphomas 6%
All Other 14%

3% Melanoma of Skin
2% Oral
31% Breast
13% Lung
2% Pancreas
11% Colon & Rectum
4% Ovary
8% Uterus
4% Urinary
6% Leukemia & Lymphomas
16% All Other

Fig. 2-1 Estimated cancer incidence by site and gender for 1996. (From Steele GD Jr et al: Clinical highlights from the National Cancer Data Base, *CA Cancer J Clin* 44:71-80, 1996; American Cancer Society: *Cancer facts and figures,* New York, 1996, The Society.)

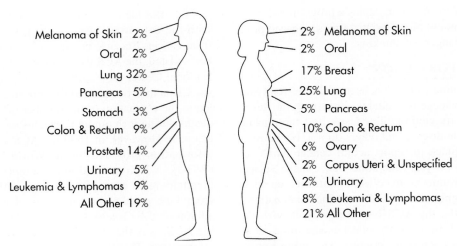

Melanoma of Skin 2%
Oral 2%
Lung 32%
Pancreas 5%
Stomach 3%
Colon & Rectum 9%
Prostate 14%
Urinary 5%
Leukemia & Lymphomas 9%
All Other 19%

2% Melanoma of Skin
2% Oral
17% Breast
25% Lung
5% Pancreas
10% Colon & Rectum
6% Ovary
2% Corpus Uteri & Unspecified
2% Urinary
8% Leukemia & Lymphomas
21% All Other

Fig. 2-2 Estimated cancer deaths by site and gender for 1996. (From Steele GD Jr et al: Clinical highlights from the National Cancer Data Base, *CA Cancer J Clin* 44:71-80, 1996; American Cancer Society: *Cancer facts and figures,* New York, 1996, The Society.)

location, or gender that is experiencing increases or decreases in the number of cancer cases. This is important because epidemiology is used to determine the way the disease can be controlled. Knowledge of the locations of cancer increases in general (or even in certain types of cancer) can help to direct which programs (prevention or treatment) are initiated. This knowledge also indicates which programs have been successful. Hospital officials are more likely to purchase specific treatment equipment if they are assured that the equipment will be in demand. In addition, with the coming of community-based care a prevention program can be geared to match the diseases most common to the community if the information is available.

Second, this information helps researchers to ask better questions. Each research project begins with a question, a **hypothesis.** If the right question is not asked, the research may be in vain. Much research of the literature and a review of scientific data must be completed before a person takes on a research project. This assures the scientist that the work will produce the desired results and will be considered valid by the scientific community.

Finally, for cancers that have no easily recognizable etiology, massive reports can help identify common factors and thus become instrumental in identifying the cause of the cancer. By being able to enter all the information collected into a computer-driven program, the scientist can sort multiple characteristics and factors to identify commonalities. An example of this is the fact that the South Atlantic states have a much higher incidence of cancers than other parts of the country. Is this due to the population being generally older in those regions, or do the lifestyles of those individuals promote cancer? Chances are good that the actual reason is a combination of the two, and to determine the real answer, scientists must consider specific cancers according to the individual's ages and lifestyles.

Other examples of the way this information is valuable can also be cited. For example, of the new cases reported in the Nation Cancer Data Base, 85.5% involved non-Hispanic, white individuals. Does this mean that these people are identified because they have better access to health care, or does it mean that they really have a higher incidence of cancer? Another set of data shows that 76.4% of the new cancers were treated at the facilities where the diagnoses were made.[7] This could have major implications for facilities considering cancer-screening programs. However, the data can also mean that only those places offering treatment really look for the disease carefully. Although the information provided by these types of databases often creates more questions than it answers, a tremendous amount of information is gained from asking these questions. As the field of radiation oncology continues to expand, the radiation therapist must be actively involved in asking these important questions and integral in providing information for the answers.

CANCER INCIDENCE

The **incidence** rate is usually referenced in a discussion on cancer. An incidence rate is the result of a comparison between the number of cancers and the number of people in a given population over a certain period.[1] This comparison presents important statistics concerning which cancers are increasing and which are decreasing in number. To have useful information, the data are often **stratified,** which means that the researcher has identified several factors and then sorts all the data according to these factors.

Approximately 30% of the population gets cancer of some form. This estimate represents only those malignancies that are not easily cured and often result in chronic illness or death. Knowing the factors involved with the development of these cancers helps health care professionals plan for diagnostic screening, educational programs, and treatment facili-

Table 2-1	National cancer data base cases by selected characteristics, 1991

Characteristics	Cases	Percent
Sex		
Male	251,638	49.6
Female	255,565	50.4
TOTAL	507,203	100.0
Age		
0-14	3,485	0.7
15-19	1,975	0.4
20-29	13,317	2.6
30-39	27,554	5.4
40-49	44,943	8.9
50-59	69,751	13.8
60-69	137,355	27.1
70-79	141,738	27.9
80 and over	67,085	13.2
Ethnicity		
Non-Hispanic white	433,882	85.5
Hispanic	13,255	2.6
Black	38,726	7.6
Asian	6,981	1.4
American Indian	766	0.2
Unknown	13,593	2.7
Region		
New England	29,434	5.8
Mid-Atlantic	66,710	13.2
South Atlantic	93,291	18.4
East North Central	85,023	16.8
East South Central	32,969	6.5
West North Central	40,071	7.9
West South Central	49,441	9.7
Mountain	25,046	4.9
Pacific	85,218	16.8
Income		
0-31,999	105,290	20.7
32,000-52,999	267,600	52.8
53,000+	99,745	19.7
Unknown	34,568	6.8

Characteristics	Cases	Percent
Percent Rural Population		
0-19	334,841	66.0
20-39	52,166	10.3
40-59	35,112	6.9
60-79	21,185	4.2
80-100	63,899	12.6
Hospital Caseload		
<150	9,982	2.0
150-499 cases	127,380	25.1
500-999 cases	212,515	41.9
≥ 1000 cases	152,239	30.0
Unknown size	5,087	1.0
Approval Category		
NCI-comprehensive	5,807	1.1
Teaching hospital	110,946	21.9
Community comprehensive	164,803	32.5
Community	145,021	28.6
Other approved	2,751	0.5
Nonapproved	77,875	15.4
Hospital Referral Status		
Diagnosed here, treated elsewhere	14,674	2.9
Diagnosed here, treated here	387,471	76.4
Diagnosed elsewhere, treated here	103,518	20.4
Unknown	1,540	0.3

From Steele GD Jr et al: Clinical highlights from the National Cancer Data Base, 1994, *CA J Clin* 44:72-73, 1994.

ties. The usual stratification factors are age, gender, ethnicity, and geographical location (Table 2-1). Some general trends are associated with each of these factors.

Age

Most types of cancer are considered chronic diseases for older persons. As the age of the population increases, generally so does the incidence of cancer. However, several cancers are exceptions to this fact. For example, acute lymphocytic leukemia is rare in patients other than the extremely young. The same is true for Wilms' tumor, which is a cancer

of the kidney.[4] One cancer (Hodgkin's disease) is considered **bimodal** in incidence. *Bimodal* refers to a cancer that has two clusters, or peaks, of incidence (one cluster at 20 to 30 years of age and another after the age of 50). Knowing the age of individuals can offer valuable information during consideration of population projections (Tables 2-2 and 2-3).

Gender

Another factor that has been important is gender. A historical review of statistics shows that a large difference has existed in male and female incidence of cancer, excluding sex-linked

Table 2-2	Mortality for the five leading cancer sites for males by age group, United States, 1990				
All ages	**Under 15**	**15-34**	**35-54**	**55-74**	**75+**
All cancer 268,283	All cancer 949	All cancer 3788	All cancer 27,005	All cancer 141,787	All cancer 94,739
Lung 91,091	Leukemia 344	Leukemia 719	Lung 8882	Lung 56,225	Lung 25,770
Prostate 32,378	Brain and CNS 248	Non-Hodgkin's lymphomas 485	Colon and rectum 2412	Colon and rectum 14,190	Prostate 19,622
Colon and rectum 28,635	Endocrine 113	Brain and CNS 441	Non-Hodgkin's lymphomas 1542	Prostate 12,423	Colon and rectum 11,842
Pancreas 12,199	Non-Hodgkin's lymphomas 66	Skin 289	Brain and CNS 1454	Pancreas 6771	Pancreas 4128
Leukemia 10,192	Connective tissue 41	Hodgkin's disease 279	Pancreas 1252	Non-Hodgkin's lymphomas 4516	Bladder 3694

From Steele GD Jr et al: Clinical highlights from the National Cancer Data Base, 1994, *Ca J Clin* 44:71-80, 1994.

Table 2-3	Mortality for the five leading cancer sites for females by age group, United States, 1990				
All ages	**Under 15**	**15-34**	**35-54**	**55-74**	**75+**
All cancer 237,039	All cancer 748	All cancer 3458	All cancer 29,041	All cancer 110,545	All cancer 93,235
Lung 50,194	Leukemia 232	Breast 643	Breast 9192	Lung 29,729	Colon and rectum 15,524
Breast 43,391	Brain and CNS 212	Leukemia 484	Lung 5417	Breast 20,096	Lung 14,924
Colon and rectum 28,895	Endocrine 89	Uterus 358	Uterus 2071	Colon and rectum 11,205	Breast 13,458
Pancreas 12,883	Connective tissue 49	Brain and CNS 301	Colon and rectum 1998	Ovary 6575	Pancreas 6376
Ovary 12,762	Bone 39	Non-Hodgkin's lymphomas 197	Ovary 1728	Pancreas 5674	Ovary 4310

From Steele GD Jr et al: Clinical highlights from the National Cancer Data Base, 1994, *CA J Clin* 44:71-80, 1994.

cancers such as those of the breast, prostate, and cervix. This factor was rather confusing to researchers who tried to link cancer to the environment because men and women have shared the environment. However, over the past few years the incidence of cancer in women has increased to the point that the difference between men and women is not extremely great. Researchers have proposed several theories to explain this increase. First, women have been smoking more over the past 20 years. Women who started smoking in the 1940s are now approaching the age at which many cancers associated with smoking are diagnosed. Second, more men have stopped smoking over the past 20 years. This has lowered not only the incidence of lung cancer for men, but also the death rate from cardiovascular disease. Finally, women over the past 30 years have taken on the lifestyles of men.[4] The pressures of work, management of a household, and interaction with the work force and all its hazards have increased cancers in women. Women are bridging the gender gap so quickly that this is no longer considered to be a major variable in cancer incidence.

Ethnicity

Ethnicity has often been identified as a definite stratification factor for cancer research. Examples of this are lower rates of cervical cancer among Jewish and Mormon women even though they live in the same communities as others. A more direct relationship is the incidence of skin cancer, which is almost negligible among African-Americans yet high and rising among white Americans. Another correlation is the lower incidence of breast cancer among Japanese women. When these women immigrate to the United States, they have a lower-than-average incidence for the cancer if their traditional diet and lifestyle are maintained. Indians have a higher incidence of gallbladder, cervical, pancreatic, and stomach cancers. Hispanics have more cancers of the stomach, cervix, gallbladder, and liver yet lower rates of breast and colon cancers. These differences among races can often be associated with socioeconomic factors, lifestyle, or culture rather than genetics; however, the variation is significant enough that stratification by race is useful in cancer research statistics.[1,4]

Geography

The last typical stratification factor is geography. Considering areas of the country or world in which certain cancers tend to cluster is useful. An example of this type of clustering is the fact that women living near the Great Lakes have a higher incidence of breast cancer. Another association is that a greater number of colon cancers are cited in the northern section of the country. One relationship that is clearer is the higher number of malignant melanoma cases in the southern regions or lower latitudes of the country. This section of the country is closer to the equator; thus sun exposure is more likely. Unfortunately, our society has become so mobile that the factor of geography is now less important. However, knowing the rates of incidence for specific localities remains essential in planning radiation oncology centers.

Prevalence

With the aging of the population, often termed the *greying of America*, the incidence of cancer is expected to rise considerably over the next decade. As for other chronic diseases that will have an effect on health care, only cardiovascular disease comes close to exceeding the magnitude of the cancer problem. In addition to the increasing number of older persons, a trend exists for increases in the number of childhood tumors. The rate of cancer in African-Americans is up 26%, whereas the rate for whites has increased only 5%. This information should be a guide in knowing the types and locations of prevention and screening programs that should be held. Fortunately, the mortality rate from cancer is appearing to level off, with the exception of lung cancer, which has steadily increased in incidence and more so in mortality.

Other cancers that are less prevalent today than in previous years are breast, prostate, and colon. Although physicians diagnose many new cases annually, these cancers are being found earlier and treatment methods are more successful than ever before. All this adds up to progress toward solving the cancer problem. Society knows more about cancer, its causes, and symptoms. As experts in the field, radiation therapists must strive to increase this awareness into the next decade.

Risks

Knowing factors that increase the chances of getting cancer enhances the opportunity to change those trends. Enough of a difference must be made to alter the **relative risks** of getting cancer. The relative risk is the likelihood that a person who has a certain risk factor will actually get the disease in question. Relative risk involves considering the chances of a person getting the cancer over those who already have it but did not have that particular risk factor.[1] For example, the number of lung cancer patients can be compared with the number of the population who smoke. Then this can be compared, using a ratio, with persons who have lung cancer in relationship to those who do not smoke. This comparison results in a number representative of the actual risk that smoking contributes to the incidence of lung cancer. The number should be 1 or greater if the factor is a significant risk for the population.

Another term often applied to risk is **attributable risks**. This concept is somewhat simpler because it considers only the number of people who have the disease minus those who did not have that particular risk factor.[1] This term is not used as often as relative risk because it does not consider that other factors not considered may have increased the incidence for all individuals in the population. Scientists must consider all the demographic information, risks factors, and number of cancers diagnosed annually to determine the actual cause for a particular cancer. Through years of research, information is now available that allows health care providers, with a certain amount of assurance, to inform the public of factors that are likely to increase the chances of getting cancer or having a recurrence of cancer.

PRIMARY CAUSES OF CANCER

As mentioned earlier, no single cause can be associated with the development of a malignancy. However, a number of general causative factors such as environment, occupation, exposure to certain viruses, heredity, iatrogenic sources, car-

Table 2-4	Risk factors for selected cancer sites

Cancer site	High-risk factors
Lung	Heavy smoker over age 50 Smoked a pack a day for 20 years Started smoking at age 15 or before Smoker working with or near asbestos
Breast	Lump in breast or nipple discharge History of breast cancer in other breast or benign breast disease Family history of breast cancer Diet high in fat Nulliparity or first child after age 30 Early menarche or menopause
Colon-rectum	History or rectal polyps or colonic adenomatosis Family history of rectal polyps Ulcerative colitis or Crohn's disease Obesity Increasing age
Uterine- endometrial	Unusual vaginal bleeding or discharge History of menstrual irregularity Late menopause (after age 55) Nulliparity Infertility, through anovulation Diabetes, high blood pressure, and obesity Age 50 to 64
Skin	Excessive exposure to sun Fair complexion, burn easily Presence of congenital moles or history of dys- plastic nevi or cutaneous melanoma Family history of melanoma Heavy smoker and drinker
Oral	Heavy smoker and drinker Poor oral hygiene Long-term exposure to the sun (lip)
Ovary	History of ovarian cancer among close relatives Nulliparity or delayed age at first pregnancy Age 50 to 59
Prostate	Increasing age Occupation relating to the use of cadmium
Stomach	History of stomach cancer among close relatives Diet heavy in smoked, pickled, or salted foods

From Baird SB et al, editors: *A cancer book for nurses,* ed 6, Atlanta, 1991, The American Cancer Society.

cinogenic agents, and even psychological disturbances are associated specifically with some cancers (Table 2-4). To understand patients and their backgrounds and to help them and their family members win the battle against the disease, radiation therapists need an appreciation for these factors.

Environmental factors

The environment has been blamed for creating many diseases in animals and plants for many years. Although people have made concerted efforts to improve the quality of the environment, many cancer-causing factors such as smog, water pollution, and natural sources of harmful substances still exist. Many of the reports of cancer incidence are based on political boundaries, states, or regions, a fact that makes a review of the statistics more difficult. However, a comparison of total cancers by type from one country to another reveals some patterns. One of the factors in the environment associated with the increase in lung cancer and possibly accountable for the fact that some non-smokers get lung cancer is radon. Several years ago much concern developed over houses built with brick containing uranium ore. As uranium breaks down, radon gas is emitted. This exposure is believed to account for about 20,000 cases of lung cancer annually. The Environmental Protection Agency recommends testing homes for radon exposure and has also developed guidelines for reducing exposure to the gas.[6]

Another environmental concern of recent years is the amount of fluoride in drinking water. Numerous studies have been conducted, yet none have proved that any significant risk is associated with fluoride in the water.[4] A certain amount of risk is associated with surface water because of various contaminants. Arsenic, lead, cadmium, and mercury are found in varying amounts in surface water today.[6] In addition, herbicides, pesticides, and insecticides in use today eventually end up in the ground water. These chemicals contribute to the incidence of cancer.

Other types of pollution include those found in and near larger cities. Smog from industries and emissions from automobiles contribute to the incidence of lung cancer. These are controllable sources of carcinogens, which are present in all environments to some degree. Government programs and regulations over the past 10 years have helped slow this process; however, the pollution in the air remains a major concern for the health of the population.

The sun is also a factor in the environmental theory of the cause of cancer. The ultraviolet light from the sun is damaging to the skin, even in small amounts.[5] This is not a new concept; however, the general population does not consider the damage a problem because primary skin cancers are easy to diagnose and often easy to treat. Although these cancers are malignant, they appear to pose no serious threat to society. Unfortunately, the same is not true for melanoma. The incidence for melanoma has significantly increased in the past few years. With the increase in the number of sunbathers and introduction of the tanning bed several years ago, the number of melanoma cases is likely to increase rapidly over the next few years. The primary damage from the sun that results in cancer occurs during the teenage years. These are the years in which the sun and tanning booths are most popular.

Industry or material	Carcinogen involved	Site of associated cancer*
Asbestos	Asbestos	Lung
Brewing	Alcohol	Liver
Commercial fishing	Ultraviolet light	Skin
Demolition	Asbestos	Lung, pleura
Furniture manufacturing	Wood dusts	Nasal passages
Glue factories	Benzene	Leukemia
Insulation	Asbestos	Lung, pleura
Ion-exchange resin production	Bis(chloromethyl) ether	Lung
Isopropyl alcohol manufacturing	Isopropyl alcohol	Nasal passages
Mineral oil	Polycyclic hydrocarbons	Lung, skin
Nickel refining	Nickel	Lung, nasal passages
Ore manufacturing	Chromium	Lung
Outdoor occupations	Ultraviolet light	Skin
Pesticides	Arsenic	Lung, skin
Petroleum production	Polycyclic hydrocarbons	Lung
Pigment manufacturing	Chromium	Lung
Rubber manufacturing	Aromatic amines	Bladder
Shipyards	Asbestos	Lung, skin
Smelters	Arsenic	Lung, skin
Uranium mining	Ionizing radiation	Multiple sites
Varnish	Benzene	Leukemia
Vinyl chloride	Vinyl chloride	Liver

Table 2-5 Occupational exposures and cancer

From Osteen RT, editor: *Cancer manual*, ed 8, Boston, 1990, The American Cancer Society, Massachusetts Division.
*All industry-related lung cancers are associated synergistically with tobacco use. Exposure to tobacco, alcohol, sunlight, and certain dietary factors is far more important in the etiology of lung cancer than are any of the exposures listed above.

Occupational factors

Reports from numerous occupational studies indicate that some workers may be at a particularly high risk for certain cancers (Table 2-5). One of the occupations identified is the mining of tar and coal. These miners have a high incidence of lung cancer. Individuals who work in rubber, plastic, dye, or paint industries have a high incidence of bladder cancer. Farmers have a high incidence of skin cancer because of sun exposure and insecticides. Individuals who work in the leather and furniture industry have a high incidence of nasal cavity cancer from exposure to dust. One occupational risk that has been documented for years is the increase in bone cancer among workers who painted radium on the faces of watches.[4] Another occupational risk that has received much interest over the past decade involves workers who are exposed to asbestos, particularly those who smoke cigarettes. A definite link exists between asbestos workers and mesothelioma (cancer of the lining of the lung) or lung cancer.[5]

Some occupations truly carry certain risks for cancers. One such occupation is that of radiation work. Theories have been proposed regarding increases in the number of leukemia cases among radiation workers. This problem originated with physicists and physicians years ago when little or no attention was given to radiation safety. A study conducted with members of the Radiological Society of North America

(RSNA) indicated a slight increase in the incidence; however, this report has not been confirmed. In a modern therapeutic setting the exposure is extremely low.

Additional controls by the Occupational Safety and Health Administration (**OSHA**) have started to have an effect on hazards associated with many radiation occupations. OSHA establishes regulations for the work place that protect the employee from damaging substances. The government requires the employer to enforce these safety practices. As new information is gained on the cause of cancer, new regulations are devised to help protect employees.

Viruses

Another theory of the cause of cancer is exposure to certain viruses. Probably one of the most notable viruses is the Epstein-Barr virus (EBV). Individuals who contract EBV (the virus responsible for mumps) have a higher incidence of nasopharyngeal cancers, Hodgkin's disease, and Burkitt's lymphoma. In Asia and Africa, many people have had hepatitis B virus, which has a direct link with cancer of the liver. Health care workers must carefully follow OSHA standards regarding the handling of blood and body fluids so that the spread of this virus is prevented. Another virus that has received much attention in recent years is papillomavirus.[5] This is a sexually transmitted virus that has a direct link with cancer of the cervix.

Probably the most prevalent example of a viral link to cancer today is the human immunodeficiency virus (HIV). As most people today know, this is the virus that is believed to be responsible for acquired immunodeficiency syndrome (AIDS). After the virus has developed into AIDS the risk of Kaposi's sarcoma, anorectal carcinoma, and other opportunistic infections increases.[5] A majority of patients who have AIDS are treated in radiation oncology departments for Kaposi's sarcoma.

Genetics

More than 200 genes have been linked to cancer.[5] Several syndromes that have genetic origins (such as Turner syndrome and cancers of the brain or neural crest) have been associated with a higher incidence of cancer. This link is believed to be caused by these syndromes that result in unstable chromosomes.[4] The instability of these chromosomes may lead to faulty synthesis of deoxyribonucleic acid and mutation into cancer cells. The research is continuing because this theory does not offer a plausible explanation for the development of cancer in some individuals. Genetic links to cancer are also seen much more in matched organs,[5] such as breasts, eyes, and kidneys.

The cancers most frequently associated with genetics are breast, retinoblastoma, and colon. For women who have breast cancer the risk is much higher if the mother or a maternal relative has also had breast cancer. Cancers that share this link tend to appear at an earlier age. Retinoblastoma has a 100% risk of cancer in a subsequent generation.[5] Breast cancer has also been strongly associated with Klinefelter syndrome,[4] which is characterized by the presence of an extra X chromosome in males.[8] Colon cancer, which has been studied for some time, also has genetic links. If a patient has familial polyposis and resultant cancer of the colon, the risk of the offspring also being affected by the disease is great.[5] In this particular situation, this knowledge has led to a steady improvement in survival rates because members of those families can be followed much closer for early detection. Therefore the foundation exists for recommending that women who have family histories of breast cancer obtain baseline mammograms at younger ages than other women and that individuals who have colon cancer in their families obtain annual screenings for the disease.

Iatrogenic factors

Some cancers are the result of treatment administered for other conditions. **Iatrogenic** origin of the cancer describes this type of condition. The definition of this word implies that misadministration of the treatment is the cause for the condition.[8] For most cancers that result from previous treatment, the damage is caused not from misadministration but from lack of knowledge. In some situations the risks are of less concern than the benefit from the treatment.

Chemotherapeutic drug therapy has made many advances over the past 20 years. At the time of the original trials with the new forms of these drugs, many people did not realize the long-term deleterious effects of the drugs. To further complicate the issue, chemotherapeutic drugs are often used with radiation. Over the years the drug and radiation dosages have been adjusted so that the long-term effects are not as prevalent. The major concern of chemotherapeutic administration is that if the reticuloendothelial system is damaged, the possibility of leukemia is much greater. One drug in particular that has a direct link with a cancer is cyclophosphamide, a chemotherapy alkylating agent. This drug has been associated with an increase in acute nonlymphocytic leukemia.[5] Other types of leukemia have occurred in patients who have been successfully treated for Wilms' tumor and Hodgkin's disease with chemotherapeutic drugs and radiation. Although a risk of a secondary cancer exists at a later time, these primary cancers would have resulted in mortality without the treatment.

As mentioned previously, another type of treatment that has the ability to create an iatrogenic condition is radiation oncology. Although radiation therapy is rarely used for non-malignant conditions, this was not always so. Approximately 50 years ago, physicians used radiation therapy to treat conditions such as acne, arthritis, plantar warts, infections, tuberculosis, tinea capitis, and enlarged thymus glands. Now other methods of treatment are available for these conditions, and experts realize that the risks associated with the treatment are not worthy of the benefit. Cancers of the head and neck, thyroid, breast, skin, and lung have developed in some patients because of this therapy. Now radiation oncology is reserved for malignant tumors in all but a few selected cases, such as heterotropic bone, arteriovenous (AV) malformations, pituitary tumors, and keloids.

Another type of iatrogenic cancer is that induced from the administration of certain chemicals. The most prevalent example of this is endometrial cancer, which occurs at puberty in the daughters of women who received diethylstilbestrol (DES) during pregnancy.[5] DES was administered to pregnant women who were at a high risk of miscarriage, but the drug is no longer used for this purpose because of its effects.

Other drug-induced cancers are breast and cervical, which have been identified in women who took large doses of estrogen for birth control. Experimentation over the years has shown that birth control can be accomplished with much lower doses of estrogen. Now this form of birth control is even suspected to reduce the incidence of breast cancer. Much discussion and future study remain to be conducted on the subject. Increased levels of estrogen for postmenopausal women has also been linked to the increased incidence of endometrial cancers.[1] Previously, women have been given this drug to lessen the effects of menopause. A review of the incidence of endometrial cancer reveals that the number of cases was much higher during the 1970s and 1980s. Since that time, postmenopausal dosages have been monitored more closely and the incidence of endometrial cancers has been on the decline.

Lifestyle

By far, the largest contributor to the incidence of cancer is lifestyle and carcinogens to which people are exposed by virtue of their lifestyles.[1] A strong association exists between lifestyle and the likelihood of developing certain cancers. Behaviors such as tobacco consumption, alcohol intake, and sexual promiscuity increase the incidence of cancer, and behavior modification must occur to reduce the risks. The stressful environment of inner cities and high-pressure positions are also contributors to the incidence of cancer. Finally, lack of education also increases the chances of getting cancer and not having successful treatment because of delayed diagnosis.[4]

Tobacco

In 1990 the incidence of lung cancer decreased slightly. This was the first time an appreciable decrease was noted for the disease.[3] The reason for the decline is that a significant number of men have stopped smoking. Unfortunately, more women are smoking, so the incidence of lung cancer has not decreased as much as health care workers would like. The primary cause of cancer deaths is lung cancer for men and women. The number of deaths from cancer of the lung is now estimated to be 30%.[1] If everyone stopped smoking today, the incidence of lung cancer would drop by over 85%.[5] Smoking increases the risk of cancer not only in smokers, but also in those around them. The Surgeon General of the United States has estimated that a person exposed to secondary smoke has a 30% greater risk of getting lung cancer.

Although lung cancer causes the greatest concern, cigarette smoking contributes to many other types of cancer. The incidence of cancers of the upper airway (such as pharyngeal, nasophyarngeal, and esophageal) are also increased in smokers. In addition to cancers directly related to the inhalation of the smoke, those of the bladder, cervix, pancreas, and kidneys are more prevalent among smokers. Other effects created by tobacco are low birth weight and traces of nicotine found in the children of parents who smoke.

Tobacco companies continue to lobby for lesser controls on smoking, and recent allegations have been made that the tobacco industry has deliberately withheld information concerning the deleterious effects of tobacco consumption. An effort has been made to decrease the amount of nicotine in cigarettes; however, this has yet to show any significant changes in the incidence of lung cancer. After a person stops smoking and is smoke free for 10 to 15 years, the risk of lung cancer equals that of a nonsmoker. In the era of health care reform, more stringent regulation of public smoking and tobacco company products is likely. One pro-

posal even suggests that nicotine be identified as a controlled substance. This will have a tremendous impact on the tobacco industry and thus the incidence of cancers associated with smoking.

Diet

In the 1970s, evidence that connected diet to the incidence of cancer began to emerge. Specifically, red meat is linked to colon cancer and a high-fat diet is linked to breast and uterine cancer.[4] Some of the research has been questioned in the past because the majority of it has been conducted in laboratories with animals and the dosages far exceeded the normal amounts for humans. Further research has indicated that certain dietary habits can increase the likelihood of cancer development.

Over the past 20 years the incidence of stomach cancer has decreased. This decrease is believed to be directly linked to the change in methods of food preparation and storage. Foods that are fried, high in preservatives, and preserved by salting or pickling contribute significantly to the risk of cancer in the digestive tract.[4] Some foods are believed to be anticarcinogens because they actually contain enzymes that can deactivate harmful substances in foods. Other studies indicate that inert substances in some foods actually slow the metabolism of the host, thus giving a greater opportunity for carcinogens to do damage.[5] The problem in pinpointing the culprit in dietary consideration is that the existence of so many variables makes segregating the specific factor difficult.

Alcohol

Alcohol consumption receives much less acknowledgment in the risks of cancer; however, 5% of deaths from cancer can be associated with alcohol.[1] The typical cancers that result from alcohol consumption are liver, mouth, pharynx, larynx, and esophagus. The association of the head and neck and esophageal cancers with alcohol consumption is further enhanced if cigarette smoking is also a factor. Although each is a carcinogen, together the effects are even more apparent. The link between the use of alcohol and cancer of the liver is connected with the presence of cirrhosis.[5] Current studies indicate that moderate alcohol consumption may actually be beneficial to the patient who has other health problems such as heart disease. Most authorities consider moderate alcohol consumption to be no more than one or two drinks daily.

Chemicals

As mentioned previously, the exposure to chemicals in the environment is considered a major source of cancer development. Hydrocarbons are present in the atmosphere and numerous additives in foods. Benzene, chromates, polyvinylchloride, and aflatoxins have all been cited as carcinogens and are present in many aspects of society.

Researchers have analyzed numerous chemical compounds in an effort to determine the common characteristic in the development of cancer. The one typical characteristic is that all carcinogenic chemicals are referred to as *electrophilic*, which means that these chemicals seek out spare electrons and then attach to them.[4] The likelihood that cancer will develop as a result of this attachment and the ensuing damage to the ribonucleic acid and deoxyribonucleic acid is quite high.

Stress

The final realm of study in the etiology of cancer is the psychological status of the host. The effect of psychological status has been implied for years; however, the actual studies are difficult to substantiate. The risk factors that can be associated with the development of cancer are childhood instability, lack of goals in life, job and marital instability, and recent loss of a loved one or significant possession. The primary concern with many of these theories is that the knowledge of the cancer can actually contaminate the psychological status of the patient, so the factor cannot be identified exclusively.[4]

Insecurity, stress, and lack of control may all be the result of learning about the disease. Studies indicate that stress and lack of family support increase the risks of cancer. One particular study (called a **prospective** study) used medical students as the subjects. A prospective study means that the factors of consideration are identified in the subjects. The individuals were followed over time and matched with the incidence of cancer that occurred in them.[4] The cancer can then be associated with the factors being considered for etiology. Though this study was prospective, most studies in this area have been **retrospective**, or after the fact. Many questions remain about whether the response was the result of the psychological status of the patient or the way the patient chose to cope with the stresses of life. Researchers are then faced with the task of differentiating between the psychological state and the adverse lifestyle.

Obviously more studies are necessary in the area of the psychological state and the development of cancer. Radiation therapists can be instrumental in conducting this type of research. Although the involvement of the therapist is always retrospective, useful investigations can still be made into the development of second cancers or progress in response to treatment and the psychological state of the patient who has cancer.

USES OF DATA COLLECTION

Knowing the cause is the most efficient way of solving any problem. This is particularly true for cancer. Statistics on cancer incidence and mortality provide understanding about the reasons that cancer exists. As this information becomes available, professionals can work toward changing factors associated with cancer, whether through education, behavior, or conditions.

Prevention

For cancers associated with diet, prevention guidelines are extremely straightforward. The individual should decrease the amount of dietary fat to 30% or less of the daily calories consumed. The amount of fruits, vegetables, and whole grains should be increased in order to have an overall gain in the amount of fiber in the individual's diet. A concerted effort should be made to limit the amount of dietary supplements and alcohol. Finally, the individual should avoid food-preparation methods that involve pickling, smoking, or curing.[5]

As discussed throughout the chapter, cigarette smoking is the most preventable cause of death from cancer. Behavior-modification and smoking-cessation programs have been extremely successful in reducing the number of smokers and lowering the incidence of cancer. The effects of smoking-cessation programs have been appreciated in the 1980s in regard to the death rate of men as a result of lung cancer (Figs. 2-3 and 2-4). Although the rate is still increasing for women, the hope is that this too will begin to decline in the next few years.

Education

Education of the general public has also been a beneficial component in reducing the incidence of cancer and thus the death rate. As a result of extensive public education programs, the death rates for persons who have cancers of the breast and prostate have decreased. As people understand the importance of screening for these cancers, the opportunity for curing the disease becomes much greater. Sun exposure causes damage to the skin, and any amount of sun exposure is harmful. However, with education the general public is beginning to understand that using sunscreens is an extremely important thing to do.

Many studies have shown that the majority of cancers are caused by environment or lifestyle. The incidence of cancer can be greatly reduced if the public is better informed about its causes. Cancer control must go beyond the treatment of the disease. Persons who know the causes of cancer have an obligation to use this knowledge with the public to bring about an overall decline in the number of cancers and earlier detection for cancer victims.

Detection

Because such good information is available about which cancers are most prevalent and the most likely cause of the cancer, reaching target populations is a much easier process. Special screening programs should be conducted in areas of higher incidence or in populations that have a greater risk.

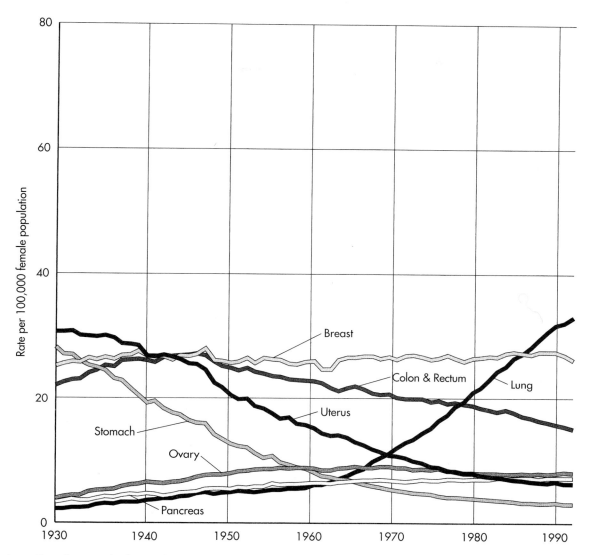

Fig. 2-3 Age-adjusted cancer death rates for selected sites, females, United States, 1930 to 1992. (From American Cancer Society: *Cancer facts and figures,* New York, 1996, The Society.)

The public must be educated about the disease, taught self-examination techniques, and informed of the likely symptoms of the disease.

The Health Insurance Plan of Greater New York conducted a study in the 1960s that demonstrated the benefits of screening for breast cancer.[5] Through screenings, more cancers were found that would not otherwise have been detected through mammograms and physical examinations. Almost all patients who have cancer of the cervix in situ survived 5 years with no evidence of disease. If the cancer has already spread to distant sites, the patient has little or no chance of survival. Cancer of the colon is diagnosed and treated with much greater success if the patient has regular screening examinations. Because no effective screening method has been found for cancer of the lung, the best method of control remains to stop smoking.

Management

Information concerning the types and trends of particular cancers will help a facility's administration to determine which type of equipment to purchase, which programs to offer, and which expansion possibilities to consider. As treatment facilities expand, the focus of the facility will naturally change. Knowing the type and number of cancers for a particular area offers an indication of which areas will require more effort and attention.

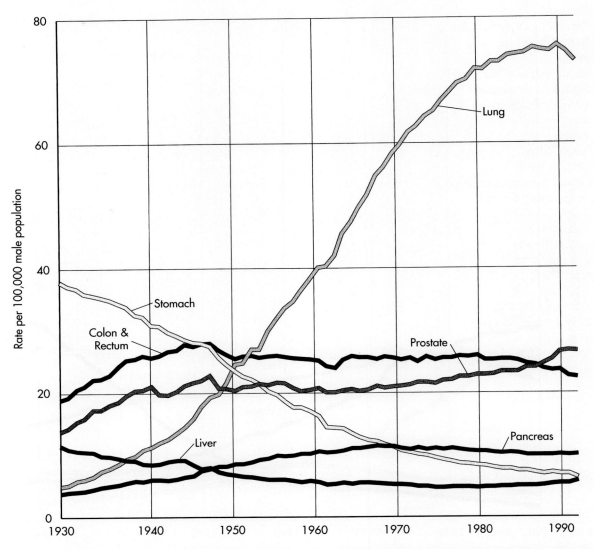

Fig. 2-4 Age-adjusted cancer death rates for selected sites, males, United States, 1930 to 1992. (From American Cancer Society: *Cancer facts and figures,* New York, 1996, The Society.)

Review Questions

Multiple Choice

1. The study of the cause of a disease is which of the following?
   a. Attributable risk
   b. Epidemiology
   c. Etiology
   d. Assigned risk
2. What is the name of the program that collects information from tumor registries throughout the country?
   a. Reporting commission
   b. SEER
   c. U.S. census
   d. OSHA
3. Which of the following is a specific benefit of collecting cancer-incidence information?
   a. Equipment purchases can be made with more assurance that the population it serves is accurate.
   b. Prevention programs can be developed in areas in which they are most needed.
   c. Data can be sorted in such a way that the most reasonable cause for the cancer can be determined.
   d. All of the above are true.

4. What does the term *stratification* mean in regard to data collection?
   a. Separation of the data into logical groups
   b. Reduction of the data to more closely examine the group
   c. Identification of the straight-line portion of the data
   d. Statistical arrangement of the data

5. In general, which age group has the highest incidence of cancer?
   a. Infants
   b. Young adults
   c. Older persons

6. What are the classifications into which cancer data is often separated for study?
   I.   Age
   II. Location
   III. Gender
   IV. Hobbies
   a. I and II only
   b. II and IV only
   c. I, II, and III only
   d. I, II, III, and IV

7. When considering the prevalence of cancer, which of the following terms describes only the likelihood that a certain population will get cancer?
   a. Attributable risks
   b. Absolute risks
   c. Relative risks
   d. Likely risks

8. A person who works in a plastics industry position has a greater incidence of getting bladder cancer later in life. This is an example of what type of cancer cause?
   a. Environment
   b. Occupation
   c. Iatrogenic factors
   d. Genetics

9. Each of the following factors are linked with medicinal benefit and cancer incidence. Which one *does not* have both correlations?
   a. Alcohol
   b. Estrogen
   c. Diet
   d. Tobacco

10. Data collected on cancer incidence can be used for which of the following purposes?
    I.   Public education
    II. Facility development
    III. Collegiate programs
    IV. Cancer prevention
    a. I, II, and IV only
    b. I, III, and IV only
    c. II, III, and IV only
    d. I, II, and III only

Questions to Ponder

1. Why is the etiological study of a specific cancer important?
2. What is the significance of a tumor registry?
3. Discuss the importance of a careful review of the environmental causes of cancer.
4. Explain *risks versus benefit* in regard to iatrogenic cancers.
5. What effect does cigarette smoking, diet, and lifestyle have on the development of cancer?

REFERENCES

1. Baird SB et al: *A cancer source book for nurses,* ed 2, Atlanta, 1991, The American Cancer Society.
2. Boring CC et al: Cancer statistics, 1994, *CA Cancer J Clin* 44:7-26 1994.
3. Garfinkel L: Cancer statistics, 1994, *CA Cancer J Clin* 44:5-6, 1994.
4. Groenwald SL, editor: *Cancer nursing: principles and practices,* Boston, 1987, Jones & Bartlett.
5. Osteen RT, editor: *Cancer manual,* ed 8, Boston, 1990, The American Cancer Society, Massachusetts Division.
6. Spitz MR, Newell G: *Recommendations for cancer prevention,* St Louis, 1992, Mosby.
7. Steele GD Jr et al: Clinical highlights from the National Cancer Data Base, 1994, *CA Cancer J Clin* 44:71-80, 1994.
8. *Taber's cyclopedic medical dictionary,* ed 17, Philadelphia, 1989, FA Davis.

The Cancer-Management Team

Diana Browning

Outline

Key terms

Biopsy
Brachytherapy
Case manager
Cesium
Chemotherapy
Cobalt 60
Definitive
Electrons
Gamma rays
Hospice
Interdisciplinary

Interstitial
Intracavitary
Iridium
Linear accelerator
Neutrons
Palliative
Protocols
Psychosocial
Radiation therapy
Simulators
X-rays

Cancer is not a single disease with one well-defined method of treatment but a group of diverse diseases that occur in all regions of the body, in males and females, and at any age. The diseases are grouped under a generic title because of similar properties and their capacity to replace normal tissue, interrupt normal systemic function, and cause death if untreated.

Because cancer is a multisystem disease, it requires an **interdisciplinary** treatment approach to achieve the best opportunity for cure or long-term palliation. The cancer-treatment team comprises the following three major modalities: (1) surgery, which is used to remove the tumor and other involved areas of tissue; (2) medical oncology, which uses pharmaceuticals (commonly called *chemotherapeutic drugs*) to shrink or eradicate the tumor; and (3) radiation therapy, which uses ionizing radiation to destroy the tumor while sparing surrounding tissue. These modalities may be used individually, sequentially, or concurrently depending on the location, pathology, and stage of the disease. The role of each modality, sequence of administration, and medical and social support of the patient during and after the course of treatment require a team approach with a predetermined rationale acceptable to the patient and all members of the team.

THE INTERDISCIPLINARY CANCER TEAM MEMBERS

A *team* has been defined as "a small number of people with complementary skills who are committed to a common purpose, set of performance goals, and approach for which they hold themselves mutually accountable."[6] The importance of each of the team members and mutual recognition of their

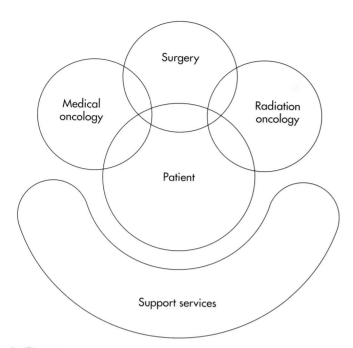

Fig. 3-1 The cancer patient receives treatment and support from multiple sources during disease management.

individual and collective skills are among the key elements of successful cancer treatment. The team leader role may change several times from one specialist to another over the course of treatment, and the patient may move between the outpatient and inpatient facilities during the continuum of care. Although members of the team providing care for the cancer patient cannot be defined in absolute terms, three major disciplines provide treatment and a wide and varying group of disciplines support the patient physically and psychologically during treatment[3] (Fig. 3-1).

Surgery

Surgery has a role in the diagnosis and treatment of many cancers. Diagnosis of a solid tumor frequently requires surgical removal of a small portion of the lesion for pathological identification and staging. Surgery is used as a primary treatment for cancer if the diagnostic work-up indicates the tumor may be removed completely without leaving residual cells that may allow the tumor to recur in the original site. With **definitive** surgery in the treatment of cancer the margins of the tissue removed during the procedure are frequently checked by pathologists before closure of the incision. This is done to ensure that the margins are clean (i.e., free of tumor cells). If pathological tests during the surgery indicate tumor cells remaining at the margins, a radical resection is performed until clean margins are reported by the pathologist. When definitive surgery is attempted and the surgeon is unable to achieve clean margins, additional therapy such as **radiation therapy** may be prescribed after the

procedure. Many standard treatment regimens now include conservative surgery to remove the tumor and adjuvant therapy such as radiation therapy and/or **chemotherapy** to treat any subclinical disease that may remain.[2]

Surgery also has a role in **palliative** treatment if a cure may not be possible but removal of the tumor may relieve symptoms or reduce the threat of invasion of vital organs. Surgery may also be used in other support roles such as the insertion of feeding tubes and a tracheotomy or colostomy for obstructive lesions.

Radiation oncology

Ionizing radiation in the form of **x-rays, gamma rays,** or fast particles such as **electrons** or **neutrons** has a role in the treatment of about half of all cancer patients. All radiation damages tissue or, in large enough dosages, kills it. The biological basis for using radiation in the treatment of cancer is the therapeutic ratio. The therapeutic ratio means that cells in different parts of the body and tumors with various histologies respond differently to radiation. Rapidly dividing cells are more susceptible to radiation damage than slowly dividing cells. A good therapeutic ratio means that the tumor cells are dividing more rapidly than the surrounding normal tissue.

To overcome the potentially limiting factor of damage to normal tissues and improve the therapeutic ratio, the radiation dosage is delivered through multiple entry points, thus intersecting at the tumor site and minimizing the dosage to normal tissue. Curative dosages of radiation therapy are delivered in multiple fractions to allow recovery of normal tissue from sublethal damage and maximize the dosage that may be administered to the tumor.[5]

Cancers in which the tumor cells grow more rapidly than surrounding normal tissues are usually the best candidates for curative radiation therapy because a favorable therapeutic ratio exists. Radiation therapy is not usually the best treatment for large, solid tumors or slow-growing tumors because they have poor therapeutic ratios. Radiation therapy may be used with adjuvant chemotherapy and surgery for irradiation of the tumor bed after removal of the tumor.

Medical oncology

Medical oncology uses chemotherapeutic agents and other drugs such as hormones and immunotherapeutic agents to treat cancer systemically. Chemotherapy is used as the primary treatment for nonsolid tumors such as leukemias and lymphomas. However, chemotherapy is more frequently used as adjuvant therapy with radiation and/or surgery for which the objective is treatment of subclinical disease. Medical oncology is the most rapidly developing cancer treatment modality and the most closely linked modality to clinical research because new agents are developed and moved into clinical trials and existing agents are refined. The effectiveness of chemotherapeutic agents is based on a principle similar to that of radiation therapy (i.e., assuming that tumor cells proliferate more rapidly than normal tissue and targeting those cells for destruction). However because chemotherapeutic agents are usually administered systemically and are not localized in the tumor region, side effects such as nausea and hair loss are induced as a result of the drug action on all rapidly proliferating cells.[1]

Clinical researches in medical oncology are continually seeking tumor- or cell-specific chemotherapeutic agents that reduce common side effects. Researchers are also investigating the role of immunotherapy in interventions such as genetic engineering and in interventions that enable the body to fight cancer (as it does infections and viruses) through the immune system.

Diagnostic and rehabilitation services

The primary members of the cancer-treatment team are supported by other teams in the management of disease. Diagnostic services include medical imaging, pathology, and laboratory medicine, all of which play major roles in the diagnosis, staging, and continuing treatment of the patient. Rehabilitation services include reconstructive surgery, physical therapy, and **psychosocial** support.

Sophisticated diagnostic imaging systems, such as computed tomography and magnetic resonance imaging, and the more routine contrast studies have key roles in the diagnosis of the location and extent of the disease. Radiographical studies provide a noninvasive evaluation of the disease and determine whether the patient is a candidate for surgery, radiation therapy, chemotherapy, or a combination of therapies. Diagnostic imaging studies also play an important role in the follow-up of patients after treatment is complete to monitor the response to treatment and recurrence or new foci of disease.

Pathological reviews of tissue samples from the tumor are critical in determining the diagnosis, grade, and histology of the tumor. This information guides the decision of the interdisciplinary team for optimal treatment.

The wide-ranging laboratory tests available for blood and body fluids provide diagnostic and staging information (especially in leukemia and lymphoma cancers) and monitor progress and tolerance of the patient to radiation and chemotherapeutic treatment.

Physical therapy, rehabilitation services, or reconstructive surgery may be needed to support the interdisciplinary cancer team because curative treatment sometimes leaves the patient with a deficit that adversely affects a return to normal life. For example, a mastectomy or extensive surgery in the head and neck area may require reconstructive procedures. Planning for this type of procedure allows the optimal chance for effectiveness.[8]

All cancer patients need access to psychosocial services to help them cope with changes in lifestyle and possible threats to life itself. As an important member of the cancer team, the social worker provides assessment, group and individual counseling sessions, and referral to more extensive psychological therapy if necessary.

THE CONTINUUM OF CARE

The continuum of care for cancer patients is difficult to diagram. The course of treatment varies for different cancers and even for different pathological conditions and stages of the same disease. Patients may loop through the continuum several times before moving to the next step.

At the time of diagnosis the aim of treatment is usually defined as *curative* or *palliative*. Curative treatment means that the objective of the planned course of treatment is eradication of the disease and the return of the patient to a normal lifestyle. A cure in cancer treatment is defined by disease-free survival after treatment rather than the apparent elimination of disease. The standard period for evaluating cure is 5 years, although this may vary according to the disease. At the time of diagnosis and staging, the cancer team makes projections regarding the probability of cure as a percentage of all cases. This information is used in discussing the prognosis with the patient. Palliative treatment means that the cancer has progressed beyond the point at which a cure can be achieved by current treatment methods. The aim of palliative treatment is the increase in quality rather than quantity of life.

The continuum of care covers the entire scope of treatment, including curative treatment, palliative treatment, pain management, hospice care, and death. Patients may start the continuum at any point. If the curative treatment is successful, the patient never reaches the palliative point. Other patients may move through the entire continuum or enter at the midpoint and continue to the end.

The overall course and sequence of therapies are decided by the cancer team and discussed with the patient at the initial work-up. However, frequent adjustments and changes may be necessary as the patient's response to treatment and the disease status is monitored. The patient must understand the need for changes in the initial plan, and the team members must remain informed and have the opportunity for input to any adjustments. Communication to the referring physician is also an important factor in the continuum of care so that the care received by patients integrates with maintenance of their general health and treatment of concurrent or chronic conditions (Fig. 3-2).

Diagnosis

The interdisciplinary management of cancer starts with the proper diagnosis of the disease. Pathological diagnosis requires microscopic analysis of tissue samples obtained by biopsy to establish histology, grade, and staging. Therefore the team must have input concerning the techniques used to obtain specimens. Surgical contamination of the tumor site during biopsy can compromise the optimal course of treatment and adversely affect the patient's prognosis. Patients should be referred to a cancer-treatment center for biopsies requiring surgical procedures so that the overall management of the disease is not compromised.

For some cancers a preliminary diagnosis may be established by diagnostic imaging procedures and the biopsy may

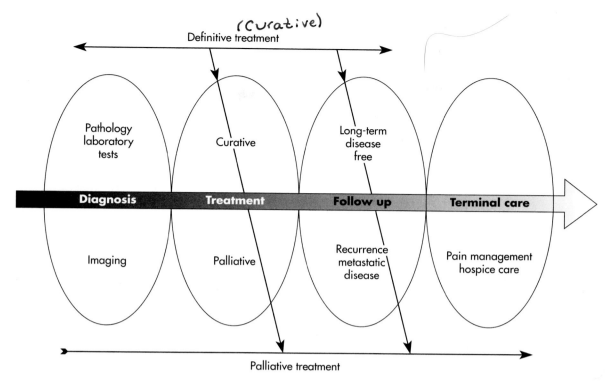

Fig. 3-2 The continuum of care in cancer management.

be performed during the surgical procedure. The extent of the surgery depends on the outcome of the pathological review of the frozen section specimen. This allows the surgeon to base the extent of surgical treatment on the findings during surgery, lymphatic involvement and local invasion, and pathological diagnosis obtained from the frozen section. Pathological examination of tissue during surgery also guarantees that the tissue removed has clean margins, the borders of the excised tissue are all normal cells, and all the cancer has been removed. Performing surgical diagnosis and treatment concurrently for deep-seated tumors means that the patient must only undergo a single operation and anesthetic, thus limiting the usual morbidity that is associated with procedures.

The interdisciplinary team managing the care of a patient with a pathological diagnosis reviews the slides and operative report at the time of initial consultation. This is done so that the diagnosis is independently confirmed and the procedure used for the biopsy is evaluated in the treatment-planning process.

Diagnostic imaging studies are an integral part of the diagnostic work-up of cancer patients. These studies interface with pathologists for localization of the tumor for biopsy and provide an assessment of the extent of the disease.

Frequently used with surgical pathology techniques for biopsies, radiography and ultrasound visually guide the surgical placement of the biopsy needle in the tumor or lesion and avoid surrounding normal structures. These procedures,

withoug a general anesthetic, obtain the tissue needed for pathological diagnosis and minimize morbidity during the diagnostic phase of the continuum of care.

Diagnostic imaging studies, including nuclear medicine scans, are used to assess the extent of the disease and evaluate the patient for metastatic disease before development of a treatment plan. The radiographs and radiologist's reports are reviewed by the interdisciplinary team as part of the work-up and are used as baseline measurements to evaluate the effectiveness of treatment and any change in patient status during follow-up.

Laboratory blood work is one of the major tools that is used in the diagnosis and staging of leukemia, and it provides valuable information for all types of lymphomas. Blood tests are also used with radiation and chemotherapy to monitor the patient's tolerance to the treatment and the progress of the disease.

A complete physical assessment of the patient is also included in the diagnostic phase of the continuum of care. This assessment is completed by nurses and physicians at the initial consultation, provides information regarding the general health status of the patient, and enables the team to predict the patient's expected tolerance of the treatment. The physical examination also alerts the team to concurrent medical conditions (such as heart disease and diabetes) that should be observed during treatment and screens the patient for other malignancies that may be asymptomatic (such as skin cancers).

Treatment planning

Treatment planning for cancer patients is the start of the interdisciplinary team process, must involve representatives from the three major treatment disciplines, and is usually accomplished by a group meeting.[3,7] The format of this meeting may vary with the organizational structure of the institution. In cancer centers in which all disciplines are represented, the planning or disposition clinic may take place immediately after the examination of the patient and the review of all diagnostic tests. In community hospitals the team members may examine the patient and review tests results at separate appointments and may meet at the tumor conference (board) to present all findings. Regardless of the forum, after the treatment objective is definitive (e.g., cure), representatives from the three treatment disciplines— surgery, radiation, and medical oncology—review each case and map out the course, modalities, and sequence of the entire treatment. For some situations in which the treatment regimens are accepted standards, little need exists for discussion and the presentation serves as a quality assurance review for the treatment plan. In more complex or unusual cases the plan is developed at the conference with input from all team members.

The interdisciplinary team conference also identifies patients who may fit the criteria for **protocols** designed to evaluate the efficacy of different methods of treatment. As technologies and drugs used to treat cancer are advanced, they are introduced into direct patient care in carefully designed protocols that test the new therapy against the current standard treatment for the particular disease. Protocols may compare the results of different regimens of the same treatment modalities. For example, one daily fraction may be compared with three daily fractions of radiation therapy, or one modality may be compared with another, as in comparing radiation therapy alone with radiation therapy and chemotherapy.

Protocols, which are stringently monitored by appropriate agencies, are used to bring advances in cancer research from the laboratory into clinical practice. In patient care institutions, all protocols that compare and evaluate different treatment methodologies must be approved by the institutional review board (IRB), which is the body responsible for all ethical questions. Typically, the IRB must review and approve the hypothesis and methodology for all protocols, whether they are designed by various national research organizations (such as the National Cancer Institute) or internally by institution staff members before implementation. In the clinical setting the protocol and possible benefits and side effects must be explained to the patient, who signs a specific consent form. Protocols can be the forerunners of standard treatment regimens, as with Hodgkin's disease, and lead to dramatic changes in expected survival. The current standard therapy for Hodgkin's disease is the result of years of carefully designed and evaluated protocols and has been implemented at many cancer centers worldwide.

Protocols are also used to bring experimental drugs into clinical use. Under the supervision of the Food and Drug Administration (FDA), pharmaceutical companies join academic research programs in health care institutions to identify diseases and their stages that may benefit from experimental drugs. Controlled studies are then conducted, the results are compared with usual expectations of the disease progression, and the value of the drug is assessed. Many drugs are tested this way, with the fully informed consent of the patient, and some evolve into standard care plans for cancer patients. The drug 5-fluorouracil (5-FU) was introduced this way. Used with radiation therapy, 5-FU is now considered part of the standard treatment for rectal cancer and is credited with significantly reducing the need for radical surgery.

After the team members agree on the overall treatment plan, it must be presented to the patient with appropriate education and the opportunity for discussion. If the patient is to receive more that one modality of treatment, concurrently or sequentially, the changing leadership of the team must be explained and provision for continuity must be included in the plan. In many cancer centers a member of the team is appointed as a **case manager** for each patient to facilitate the treatment and make sure that all needs are met. In some programs the patient is educated to fulfill the case manager role and actively participate in treatment planning and delivery. The coordination function must be addressed in the treatment-planning process so that the support and guidance necessary to the patient are defined and available through the entire continuum of care.

An important part of the treatment-planning component of the continuum is patient education, which provides the patient with an overall assessment of the disease, a realistic prognosis, and a description of the planned course of treatment with expected side effects. Many cancer centers have developed educational tools for patients, including videotapes and information brochures, to ensure that information is uniformly provided and accessible for review.

Treatment delivery

As the patient moves through the continuum of care and into administration of the planned courses of treatment, the number of caregivers increases and team communication becomes even more important. The treatment prescribed by the team must be clear to health care professionals responsible for administration, and the disease, stage, and prognosis for the patient must be accurately communicated to ensure patient confidence in the education and information provided. Therapists administering the radiation treatment must understand the overall treatment plan, their role in delivery, and the patient's expectations. The caregivers must monitor the patient's physical reactions to the treatment and treat the side effects as necessary and in accordance with the education provided to the patient. Any adjustment made while the treatment is in progress must be discussed with the interdisciplinary team members and the patient to ensure that the change complements the original plan.

Patient support

During the entire continuum of care the patient needs access to support care personnel who are also members of the interdisciplinary team to help with all aspects of the treatment. The team should include all support groups necessary for the patient. The most common members are the nutritionist, pharmacist, physical and occupational therapist, social worker, psychologist or psychiatrist, patient advocate, and chaplain.

Nutritional support is important in all cancer therapies but especially if the treatment or disease make adherence to a balanced diet difficult for the patient. Nutritional education is important for patients receiving radiation therapy treatment and enables them to anticipate reactions that may make eating and maintaining an adequate nutritional status throughout treatment difficult. Patients treated for head and neck cancers may suffer acute mucosal reactions, which make eating extremely painful. The nutritionist enables the patient to anticipate the onset of reactions and obtain foods that provide adequate caloric intake and do not aggravate the mucosal tissues in the mouth and esophagus. Radiation therapy to the abdominal and pelvic regions can cause nausea and diarrhea, but the nutritionist can recommend bland foods that assist in toleration of these side effects.

Patients receiving systemic chemotherapy often have side effects such as nausea, vomiting, and hair loss. Nutritional support is important to maintain caloric intake for these patients. The pharmacist also has an important role in supporting the prescription of antiemetic drugs and monitoring their administration and effectiveness so that the patient can tolerate the drug therapy. In many cancer centers the pharmacist is a member of the cancer-care team for medical oncology and supports the physician in prescribing chemotherapeutic agents and the patient with administration of antiemetic and other prescriptions.

Physical therapy or other rehabilitative support may be necessary during or after treatment to help return patients to their former lifestyles and activities. For example, patients who have had mastectomies for breast cancer and are referred for radiation therapy need a range-of-motion assessment and may be recommended for concurrent physical therapy to restore or maintain arm movement.

Although the cancer-care team can define the physical supportive care required for toleration of treatment, patients and their families also have financial, logistical, and psychosocial support needs that must be addressed. Social work can bridge the gap between patients and cancer teams in identifying and meeting these needs.

Logistical or financial concerns often compromise patient compliance with treatment recommendations. Financial support for the family during hospitalization of the patient or daily transportation to the cancer center may seem to be insurmountable problems as the patient comes to terms with a diagnosis of cancer.[11] Social workers can provide patients with information regarding local agencies that provide housing, financial support, and transportation; facilitate access to these services; and act as patient advocates.

Social workers also provide patients with psychological support over the entire continuum of care. This support can take many forms. Group discussions moderated by the social worker are often extremely helpful because they provide forums for comparison of treatment side effects and coping mechanisms.[11] Group meetings often help patients overcome frequent feelings of isolation from their families and friends. Support groups for the family are also used as forums for discussion of fears, guilt, and anger that result from the serious illness of a family member.

Cancer networks, which link patients undergoing treatment with individuals who have previously been treated for the same disease, can also be important support mechanisms because they provide avenues for discussion of the long-term sequelae of treatment and validation of the disease prognosis. Several major cancer centers have established these networks, which bring people together from diverse regions of the country for discussions of some of the rare types of cancer. These cancer centers also sponsor annual meetings allowing cancer patients to meet, to celebrate their successes, hear reports on treatment and research initiatives, and mourn patients who did not succeed in overcoming their diseases.

Pediatric patients make up a relatively small proportion of the overall population diagnosed with cancer each year, but their support needs are unique and provide significant challenges to the cancer team. Nutritional support and physical therapy are as important for children as for adults, but the psychosocial needs are different. Maintaining as normal a lifestyle as possible for their patients is a goal of most pediatric oncology programs. If possible, children should stay in school or their homes and receive outpatient treatment. Many cancer centers offer evening appointments for chemotherapy so that the school day is not interrupted. For children who are inpatients, school classes are given in hospital settings, and child life specialists organize play therapy sessions and other activities.[15]

The psychosocial needs of pediatric patients and their families are also extremely different from those of adult patients, and the social worker provides access to services that help the child and family understand the diagnosis and possible implications to their lives. Special skills are necessary in helping pediatric patients come to terms with potentially life-threatening aspects of cancer, cope with treatment regimens, and maintain stable lifestyles.

THE RADIATION ONCOLOGY TEAM

Just as the cancer team is made up of members from many different disciplines, including radiation oncology, the radiation oncology team comprises many specialists working together to treat the patient. Teamwork is as important in the successful delivery of radiation therapy as it is in overall cancer management. The team may vary with the disease, treatment methodology, and prognosis, but it always includes the

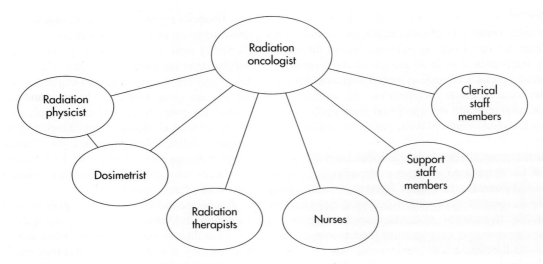

Fig. 3-3 The radiation oncology team.

following members: radiation oncologist, radiation physicist, radiation therapist, dosimetrist, and nurses (Fig. 3-3).

The radiation oncologist is the physician member of the team and works with the interdisciplinary cancer team to determine the optimal treatment for each patient. This person accepts responsibility for prescribing and administering the radiation therapy as part of the overall plan. After medical school a radiation oncologist completes a 4-year residency training program that provides education in all aspects of cancer as a disease, including the physical and radiobiological bases for radiation therapy and the technology of equipment used for treatment. All states require licensure of physicians in their specialties. The radiation oncologist is responsible for prescribing the appropriate treatment modality, energy, and dosage; localizing and defining the extent of the tumor volume; approving the treatment plan; supervising the administration of the treatment; evaluating the response to treatment; and providing long-term follow-up of the patient relative to the treatment and disease.

The radiation physicist provides many of the support services to the radiation oncologist that facilitate radiation therapy. A radiation physicist usually has a graduate degree in medical physics and frequently completes a doctoral degree. Many states require licensure of medical radiation physicists. Physicists are responsible for the maintenance and calibration of the equipment used to deliver radiation therapy, development of treatment plans and dosage calculations, manufacturing of beam-shaping devices, and administration of complex treatment techniques. In addition, physicists are available to consult with radiation oncologists on unusual cases.

The radiation therapist is the team member responsible for the localization of the tumor volume, simulation of the treatment plan, and administration of the prescribed course of radiation therapy. Radiation therapists complete accredited educational programs that provide an understanding of can-

cer, the biological basis for radiation oncology, and the technology of the equipment. These educational programs also provide the necessary competencies to administer the prescribed course of treatment. Graduates of these programs take a national certifying examination that documents competency, and many states require licensure. Radiation therapists operate radiation-treatment units and administer treatment to patients as prescribed by radiation oncologists. Over the course of radiation therapy the patient meets with the radiation therapist every day for treatment over long periods, sometimes up to 7 weeks.[4] This gives the therapist a unique opportunity to observe the patient and provide the physician, nurse, or other support staff members with evaluations that may assist in management of the disease. The therapist frequently gains an understanding of the patient's psychosocial needs that may not have been acknowledged by the social worker and can suggest appropriate referrals to help the patient and family cope with the stress of cancer.

The dosimetrist works with the physicist, radiation oncologist, and radiation therapist to develop a treatment plan that allows administration of the prescribed dose of radiation to the tumor volume. Dosimetrists may be physicists or radiation therapists with on-the-job training but increasingly are graduates of dosimetry training programs. National certification of dosimetrists is available, but state certification is not currently required in this developing profession. The dosimetrist uses the treatment-planning computer systems, the localization and simulation radiographs, and if appropriate, the computed tomography scans to develop a treatment plan that delivers the prescribed dose of radiation to the tumor volume and keeps the dose to the surrounding normal tissue at an acceptable level. Dosimetrists work with radiation oncologists on plans for external beam radiation therapy and **brachytherapy** and with radiation therapists to calculate and monitor treatment parameters for the prescription.

Nurses fill many roles in the radiation oncology team. Clinic nurses work with radiation oncologists during the initial consultation and assessment of patients referred for radiation therapy. They educate patients before the start of treatment and evaluate and monitor the response to treatment during weekly management visits. Research nurses work with radiation oncologists to recruit patients to clinical protocols, obtain necessary consent forms, monitor compliance, and assess the patient during treatment to collect data for evaluation of the protocol. Oncology nurse specialists work with radiation oncologists and nurses to extend the role of the physician and provide additional support for the patient. The advanced training of clinical nurse specialists enables them to conduct the initial consultation screening of patients, provide recommendations to physicians, function as case managers for patients in the interdisciplinary cancer team and radiation oncology team, and conduct long-term follow-up clinics.

The radiation oncology team needs administrative support to facilitate the continuum of care. The administrative team makes patient appointments with the radiation oncologist and with necessary diagnostic and consultative services, obtains medical records and diagnostic test results for patients, and orders supplies for clinic and treatment areas. The radiation oncology team also contains many of the previously discussed patient-support personnel, who provide for the needs of patients as they receive radiation therapy.

Interactive roles

The radiation oncology team can be defined in many ways depending on the size of the staff, the number of patients under treatment, and the number of treatment units. In large departments in which the radiation oncologists subspecialize, the team may be based on the disease site (e.g., breast, head and neck). In smaller departments the team may be defined by the treatment unit. Coordination of the team is essential for a smooth and seamless patient service flow.[4] Although the radiation oncologist may function as the team leader, all team members must be recognized for their contributions to the service flow. The focus of the team must be on the patient, and the procedures and policies should add value and facilitate the service flow. Regular team meetings, which often take the form of weekly chart rounds, provide forums for discussion of each patient, opportunities for review and assessment of the treatment plan, and discussions of necessary adjustments or changes. [3,7]

Equipment

For administering treatment, radiation oncology uses two principle techniques (external beam radiation therapy and brachytherapy), both of which require sophisticated equipment to produce the radiation in a variety of energies and modalities. Over the years that radiation oncology has developed into one of the major modalities in the treatment of cancer, many different technologies for producing radiation have

undergone experimentation in the laboratory and clinical area. **Linear accelerators,** which provide multiple energies in photons and electrons, are the primary technology currently used for external beam radiation therapy. **Cobalt 60** treatment units are also used at locations that require low-energy photon beams, and orthovoltage and superficial units have a role in treating skin cancers.

Simulators are diagnostic radiography units mounted on gantries that mimic the treatment unit's entire range of motion. They can be used to localize the tumor volume and simulate the planned treatment technique by using fluoroscopy and diagnostic quality radiographs.

Brachytherapy is the term used for **intracavitary** or **interstitial** treatment, in which radioactive sources are placed directly into the tumor volume to deliver the prescribed dose. The sources (commonly **cesium, iridium,** or gold) are placed in a naturally occurring body cavity or implanted directly into the tissue through the use of catheters or needles and are capable of delivering a highly localized dose.

All radiation therapy equipment is installed in appropriately shielded rooms with controlled access systems, and radioactive sources are stored in shielded safes. All equipment is operated under the direction of a radiation safety officer and in accordance with state and federal regulations.

Patient education

Cancer is widely perceived as a life-threatening disease, and the idea of radiation and radioactivity is often frightening to the public. Therefore patient education is a key responsibility of the entire team. Although the education of the patient is usually divided along the service flow, all team members should be prepared to answer any questions from patients or refer them to the appropriate member. Patient handbooks, videos, and group and one-on-one teaching sessions are common methods of giving patients information regarding their diseases and treatment courses. The informed consent that the patient signs before treatment provides the radiation oncologist with the opportunity to outline expected side effects and discuss all possibilities, however remote. Video is an excellent medium for explaining the size and complexity of treatment units to patients before they enter the treatment room, thus reducing their anxiety. A brochure can provide written confirmation of an oral teaching session so that the patient can review the information under less stressful conditions.

THE ROLE OF THE PATIENT IN THE CANCER TEAM

The growth of consumer awareness in the United States over the past decade has affected the health care delivery system. Patients are increasingly reluctant to accept the recommendation of physicians for treatment without discussion of the disease, prognosis, and available alternatives. This attitude has been fostered by many indemnity insurance programs and health maintenance organizations, which require members to get second opinions before reimbursements are approved for major medical procedures. This consumer awareness has been especially militant in patients with breast cancer, a disease for which media coverage has been extraordinary concerning available treatment options.

Patients are asking more questions and being more active in planning and administering their own treatment and therapies. Cancer patients are demanding all available options, seeking centers that have access to experimental therapies, participating in clinical protocols, and making quality-of-life decisions based on the prognosis. The cancer-management team must recognize the right of patients to receive all the information regarding their diseases, treatment options, and recommendations and must assist them in making decisions. Education of the team regarding patient rights is important and a major concern of many institutional ethics committees.

The cooperative model

Many health care institutions across the country are experimenting with patient-centered care models in which the objective is to improve patient and staff satisfaction and outcomes. The Planetree Program was developed in the late 1970s as a resource center and library to provide patients with health care information and encourage patient and family involvement in health care decisions.[10] Planetree developed an extension of this program, an innovative hospital project in which the patient was considered a member of the team and participated in the treatment planning. The hospital unit was remodeled to provide a more homelike atmosphere in which the family members could participate in the patient's care. Although this program has been considered successful in terms of patient satisfaction outcomes and nursing staff involvement, not every patient is willing to achieve the level of knowledge necessary to participate in treatment decisions. Aspects of the Planetree model are being incorporated into many of the patient-focused care projects, and the importance of educating the patient as a health care consumer is now widely recognized.

Advance directives and living wills

Advance directives and living wills allow individuals to make personal care decisions regarding the use of extreme measures, including life-support systems, before the need is even identified. Many healthy individuals are completing these documents so that their wishes are known in the event of an accident or life-threatening illness. As they become more educated about their diseases, many cancer patients are making advance decisions regarding the final outcome of their treatment rather than allowing the responsibility for these decisions to fall on family members. Patients have the security of knowing that their wishes will be carried out and their families will not have to make these decisions without knowing the patients' wishes. Patient education regarding the usual progression of the disease, the treatment options at

each stage, and the associated quality of life is essential so that decisions can be made rationally and in accordance with accepted ethical practices and the patient's beliefs. The social work departments of many hospitals (with the ethics committee and risk management) have developed information on advance directives and living wills that can be provided to patients who have potentially life-threatening illnesses.

Hospice care and pain management

For situations in which the disease progression requires palliative treatment and the patient may be terminally ill, care for the patient and family is often provided by a hospice. Hospice care is extended to the entire family and provided until the conclusion of the mourning process.[17] Hospice care becomes part of the continuum of care provided by the cancer-management team as the patient progresses beyond the point that treatment intervention can extend the quantity or improve the quality of life. The objective then becomes the comfort of the patient, relief of pain and other symptoms, and acceptance of death by the patient and family. Moving into hospice care is often more difficult for the cancer team and family than for the patient because the move is acknowledgment that no further treatment can be given. Patients who have moved into the acceptance stage of the disease and are ready for hospice care may be distressed if their families resist this transition.

Hospice care can be a service in the patient's home or in a facility that provides inpatient care. Some patients are more comfortable in their own homes, and their families are able to care for them with help from hospice programs. Because they do not want to feel that they are disrupting the lifestyles of their families, other patients prefer inpatient units. The inpatient hospice also provides support through interaction with other patients and their families and a staff accustomed to caring for the needs of terminally ill patients.[12]

Pain management is an essential tenet of the hospice philosophy. To contemplate the end of their lives with dignity, patients must be free of pain. Terminally ill patients do not have to worry about addiction to drugs as a long-term problem, and narcotics can be prescribed in the most effective manner. Management of pain in the hospice setting requires a team approach among the nurse, physician, and pharmacist. Professional education is essential to address concerns and misconceptions of staff members, the patient, and the family regarding analgesics and narcotics. Daily assessment is required to evaluate the patient's response to medication and adjust the dosage of drugs as necessary.[18]

THE TEAM CONCEPT IN HEALTH CARE

The concept of cross-functional, process-oriented teams organized by product rather than function has been developing in industry throughout the 1980s as part of the restructuring and reengineering initiatives required to remain competitive in the global marketplace.[13,16] As a result of these initiatives, manufacturing companies that have successfully made this operational and cultural transition have emerged as horizontal organizations focused on their customers and product needs.

The same pressures that caused these changes in industry are now affecting health care. The continually rising cost of health care in the national economy is pressuring the government to explore reform options and motivating employers to look for ways to reduce and control costs of employee benefits. As a result, health care providers, whose organizations have been traditionally hierarchical and bureaucratic, are looking to successful industries as models of reform. The two most frequently used models are based on the recognition of the patient as a consumer or customer of the health care product and the reorganization of health care providers into product-oriented teams.

The concept that is difficult for physicians and other health care providers to embrace is the recognition of the patient as a customer who has expectations of the product quality. The medical profession has tended to define quality in terms of the provider's qualifications and the technology available. The public had little knowledge of medicine and accepted physicians' definitions of quality and recommendations for treatment without question. As technology has become more complex and medical procedures able to change the outcomes of many previously fatal conditions or injuries, the media has educated the population as never before. The ethical questions of medicine (such as those that arise from transplant surgery, neonatal medicine, and life-support capabilities) are frequently and openly debated in newspapers and on radio and television talk programs. Although these issues are the extremes of medical care, their open discussion has given patients the vocabulary and basic knowledge to ask questions regarding their own care and evaluate the information according to their personal values.

In addition, the mobility of the population and increase in the number of medical practices have provided a range of choice in physicians that was not available 25 years ago. This has led to patient choice of physician based on location, accessibility, and other customer-service factors rather than qualifications and technology. Physician practices and hospitals (especially those in academic settings) have been slow to recognize consumer standards that a better educated public is applying to the selection of health care providers.

The recognition of the patient as a customer with many choices in the selection of health care products has led to the application in the medical field of many of the customer-focused, product-team initiatives that have proved successful in industry. Although application of these techniques is relatively easy in private practice offices where the product is well defined (e.g., outpatient pediatric visits), the application becomes more complex in the interdisciplinary ambulatory practice and hospital.

The most successful of these initiatives in the hospital setting has been generically termed *patient-focused care* and concentrates on the processes necessary to provide patient-

care services in an inpatient unit. The overall objective of patient-focused care is to provide a team approach to provision of services by cross-trained, multifunctional personnel who are totally responsible for a small number of patients. Several models have been implemented in hospitals across the country. The Care 2000 and ProACT models are among the most frequently documented.[9,14] The models documented in the literature demonstrate increases in patient and employee satisfaction.

The team goals and objectives identified for the patient-focused care projects apply equally to service of patients who have diseases requiring the interaction of specialists from several functional groups. Many hospitals, clinics, freestanding medical facilities, and physician practices are evaluating their published mission statements, operational processes, and structures to ensure that their services, or products, meet the needs of their patients, or customers, and support a team approach to the delivery of these services.

Physicians involved in the provision of cancer care (more than many other medical specialties) have long recognized the need for a team approach to the management and treatment of the disease and have developed strategies that overcome structural and organizational barriers. Because no well-established paths for referral of cancer patients to an interdisciplinary practice existed, tumor conferences (boards) were established in hospitals to bring the various specialists together. These conferences provided opportunities for the presentation of cases, discussion of management strategies, and agreement on the modality and sequence of treatment.[7]

Because of tumor conference discussions, acceptable treatment regimens based on disease site and stage became standard practice and patient referral patterns based on these regimens were established. The role of the tumor conference changed and was used to discuss cases that did not fit into a standard regimen of care. The initial objectives of the tumor conferences were educational and typically took place in teaching hospitals. The value of the tumor conference as a forum for interdisciplinary discussion of cancer treatment options led to its migration to community hospitals. As tumor conferences became active in community hospitals, and cancer specialists from teaching institutions visited regularly, a mechanism for referral of complex cases to the major cancer centers developed.

During the 1970s, community hospitals and physician groups began to consolidate cancer care into oncology practices, thus usually combining radiation and medical oncology in a single location with referral patterns to and from surgeons specializing in cancer. These cancer centers provided predominantly outpatient care, although access to a hospital for inpatient care was essential and facilitated interdisciplinary practice for physicians treating cancer. These practices are being refined in the patient-focused care model, thus providing quality care in a convenient location with access to a full interdisciplinary team for diagnosis, planning, and administration of treatment.

SUMMARY

Cancer is not one disease but a group of diseases that range from the usually curable to the usually terminal and that require a team approach for optimal management. The cancer team is made up of the three major treatment modalities, each of which is a team within a team. The interdisciplinary team comprises the surgery, radiation oncology, and medical oncology teams. The cancer team consults to provide the optimal treatment plan for each patient based on disease, stage, and prognosis and participates in the management of the patient's treatment over the entire continuum of care. Support services become members of the team as needed to help the patient tolerate treatments, manage symptoms, and cope with physical and psychological effects of cancer. Patients are provided with information enabling them to participate in team discussions that result in treatment decisions and dispositions along the continuum of care.

Review Questions

Multiple Choice

1. To achieve the best opportunity for long-term cure or palliation in treating cancer, which of the following approaches needs to be employed?
   a. Interdisciplinary
   b. Generic
   c. Local and regional
   d. Sequential
2. Overall, the cancer-management team's role in disease management entails which of the following?
   I. Maintenance of quality of life
   II. Cessation of disease proliferation
   III. Provision of effective patient education
      a. I and II
      b. I and III
      c. II and III
      d. I, II, and III
3. In the management of cancer, which of the following do medical imaging, pathology, and laboratory medicine provide?
   a. Disease staging
   b. Diagnosis
   c. Both of the above
   d. Neither of the above
4. The entire scope of treatment that a cancer patient receives from curative treatment, palliative treatment, pain management, and death is covered by which of the following?
   a. Patient assessment
   b. Continuum of care
   c. Referring physician
   d. None of the above
5. Usually accomplished through interactive meetings, effective cancer-treatment planning must involve representatives from which of the following?
   I. Surgery
   II. Chemotherapy
   III. Radiation therapy
      a. I and II
      b. I and III
      c. II and III
      d. I, II, and III
6. Which of the following is true regarding protocols?
   a. They bring advances in cancer research into clinical practice.
   b. They must be ethically sound.
   c. They may be forerunners of standardized treatment regimens.
   d. All of the above are true.
7. Before the need is identified, individuals can make personal decisions regarding the use of life support in their care through which of the following?
   a. Advance directives
   b. Living wills
   c. Both of the above
   d. Neither of the above
8. Patient-focused care does which of the following?
   a. Uses a team of cross-trained, multicompetent practitioners
   b. Focuses on patient and employee satisfaction
   c. Both of the above
   d. Neither of the above

True or False

9. The cancer management team, including the radiation therapist, must know and be able to effectively communicate all information regarding disease-treatment options to patients undergoing treatment.
   True _____ False _____
10. Today, cancer centers typically provide full-service treatment options to patient in convenient locations, including access to a full interdisciplinary team for diagnosis, planning, and treatment administration.
   True _____ False _____

Questions to Ponder

1. Discuss the three major disciplines used in the treatment of cancer and the role of each in disease management.
2. Differentiate between curative- and palliative-treatment objectives and their place in the continuum of care.
3. Clinical protocols advance cancer-treatment techniques. Discuss the various ways this may be demonstrated.
4. Identify three of the support services commonly available to cancer patients. Describe their relationship to disease management and quality of life.

5. Identify the members of the radiation oncology treatment team and the skills that each member contributes to the treatment plan.
6. Describe the importance of patient education in cancer treatment and interactions with the patient that lead to an informed consent for treatment.
7. Differentiate between the delivery of external-beam and brachytherapy radiation therapy.

REFERENCES

1. Cooper MR, Cooper MR: Principles of medical oncology. In Holleb AI, Fink DJ, Murphy GP, editors: *American Cancer Society textbook of clinical oncology,* Atlanta, 1991, American Cancer Society.
2. Eberlein TJ, Wilson RE: Principles of surgical oncology. In Holleb AI, Fink DJ, Murphy GP, editors: *American Cancer Society textbook of clinical oncology,* Atlanta, 1991, American Cancer Society.
3. Fountain MJ: Key roles in issues of the multidisciplinary team, *Semin Oncol Nurs* 19:25-31, 1993.
4. Harris EL: Offer the compassion and hope your patients so desperately need, *Rad Therapist* 3:63-64, 1994.
5. Hendrickson FR, Withers HR: Principles of radiation oncology. In Holleb AI, Fink DJ, Murphy GP, editors: *American Cancer Society textbook of clinical oncology,* Atlanta, 1991, American Cancer Society.
6. Katzenbach JR, Smith DK: The discipline of teams, *Harvard Business Review* pp 111-112, March/April 1993.
7. Kerstetter NC: A stepwise approach to developing and maintaining an oncology multidisciplinary conference, *Cancer Nurs* 13:216-220, 1990.
8. King GE, Lemon JC, Martin JW: Multidisciplinary teamwork in the treatment and rehabilitation of the head and neck cancer patient, *Tex Dent J* pp 9-12, June 1992.
9. Luckenbill B, Crabtree JL, Tonges M: Restructured patient care delivery: evaluation of the ProACT model, *Nurs Econ* 8:36-44, 1990.
10. Martin DP et al: The Planetree model hospital project: an example of the patient as partner, *Hosp Health Services Admin* 35:591-601, 1990.
11. McKenna RJ: Supportive care and rehabilitation of the cancer patient. In Holleb AI, Fink DJ, Murphy GP, editors: *American Cancer Society textbook of clinical oncology,* Atlanta, 1991, American Cancer Society.
12. McWilliam CL, Burdock J, Wamsley J: The challenging experience of palliative care support-team nursing, *Oncol Nurs Forum* 20:779-785, 1993.
13. Meyer C: How the right measures help teams excel, *Harvard Business Review* pp 95-103, May/June 1994.
14. Ollier C: Ambitious' Care 2000 initiative decentralizes work processes at San Diego's Mercy Hospital and Medical Center, *Strategies Healthcare Excellence* 5:1-12, 1992.
15. Pinkerton CR: Multidisciplinary care in the management of childhood cancer, *Br J Hosp Med* 50:54-59, 1993.
16. Sashkin M, Sashkin MG: *The new teamwork: developing and using cross-function teams,* New York, 1994, American Management Association.
17. Stoddard S: *The hospice movement: a better way of caring for the dying,* New York, 1978, Random House.
18. Williams A et al: Models of health care delivery in cancer pain management, *Oncol Nurs Forum* 19(suppl):20-26, 1992.

4

The Ethics and Legal Considerations of Cancer Management

Janet M. Salzmann

Outline

Key terms

Analytical model
Assault
Autonomy
Battery
Beneficence
Civil law
Collegial model
Consequentialism
Contractual model
Covenant model
Deontology
Doctrine of foreseeability
Doctrine of personal liability
Doctrine of res ipsa loquitur
Doctrine of respondeat superior
Engineering model
Ethics

False imprisonment
Incident
Informed consent
Invasion of privacy
Justice
Legal concepts
Legal ethics
Libel
Medical record
Moral ethics
Negligence
Nonmaleficence
Priestly model
Risk management
Scope of practice
Slander
Tort law
Virtue ethics

In radiation therapy, ethical issues arise daily in dealing with other health care professionals, patients, and families. In this fast-paced, changing world of health care, radiation therapists and students must be well versed in ethics and legal considerations of cancer management. The radiation therapist deals with patients who have specific needs related to their attempts to control catastrophic diseases taking over their lives and the lives of those close to them. Defining the roles and responsibilities of the radiation therapy student, the practicing radiation therapist, and other members of the radiation oncology team as they care for their patients is extremely important. In addition to developing technical skills necessary to practice in the profession, members of the radiation oncology team must develop an understanding of the basic theories regarding ethics, patients' rights, the scope of practice for radiation therapists, and the code of ethics for radiation therapy. The medical-legal aspects of informed consent, record keeping, and confidentiality are also important.

Radiation therapy has a code of ethics to guide students and therapists in professional conduct (see the box on p. 39). However, the code does not list all principles and rules but only those that constitute the heart of ethically sound professional practice. A code of ethics serves two major functions: education and regulation. It educates persons in the profession who do not reflect on ethical implications of their actions unless something concrete is before them. It also educates other professional and lay groups concerning ethical standards expected of a given profession.[12] Understanding ethical concepts and legal issues and developing interpersonal skills through the study of the material in this chapter

Code of Ethics for Radiation Therapists

- The radiation therapist advances the principal objective of the profession to provide services to humanity with full respect for the dignity of mankind.
- The radiation therapist delivers patient care and service unrestricted by concerns of personal attributes or the nature of the disease or illness and nondiscriminatory with respect to race, color, creed, sex, age, disability, or national origin.
- The radiation therapist assesses situations; exercises care, discretion, and judgment; assumes responsibility for professional decisions; and acts in the best interest of the patient.
- The radiation therapist adheres to the tenets and domains of the scope of practice for radiation therapists.
- The radiation therapist actively engages in lifelong learning to maintain, improve, and enhance professional competence and knowledge.

Modified from the American Society of Radiologic Technologists: *The code of ethics for radiation therapists,* Albuquerque, 1993, The Society.

enables student therapists and practicing radiation therapists to care for their patients humanely and compassionately.

ETHICAL ASPECTS OF CANCER MANAGEMENT
Definitions and terminology

Webster's New Collegiate Dictionary[13] defines **ethics** as (1) the discipline dealing with what is good and bad, moral duty, and obligation; (2) a set of moral principles or values; (3) a theory or system of moral values; and (4) the principles of conduct governing an individual or a group <professional>. Ethics for the individual derives from the person's experiences, teachings, and values. The individual gathers an understanding of right and wrong from the cumulative experiences of life and develops patterns of approaching situations in which the complexities of right and wrong must be addressed.[14]

In the study of ethics a person must distinguish between **moral** and **legal ethics.** Morality has to do with conscience. It is a person's concept of right or wrong as it relates to conscience, God, a higher being, or a person's logical rationalization. *Morality* can be defined as fidelity to conscience. **Legal concepts** are defined as the sum of rules and regulations by which society is governed in any formal and legally binding manner. The law mandates certain acts and forbids other acts under penalties of criminal sanction. The law is primarily concerned with the good of a society as a functioning unit.[7]

In dealing with ethical issues in cancer treatment, health care professionals should consider bioethics, which is based on four underlying principles: **beneficence, nonmaleficence, autonomy,** and **justice.** Beneficence calls on health care pro-

fessionals to act in the best interest of patients, even at some inconvenience and sacrifice to themselves. Nonmaleficence directs professionals to avoid harmful actions to patients. Autonomy emphasizes that patients are independent actors whose freedom to control themselves is to be respected. Justice asks persons to ensure that fairness and equity are maintained among individuals.[10]

Ethical theories and models

Many persons believe that ethics simply means using common sense. Therefore a value system and appropriate behavior should be factors in any health care professional. However, ethical problem solving begins with an awareness of ethical issues in health care and is the sum of ethical knowledge, common sense, personal values, professional values, practical wisdom, and learned skills.[11] Although an individual's personal system of decision making may be developed from values and experiences, it generally involves some understanding and application of basic principles common to formal ethics.[14]

Ethical theories can be divided into the following three broad groups: (1) **consequentialism,** (2) **deontology,** and (3) **virtue ethics.** Consequentialism, or the theory of utility, evaluates an activity by weighing the good against the bad or the way a person can provide the greatest good for the greatest number. Deontology uses formal rules of right and wrong for reasoning and problem solving. A few grey areas exist in this theory, which make it difficult to use in our society because varieties of life experiences make formal rules of right and wrong impossible to define. Virtue ethics is the use of practical wisdom for emotional and intellectual problem solving. Practical reasoning, consideration of consequences, rules established by society, and effects that actions have on others play important parts in applying the theory of virtue ethics. This approach to problem solving serves the health care professional by integrating intellect, practical reasoning, and individual good.[11]

Models for ethical decision making involve different methods of interactions with the patient. The **engineering,** or **analytical, model** identifies the caregiver as a scientist dealing only in facts and does not consider the human aspect of the patient. The engineering model is a dehumanizing approach and is usually ineffective.[11] For example, with the engineering model the radiation therapist considers the patient only a lung or brain rather than an individual who has thoughts and feelings. This type of approach in the care of cancer patients is cold, unfeeling, and extremely inappropriate.

The **priestly model** provides the caregiver with a godlike, paternalist attitude that makes decisions *for* and not *with* the patient. This approach enhances the patient's loss of control by giving the caregiver not only medical expertise, but also authority about moral issues.[11] An example of this model is the therapist or student forcing a patient to comply with planning or treatment procedures regardless of the patient's pain or discomfort because the physician ordered it or because the disease is known to respond to treatment. Patients must be allowed to make decisions about their compliance to treatment.

The **collegial model** presents a more cooperative method of pursuing health care for the provider and patient. It involves sharing, trust, and consideration of common goals. The collegial model gives more control to the patient while producing confidence and preserving dignity and respect.[11] For example, the therapist takes the extra time required to get acquainted with patients and listen to their needs. This knowledge enables the therapist to help patients cooperate with demands of positioning for planning and treatment. The collegial model takes time and is crucial to the humane treatment of cancer patients.

The **contractual model** maintains a business relationship between the provider and patient. A contractual arrangement serves as the guideline for decision making and meeting obligations for services. With a contractual arrangement, information and responsibility are shared. This model requires compliance from the patient; however, the patient is in control of the decision making.[11] The contractual model is best represented by the process of informed consent. Complete information is given and explained thoroughly, and the patient makes decisions.

The **covenant model** recognizes areas of health care not always covered by a contract. A covenant relationship deals with an understanding between the patient and health care provider that is often based on traditional values and goals.[11] The covenant model is demonstrated by a patient trusting the caregiver to do what is right. This trust is often based on previous experience with health care, particularly cancer care procedures and treatment.

The role of the radiation therapist in regard to ethical decision making involves the application of professionalism, the selection of a personal theory of ethics, and the choice of a model for interaction with the patient. The difficulties encountered are the result of constant changes in health care, patient awareness, and evolving growth of radiation therapy in a highly technical and extremely impersonal world of health care.[11]

Patients should actively participate in their own care. Patients' awareness of their rights, their needs, and the availability of the many treatment options provides opportunities and complications. The American Hospital Association has published *A Patient's Bill of Rights*[11] (see the box on p. 41), and every medical institution has the responsibility to make this document available to its patients. Each patient's responsibility for the treatment process grows with patient education.[11]

PATIENT AUTONOMY AND INFORMED CONSENT

Cancer remains one of the most dreaded diseases and often evokes images of death, disfigurement, intolerable pain, and suffering. Approximately 30 years ago, the central ethical

issue in caring for the cancer patient was whether to tell the patient the truth that the diagnosis was cancer. Today, advancements in treatment, surgery, chemotherapy, and radiation therapy have resulted in longer periods of remission, improved survival, and even cure. This has generated more complex ethical issues.[10] More than half of all cancer patients ultimately need radiation therapy. The physician and patient must weigh the benefits of therapy against possible complications.[2]

The health care professional's ability to listen to patients sensitively, grasp the patient's truth, and honor that truth is indispensable, even across social, cultural, and age barriers. To be effective and supportive, physicians and caregivers must in a sense be masters of each patient's personal language. This ability to listen and communicate is an extremely important clinical skill that must be learned, preferably from experts. Mastery of listening and communicating should be highly valued.[8]

Truth telling, which is required for informed consent, is an extremely curious principle. Persons have been taught from early childhood to tell the truth, but doing so is often extremely difficult and sometimes even seems wrong. Not long ago, lying to a patient about the cancer diagnosis was the norm. Caregivers believed that telling the truth would be destructive and that patients preferred ignorance of their conditions. Studies over the years, however, have conclusively documented that cancer patients want to know their diagnoses and do not suffer psychological injuries as a result of knowing.[10]

The claim that each person is free to make life-directing decisions is often known as the *autonomy principle*. The concept of autonomy, understood in this sense, is crucial to ethics. Without some sense of autonomy, no sense of responsibility exists, and without responsibility, ethics is not possible.[15] In conventional cancer therapy, patient autonomy is protected further by the practice of **informed consent.** The

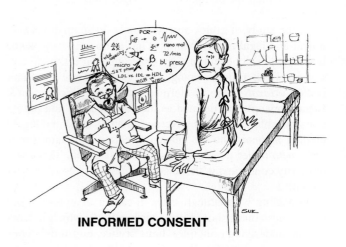

INFORMED CONSENT

A Patient's Bill of Rights

1. The patient has the right to considerate and respectful care.
2. The patient has the right to obtain from the physician complete current information concerning the diagnosis, treatment, and prognosis in terms the patient can be reasonably expected to understand. When it is not medically advisable to give such information to the patient, the information should be made available to an appropriate person in the patient's behalf. The patient has the right to know, by name, the physician responsible for coordinating care.
3. The patient has the right to receive from the physician information necessary to give informed consent prior to the start of any procedure and/or treatment. Except in emergencies, such information for informed consent should include but not necessarily be limited to the specific procedure and/or treatment, the medically significant risks involved, and the probable duration of incapacitation. Where medically significant alternatives for care or treatment exist or when the patient requests information concerning medical alternatives, the patient has the right to such information. The patient also has the right to know the name of the person responsible for the procedures and/or treatment.
4. The patient has the right to refuse treatment to the extent permitted by law and to be informed of the medical consequences of this action.
5. The patient has the right to every consideration of privacy concerning the medical care program. Case discussion, consultation, examination, and treatment are confidential and should be conducted discreetly. Those not directly involved in care must have the permission of the patient to be present.
6. The patient has the right to expect that all communications and records pertaining to care should be treated as confidential.
7. The patient has the right to expect that within its capacity a hospital must make reasonable response to the request of a patient for services. The hospital must provide evaluation, service, and/or referral as indicated by the urgency of the case. When medically permissible, a patient may be transferred to another facility only after the patient has received complete information and explanation concerning the needs for and alternatives to such a transfer. The institution to which the patient is to be transferred must first have accepted the patient for transfer.
8. The patient has the right to obtain information as to any relationship of the hospital to other health care and educational institutions insofar as care is concerned. The patient has the right to obtain information as to the existence of any professional relationships among individuals, by name, who are treating the patient.
9. The patient has the right to be advised if the hospital proposes to engage in or perform human experimentation affecting care or treatment. The patient has the right to refuse to participate in such research projects.
10. The patient has the right to expect reasonable continuity of care. The patient has the right to know in advance what appointment times and physicians are available and where. The patient has the right to expect that the hospital will provide a mechanism whereby the patient is informed by the physician or a delegate of the physician of the patient's continuing health care requirements following discharge.
11. The patient has the right to examine and receive an explanation of the bill regardless of source of payment.
12. The patient has the right to know what hospital rules and regulations apply to personal conduct as a patient.

Courtesy American Hospital Association.

American Medical Association's principles of medical ethics imply the following about informed consent: a physician shall be dedicated to providing competent medical service with compassion and respect for human dignity, shall deal honestly with patients and colleagues, and shall make relevant information available to patients. Patients should be informed and educated about their conditions, should understand and approve their treatments, and should participate responsibly in their own care.[2] The basic elements of informed consent are called *patients' rights to know* and participate in their own health care. Informed consent is a doctrine that has evolved sociologically with the changing times.

Every patient is entitled to informed consent before any procedure is performed.[7] To give informed consent, the patient must be informed of the following[2]:

1. The nature of the procedure, treatment, or disease
2. The expectations of the recommended treatment and the likelihood of success
3. Reasonable alternatives available and the probable outcome in the absence of treatment
4. The particular known risks that are material to the informed decision about whether to accept or reject medical recommendations

Competency refers to the minimal mental, cognitive, or behavioral ability or trait required to assume responsibility. Generally the law recognizes only decisions or consents made by competent individuals. Persons over the age of 18 are presumed to be competent; however, this may be disputed with evidence of mental illness or deficiency. If the individual's condition prevents the satisfaction of criteria for competency, the person may be deemed incompetent for the purpose of informed consent. Mental illness does not automatically render a person incompetent in all areas of functioning. Respect for autonomy demands that individuals, even if they are seriously mentally impaired, be allowed to make decisions of which they are capable. Minors are not considered legally competent and therefore require the consent of parents or designated guardians.[2]

The rule directing that a patient may not sign a document or give informed consent for a procedure after being medicated was established to protect the person going to surgery. Persons who have been premedicated for procedures are considered incompetent. However, persons experiencing intractable pain may be incapable of exercising autonomy until after they are medicated and pain free or experiencing pain control.[14]

The responsibility for obtaining informed consent from a patient clearly remains with the physician and cannot be delegated. The courts believe that a physician is in the best position to decide which information should be disclosed for a patient to make an informed choice. The scope of disclosure in any situation is a physician's responsibility. Some states, however, also have legislative standards or state statutes that articulate the information the physician needs to tell a patient.[2]

Often a third person (a health care provider) is present during the informed consent session because patients are reluctant to question their physicians but will likely question the witness. The witness can then inform the physician about the patient's lack of understanding. The third party signature is merely an attestation that the informed consent session took place and the signature on the document is the patient's.[2] The patient must be able to understand the information as presented, and no attempt must be made to influence the decision. General agreement exists that informed consent is an active, shared decision-making process between the health care provider and patient.

Confidentiality

A struggle exists in medical practice between confidentiality and truthfulness. According to Garrett, Baillie, and Garrett,[3] truthfulness is summarized in two commands: "Do not lie and you must communicate with those who have right to the truth." Truthfulness must not be the only consideration in discussing patients' rights and caregivers' obligations to patients. One of the major restrictions a health care profession imposes is strict confidence of medical and personal information about a patient. This information cannot be revealed without the direct consent of the patient's physician.

Breach of confidence is one of the major problems encountered in providing patient care and can result in legal problems. Information should not be discussed with other department personnel, except in the direct line of duty if it is requested from one ancillary department to another or with nursing service to meet specific medical needs. In the radiation therapy setting, staff members must be especially careful not to discuss patients in hallways or around the treatment area unless the discussion is directly related to the treatment. Staff members should never discuss information with their own families or friends, even in the most general terms, because doing so is a violation of the patient's rights. The patient's treatment chart should be kept in a secure area, inaccessible to anyone not involved in the treatment. Confidentiality issues must be stressed in every educational program at every opportunity.[4]

State laws requires some exceptions to confidentiality. These exceptions may include particular types of wounds, certain communicable diseases, and abuse.[11] Subject to state law, confidentiality may be overridden when the life or safety of the patient is endangered such as when knowledgeable intervention can prevent threatened suicide or self-injury. In addition, the moral obligation to prevent substantial and foreseeable harm to an innocent third party usually is greater than the moral obligation to protect confidentiality.[11]

Roles of other health care team members

Patients and families dealing with cancer may be suddenly thrust into a new and potentially threatening world of blood tests, scans, and specialists. A family physician or internist who is familiar with the patient's history and has established a trusting relationship with the patient can be a key member of the cancer-management team. This physician can help the patient and family make appropriate treatment decisions and can act as a liaison between the patient and other people involved in the evaluation and treatment. If a patient does not have a physician to act as an advocate at the time of the cancer diagnosis, a physician should quickly be chosen to serve in this capacity through the course of the illness.[1]

In most situations, other health care professionals are available to help patients cope with the emotional effects of cancer. Nurses who spend much time at a patient's bedside can provide important information to the patient and physician. Social workers are invaluable in assessing the level of a family's psychological distress and its capacity to cope with the illness.[1] Community resources such as veteran patient programs (e.g., Reach to Recovery) that involve people who have coped with cancer in their own lives can provide valuable information and help reassure patients and their families. The local clergy may be able to provide spiritual guidance based on their knowledge of a particular patient's and family's needs.[1] The responsibilities of radiation therapists are shown in the box on pp. 43-44.

The Scope of Practice for the Radiation Therapist

The American Society of Radiologic Technologists (ASRT) developed and published the **scope of practice** for the field of radiation therapy. It is imperative that every student therapist and every radiation therapist practicing their profession be knowledgeable regarding the scope of practice. It is the defining document to guide us through our day-to-day responsibilities as radiation therapists caring for our patients.

The structural elements of radiation therapy technology as a health profession in the contemporary health care delivery system in the United States include the following:

- A cognitive base
- A structured curriculum
- A professional credential
- A code of ethics
- Clinical practice autonomy
- Self-governance

The history of these elements combines in a complex structure that can be traced across historical time spans and contemporary functional boundaries. For example, in the history of radiography, radiation therapy was at one time an area of responsibility of the radiographer. This is no longer true today.

Curriculum of the discipline contains elements of physics, psychology, patient care, and pathology, among others, that cross horizontally through several medical specialties. The professional curriculum incorporates didactic and clinical elements and basic sciences that are reflective of contemporary practice in radiation therapy. The content and structural learning experiences facilitate attitudes and skills that prepare graduates to demonstrate a commitment to patient care and continued personal and professional development.

Description of the Profession

Radiation therapy is the art and science of treatment delivery to individuals to restore, improve, and enhance performance; diminish or eradicate pathology; facilitate adaptation to the diagnosis of malignant disease; and promote and maintain health. Since the major focus of radiation therapy is the delivery of prescribed dosages of radiation to individuals from external beam and/or brachytherapy radiation sources or hyperthermia units, the radiation therapist's concern is with those factors that influence radiation dose delivery, individual well-being, and responsiveness to treatment, as well as those factors serving as barriers or impediments to treatment delivery.

The practice of radiation therapy is performed by competent radiation therapists who deliver care to the patient in the therapeutic setting and are responsible for the simulation, treatment planning, and administration of a prescribed course of radiation therapy and/or hyperthermia. Additional related settings where radiation therapists practice include education, management, industry, and research.

Professional Credential

The initials RT(T) (ARRT) indicate a registered technologist in radiation therapy and certification as a radiation therapist by the American Registry of Radiologic Technologists.

Scope of Practice

The curriculum base for a radiation therapist is that outlined in the ASRT Professional Curriculum for Radiation Therapy. Education program standards are those defined in the Essentials and Guidelines of an Accredited Educational Program for the Radiation Therapist. Radiation therapy professional educational programs prepare the radiation therapist to but are not limited to the following:

1. Provide radiation therapy services by contributing as an essential member of the radiation oncology treatment team through provision of total quality care of each patient undergoing a prescribed course of treatment
2. Evaluate and assess treatment delivery components
3. Provide radiation therapy treatment delivery services to cure or improve the quality of life of patients by accurately delivering a prescribed course of treatment
4. Evaluate and assess daily the physiological and psychological responsiveness of each patient to treatment delivery
5. Maintain values congruent with the profession's code of ethics and scope of practice as well as adhere to national, institutional, and/or departmental standards, policies, and procedures regarding treatment delivery and patient care

Domains of Practice

DOMAIN: ORGANIZATIONAL AND WORK ROLE COMPETENCIES
1. Coordinate and meet multiple patient needs and requests: set priorities
2. Participate effectively in a therapeutic team approach to provide optimal therapy
3. Adapt to contingency planning in response to variables that influence workload and/or schedule
4. Maintain a flexible stance toward patients, visitors, and staff, as well as technology and bureaucracy
5. Coordinate daily activities so as to devote complete attention to all necessary tasks involved in treatment delivery

Modified from the American Society of Radiologic Technologists: *The scope of practice for radiation therapists,* Albuquerque, 1993, The Society.

Continued.

The Scope of Practice for the Radiation Therapist—cont'd

DOMAIN: ADMINISTERING AND MONITORING
RADIATION THERAPY TREATMENTS

1. Implement and deliver a planned course of treatment
2. Administer treatment accurately and safely: monitor and report untoward effects, reactions, therapeutic responses, and incompatibilities
3. Withhold treatment when conditions warrant and consult with a radiation oncologist before proceeding
4. Participate in total quality management system to ensure safe and accurate patient care
5. Detect equipment malfunctions and take appropriate action
6. Accurately document details of treatment procedures and maintain daily treatment records
7. Apply principles of radiation protection at all times
8. Take appropriate action with regard to real or potential radiation hazards
9. Understand the function of equipment, accessories, treatment methods, and protocols and apply such knowledge appropriately
10. Simulate and plan a course of treatment by defining and identifying tumor volume, target volume, and treatment volume as directed and prescribed by the radiation oncologist
11. Construct and/or prepare immobilization devices, beam directional devices, and the like that facilitate treatment delivery
12. Perform daily and periodic quality assurance checks and related tasks as appropriate
13. Perform dosimetric calculations and treatment planning procedures
14. Monitor doses to normal tissues within the irradiated volume to ensure that tolerance levels are not exceeded
15. Prepare and/or assist in the preparation and use of brachytherapy sources

DOMAIN: CAREGIVING

1. Create a climate for and establish a commitment to healing and/or improving quality of life
2. Provide comfort measures and facilitate the preservation of patient self-image and dignity
3. Serve as a source of support and encouragement for each individual patient and family
4. Provide patient education in order to maximize patient compliance with the plan of care and provide family education as needed
5. Monitor and interpret patient side effects and/or complications in order to create a management strategy that fosters prevention, healing, and comfort

6. Monitor the patient's physical and psychological response to treatment and refer the patient for appropriate management when indicated
7. Detect, document, and report significant changes in patient conditions
8. Understand the particular demands and experiences of a pathological illness and anticipate related patient care needs
9. Participate in patient follow-up, statistical reporting programs, and clinical research
10. Practice techniques that prevent the spread of disease to provide a safe environment for patients, staff, and self
11. Provide basic patient care
12. Practice basic techniques of venipuncture and the administration of contrast media
13. Prepare patients for procedures to gain desired results and minimize anxiety
14. Work to make culturally avoided aspects of an illness approachable and understandable

DOMAIN: EFFECTIVE MANAGEMENT OF RAPIDLY
CHANGING SITUATIONS

1. Perform skillfully in extreme, life-threatening emergencies; rapid grasp of a problem; contingency management; rapid matching of demands and resources in emergency situations involving patient or equipment applied in treatment delivery
2. Identify and manage a patient crisis until physician assistance is available
3. Take appropriate action in case of fire or other emergency situations to provide a safe environment for patients, visitors, and staff
4. Assist in the rehabilitation process or the loss of ability to provide self-care as a patient's lifestyle changes

DOMAIN: PROFESSIONALISM

1. Demonstrate respect for confidentiality of medical records and privileged knowledge.
2. Demonstrate respect for the Patient's Bill of Rights
3. Share expertise and knowledge with students and others while respecting their needs and rights.
4. Pursue appropriate continuing education
5. Apply the profession's code of ethics in all aspects of practice
6. Adhere to any applicable standards, policies, and procedures
7. Refrain from practicing procedures for which appropriate training and/or education has not been obtained

DYING PATIENTS AND THEIR FAMILIES

Care for the dying patient and family has changed dramatically over the years with improvements in technology. The evolution of terminal care changed curing to caring, beginning with the publication of Dr. Elizabeth Kübler-Ross' book *On Death and Dying.*[6] Because they deal daily with terminally ill patients, radiation therapists and their students must explore questions concerning patients' rights, refusal of treatment, and quality of life and must understand the emotional state of cancer patients. A basic fear of dying is present in all humans. Patients fear the diagnosis, the treatment, the disease, and the death associated with it.[9]

Although the final stage of a terminal illness is obvious, its beginning is less well defined. At some point during the treatment of patients who have metastatic cancer, the focus of management shifts from aggressive therapy to palliative care, from efforts to suppress tumor growth to attempts to control symptoms. Signals that the goals of treatment need to be changed include the recognition of the tumor's progression, the failure of therapy to control the disease, the patient's deteriorating strength, and the patient's loss of interest in pursuing previously important objectives and pleasures. Rarely is this decision a difficult one; rather, it reflects the natural acceptance of the inevitability of patients' deaths on the part of families, caregivers, and patients themselves.[1]

Over the past decade, people in many countries have come to accept the notion that aggressive life support (i.e., prolonging life to the bitter end) is frequently not the right action to take. The ethic of allowing terminally ill patients to die with dignity has evolved. In recent years the concept of the individual's right of self-determination has been central in the resuscitation issue. The medical and legal communities have recognized that self-determination is no more than an extension of the patient's right of informed consent. Physicians in the past were placed in an extremely uncomfortable position of wanting to comply with the patient's wishes to die in peace and dignity but fearing a malpractice suit by family members for failing to do all that should, could, or might have been done to resuscitate the dying patient. The response to this dilemma was the living will. The purpose of the living will is to allow the competent adult to direct the course of a possible future medical condition when the individual might no longer be competent by reason of illness. The living will concept assumes that the individual who executes the directive does the following:

1. Demonstrates competency at the time
2. Directs that no artificial or heroic measures be undertaken to preserve the patient's life
3. Requests that medication be provided to relieve pain
4. Intends to relieve the hospital and physician of legal responsibility for complying with the directives in the living will
5. Has the signature witnessed by two disinterested individuals who are not related, are not mentioned in the will, and have no claim on the estate[2]

In practice, actions to carry out a living will may involve withholding or discontinuing interventions such as respirator support, chemotherapy, surgery, and even assisted nutrition and hydration.[8] The decision to withhold curative therapy is based on the conclusion that the course of the patient's disease is irreversible and extraordinary measures to sustain life are not in the patient's best interest. To nullify the routinely mandatory order for cardiopulmonary resuscitation in the event of a cardiac arrest, many hospitals require the physician in charge of a terminal care patient to issue a specific DNR (do not resuscitate) order. Plans for the patient's death, including issuance of the DNR order, should be made soon after the issue has been discussed with the patient and family. In most situations, patients and their families are relieved to know that every effort will be made to maintain the patient's comfort and the death will be peaceful.[1] All hospitals must have written policies and procedures describing the way patients' rights are protected at their institutions.

Hospice care

In the Middle Ages a hospice was a way station for travelers. Today a hospice represents an intermediate station for patients with terminal illnesses. The hospice movement began with programs to provide palliative and supportive care for terminally ill patients and their families. Hospice services include home, respite, and inpatient hospital care and support during bereavement. In addition to providing 24-hour care of the patient, the goal of hospice care is to help the dying patient live a full life and to offer hope, comfort, and a suitable setting for a peaceful, dignified death. The hospice team assists family members in caring for the patient by providing physical, emotional, psychological, and spiritual support. Several types of hospices are available, including freestanding facilities, institutionally based units, and community-based programs.[1]

Patients may enter the hospice on their own or may be referred by family members, physicians, hospital-affiliated continuing-care coordinators and social workers, visiting nurses, friends, or clergy. Although admission criteria vary, they usually include the following: a terminal illness with an estimated life expectancy of 6 months or less; residence in a defined geographical area; access to a caregiver from immediate family members, relatives, friends, or neighbors; and the desire for the patient to remain at home during the last stage of the illness. On the initial assessment visit a member of the hospice team obtains the patient's medical history and emotional and psychosocial histories of the patient and family and discusses nursing concerns. After the program begins, team members meet regularly to review the care plan for each patient and put into effect and supervise services for the patient and family.[1]

Most families prefer home care for dying relatives if they can rely on the supportive environment offered by a hospice. Institutionalization is perceived as impersonal and impractical, and acute care hospitals are not designed for the long-term care of terminal patients. A private home can be transformed to accommodate the level of care required, and nurses can instruct family members in physical care techniques, symptom management, nutrition, and medications. After the patient and family are made to feel confident and capable of managing the physical care, they can begin to address the emotional and spiritual issues surrounding death. During a patient's terminal illness, many problems arise, some of which test the hospice team's ingenuity and endurance. In general, however, simple remedies, common sense, good nursing care, preventive medicine, and generous use of analgesia should be used to help reduce the suffering of the patient.[1]

MEDICAL-LEGAL ASPECTS OF CANCER MANAGEMENT
Definitions and terminology

Radiation therapists need to perform their duties with little thought of situations that may result in legal actions against them or the facilities in which they work. As consumers become more aware of the standards of care that they should receive and more cognizant about seeking legal compensation, health care professionals must become more knowledgeable about legal definitions concerning the standard of care.[7]

The type of law that governs relationships between individuals is known as **civil law.** The type of law that governs rights between individuals in noncriminal actions is called **tort law.** Torts are not easy to define, but a basic distinction is that they are violations of civil, as opposed to criminal, law. Tort law is personal injury law. The act may be malicious and intentional or the result of negligence and disregard for the rights of others. Torts include conditions for which the law allows compensation to be paid an individual damaged or injured by another. The two types of torts are those resulting from intentional actions and those resulting from unintentional acts.[7] Health care providers incur duties incidental to their professional roles. The law does not consider the professional and patient to be on equal terms; greater legal burdens or duties are imposed on the health care provider.[2]

Several situations exist in which a tort action can be taken against the health professional because of deliberate action. Intentional torts include civil assault, civil battery, false imprisonment, libel, slander, and invasion of privacy.

Assault is defined as the threat of touching in an injurious way. If patients feel threatened and believe they will be touched in a harmful manner, justification may exist for a charge of assault. To avoid this, professionals must always explain what is going to happen and reassure the patient in any situation involving the threat of harm.[7]

Battery consists of touching a person without permission. Again, a clear explanation of what is to be done is essential. If the patient refuses to be touched, that wish must be respected. Battery implies that the touch is a willful act to harm or provoke, but even the most well-intentioned touch may fall into this category if it has been expressly forbidden by the patient. This should not prevent the therapist from placing a reassuring hand on the patient's shoulder as long as the patient has not forbidden it and the therapist does not intend to harm or invade the patient's privacy. However, a procedure performed against a patient's will may be construed as battery.[7]

False imprisonment is the intentional confinement without authorization by a person who physically constricts another with force, threat of force, or confining clothing or structures. This becomes an issue if a patient wishes to leave and is not allowed to do so. Inappropriate use of physical restraints may also constitute false imprisonment. The confinement must be intentional and without legal justification. Freedom from unlawful restraint is a right protected by law. If the patient is improperly restrained, the law allows redress in the form of damages for this tort. The proof of all elements of false imprisonment must be established to support the claim that an illegal act was done. If they are dangerous to themselves or others, patients may be restrained. An example of false imprisonment is a therapist using restraints on a patient without informing the family, particularly if a child is involved.[7]

Libel is written defamation of character. Oral defamation is termed **slander.** These torts affect the reputation and good name of a person. The basic element of the tort of defamation is that the oral or written communication is made to a person other than the one defamed. The law recognizes certain relationships that require an individual be allowed to speak without fear of being sued for defamation of character. For example, radiation oncology department supervisors who must evaluate employees or give references regarding an employee's work have a qualified privilege. Radiation therapists can protect themselves from this civil tort by using caution while conversing in the hearing of patients and their families.[7]

Invasion of privacy charges may result if confidentiality of information has not been maintained or the patient's body has been improperly and unnecessarily exposed or touched. Protection of the patient's modesty is vital during simulation, planning, and treatment procedures.[7] Maintaining that privacy is extremely important in regard to video monitors in treatment areas. No one should ever be in the viewing area except necessary staff members.

An unintentional injury to a patient may be negligent. **Negligence** refers to neglect or omission of reasonable care or caution. The standard of reasonable care is based on the doctrine of the reasonably prudent person. This standard requires that a person perform as any reasonable individual of ordinary prudence with comparable education and skill and under similar circumstances. In the relationship between a professional person and a patient an implied contract exists to provide reasonable care. An act of negligence in the con-

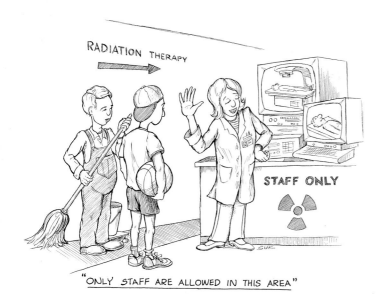

RADIATION THERAPY

STAFF ONLY

"ONLY STAFF ARE ALLOWED IN THIS AREA"

text of such a relationship is called *malpractice*. Negligence, as used in malpractice law, is not necessarily the same as carelessness. A person's conduct can be considered negligent in the legal sense if the individual acts carefully. For example, if a therapist without prior education attempts a procedure and does it carefully, the conduct can be deemed negligent if harm results to the patient.[7]

LEGAL DOCTRINES
Doctrine of personal liability

Radiation therapists should be concerned about the risk of being named as defendants in medical malpractice suits. Things can go wrong, and mistakes can be made. The legal responsibility of the radiation therapist is to give safe care to the patient.

The fundamental rule of law is that persons are liable for their own negligent conduct. This is known as the **doctrine of personal liability** and means that the law does not permit wrongdoers to avoid legal liability for their own actions even though someone else may also be sued and held legally liable for the wrongful conduct in question under another rule of law. Although they cannot be held liable for actions of hospitals or physicians, therapists can be held responsible and liable for their own negligent actions.[7]

Doctrine of respondeat superior

The **doctrine of respondeat superior** ("let the master answer") is a legal doctrine that holds an employer liable for negligent acts of employees that occur while they are carrying out orders or serving the interests of the employer. As early as 1698, courts declared that a master must respond to injuries and losses of persons caused by the master's servants. The nineteenth century courts adopted the phrase *respondeat superior*, which is founded on the principle of

social duty that all persons, whether by themselves or by their agents or servants, shall conduct their affairs in a manner not to injure others.[7] This principle is based on the concept that profit from others' work and the duty to select and supervise employees are joined in liability.[2]

Doctrine of res ipsa loquitur

In a malpractice action for negligence the plaintiff has the burden of proving that a standard of care exists for the treatment of the medical problem, the health care provider failed to abide by the standard, this failure was the direct cause of the patient's injury, and damage was incurred. If the alleged negligence involves matters outside general knowledge, an acceptable medical expert must establish these criteria. A long-accepted substitute for the medical expert has been the **doctrine of res ipsa loquitur**,[4] which means "the thing speaks for itself." Courts have decided to resolve the problem of expert unavailability in certain circumstances by applying res ipsa loquitur, which requires the defendant to explain the events and convince the court that no negligence was involved.[2]

Doctrine of foreseeability

The **doctrine of foreseeability** is a principle of law that holds an individual liable for all natural and proximate consequences of negligent acts to another individual to whom a duty is owed. The negligent acts could or should have been reasonably foreseen under the circumstances. A simple definition is persons reasonably foreseeing that certain actions or inactions on their part could result in injury to others. In addition, the injury suffered must be related to the foreseeable injury. Routine radiation therapy equipment checks are important in overcoming this doctrine.[7]

RISK MANAGEMENT

Conceived little more that a decade ago, the concept of risk control, or **risk management**, was believed to be the key element in loss prevention from adverse medical incidents. Risk management links every quality-improvement program with measurable outcomes necessary to determine overall effectiveness. Effectiveness here means success in reducing patient injury. An acute care hospital or medical center has the duty to exercise such reasonable care in looking after and protecting the patient. The legal responsibility of any health care practitioner is safe care. Risk management, which is a matter of patient safety, is the process of avoiding or controlling the risk of financial loss to staff members and the hospital or medical center. Poor quality care creates a risk of injury to patients and leads to increased financial liability. Risk management protects financial assets by managing insurance for potential liability by reducing liability through surveillance. It identifies actual and potential causes of patient accidents and implements programs to eliminate or reduce these occurrences.[7]

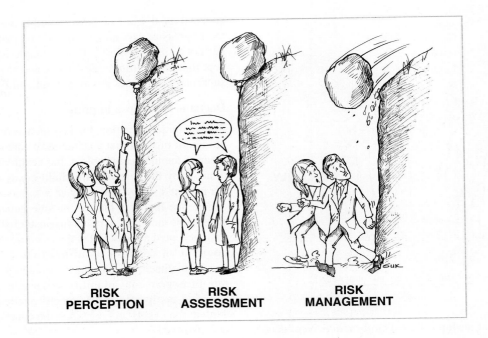

RISK PERCEPTION   **RISK ASSESSMENT**   **RISK MANAGEMENT**

Hospital liability and malpractice insurance, also known as *patient liability insurance,* is intended to cover all claims against the hospital that arise from the alleged negligence of physician staff members and employees. Many have discussed whether radiation therapists should carry malpractice insurance. In making that decision, persons must determine the extent of provisions for malpractice coverage in their institutions. According to the doctrine of respondeat superior, the employer is liable for employees' negligent acts during work. The authority and responsibility of a physician supervising and controlling the activities of the employee supercede those of the employer according to the doctrine of the borrowed servant. Regardless of the way these legal doctrines may be applied, the fundamental rule of law that every therapist should clearly know and understand is the doctrine of personal liability; persons are liable for their own negligent conduct. A wrongdoer is not allowed to escape responsibility even though someone else may be sued and held legally responsible. In some situations, hospital insurers who paid malpractice claims have successfully recovered damages from negligent employees by filing separate lawsuits against them.[7]

Hospital employees are instructed to report any patient injury to administration through the department manager. An incident report is routinely used to document unusual events in the hospital. An **incident** is defined as any happening that is not consistent with the routine operation of the hospital or the routine care of a particular patient. It may be an accident or a situation which could result in an accident.[11] Hospitals use incident reports in their accident-prevention programs to advise insurers of potential suits and prepare defenses against suits that might arise from documented incidents. Incident reports should be prepared according to the institution's published policies and procedures. An incident report is no place for opinion, accusation, or conjecture; it should contain only facts concerning the incident reported.[2]

MEDICAL RECORDS

The radiation oncology **medical record** is used to document chronologically the care and treatment rendered the patient. All components of the patient's evaluation and cancer must be documented in the radiation oncology record. The format usually includes the following: a general information sheet listing the names of pertinent relatives, follow-up contacts, family physicians, and persons to notify in an emergency; an initial history and findings from the physical examination; reports of the pathology examinations, laboratory tests, diagnostic imaging studies, and pertinent surgical procedures; photographs and anatomical drawings; medications currently used; correspondence with physicians and reimbursement organizations; treatment set-up instructions; daily treatment logs; physics, treatment planning, and dosimetry data; progress notes during treatments; summaries of treatment; and reports of follow-up examinations. These radiation oncology records must be maintained and secured in the department separate from hospital and clinic records to ensure ready access at any time.[5]

Medical record entries should be made in clear and concise language that can be understood by all professional staff members attending the patient. Handwritten entries must be legible. An illegible record is worse than no record because it documents a failure by staff members to maintain a proper record and may severely weaken a hospital's or physician's defense in a negligence action. Entries should be typed or made in ink, and persons making entries should identify themselves clearly by placing their signatures after each entry. The hospital and physician should be able to determine who participates in each episode of patient care.[2] Entries should be made daily by the therapist operating the treatment machine. Any other therapist involved in that day's treatment of a patient should also check the entry for accuracy and initial the record.

Medical records are sometimes used by staff members to convey remarks inappropriate for a patient's chart. The following are examples of entries that should never be made:

- "This is the third time therapist X has been negligent."
- "Dr. A has mistreated this patient again."
- "This patient is a chronic complainer and a nuisance."

Such editorial comments are inevitably used against the physician and hospital in any negligence action filed by the patient. In addition, as the trend moves toward access by patients to their own medical records, patients are more likely to read and react with hostility to such comments.[2]

The general rule is to avoid the need for making corrections, but because humans are not perfect, corrections must be made from time to time. A staff member should simply draw a line through an incorrect entry because doing so leaves no doubt about which item has been corrected. The staff member should initial the correction, enter the time and date, and insert the correct information. Mistakes in the chart should not be erased because doing so may create suspicion concerning the original entry.[2]

Radiation therapists under the direct supervision of the radiation oncologist and medical physicist carry out daily treatments. All treatment applications must be described in detail (orders) and signed by the responsible physician. Likewise, any changes in the planned treatment by the physician may require adjustment in immobilization, new calculations, and even a new treatment plan. Therefore the therapist, physicist, and dosimetrist must be notified.[5]

SUMMARY

In addition to the development of technical knowledge and skills, the foundation of radiation oncology includes standards of conduct and ideals essential to meeting emotional and physical needs of patients. Radiation therapists must first view their profession as more than a job. Student therapists should not pursue a simple goal to just pass a series of examinations and eventually the registry or earn a degree. Student therapists should set goals that establish them as professionals. An ideal professional has superior technical knowledge

and works in harmony and cooperation with peers, physicians, and other health care personnel. With the appropriate educational background and determination to excel, a person can practice professionalism and achieve technical excellence. The patient, health care system, and therapist benefit, and the result is a large number of individuals working together to achieve the best possible treatment and care for their patients.[4]

Case Studies

CASE I

As a student therapist, Susan observes many clinical situations. She is assigned to a treatment area that has an extremely high volume of patients. Susan observes that a staff member has treated a patient without an important treatment device in place. When she approachs the staff member about the situation, he mumbles something about the patient being palliative. Obviously the treatment error needs to be corrected. How does Susan ethically and professionally handle this issue that her conscience dictates be addressed? Is this an ethical or legal issue?

CASE II

Sam is a staff radiation therapist in a large center. He has a patient on his treatment schedule who is uncooperative and verbally abusive to the staff members. It is time for the patient's treatment, but once in the treatment room he is refusing to cooperate by getting into the position required and holding still. Sam knows the patient is uncomfortable and needs the treatment to relieve symptomatic disease. Should Sam restrain the patient and force him to have the treatment? What legal and ethical considerations are involved in Sam's final decision?

CASE III

Mrs. Smith is a 50-year-old mother with three adult children. She has been admitted to the hospital for tests to rule out cancer. While the tests are being processed, her husband and children meet with the doctor and ask him not to tell Mrs. Smith if the results are malignant. They tell him that she is afraid of cancer and that if she is given the diagnosis, she will become severely depressed and give up all desire to live. The physician is not comfortable with this request, but the family insists. The physician reluctantly agrees. What ethical and legal concepts are implicated in the family's request and physician's decision to comply with it?

Review Questions

Multiple Choice

1. Which of the following does not govern ethics?
   a. Professional codes
   b. Popular science
   c. Patient's Bill of Rights
2. Which of the following rights does legal ethics include?
   a. Life
   b. Liberty
   c. Medical care
   d. All of the above
3. Moral ethics are based on which of the following?
   a. Right and wrong
   b. Institutions
   c. Legal rights
   d. Codes
4. Which of the following is an ethical characteristic?
   a. Justice
   b. Individual freedom
   c. Egoism
   d. Confidentiality

5. Professional ethics deals with personal character and which of the following factors that identifies professionals as caring and capable persons?
   a. Professional expertise
   b. Chosen profession
   c. Moral character
   d. All of the above
6. Confidentiality, truth telling, and benevolence are which of the following?
   a. Ethical principles
   b. Legal rights
   c. Ethical characteristics
7. A tort falls under which of the following?
   a. Criminal law
   b. Statutory law
   c. Civil law
   d. Common law
8. *Res ipsa loquitur* means which of the following?
   a. "Things speak for themselves"
   b. "The thing speaks for itself"
   c. "Do no harm"
   d. "The things speak for themselves"

Questions to Ponder

1. What does deontology emphasize?
2. Discuss the difference between legal and ethical, and describe a situation in which the two may be in conflict.
3. Discuss and compare the analytical and covenant models of ethical decision making. Discuss the way these models may be used in your profession and by whom.
4. What components are involved in ethical decision making for the radiation therapist?
5. Discuss the required elements that make up an informed consent.

6. Explain the purpose of the scope of practice as it pertains to your performance as a radiation therapist.
7. Compare and discuss the different settings available in hospice care.
8. Discuss the differences in assault and battery. What kind of action can be taken in response to either of these?
9. Analyze the difference between negligence and carelessness. Can careful behavior still result in a charge of negligence? Describe such an instance.
10. Explain the purpose of a medical record, and note the components of a complete radiation oncology record.

REFERENCES

1. American Cancer Society, Massachusetts Division: *Cancer manual,* ed 8, 1990, The Society.
2. American College of Legal Medicine: *Legal medicine: legal dynamics of medical encounters,* ed 2, St Louis, 1991, Mosby.
3. Garrett T, Baillie HW, Garrett R: *Healthcare ethics and principles and problems,* ed 2, Englewood Cliffs, NJ, 1993, Prentice Hall.
4. Gurley LT, Callaway WJ: *Introduction to radiologic technology,* ed 3, St Louis, 1992, Mosby.
5. Inter-Society Council for Radiation Oncology: *Radiation oncology in integrated cancer management,* United States, 1991, The Council.
6. Kübler-Ross E: *On death and dying,* New York, 1969, Macmillan.
7. Parelli RJ: *Medicolegal issues for radiographers,* ed 2, Dubuque, Iowa, 1994, Eastwind.
8. Roy DJ: Ethical issues in the treatment of cancer patients, *Bull World Health Organ* 67(4):342, 1989.
9. Slaby AE, Glicksman AS: *Adapting to life threatening illness,* New York, 1985, Praeger.
10. Smith DH, McCarty K: In the care of cancer patients, *Primary Care Cancer* 19:26-27, 822, 1992.
11. Towsley D, Cunningham E: *Biomedical ethics for radiographers,* Dubuque, Iowa, 1994, Eastwind.
12. Warner S: Code of ethics: professional and legal implications, *Radiol Technol,* p. 485, Dec 1981.
13. *Webster's new collegiate dictionary,* Springfield, Mass, 1976, G & C Merriam.
14. Winter G, Glass E, Sakurai C: Ethical issues in oncology nursing practice: an overview of topics and strategies, *Oncol Nurs Forum* 20:21-34, 1993.
15. Wright R: *Human values in health care: the practice of ethics,* New York, 1987, McGraw-Hill.

The Cancer-Management Perspective

Historical Overview of Cancer Management

Cathy Quane-Smyth

Outline

Key terms

EARLY METHODS OF CANCER TREATMENT

 The treatment of cancer throughout history is a reflection of the way medical science of the time viewed the disease process as a whole and in a more general sense the way contemporary thought dealt with issues of life and death. From its earliest recognition as a disease, cancer has inspired strong emotions in patients and healers and thus affected treatment approaches.

Ancient medicine

In the fifth century BC, Hippocrates described several types of malignant disease. He reserved the term *karkinos* (from the Greek verb meaning "to spread out") for open, ulcerating tumors, especially those of the breast.[7] This type of tumor could be operated on, he felt, but with a "hidden" disease (i.e., internal extension) treatment would only hasten death. The surgical technique described by the Greeks and by Egyptians a thousand years earlier was excision with a knife and cauterization with a hot iron.[4]

Galen, physician to Emperor Marcus Aurelius in the second century AD, wrote extensively about cancer and described many types in detail. He subscribed to the humoral theory of disease, which held that an imbalance of four humors, or fluids, of the body caused illness. Cancer, he believed, was the result of an excess of black bile, or melancholia. Therefore Galen favored a more systemic approach to the treatment of tumors and prescribed diet modifications and purgatives to his patients to eliminate harmful substances.[9] Unfortunately, Galen's anatomical theories were derived from animal studies and he postulated that human anatomy was no different.

The Middle Ages

In the Dark Ages the spirit of inquiry that characterized the ancient Greeks' approach to medicine was replaced by a fatalistic belief in the divine origin of illnesses. The medical writings that survived from classical times, especially those of Galen concerning anatomy, were accepted as indisputable and considered doctrine by the increasingly powerful Roman Catholic Church. Investigations and experiments that threw any of Galen's conclusions in doubt were dismissed by the intellectual and religious hierarchy.[12] This naturally had a chilling effect on the practice of medicine, and few advances if any were made in the treatment of cancer. In addition, interest in cancer and probably the incidence of cancer waned as leprosy and plague spread throughout the world during the Middle Ages.

Scientific revival

Not until the **scientific revival** of the sixteenth century did the investigation and treatment of cancer make a resurgence. Anatomists such as Velasius and later William Harvey challenged and refuted Galen's anatomical theory and opened the door to modern cancer surgery.

In the seventeenth century, Marcello Malpigi made a detailed study of the lymphatic system that provided a rational basis for lymph node dissections in cancer surgery, especially in mastectomies. Jean Louis Petit, an eighteenth century surgeon, laid the foundations for modern breast surgery by excising adjacent lymph nodes and attempting skin-preservation techniques. The first successful colostomy to relieve an obstruction in a patient with rectal carcinoma was performed in 1797.[9]

RELEVANT MEDICAL ADVANCES

Tremendous advances in science and medicine occurred in the nineteenth century, especially in the closing decades. Many of these advances had great effects on cancer management.

Anesthesiology

In 1846 ether **anesthetic** was used for the first time to remove a tumor. Before this, the only pain medications surgeons could offer cancer patients on whom they operated were soporifics (sleep-inducing agents) such as alcohol or hypnotic analgesics such as opium and its derivative, morphine. These drugs reduce the level of perception but do not block sensation. Therefore the use of ether, a true anesthetic, was a major breakthrough. It allowed patients to withstand complex procedures and somewhat reduced the dread of cancer surgery.

Asepsis

The effect of Joseph Lister's advocacy of **asepsis** in surgery can hardly be exaggerated. Although a **germ theory** of infection had been proposed many centuries before, Lister was the first to demonstrate the clinical superiority of asepsis in surgery and the benefits of using antiseptic agents in hospital wards. The high postsurgical death rates from infection began to drop, and for the first time an operation involving the abdomen had some chance of success. Because surgery was the only real choice in the treatment of cancer in the nineteenth century, this great improvement in surgical technique was important for the history of cancer management. Asepsis, however, was not universally and immediately accepted and did not always eliminate postsurgical infections. Until the use of antibiotics became routine, cancer surgeries involving internal organs could not be expected to do more good than harm. The medical profession could not overturn the public's perception that a diagnosis of cancer was a death sentence; it was painfully close to the truth.[11]

Advances in physics

Other advances in science during this time also affected later cancer treatment. The late nineteenth century was a period of great experimentation in electricity, magnetism, and fluorescence. The experiments of Ohm, Faraday, Maxwell, Crookes, Thompson, and others made possible in 1895 Roentgen's discovery of x-rays, which were soon used in a new approach to the treatment of cancer.

However, the typical physician of this era had few weapons to combat cancer. Doctors' attitudes toward malignant disease had not changed significantly since the time of Hippocrates, who stated that treating advanced cancers did more harm than good.

Because of this and the beginning of the advertising age in the late nineteenth century, sellers of patent medicines who claimed to cure a broad spectrum of diseases, including cancer, flourished. These nostrums offered hope of a speedy and painless cure for those frightened to trust physicians who held out little encouragement. Most of these "cures" were blatantly fraudulent and successful only in making fortunes for persons who sold them.

Popular fears about cancer in the late nineteenth century were fueled by the suffering and death of Ulysses S. Grant from cancer of the head and neck. A former president and victorious general, Grant was one of the most famous and respected men of his time. Newspaper accounts of his steady decline made evident the helplessness of medical practice in treating cancers.[11] Cancer began to rival tuberculosis as the most feared disease.

CONTEMPORARY CANCER MANAGEMENT

Cancer management today consists of the three established modalities: surgery, radiation therapy, and medical oncology. It also involves the newest and most experimental treatment approach, biotherapy.

Surgery

Surgery is the oldest direct method of treating cancer, and for most of history, it was the only means available. Historical developments in surgery and improvements in medical education and standards of practice led to greater confidence of cancer surgeons, who felt that the awful scourge of cancer might be controlled by more extensive surgeries. These extensive procedures became medically possible as aseptic techniques became universally adopted, knowledge of cancer spread patterns increased, and postsurgical care improved.

Developments in surgery for breast cancers clearly demonstrate this new attitude toward cancer surgery. As mentioned, documentation on surgical procedures for breast cancers exists far back in medical history. In 1867 an English surgeon named Charles Hewitt Moore published an article in which he stated that current surgeries were inadequate because of the patterns of invasion in breast cancer, and this was the reason patients had recurrent disease. The era of increasingly extensive procedures for controlling cancers of the breast had begun. Surgeons throughout the world routinely began to remove the pectoral fascia and axillary contents.[9]

From 1890 to 1907, William Halsted, a Baltimore surgeon, documented over 250 patients whose breast cancers he had treated by removing the pectoralis muscle and axillary contents in one piece. He performed even larger surgeries on some patients. "He sometimes removed part of the chest wall and traced out the routes of metastases to the bones. Sometimes, he said, amputation at the hip might be necessary."[9] The radical procedure that bears his name was widely used into the 1970s.

This approach is based on the belief that breast cancer spreads in an orderly progression and aggressive local intervention can stay one step ahead until the cancer is eradicated.[8] That supposition has been seriously challenged in recent years and has led to the use of far more conservative surgeries in combination with other modalities. In the early decades of the twentieth century, however, Halsted's approach seemed to offer the best hope of success. At the time Halsted was perfecting his surgical technique, no other satisfactory options existed in treating cancers. Radiation therapy was in its developmental stages, and cancer chemotherapy had yet to be developed.

Improvements in surgical techniques were demonstrated in other anatomical sites. The first successful pneumonectomies and lung lobectomies were performed in the 1930s. Pancreatectomies were also initiated at this time and progressed in scope to the Whipple operation in which neighboring organs were also removed. Radical head and neck surgeries also became technically possible. However, although these operations were performed with great expertise, surgical skill alone was not sufficient to improve survival statistics. Surgery, as Hippocrates stated, was a reasonable option in localized cancers but could not eradicate those that had spread. Improved techniques certainly extended the scope of surgery to new frontiers, but disseminated cancers ultimately eluded the surgeon's knife and these "heroic" surgeries often caused pain and disfigurement without significantly extending life. This recognition of surgery as a valuable tool in the cure of localized cancers led to public information campaigns that encouraged people who had warning signs of cancer to seek early medical attention.

In recent times the availability of other treatment options and revised ideas as to metastatic behavior of various cancers has caused a shift in focus. Surgery is without doubt the first line of treatment for most localized cancers of the gastrointestinal tract and early cancers in some other sites. However, criteria of operability that address the risk-benefit relationship and quality-of-life issues are established for most organ sites. Surgery now is usually an important factor in a combined-modality approach.

Radiation therapy

Unlike surgery, radiation therapy's beginning as a cancer modality has a definite date. Building on the electricity and cathode ray experiments of other late nineteenth century scientists, Wilhelm Roentgen discovered x-rays in 1895. The diagnostic possibilities of x-rays were recognized first, but in a surprisingly short time, their potential as a new approach to the treatment of cancer was also realized. Soon after this the discovery of radium attracted even greater attention in the popular press. At the same time, treatments with electricity, light, and various elements were being touted as potential cures, but hopes for them were short lived and led to disappointment. One cancer historian writes, "This pattern was particularly clear in the United States, where it mirrored a tendency of American culture to embrace whatever was new, especially if it seemed to rest on advanced science and technology."[11]

Unrealistic expectations of the benefits of radiation led to early fears that it too would be a short-lived phenomenon, arousing high expectations doomed to disappointment. Early claims for the curative properties of radium were wildly optimistic. In addition to being a cure for cancer, radium was hailed as a restorer of youth and vigor.[11] Inevitably, disappointment followed such extravagant claims, and radiation therapy took some time to develop into a science that could fill a realistic role in cancer management.

The development of radiation therapy as an important discipline was greatly facilitated by the establishment of a unit of exposure. An exact amount of radiation being generated or administered is taken for granted, but a unit of measurement was not accepted until the late 1920s. Until this time, quantities were estimated in various ways but no universally accepted method existed by which amounts could be standardized. Therefore comparison of results was impossible. The adoption of the roentgen as the unit of exposure took place at the Stockholm Congress of 1928.[14] The use of the roentgen was a great stride forward but of somewhat limited use in radiation therapy because it measured exposure rather than dose, was measured only in air, and was valid only for energies up to 3 MeV. The acceptance in 1953 of the rad as the unit of absorbed dose overcame these limitations and became the standard unit in radiation therapy.[1] In the 1980s the gray, which equals 100 rads, was adopted as the new unit of absorbed dose.

In the late 1920s the work of Seitz and Wintz led to the use of small daily doses rather than large single doses. In 1930, Coutard expounded the principle of protracted fractionation, which is still the basis for current fractionation schedules.[14]

The evolution of equipment from modified diagnostic tubes to the modern linear accelerators has also contributed to radiation therapy's acceptance as a major modality. Early orthovoltage units operated in the kilovoltage range and caused serious problems with skin reactions, high absorption to bone, and poor delivery of a dose to deep-seated lesions. Complex field arrangements were devised to minimize these problems, but many patients experienced severe acute reactions such as burns and ulcers, and more important, late and irreversible reactions such as necrosis of skin and bone. Radiation therapy developed a somewhat sinister reputation, and radiation therapists today may encounter patients who are frightened of developing radiation burns and need reassurance that most skin reactions are quite mild.

Megavoltage treatment units in radiation therapy began with the installation of the first cobalt 60 unit in Canada in 1951. Until the 1970s and into the 1980s in many areas of the United States, the cobalt 60 unit was the most common treatment unit, capable of delivering a relatively high energy beam and famed for its reliability and lack of down time.

Approximately 1 year after the introduction of the cobalt unit the first medical linear accelerator was installed at the Radiation Research Center at the Hammersmith Hospital in London.[13] Both of these units, which operate in the megavoltage energy range, have skin-sparing properties (i.e., the point of maximum dose is below the skin). These units do not deliver higher doses to bone, and the percentage of the beam arriving at points deep in tissue is far superior to that of early treatment units. Therefore many technical problems associated with treatment in the orthovoltage range were solved by the introduction of these units.

Over the last 20 years a gradual shift to the use of linear accelerators has taken place in the United States. Linear accelerators have advantages over cobalt units in that personnel are not exposed to leakage, higher-energy beams can be generated, and field edges are sharply demarcated with little penumbra. An additional advantage is that many linear accelerators can treat in the electron mode, thus making them quite versatile.

The use of sophisticated simulation techniques, the introduction of computed tomography (CT) treatment planning, the increasing emphasis on quality improvement, and the recent introduction of multileaf collimation and conformal therapy in some centers have brought modern radiation therapy to a high level of technical sophistication. Radiation therapy has made great progress toward the goal of maximizing damage to tumor cells while minimizing damage to normal tissue. However, radiation therapy remains a local modality, which like surgery, is most effective at destroying tumors detected early and not yet disseminated.

Medical oncology

Chemotherapy can be defined as "the search for, and the investigation and application of, chemical compounds which may be employed to control disease processes by depression or destruction of pathogenic organisms or abnormal cells."[6] These last three words were added to an older notion of the nature of chemotherapy to accommodate the relatively recent innovation of the treatment of neoplastic disease with various chemical compounds. This discipline is now referred to as *medical oncology.*

The chemotherapeutic approach to the treatment of disease in general begins with the work of Paul Ehrlich in the late nineteenth century. Previously, accidental discoveries led to the treatment of various illnesses with drug remedies. For example, the use of quinine was derived from tree bark to treat malaria. However, no one understood the nature of the drug or its specific action against disease.

Ehrlich investigated the chemical structure of various compounds and their actions on specific diseases. In 1910 his work culminated in the preparation of the drug salvarsan, which was the first synthetic compound effective against a human parasite. In the decades that followed, chemotherapy made dramatic progress against various bacterial and protozoan diseases. Chemotherapy was established as a first-line defense against many diseases. Ehrlich attempted research into a chemotherapeutic approach to cancer medicine but was pessimistic about the results. Although Ehrlich discovered the first alkylating agent, many years would pass before its effects on cancer would be studied.[6]

A famous accident spurred interest in antineoplastic chemotherapy. A ship carrying the chemical weapon mustard gas exploded in a harbor in Italy in 1943. Autopsies of the victims demonstrated a powerful white blood cell suppression. Secret research during World War II became medical research later, and many alkylating and antimetabolite agents were tested with some dramatic results in controlling childhood leukemias.[11] Enormous amounts of government monies were spent on the testing of hundreds of thousands of drugs. During the 1950s and for many years after, medical science was extremely optimistic that chemotherapy was the ultimate answer for cancer control. The stunning successes of chemotherapeutic approaches to other diseases such as polio and many infectious diseases fueled hopes that cancer-specific drugs would be equally successful.

To a limited extent, the optimism was justified. Medical oncology has made significant contributions to the cure of leukemias and lymphomas and the fulfillment of an important role as an adjunct to other modalities. However, these drugs, like surgery and radiation therapy, have drawbacks. In many situations, the limitations are due to toxic effects on patients. Many antineoplastic drugs are carcinogenic. Resistance to drugs is another problem. The use of a combination of chemotherapeutic drugs has reduced the negative effects of these factors to some extent.[2]

The development of a combination of drugs considered active against a specific cancer is an arduous process. Investigating and developing a single agent and having it approved for human trials requires much time and considerable resources. To assess the effectiveness of several drugs used together is geometrically more difficult and expensive. In recent times, in vitro studies and computer models have been used to predict effectiveness and levels of toxicity.

Half a century has passed since the initial experimentation in cancer chemotherapy. This makes cancer chemotherapy a relative newcomer in cancer management. Room exists for more research and experimentation in this modality, especially in the area of solid tumors.

Biotherapy

In the late 1960s, research began on an approach to cancer management fundamentally different from the traditional methods of surgery, radiation therapy, and chemotherapy. Rather than using external agents to eradicate a malignancy, **immunotherapy** (as this approach was originally termed) focuses on identifying ways to stimulate hosts' own defenses to repress the neoplastic process. The principles underlying this approach have been summarized as follows[3]:

1. Tumor cells are inherently different from the normal cells from which they are derived.
2. Some of these differences can be recognized by the host immune system.
3. This recognition process, when optimal, may develop into a tumor rejection response by the host.

Immunotherapy initially involved the use of nonspecific agents such as BCG (bacille Calmette-Guérin), which might activate natural killer cells in the host to destroy tumor cells. Recently this approach has increased in scope to include other biological modifiers, so the term *biotherapy* is now considered more inclusive and descriptive than immunotherapy. *Biotherapy* is defined as "treatment with agents derived from biologic sources and/or affecting biologic response."[15]

Immunology and genetics are on the cutting edge of modern research, but the first notion that cancer patients' own bodies could be stimulated to fight their diseases came a century ago. William Coley, a New York physician, became interested in the records of a patient with a supposedly incurable bone cancer. The patient was infected with erysipelas, a virulent strep infection. After enduring high fever, chills, and malaise, the patient recovered from the infectious condition and his bone tumor dramatically regressed. The patient lived many years free of malignant disease and died of an unrelated cause.[10]

This so intrigued Coley that he began to treat patients by using mixed bacterial vaccine. Sometimes impressive results were achieved, but inducing and controlling the erysipelas was difficult. Also difficult, based on the medical knowledge of the time, was evaluating whether the bacteria itself or the resulting high fever was responsible for the beneficial effects. After Coley's death, this treatment method was largely abandoned, but it was a historical precedent to modern biotherapy.

In the recent history of biotherapy a shift has occurred from the basic concepts of immunotherapy to the use of purified and specific biological products with antineoplastic activity. The development of hybridoma technology allows the production of **monoclonal antibodies,** which are substances that can specifically target tumor-associated antigens existing on cancer cells.[5]

The rapid increase in the knowledge of human genetics and immune response in the 1980s has fueled interest in biotherapy and established it as a promising approach to future cancer management.

Review Questions

Multiple Choice

1. What was the earliest modality used in the treatment of cancer?
   a. Surgery
   b. Radiation therapy
   c. Medical oncology
   d. Biotherapy
2. Ether anesthesia was first used in which century?
   a. Seventeenth century
   b. Eighteenth century
   c. Nineteenth century
   d. Twentieth century
3. Who discovered x-rays?
   a. Crooks
   b. Halstead
   c. Ohm
   d. Roentgen
4. Joseph Lister is associated with which of the following?
   a. Radical cancer surgery
   b. Surgical antisepsis
   c. The development of anesthesia
   d. Chemotherapy
5. What was the first megavoltage radiation therapy unit to be widely used in the United States?
   a. Orthovoltage
   b. Cobalt 60
   c. Linear accelerator
   d. Betatron

Questions to Ponder

1. How has a greater understanding of the metastatic process affected the way cancer is treated?
2. Why was the adoption of a unit to measure exposure so crucial to the development of radiation therapy?
3. What factors have contributed to advances in cancer management in the last century?
4. What is the fundamental difference between biotherapy and the other cancer-treatment modalities?
5. What do you think will be the next breakthrough in cancer management?

REFERENCES

1. Bentel G: *Radiation therapy planning,* New York, 1993, McGraw-Hill.
2. Carter S: *Chemotherapy of cancer,* ed 3, New York, 1987, John Wiley & Sons.
3. Carter S: *Principles of cancer treatment,* New York, 1982, McGraw-Hill.
4. DeMoulin D: *A short history of breast cancer,* Boston, 1983, Martinus Nijhoff.
5. DeVita VT et al: *Cancer principles and practice of oncology,* Philadelphia, 1985, JB Lippincott.
6. Goldin A: *Advances in chemotherapy,* New York, 1964, Academic Press.
7. Henschen F: *The history and geography of diseases,* New York, 1966, Delacorte Press.
8. Lawrence PF: *Essentials of general surgery,* ed 2, Baltimore, 1992, Williams & Wilkins.
9. Meade R: *An introduction to the history of general surgery,* Philadelphia, 1968, WB Saunders.
10. Moss RW: *The cancer industry: unravelling the politics,* New York, 1989, Paragon House.
11. Patterson JT: *The dread disease,* Cambridge, 1987, Harvard University Press.
12. Sheldon H: *Boyd's introduction to the study of disease,* ed 11, Philadelphia, 1988, Lea & Febiger.
13. Stryker J: *Clinical oncology for students of radiation therapy technology,* St Louis, 1992, Warren H Green.
14. Walter J, Miller H: *A short textbook of radiotherapy,* Boston, 1969, Little, Brown.
15. Young C: *The year book of oncology,* St Louis, 1991, Mosby.

6

Principles of
Pathology

J.H. Hannemann

Outline

Key terms

Cell cycle
Chromosomes
Cytoplasm
Endoplasmic reticulum
Genome
Golgi apparatus
Lysosomes
Mitochondria
Nuclear membrane
Nucleoli
Nucleoside
Nucleotide

Nucleus
Oncogene
Organelle
Peroxisomes
Polypeptides
Protein
Ribosome
Transcription
Translation
Tumor-suppressor gene
Vacuoles

Pathology is the branch of medicine devoted to the study and understanding of disease. More precisely, the discipline seeks to understand the effect of disease on the function of the human organism at all levels and relate functional alterations to changes perceived at the gross anatomical, cellular, and subcellular levels. This chapter considers briefly the history and evolution of the pathology of cancer,[13] discusses the cellular theory of disease, and examines the physiology of the neoplastic process. In addition, some of the practical aspects of establishing a pathological diagnosis and using that information to classify and treat cancer are considered. Finally, this chapter provides an overview of subcellular molecular biology and its emerging effect on cancer.

Although the theory of disease and methods by which disease processes are studied have changed dramatically, humans have pursued these issues one way or another for well over 2000 years. The unifying if unspoken premise behind these pursuits has been the notion that every observed effect must have a corresponding cause. Historically, the link between cause and effect was often far from accurate but the hypothesis drove the process forward.

Whereas diseases (mostly ascribed to the intervention of the gods) became manifest during imbalances, a healthy physiological state was the result of a harmonious balance between the humors. Therapeutic intervention was prescribed after a careful physical examination and observation had identified the type and extent of the perceived imbalance. These gross anatomical observations and recordings represent the earliest beginnings of the discipline now identified as pathology.

As time passed, perceptions slowly changed. During the Middle Ages, semiscientific observations continued to be made and recorded, but evolution of the theory of disease was stagnant, and treatment was based mostly on superstition or witchcraft. Prevailing theory and recorded observations were not considered at odds until the sixteenth and seventeenth centuries. After these contradictions were recognized and old ideas challenged, the understanding of disease began to move rapidly forward assisted by new technology that opened unimaginable frontiers.

The introduction of the microscope in the early seventeenth century made possible the observation of unicellular human anatomy, thus propelling pathology from its infancy into its childhood. This also made possible correlations between clinical manifestations of disease and gross anatomical findings and between gross pathology and microscopic observations. These correlations were further developed and refined during the eighteenth and nineteenth centuries as physicians began to comprehend the roles individual organs played in the expression of illness and began to introduce new theories of disease and refine old ones. Practical application of these theories resulted in the development of the first scientifically sophisticated treatment of many diseases. A logarithmic growth has taken place in the twentieth century in medical technology and understanding of disease processes.

Since 1970, another great advancement has been made to understand more completely the physiology of disease. This movement into an unfamiliar and even smaller microcosm has revealed the world of molecular biology, in which disease may be studied at a subcellular level not previously appreciated. This advancement, which has permitted study and observation of function at the molecular level, is at least as great as the development in the seventeenth century that refocused observations from the gross anatomical to the cellular level. The rate at which knowledge is expanding in molecular biology is so fast that only a regular review of the current scientific literature on the subject can provide up-to-date information. This chapter offers an overview of molecular biology and related enterprises to help the student or practitioner of radiation therapy understand vistas that lie ahead.

CELLS AND THE NATURE OF DISEASE

Every clinical disease has its inception with some kind of cellular injury or malfunction that ultimately is expressed at the molecular level of cellular function. To understand this chapter, the reader should be familiar with basic principles of elementary mammalian biology. A general understanding of the structure and function of the mammalian cell, including the several organelles (nucleus, endoplasmic reticulum, ribosomes, Golgi apparatus, mitochondria, lysosomes, peroxisomes, and vacuoles) and plasma membrane, is particularly important. Details of cellular form and function may be obtained from any modern textbook of general biology.

Cells differ greatly concerning functions they perform; however, they have certain characteristics in common. All cells share the ability to produce energy and maintain themselves in a state of normal function by elaborating a vast array of proteins and macromolecules that facilitate adaptation to physiological or pathological stress. As long as cells can maintain themselves in the range of normal function, they exist in a state of homeostasis. The homeostatic state represents a set of circumstances in which cellular processes associated with life proceed normally and in accordance with the function genetically assigned to that cell. In a typical cell, these functions include processes that provide nutrition, protection, communication, and sometimes mobility and reproduction. All these processes are facilitated by the hundreds of macromolecules produced by each cell. Under prolonged or acute physiological stress, this homeostasis may be maintained only with great difficulty. When a cell's adaptive mechanisms fail, changes in cellular structure become identifiable and a pathological or disease state ensues.

Changes in cellular structure can usually be seen under the microscope and may be broadly divided into two categories: irreversible and reversible. Irreversible changes represent cellular death or changes that eventually prove lethal to the cell. Changes representing reversible injury are consistent with cell survival if the precipitating cause is corrected. Dead cells are recognized under the microscope because enzymes begin to destroy them. These enzymes may be derived from the dead cell itself, or they may originate in other scavenging cells such as macrophages. Enzymatic action obliterates cellular detail. Irreversible changes signaling incipient cell death appear as a series of color alterations in typical cellular staining patterns and irregularities in the structure of the cell's nucleus. The nucleus under such circumstances may become fragmented, shriveled, or enzymatically destroyed. The changes of reversible cell damage may be more subtle. They arise from internal loss of power caused by respiratory embarrassment. Cellular swelling is the hallmark of reversible damage and occurs as the damaged cellular membrane fails to regulate properly the concentration of sodium in the cell. As a consequence, water passes across the membrane to produce swelling. Swelling is followed by morphological changes in the intracellular organelles and a decrease in the pH of the cell that can be identified by the application of special cellular stains. The radiation therapist must recognize that all these changes, whether reversible or irreversible, may occur in malignant and normal cells.

These changes in cellular form and function that represent a departure from homeostasis do not occur in a vacuum. They occur instead in the context of the aggregate physiology of the organism and therefore are subject to monitoring and response. In broad terms the monitoring of and response to tissue damage is called the *inflammatory reaction.*[11] Its clinical features have been known since antiquity and described as rubor, calor, tumor, and dolor (i.e., redness, warmth, swelling, and pain). Although the clinical syndrome has not changed since Celsius described these cardinal features in the first century AD, much more is known about its purpose and physiology.

The inflammatory response is a complex, immunochemical reaction initiated by normal cells that have been injured or damaged. It has implications for the defense of the organism and repair of the injury or damage that initially provoked the reaction. The reaction may be intense or subdued depending on the magnitude and nature of the precipitating stimulus. If the reaction evolves completely over a few hours or days, it is acute. If it persists for longer periods, it is chronic. In either situation, the features of the reaction account for the well-known cardinal signs.

Inflammation begins as local vascular dilatation that permits an increase in blood flow to the affected tissue. The increase in blood flow accounts not only for the redness and warmth that accompany inflammation, but also for increases in intravascular pressure and permeability of the vascular membrane. These changes in pressure and permeability expedite the escape of fluid into the interstitial space to produce swelling. This interstitial fluid, which escapes through gaps between the endothelial cells lining small veins, is mostly water-rich in proteins, polypeptides, and other low-molecular-weight substances called *inflammatory mediators* or *cytokines*. These latter substances, thought to be by-products of tissue injury, seem to play a role in nerve stimulation and pain production.

Many white blood cells, mostly neutrophils and other phagocytes, escape the vascular compartment with this fluid. These cells destroy bacteria and other microorganisms, neutralize toxins, and enzymatically destroy dead or dying tissue. When this phagocytic response accomplishes its physiological objectives, it promotes the ingrowth of new capillaries and fibroblasts, which in turn facilitate tissue repair and a return to homeostasis. Tissue damage or injury initiates the cascade of events that constitute the inflammatory response. Without such an initiator, inflammation does not occur.

Many agents cause tissue damage leading to an inflammatory response. Among the most common agents are hypoxia, microbial infections, ionizing radiation, chemicals, allergic or immune reactions, and cancer.

The most common cause of tissue damage is hypoxia. Oxygen deprivation renders a living cell incapable of manufacturing energy. When insufficient energy is present to sustain the cell, intracellular organelles fail, the integrity of the cellular membrane is lost, and death results. Local hypoxia commonly results from vascular occlusive disease and trauma. Vascular occlusive disease is classically seen in acute myocardial infarction. Trauma is present, for example, in skin flap necrosis secondary to vascular damage at the time of a radical mastectomy. The radiation therapist sees generalized hypoxia as a result of cardiorespiratory embarrassment secondary to acute compression of the superior vena cava caused by lung cancer. If not promptly corrected, hypoxia of this magnitude results in death rather than localized tissue

destruction and an ensuing inflammatory reaction. Similarly, other causes of generalized hypoxia such as carbon monoxide or cyanide poisoning, which prevent oxygen transport or use at the cellular level, do not involve inflammation.

Infections produced by bacteria and other microbes represent the most widely recognized cause of inflammation and commonly occur in patients undergoing radiation therapy. The many mechanisms of injury produced by microorganisms are complex and beyond the scope of this discussion; however, the bacterial cellulitis produced by minor injury to the edematous arm of a breast cancer patient who has undergone a radical mastectomy, an axillary lymph node dissection, and radiation therapy is often dramatic. Such an infection is frequently accompanied by all the cardinal signs of inflammation.

For the radiation therapist the most obvious and frequently seen cause of tissue damage is ionizing radiation. Radiation is an agent of tissue damage used medically in a sophisticated fashion to achieve carefully delineated objectives. The primary objective is to lethally damage all cancer cells in a predefined volume of tissue, thus rendering the surviving normal tissue free of neoplastic disease. In pursuit of this objective, some damage is inevitably inflicted on normal tissues incorporated in the radiation portal. Such damage, whether to normal or neoplastic tissue, elicits an inflammatory response. In patients undergoing radiation therapy, this response may be intense and easily identified. More often it is subtle or in deep tissues and not obvious.

Tissue damage produced by the use of chemicals or drugs is frequently encountered clinically. The list of agents responsible for such damage is long, and the mechanisms of injury are numerous. As with ionizing radiation, the judicious administration of certain chemotherapeutic agents may result in tissue destruction, thus having a tangible benefit for the patient. Chemical damage to superficial tissue may be observed after inadvertent extravascular extravasation of some chemotherapeutic agents. These extravasations provoke an intense local inflammatory response. Moreover, the application of some dermatological agents to the skin of patients undergoing radiation therapy may contribute to an easily seen inflammatory reaction in and beyond the radiation portal.

Immune reactions protect the host organism from biological agents. These agents or antigens may be encountered in the external environment of the host or generated less frequently internally. Under normal circumstances the intensity of the reaction confirms it to be a powerful mechanism of protection and tissue repair. Nevertheless, the reaction is often cytolytic and results in tissue damage. The normal immune reaction is subject to complex physiological monitoring and control that promote the reaction's resolution when it is no longer a benefit to the host. Sometimes, however, when the reaction is caused by the presence of internally produced antigens, it can be a force that is destructive rather than beneficial to the organism.

A final and perhaps less obvious cause of tissue damage is neoplastic growth. One of the hallmarks of malignant tumors is local invasion and destruction of normal tissue. This destruction is accompanied by an inflammatory reaction that is usually of low intensity but microscopically identifiable. Occasionally the classical signs of inflammation may be encountered in clinical malignancies. Inflammatory breast cancer typically exhibits to a striking degree the four cardinal signs of inflammation but is unaccompanied at the microscopic level by typical inflammatory cells, thus emphasizing once more the role of tissue damage rather than macrophages in provoking the inflammatory response.

The six important causes of cell damage (radiation, hypoxia, chemicals, microorganisms, immunological reactions, and neoplasms) often share a final common pathway in the production of their damage. This pathway leads to the formation of free radicals, which are highly reactive molecular species that are usually intermediary products of oxygen metabolism. Free radicals, which may be produced directly by agents such as ionizing radiation or indirectly by enzymatic reactions in tissue, are destructive to nucleic acids and other vital cellular components.

THE PATHOLOGY OF NEOPLASMS
Neoplastic diseases

Of the diseases that afflict mankind, cancer is of major importance. In the United States, it claims more lives than any disorder except cardiovascular disease. Furthermore, it is the primary disease with which radiation therapists deal. Accordingly, an understanding of the pathology of neoplastic disease is vital to therapists in the performance of their jobs and in their quests for professional maturity.

The term *cancer* applies to many different disease processes that seem to share some common characteristics. In fact, over 100 types of cancer have been recognized and categorized.

The term *neoplasia* (meaning "new growth") applies to an abnormal process resulting in the formation of a neoplasm or tumor. In the neoplastic process, this new growth occurs beyond the limits of the normal growth pattern. The distinction between normal and neoplastic growth is usually though not always well-defined and easily recognizable. Therefore the process of neoplasia can be appreciated as one of disordered growth.

Vast differences exist in the clinical implications of these abnormal growths. Some of these growths are benign, whereas others are malignant. These descriptive terms characterize the behavior of the tumor in its biological setting and the microscopic pattern observed by the pathologist. Actually, the correlation of the latter with the former over extended periods allows the pathologist initially to establish the diagnosis of neoplastic disease and comment accurately regarding its probable clinical course.

For the patient the first and most important distinction between benign and malignant tumors involves the prognosis. Benign neoplasms seldom pose any threat to the host, even if left untreated. Several glaring inconsistencies notwithstanding, benign tumors usually carry descriptive names that end simply with *-oma*. These tumors tend to grow slowly and be composed of cells often appearing similar to the normal cells from which they arise. The size of benign tumors may persistently increase or inexplicably halt at a certain point. A benign tumor is usually surrounded by a distinct capsule of fibrous tissue that facilitates surgical removal if treatment is necessary. Though often large, these tumors do not invade surrounding tissue to produce direct destruction, nor do they spread distantly to produce metastases.

However, characteristics of malignant tumors, which as a class are referred to as *cancers,* are much different. Cancers generally pose a serious if not fatal threat to the host. Therefore they are seldom left untreated after discovery. This class of tumors has two large subcategories (carcinoma and sarcoma) that designate the tissue of tumor origin. Cancers tend to grow rapidly, doubling in size over periods ranging from a few days to several months. They are composed of cells with microscopic characteristics decidedly different from normal cells that make up the tissue of origin. In fact, cancers may be so bizarre that they bear little if any resemblance to these cells. As cellular detail becomes more bizarre the cell is said to be poorly differentiated compared with tumor cells more closely resembling the cells of origin and are said to be well differentiated. Growth is incessant and proceeds with invasion and destruction of nearby tissues. The speed of growth correlates roughly with the differentiation of the cells (i.e., well differentiated cancers tend to grow more slowly than poorly differentiated ones). A true limiting fibrous capsule of the type in benign tumors is lacking. Distant spread, or metastasis, of the cancer results from malignant cells gaining access to blood and lymphatic channels. Not all such cells survive to colonize distant tissues. The metastatic process is only partially understood but clearly more complex than the passive transport of cancer cells through nearby lymphatics or veins. Most cells gaining access to vascular channels never produce viable deposits of tumor cells in regional lymph nodes or more distant tissues. Instead, they are immunologically destroyed by internal surveillance mechanisms. Cancer cells arising in certain organs have a predilection for metastases to specific sites (i.e., cancers of the prostate and breast have a tendency to metastasize to bone). This specific metastatic potential is influenced by the biochemical interaction between proteins and polypeptides produced by both the tumor cells and the cells' populating sites of potential colonization. (See Table 6-1 for a comparison of characteristics of benign and malignant tumors.)

Because benign tumors often require no treatment and have few radiotherapeutic implications, this chapter does not consider further their pathological characteristics. Instead, subsequent attention is given to cancers, and their pathological implications are considered from several points of view.

The term *cancer* in common usage applies to the entire spectrum of malignant neoplastic processes. Cancers are

Table 6-1	Characteristics of benign and malignant tumors		
Characteristic		**Benign**	**Malignant**
Growth rate		Slow	Rapid
Mitoses		Few	Many
Nuclear chromatin		Normal	Increased
Differentiation		Good	Poor
Local growth		Expansive	Invasive
Encapsulation		Present	Absent
Destruction of tissue		Little	Much
Vessel invasion		None	Frequent
Metastases		None	Frequent
Effect on host		Often insignificant	Significant

From Damjanov I, Linder J: *Anderson's pathology*, ed 10, St Louis, 1995, Mosby.

broadly divided into carcinomas and sarcomas. The term *carcinoma* refers to a malignant tumor taking its origin from epithelial cells, which are widespread and generally considered to be cells that line surfaces. As such, epithelial cells cover most external surfaces, line most cavities, and form glands. From a functional standpoint, therefore, epithelial cells are protective, absorptive, or secretory. Because they are so widely distributed and metabolically active, epithelial cells give rise to a wide variety of tumor types that comprise the majority of solid tumors encountered in clinical practice. Carcinomas tend to invade lymphatic channels more often than blood vessels; therefore metastases are frequently found in lymph nodes. The designation of carcinoma by the pathologist may be modified by a preceding phrase or prefix further identifying the tissue of origin. For example, a cancer arising from cells lining the upper air and food passages may be designated a *squamous cell carcinoma* to identify further the nature of the epithelial surface from which the cancer arose. Similarly, a cancer with its origin internally in an organ such as the pancreas (for which surfaces are difficult to imagine) is designated an *adenocarcinoma* to indicate origin from the secretory epithelium that lines the individual pancreatic glands.

In contrast, the term *sarcoma* describes a neoplasm arising from cells other than those forming epithelial surfaces. From a practical point of view, these cells reside in connective tissue or the nervous system. Though such cells constitute the majority of the body by weight, they spawn relatively few malignant neoplasms. Sarcomas tend to metastasize via blood vessel invasion. This accounts for the frequent appearance of metastatic sarcoma in the lungs. Sarcomas may also carry a pathological prefix designating more precisely the tissue of tumor origin. For example, a malignant tumor arising in bone is termed an *osteosarcoma,* one arising in cartilage is termed a *chondrosarcoma,* and one originating from fat cells is termed a *liposarcoma* (see Table 6-2 for comprehensive nomenclature).

In describing carcinomas or sarcomas the pathologist provides additional commentary about the nature of the neo-plasm. This commentary is designed to provide guidance in prognostication and treatment. In gross anatomical pathology, commentary is made about the size of the cancer and its apparent extent in tissues received from the surgeon. For example, a cancer of the kidney may be noted to have invaded the renal vein, a portion or all of which has been submitted to the pathologist along with the cancer. Co-morbid changes in surrounding normal tissues such as abscess formations that might accompany perforated cancers of the colon are noted.

After examination under the microscope, cancer cells that exhibit no differentiation are called *anaplastic.* Similarly, the term *pleomorphic* describes the great variability in size and shape of these undifferentiated tumor cells. Nuclear abnormalities in cancer cells occur regularly. The nuclei of cancer cells may be assigned designations such as *hyperchromatic, clumped, undergoing mitoses,* and *containing prominent nucleoli.* These designations suggest circumstances that reflect malignant degeneration of cells.

Etiology

With so much descriptive terminology, it is perhaps surprising that so little is known about the causes of cancer. That unfortunate set of circumstances is, however, in rapid transition as a result of many advances in molecular biology. Nonetheless, the causes of cancer as presently understood are physiologically naive, incomplete, and more associative than precise. For example, some cancers are associated with exposure to certain chemicals such as those in tobacco smoke. Other cancers are associated with exposure to ionizing radiation in small-to-moderate doses. Still others are associated with viral infections. These associations are useful in describing possible risk factors in the environment, but they remain imprecise in elucidating molecular mechanics of carcinogenesis that allow useful therapeutic intervention.

Chemical carcinogenesis has been accepted as a clinical reality for many decades and was first suggested over 200 years ago.[14] In the mid eighteenth century in England, Percivall Pott noted an association between scrotum cancer and the work done by chimney sweeps. In the early part of the twentieth century, this association between cancer and products of hydrocarbon combustion was confirmed in Japan by Yamagiwa and Ichikawa, who were able to induce cancers in the skin of laboratory animals by the chronic application of coal tar. Since that time, hundreds of chemicals that play roles in cancer induction have been identified and isolated.

Chemical carcinogenesis is not a simple process that proceeds in a linear fashion from point A to point B. Instead, it is a complex process in which interplay with other mechanisms of cancer induction is likely if not probable. The rate and intensity of these processes varies from one tumor system to the next. Chemical carcinogens are mutagens (i.e., they can cause unusual changes in the deoxyribonucleic acid [DNA] of cells they attack). Most chemical carcinogens are compounds containing atoms deficient in electrons and therefore chemically active in the relatively electron-rich

Table 6-2	Nomenclature of benign and malignant tumors		
Cell or tissue of origin	**Benign**	**Malignant**
Tumors of epithelial origin		
Squamous cells	Squamous cell papilloma	Squamous cell carcinoma
Basal cells	—	Basal cell carcinoma
Glandular or ductal epithelium	Adenoma	Adenocarcinoma
	Papillary adenoma	Papillary adenocarcinoma
	Cystadenoma	Cystadenocarcinoma
Transitional cells	Transitional cell papilloma	Transitional cell carcinoma
Bile duct	Bile duct adenoma	Bile duct carcinoma (cholangiocarcinoma)
Islets of Langerhans	Islet cell adenoma	Islet cell carcinoma
Liver cells	Liver cell adenoma	Hepatocellular carcinoma
Neuroectoderm	Nevus	Malignant melanoma
Placental epithelium	Hydatidiform mole	Choriocarcinoma
Renal epithelium	Renal tubular adenoma	Renal cell carcinoma (hypernephroma)
Respiratory tract	—	Bronchogenic carcinoma
Skin adnexal glands		
Sweat glands	Syringoadenoma; sweat gland adenoma	Syringocarcinoma, sweat gland carcinoma
Sebaceous glands	Sebaceous gland adenoma	Sebaceous gland carcinoma
Germ cells (testis and ovary)	—	Seminoma (dysgerminoma)
		Embryonal carcinoma, yolk sac tumor
Tumors of mesenchymal origin		
Hematopoietic/lymphoid tissues	—	Leukemias
		Lymphomas
		Hodgkin's disease
		Multiple myeloma
Neural and retinal tissue		
Nerve sheath	Neurilemoma, neurofibroma	Malignant peripheral nerve sheath tumor
Nerve cells	Ganglioneuroma	Neuroblastoma
Retinal cells (cones)	—	Retinoblastoma
Connective tissue		
Fibrous tissue	Fibroma	Fibrosarcoma
Fat	Lipoma	Liposarcoma
Bone	Osteoma	Osteogenic sarcoma
Cartilage	Chondroma	Chondrosarcoma
Muscle		
Smooth muscle	Leiomyoma	Leiomyosarcoma
Striated muscle	Rhabdomyoma	Rhabdomyosarcoma
Endothelial and related tissues		
Blood vessels	Hemangioma	Angiosarcoma
		Kaposi's sarcoma
Lymph vessels	Lymphangioma	Lymphangiosarcoma
Synovia	—	Synoviosarcoma (synovioma)
Mesothelium	Benign mesothelioma	Malignant mesothelioma
Meninges	Meningioma	
Uncertain origin	—	Ewing's tumor
Other origins		
Renal anlage	—	Wilms' tumor
Trophoblast	Hydatidiform mole	Choriocarcinoma
Totipotential cells	Benign teratoma	Malignant teratoma

From Damjonov I, Linder J: *Anderson's pathology,* ed 10, St Louis, 1995, Mosby.

milieu that characterizes ribonucleic acid (RNA), DNA, and their products. Many of these chemicals occur naturally, but some are synthetic. Most of them require metabolic activation to assume their carcinogenic statures. Their action is thus somewhat indirect compared with a few compounds such as chemotherapeutic alkylating agents that can directly induce neoplasia. The number of chemical carcinogens is great. Some of the more important ones include polycyclic hydrocarbons produced by the combustion of fossil fuels and tobacco, alcohol, asbestos, nickel compounds, vinyl chloride, and nitrosamines and aflatoxins, both of which may be found in food.

Any of these chemical compounds may react with the DNA of a normal cell to produce a mutation. Having undergone such a mutation, a cell is not necessarily committed to neoplasia. Many mutations are not carcinogenic and more important are likely to be detected by cellular surveillance mechanisms that lead to their detection and repair. Some mutations, however, produce strategic damage sufficient to have potential neoplastic consequences. The chemical compound provoking such a mutation is called an *initiator;* the cell has undergone initiation. Initiation only conveys new potential to the cell; it does not produce an immediate cancer. In fact, the time between the initiating event and clinical appearance of the tumor may be many years or decades. The time between the two events is termed the *latent period.* During the latent period, initiated cells may appear normal under the microscope. At the same time, they may display subtle changes in their capacity to respond to mechanisms that usually regulate cell growth. Programmed cell death, or apoptosis, may not occur as it normally does, cellular differentiation may become irregular, and the action of another group of chemicals (called *promoters*) may influence cellular growth. Promoters are seldom carcinogens but have the effect of hastening and intensifying abnormal growth characteristics set in motion by the initiator. As a result, cell division accelerates beyond that normally seen under the influence of the initiator alone to produce a clone of cells displaying increased metabolic activity and early abnormal growth characteristics. In this clone, genetic evolution continues to produce occasional cells that behave more like those of a clinical malignancy. These cells in turn become ascendant and produce daughter cells with even more aggressive features. Whether or not they are augmented by the action of promoters, all these phenomena, which are set in motion by the initiator, culminate in the development of a clinical malignancy if given sufficient time.

The physiologist Francis Peyton Rous first demonstrated viral carcinogenesis in 1911.[9] He induced the growth of soft-tissue sarcomas in a strain of normal chickens simply by injecting the chickens with a cell-free filtrate made from a tumor in another bird of the same strain. Unfortunately, the importance of this experiment was not immediately recognized because the entire sequence could not be reproduced in mammals. Moreover, because the particulate nature of

viruses was not comprehensively understood at that time, Rous' experiment was relegated to the realm of curiosity. In a few years, Twort and d'Herelle significantly advanced the scientific understanding of cell-free filtrates by presenting data documenting the true nature of viruses as small packets of genetic material having the capacity to infect and sometimes destroy living cells. Twenty years later, R.E. Shope and J.J. Bittner, working independently, reported viral tumor induction in rabbits and mice, thus inviting more understanding to viral carcinogenesis in mammals.

In scientific laboratories today, many mammalian cell systems exist in which viral tumor induction can be demonstrated. In humans, no specific cancers have been shown to be caused by a viral agent acting alone. However, scientists have discovered strong associations between several cancers and specific types of viruses.

As suggested by Twort and d'Herelle, viruses are simply small packets of genetic material enclosed in capsules. This genetic material may be DNA or RNA, but with either the virus is an obligate parasite in need of a living cell to infect to reproduce itself. Some viruses can infect many kinds of cells in one or several species. For example, the rabies virus can infect rodents, dogs, and humans. Other viruses exhibit great specificity and can infect only certain cells in a single species. Regardless of the range of potential hosts, infection occurs after the genetic material in the virus gains access to the host cell. Inside the host cell, the viral **genome** assumes command of cellular function to replicate itself. In acute viral infections, this replication is rapid and not only produces hundreds of viral copies, but also destroys the infected cell. The process is more subtle in tumor-producing or tumor-associated viral infections. Instead of destructively commandeering cell function to rapidly reproduce itself, the virus strategically inserts its genetic material into chromosomes of the host cell in such a way to promote cell proliferation. Sometimes this proliferation occurs as a direct result of the viral infection and quickly assumes the hallmarks of malignancy as it does in the Rous chicken sarcoma. At other times the proliferation may not become manifest without a series of additional events that finally trigger malignant cell growth. This process is more likely in human tumors that have viral associations. In other situations the virus achieves its goal of replication because its incorporated genome participates in the reproductive cycle of the host cell. If the host cell infected with the viral genome is a germ cell in the ovary or testes, the potential for transmission of the viral DNA from one generation to the next is obvious.

Genes of viral derivation that have become incorporated into chromosomes of the host cell and are concerned with the regulation of cell growth are called viral *oncogenes.* A few human cancers are associated with certain viral infections. The four common viruses widely distributed in nature and implicated in human neoplasia are the Epstein-Barr (EBV), the human papilloma (HPV), the hepatitis B (HBV), and the human T-cell leukemia, type I (HTLV-I) viruses.

EBV causes acute infectious mononucleosis. This virus has a predelicton for lymphocytes. In some of the lymphocytes the genome of the virus may persist after the acute infection has resolved. Cell lines established from tumors in patients with Burkitt's lymphoma, immunoblastic lymphoma, and nasopharyngeal cancer frequently harbor this virus.

HPV is ubiquitous among higher vertebrates. Dozens of types have been recognized and recently classified. These viruses are associated with a variety of neoplasms ranging from simple warts to invasive cancer of the uterine cervix and probably play a role as initiator or promoter in a host of additional cancers arising from squamous cell epithelium.

HBV is endemic in Africa and Asia, continents in which chronic hepatitis is a major cause of mortality. In these same areas the incidence of hepatocellular carcinoma among those infected with HBV is many times that of uninfected persons. The transitional cascade from HBV infection to the development of hepatocellular carcinoma is complex and remains to be completely elucidated. However, the epidemiological evidence for an association between the two is overwhelming.

HTLV-I is endemic in Japan, Africa, and the West Indies and is an example of a retrovirus that plays a causal role in the development of human malignancy. Retroviruses are RNA viruses that uniquely carry their own enzyme systems. After invasion of a host cell, this enzyme (reverse transcriptase) allows retroviruses to transcribe their own RNA into DNA, which is then inserted into chromosomes of the host cell. This transcription is necessary because DNA (not RNA) is the functional material of genes.

Though each of these four viruses is associated with human cancer in a significant way, they all require the operation of cofactors to permit neoplastic expression. Complex pathological interactions are required to defeat the function of normal cells programmed to prevent carcinogenesis.

The majority of cancers seem to arise spontaneously for reasons poorly understood (i.e., they are not induced by pure chemical nor pure viral mechanisms). Such cancers are considered to be caused by environmental factors. Of course, chemicals and viruses are constituents of the environment, so the classification is somewhat contrived. Nonetheless, among environmental factors that can cause cancer, few are better documented than radiant energy. Ionizing radiation has been known for decades to be carcinogenic.[7] The increased incidence of cancer in radiation workers and survivors of atomic bombing is legendary. Most of the radiation workers, whose exposure was chronic, received many small doses of radiation over long periods and subsequently developed cancers of hematological origin (i.e., leukemias and lymphomas). In contrast, atomic bomb survivors received single large doses of whole-body radiation, which in addition to hematological malignancies, induced solid tumors of the thyroid, breast, colon, and lung. All these cancers became manifest after latent periods ranging from a few years to several decades. These long, latent periods suggest that many cofactors are operative in radiation carcinogenesis.

Similar latent periods occur in cancers induced by ultraviolet radiation. Sunlight (the principle environmental source of ultraviolet radiation) has been implicated in the induction of all common cancers of the skin (i.e., basal cell carcinoma, squamous cell carcinoma, and malignant melanoma). These cancers arise only in skin lacking protective melanin pigment and therefore rarely occur in African-Americans.

The mechanism by which radiant energy causes cancer is linked to its action as a mutagen. Energy absorbed by the cell's nucleus results in damage to the genetic material in the chromosomes, thus producing rearrangement or breakage in the strands of DNA. As in other situations that cause damage to DNA, intracellular mechanisms attempt to promote repair. When repair is incomplete in a cell surviving the radiation insult the derangement of the genetic material may be perpetuated in much the same way that the incorporated genetic material of the virus is replicated by cells surviving viral infections. During the ensuing latent period, these altered cells are subject to the action of the entire spectrum of carcinogens and may eventually, under proper circumstances, exhibit neoplastic growth.

ESTABLISHING A PATHOLOGICAL DIAGNOSIS

Little if any reason exists to treat cancer without first establishing a pathological diagnosis. This entails the recovery of cells that the pathologist can identify as malignant.[3] The probable nature of an anatomical abnormality detected in the clinic on physical examination or identified on any of the several imaging studies commonly used in modern medicine can be predicted with considerable accuracy. However, verification of the clinical suspicion usually has significant therapeutic implications for the patient and physician and satisfies minimally the standards required medicolegally before a full-scale assault on cancer can be recommended or planned. More important, the clinical suspicion is sometimes incorrect, thus resulting in major modification of the proposed treatment program. For example, carcinoma of the lung is a disease that can be diagnosed with great regularity before any cells are recovered for examination. By careful consideration of all other available information (including age, symptoms, signs, smoking history, blood tests, and results of imaging studies such as radiographs and computed tomographic scans), a malignancy of the lung can be diagnosed without much uncertainty. The conclusion might be made that little else is required. However, four common types of lung cancer exist, and the ability of the previously mentioned determinants to discriminate among them is considerably more limited than their ability to simply suggest the presence of a pulmonary malignancy. Each of the four types of lung cancer has its own clinical and biological characteristics, and these characteristics determine the best treatment and influence the outcome. Accordingly, recovering tumor cells for study to make appropriate recommendations to the patient becomes extremely important. The likely outcome of tissue recovery is only the documentation of a specific type of lung cancer, but the implications could be enormous for all concerned if the typical lung cancer turns out to be something else (i.e., a metastatic cancer or even a benign tumor). Pathologists are not always correct, but their tools for establishing a diagnosis of malignancy are the most powerful available in the medical armamentarium.

The acquisition of living cells to establish a diagnosis of malignancy is obviously a maneuver that is invasive or requires internal encroachment on the site harboring the tumor. This intrusion may be major or minor. The three procedures most commonly used to make a diagnosis of cancer (listed in ascending order of invasiveness) are (1) recovery of exfoliating cells, (2) fine-needle aspiration of malignant cells, and (3) open biopsy of the tumor. Attention to detail is necessary to obtain consistently good results from any of these procedures. The diagnosis depends on submitting to the pathologist representative portions of the tissue suspected of being cancerous. If inadequate samples are submitted, unfortunate inaccuracies in diagnosis are inevitable.

Exfoliative cytology is the study of single cells obtained from various surfaces or secretions shed by the tumor. The foremost example of exfoliative cytology is the Papanicolaou smear, which is made for the early detection of cancer of the cervix and uterus. The usefulness of this technique has been proved over several decades.

Fine-needle aspiration is another recovery technique that results primarily in the acquisition of single cells. These cells are recovered through a fine needle inserted directly into the tumor. Because the needles are of small caliber, they can traverse most normal tissue without causing damage and therefore bring remote and relatively inaccessible tumors such as cancer of the pancreas in easy range.

Open biopsy (the most invasive of the three recovery procedures) is accomplished under direct vision. The tumor is surgically removed totally or partly.

Each of these procedures has its own set of variations, and some overlap of procedures is present from one to another. For example a biopsy may be incisional with removal of only a piece of the tumor or excisional with removal of the entire tumor. Likewise, an incisional biopsy may be accomplished through a large bore needle.

The tissue sample becomes the responsibility of pathologists who direct laboratory analysis of the specimen along several different pathways. Most important is the preparation of the sample for examination and study under the light microscope. This is usually accomplished by fixing the tissue or preserving its existing form and structure by immersing it in a solution such as formalin.

Specimens of solid tissue are fixed and then placed in hot, liquid paraffin. After the paraffin cools and hardens, the tissue can be cut in extremely thin slices by a machine called a *microtome*. These slices are placed on glass slides, which are then immersed in an organic solvent, thus dissolving the paraffin. The resulting tissue sections may be treated with any of a vast number of stains to demonstrate specific features of cellular detail. Using the microscope, pathologists search for evidence of malignancy previously mentioned in this chapter.

Specimens of exfoliating cells or those obtained by fine-needle aspiration are smeared thinly on microscopic slides before being appropriately fixed and stained. In these preparations of single cells, attention is given not only to the size and shape of individual cells, but also to the specific features of the nucleus and cytoplasm. Cells lacking uniformity of size, shape, and nuclear configuration may be suggestive of malignancy.

In tissue sections, departures from cellular and nuclear uniformity are also abnormal. In addition, the presence of a malignant tumor usually disturbs normal tissue architecture.

This disturbance is the result of malignant cells invading and destroying surrounding tissue. Some of this invasion may be into blood or lymph vessels, therefore suggesting the metastatic potential of the tumor. However, no single microscopic abnormality is sufficient to establish the diagnosis of cancer in all instances. The job of pathologists often entails a highly complex and relatively subjective discrimination among a host of biological variables, which together are predictive of the behavior of the process that is under study. Fortunately, pathologists have other tools to assist in this estimation. Among these tools is the flow cytometer, which is a piece of sophisticated electronic equipment that facilitates the extremely rapid passage of cells in suspension through a laser beam and past an array of detectors. These detectors analyze individual cells for predetermined characteristics such as size, DNA content, surface markers, cell-cycle position, and viability. In carefully selected test samples, abnormal DNA content, variation in cell size, and irregular cell-surface markers can furnish additional evidence of malignancy, identify incomplete responses to therapy, or document early tumor recurrence after treatment. As the molecular biology of the cancer cell is dissected and understood, additional techniques to assist the pathologist in determining the parameters of cell growth have been and continue to be developed. A detailed discussion of this new pathology is beyond the scope of this chapter. However, some of these innovative approaches are referenced in this chapter in the section on the biology of the cancer cell.

CLASSIFYING CANCER

The classification of neoplastic diseases is far from an exact science. Published systems of classification are intended as communication guidelines for those involved in cancer management rather than absolute frames of reference for the pathologist. Virtually all these systems contain many inconsistencies that lack rational explanation but over decades have become entrenched in medical jargon. Only time and experience will convey to the inquisitive radiation therapist an understanding of the full spectrum and meaning of these inconsistencies.

For better or worse, classification systems consist of a potpourri of terms derived from observations regarding the origin, function, site, and clinical behavior of the tumor. To the corresponding disarray created by such a system are added numerous eponyms, or proper names, the meanings of which simply require memorization. Of the several bases for classification, those relating to biological behavior and tissue of origin are most important. Accordingly, the previously noted nomenclature defining malignancy and the distinction drawn between carcinomas and sarcomas is significant. Malignant behavior is designated by the use of the latter two terms. The tissue of origin in carcinomas is epithelial tissue, whereas in sarcomas the tissue is nonepithelial. In addition to those specifications, modifiers describing the organ of origin or aspects of function may be used. However, they are often superfluous. Finally, inconsistencies and eponyms plague newcomers to oncology. With time and experience, these persons understand that melanoma and hepatoma, though seemingly benign, are really malignancies and Hodgkin's disease is akin to lymphomas and leukemias.

In describing the histopathology of various cancers, the pathologist not only assigns the tumor to one of the previously mentioned subsets, but also assigns to that particular tumor a grade and sometimes a stage. Tumor grade and stage are intended to serve as indices of outcome and are therefore of clinical importance.

Tumor grade is a specification that describes the apparent aggressiveness of the cancer as determined by cytologic and morphological criteria. High-grade tumors are apt to be more aggressive than low-grade tumors. Now in common usage is a system that assigns a numeric value from one to three. Tumors with low numeric designations are likely to be well-differentiated, of lower metastatic potential, and easier to control. Conversely, grade three, or high-grade, tumors appear poorly differentiated, may metastasize early, and may be extremely difficult to control.

Tumor stage is a description of the extent of the tumor at the time of diagnosis. Staging may be clinical, pathological, or a combination of elements of both. Clinical stage is assigned on the basis of physical examination with or without the assistance of certain imaging studies depending on the tumor. It is based on recognition of tumor size, invasiveness, and local or distant metastases. The clinical staging of a cancer may be verified and therefore converted to a pathological stage by recovering for study under the microscope appropriate tissue from one or more sites. A more advanced stage of disease generally implies a worse prognosis. High-grade tumors are likely to be more advanced in stage at the time of diagnosis than low-grade tumors. Most of the time, however, the principle determinate of prognosis is the stage of disease rather than the grade.

Presently, two staging systems predominate. The first of these (the AJCC system) was developed by the American Joint Committee for Cancer Staging and End Results Reporting and represents the ongoing work of a consortium of specialty societies in American medicine. The other (the IUCC system) is the work of an international agency known as the *International Union Against Cancer.* The two systems bear similarities and employ the basic elements of TNM staging introduced over 50 years ago by Pierre Denoix. The TNM system specifies the extent or stage of a cancer by considering three categories: the primary tumor (T), the regional lymph nodes (N), and distant metastatic disease (M). In staging a particular tumor the initial of each category is given a numerical subscript designating the extent of disease found in that anatomical compartment. For example, an early breast cancer of less than 2 cm in diameter that has spread neither locally nor distantly is assigned a stage of $T_1N_0M_0$. These staging systems have many permutations and variations with unique meanings regarding tumors of specific sites.

BIOLOGY OF THE CANCER CELL

Considering the cancer cell an absolute biological renegade wreaking havoc on one system after another is tempting. This temptation is resisted, however, by recalling that to exist as an entity at all the cancer cell must participate in some of the same biological processes sustaining the many normal cells around it.[5] Consequently, the biology of the cancer cell is best examined in the context of normal cellular function by noting deviations from normal function that cancer cells display.

Cells are diverse in size, shape, and function. Nevertheless, they have many common elements (Fig. 6-1). All mammalian cells are surrounded by a cell wall, or plasma membrane. All processes of life occur inside that membrane or on its surface and are accomplished by many specialized components called **organelles.** Within the plasma membrane is the **nucleus** of the cell containing the genetic material DNA that directs cellular metabolism. DNA is the material from which genes are made. Individual genes, which may number in the hundreds of thousands, are normally assigned specific positions or loci on protein structures called **chromosomes.** The cell nucleus also contains one or more **nucleoli,** which are organelles that facilitate **ribosome** assembly. A **nuclear membrane** encloses the nucleus. Between the nucleus and outer cell wall is a substance known as **cytoplasm,** which is a conglomerate of semiliquid material called *cytosol* and numerous extranuclear organelles. Woven throughout the cytoplasm is a filamentous membrane called the **endoplasmic reticulum,** which is continuous with the nuclear membrane and houses the ribosomes. Ribosomes are important organelles responsible for protein synthesis. Other important cytoplasmic organelles include the **Golgi apparatus, lysosomes, peroxisomes, vacuoles,** and **mitochondria.** The Golgi apparatus is important in the storage and management of intracellular chemical substances. Lysosomes play a role in intracellular digestion. Peroxisomes harbor specific enzyme systems, facilitating certain metabolic processes, and vacuoles function in cytoplasmic storage. Mitochondria are the intracellular factories that produce adenosine triphosphate (ATP) from sugar and other organic fuels. ATP in turn is the source of energy that drives intracellular metabolism. Under ordinary circumstances, these components of the normal cell function together to maintain equilibrium, promote

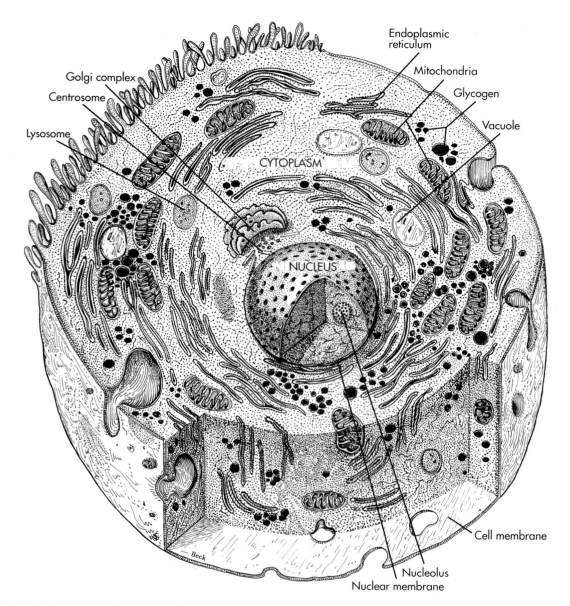

Fig. 6-1 A stylized representation of a typical cell. Note the membranes that enclose the cell proper and nucleus respectively. A typical cell contains numerous organelles, among which the endoplasmic reticulum, Golgi apparatus or complex mitochondria, and lysosomes are prominent. The ribosomes, themselves important organelles, are represented by the many dots bordering the endoplasmic reticulum. (From Anthony CP, Kolthoff NJ: *Textbook of anatomy and physiology,* ed 9, St Louis, 1974, Mosby.)

growth, and facilitate proliferation. All this occurs at one or more points during the cell cycle.

Classically, the **cell cycle** is the observable sequence of events pursued during the life span of a dividing cell.[2] The cycle is chronologically divided into four distinct phases: G_1, S, G_2, and M (Fig. 6-2). G_1 is the period before the duplication or synthesis of DNA in the nucleus. This phase is extremely variable in length and may be indistinguishable from G_0, in which living cells are fully functional but simply not programmed for mitosis. The S phase is the period during which nuclear DNA is synthesized and chromosomes

are duplicated. The G_2 phase of the cell cycle commences after DNA synthesis is complete and continues until the cell begins to divide during the M phase. During G_2, G_1, and S, the cell is growing, producing proteins and organelles, and discharging its metabolic responsibilities. The shortest phase of the cell cycle is M, during which mitosis occurs. Whereas other phases may be measured in days or weeks, mitosis usually occurs in about 2 hours. With completion of mitosis, two identical daughter cells have been made. They in turn enter G_1 to repeat the same sequence of events that led to their production.

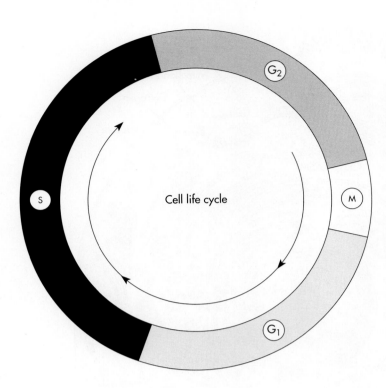

Fig. 6-2 The cell cycle. Note that compartment G contains a subpopulation of cells in phase G_0. These cells are indistinguishable from cells in G_1 but are not programmed for mitosis and therefore will not enter S with other cells in G_1. (From Anthony CP, Kolthoff NJ: *Textbook of anatomy and physiology,* ed 9, St Louis, 1974, Mosby.)

During G_1 the young daughter cell grows (i.e., increases in mass) and undergoes differentiation, or the expression of structural and functional specialization. The cell may prepare to proliferate or divide once more, but G_1 is usually a point of restraint in cellular proliferation. Ordinarily, proliferation and differentiation are closely controlled by interrelated physiological processes. They also tend to be reciprocal (i.e., the greater the differentiation, the less proliferation). When these complex, cell-cycle–related, intracellular mechanisms break down, reciprocity may be expressed in the uncontrolled proliferation of poorly differentiated cells.

Ultimately, these processes are controlled by molecular events predetermined by gene expression. Through the study and understanding of gene expression, molecular biology has evolved and dramatically expanded over the last 2 decades, and molecular biology has contributed greatly to the understanding of normal and malignant cells. (For a detailed discussion of gene form and function, refer to a standard college textbook of biology.)

Genes that line chromosomes are composed of DNA, which is composed of a series of deoxyribonucleotides.[15] **Nucleotides** in general have three chemical components: a phosphate group, a molecule of sugar containing five carbon atoms, and a nitrogenous base. The phosphate group is not variable in nucleotides, but without it a nucleotide becomes a compound known as a **nucleoside.** The five-carbon sugar may be deoxyribose or ribose, depending on whether the nucleic acid is DNA or RNA. Five nitrogenous bases—adenine, guanine, thymine, cytosine, and uracil—are in nucleotides. Adenine, guanine, thymine, and cytosine are in DNA. In RNA, uracil substitutes for thymine.

DNA is arranged in two complimentary strands configured in the shape of a double helix (Fig. 6-3). Nucleotides are present in a specific and unique sequence as far as nitrogenous bases are concerned. These bases connect the two strands of DNA and are complementary because chemical bonds that can form between the nitrogenous bases are exclusive. Adenine on one strand can combine only with thymine on the other. Similarly, guanine can combine only with cytosine. As a result, each strand bears in its structure the blueprint necessary to precisely reproduce the other strand. In the cell cycle during synthesis the strands are separated and each serves as a template to reproduce its complementary image; thus, genetic replication is accomplished.

Proteins are the building blocks of life. They provide form and function for the organism and regulate growth and metabolism. Proteins are complex molecules composed of **polypeptides.** It is at the polypeptide level that the genetic expression has its impact, for it is the unique sequencing of the nucleotides along the length of a strand of DNA which determines the polypeptide configuration of all of the body proteins. Peptide information is encoded along the DNA strand in words called *codons.* Each codon is three nucleotides in length and represents a specific amino acid. Amino acids are the molecules from which peptides are made. Between meaningful codons are series of nucleotides that are nonsense (i.e.,

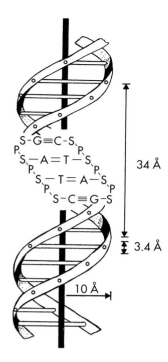

Fig. 6-3 A schematic representation of the DNA double helix. (S = the five-carbon sugar deoxyribose; P = phosphate group; G = guanine; C = cytosine; A = adenine; T = thymine). Note the sugar-phosphate backbone of each strand. The link between strands is uniquely accomplished by nitrogenous bases that form appendages of the backbone. (From Boyd CM, Dalrymple GV: *Basic science principles of nuclear medicine,* St Louis, 1974, Mosby.)

they do not represent anything). These stretches of nonsense are called *introns;* meaningful stretches are known as *exons.* RNA facilitates the transition from the code of DNA sequencing and codons to the structure of polypeptides and a protein molecule. In a process called **transcription,** enzymes in the cell nucleus facilitate the transfer of information from a strand of DNA to a strand of RNA. This particular type of RNA is called *messenger RNA* (mRNA.) To become functional, this message-bearing strand of RNA undergoes splicing, during which the introns are excised. This excision results in a strand of RNA that contains only meaningful codons. After the splicing is complete, the mRNA leaves the nucleus for ribosomes in the cytoplasm.

Ribosomes are the site of **translation** at which the message borne by the mRNA is apprehended by another type of RNA termed *transfer RNA* (tRNA) and is restated in the language of peptides. Transfer RNA is the form of RNA that transfers amino acids from the cytoplasm to the ribosome. In the sequence prescribed by the incoming mRNA the tRNA supplies the ribosome with the specific amino acids to construct the required polypeptide. As the polypeptide grows in length, it begins to assume the three-dimensional configuration characteristic of the protein being constructed. After the required number of amino acids have been assembled and the

three-dimensional folding and coiling has been completed, the resulting molecule may be a functional protein. In some situations the resulting protein undergoes enzymatic modification; in others, no such modification is required. In either situation, the result is a functional protein whose structure was determined by a unique sequence of nucleotides in the nucleus of the cell.

If the evident function of this newly made protein is to regulate cell growth by suppressing uncontrolled proliferation, such a protein is the product of a **tumor-suppressor gene.** Conversely, if the evident function is to accelerate cell growth, the responsible gene is termed an **oncogene** or perhaps its precursor, a protooncogene.[12] Tumor-suppressor genes and oncogenes are found in the normal genome. When both are properly located on the correct chromosome and accurately configured, cell growth and division proceed normally insofar as they are influenced by these proteins. If the genes become altered in location or configuration, the delicate balance between the proteins suppressing cell growth and those augmenting it may be destroyed.

DNA rearrangement occurs through mutations.[8] This rearrangement produces corresponding alterations in the resulting protein. In terms of neoplastic change the genes most sensitive to mutation are oncogenes and tumor-suppressor genes. Oncogenes may be of viral derivation or part of the normal genome. In either situation, they have the potential to trigger malignant growth. Protooncogenes have similar potential but require some modification, usually by mutation, to function as oncogenes. Mutations may result in several types of genetic aberration, including gene amplification, chromosome translocation, gene transposition, and point mutations.

After mutation, gene amplification occurs when DNA replication becomes selective, thus resulting in overproduction and therefore overexpression of any gene. Amplification of an oncogene results in augmentation of cell growth. The *erb*B-2 oncogene is often amplified in breast cancer, enhancing cell growth by elaboration of a protein that induces a favorable hormonal environment.

Chromosome translocation results from mutations that cause chromosome breakage. The broken fragments may be juxtaposed from one chromosome to another and function abnormally. They may also facilitate oncogene expression. Translocations are frequently encountered in hematological malignancies such as chronic myelogenous leukemia.

Gene transposition is caused by a mutation that results in the transfer of a segment of DNA from one locus to another on the same chromosome. Such a move may alter protein production and the level of gene expression.

Point mutations occur in a limited segment of the DNA strand and affect from one to several nucleotide pairs. Point mutations are characterized by two processes: (1) substitution and (2) insertion and deletion. The commonly used chemotherapeutic agent 5-fluorouracil is a substitution mutagen. It resembles the nitrogenous base thymine and therefore may pair with adenine at the time of DNA replication. If mutant pairing occurs in an exon rather than an intron, the meaning of the affected codon may be altered and an inappropriate amino acid inserted into the polypeptide chain. When this occurs at a critical point in the protein molecule, subsequent function may be significantly altered.

A mutation characterized by an insertion or deletion has the potential to be much more detrimental than a mutation characterized by substitution. Insertion or deletion mutations occur when one or more nucleotides are inserted into or deleted from a DNA strand. This changes the length of the strand and may scramble the three-unit codons in such a way to make them uninterpretable. Mutations that affect oncogenes or tumor-suppressor genes may result in the production of proteins having altered functional capabilities. A single mutation seldom if ever results in the complete transformation of a normal cell to one that possesses all the characteristics of a cancer. Rather, the process of total transformation is usually accomplished over many years as a result of a cascade of mutations, each of which contributes to the destabilization of delicate mechanisms that regulate cell growth.

The pathology and pathophysiology of cancer are medical disciplines undergoing rapid expansion. Investigations of the molecular biologist have created a new understanding of the basic processes of life. With the discovery of each new gene and its protein product comes the potential to fit yet another piece into the biological puzzle of cancer and its clinical management. To keep abreast of these developments the reader should monitor any of the several scientific publications devoted to providing understandable updates about cancer research.

Review Questions

Multiple Choice/Matching

1. For each item below, select the term that best describes it. Each term may be selected once, more than once, or not at all.
   I. Codon   II. Exon   III. Intron   IV. Protein
   a. Oncogene
   b. A genetic word
   c. Nonsense
   d. Preserved during splicing
   e. Does not undergo transcription

2. For each item below, select the term that is most closely related etiologically. Each term may be selected once, more than once, or not at all.
   I. Radiant energy   II. Epstein-Barr virus
   III. Polycyclic hydrocarbons   IV. Asbestos
   a. Large cell lung cancer
   b. Malignant melanoma
   c. Transitional cell carcinoma of the bladder
   d. Infectious mononucleosis
   e. Burkitt's lymphoma
   f. Basal cell carcinoma of the skin

3. All but which one of the following are characteristic of cancer?
   a. Metastases
   b. Blood vessel invasion
   c. Rapid growth rate
   d. Encapsulation
   e. Poor differentiation

4. The study of cells by flow cytometry is not useful in defining which of the following?
   a. Physiological function
   b. DNA content
   c. Cell-cycle position
   d. Surface markers
   e. Viability

5. Cellular transformation from benign to malignant may result from all but which of the following?
   a. Mutation
   b. Initiation
   c. Promotion
   d. Apoptosis
   e. Latency

True or False

6. Identify the following statements as true or false.
   a. The nucleoli, endoplasmic reticulum, Golgi apparatus, and plasma membrane are all examples of organelles.
   True _____   False _____
   b. The shortest phase of the classic cell cycle is G_0.
   True _____   False _____
   c. An inflammatory reaction is always initiated by tissue injury.
   True _____   False _____
   d. Malignant neoplasms arising from epithelial surfaces are termed *carcinomas.*
   True _____   False _____

e. The only difference between DNA and RNA is in the structure of the five-carbon sugar.
   True _____   False _____
f. Cellular characteristics as seen under the microscope seldom help determine prognosis in a patient.
   True _____   False _____
g. Sarcomas are more likely than carcinomas to spread via the bloodstream.
   True _____   False _____
h. No virus has yet been proved to cause cancer in humans.
   True _____   False _____
i. General anesthesia is almost always necessary to recover enough tissue to establish a diagnosis of cancer.
   True _____   False _____
j. When present in the human genome an oncogene eventually leads to the development cancer.
   True _____   False _____

Fill in the Blank

7. The nitrogenous bases in DNA are _____, _____, _____, and _____, whereas in RNA they are _____, _____, _____, and _____.
8. A nucleotide is composed of _____, _____, and _____ and differs from a nucleoside, which is composed of _____ and _____.
9. Three methods of recovering cells to establish a diagnosis of cancer are _____, _____, and _____.

Questions to Ponder

1. What factors influenced historically the understanding of disease?
2. What is homeostasis?
3. Briefly discuss the metastatic process of malignant neoplasms.
4. Why is staging cancer important?
5. Describe the structure of DNA.

REFERENCES

1. Baserga R: Principles of molecular cell biology of cancer: the cell cycle. In De Vita VT Jr, Hellman S, Rosenberg SA, editors: *Cancer: principles and practice of oncology,* ed 4, Philadelphia, 1993, JB Lippincott.
2. Bonfiglio TA, Terry R: The pathology of cancer. In Rubin P, editor: *Clinical oncology,* ed 7, Philadelphia, 1993, WB Saunders.
3. Campbell NA: *Biology,* ed 3, Riverside, Calif, 1993, Benjamin/Cummings Publishing.
4. Hall EJ: Principles of carcinogenesis: physical. In De Vita VT Jr, Hellman S, Rosenberg SA, editors: *Cancer: principles and practice of oncology,* ed 4, Philadelphia, 1993, JB Lippincott.
5. Henshaw EC: The biology of cancer. In Rubin P et al, editors: *Clinical oncology,* ed 7, Philadelphia, 1993, WB Saunders.
6. Howley PM: Principles of carcinogenesis: viral. In De Vita VT Jr, Hellman S, Rosenberg SA, editors: *Cancer: principles and practice of oncology,* ed 4, Philadelphia, 1993, JB Lippincott.
7. Madri JA: Inflammation and healing. In Kissane JM, editor: *Anderson's pathology,* ed 9, St Louis, 1990, Mosby.
8. Perkins AS, Vande Woude GF: Principles of molecular cell biology of cancer: oncogenes. In De Vita VT Jr, Hellman S, Rosenberg SA, editors: *Cancer: principles and practice of oncology,* ed 4, Philadelphia, 1993, JB Lippincott.
9. Sheldon H: *Boyd's introduction to the study of disease,* ed 11, Philadelphia, 1992, Lea & Febiger.
10. Shields PG, Harris CC: Principles of carcinogenesis: chemical. In De Vita VT Jr, Hellman S, Rosenberg SA, editors: *Cancer: principles and practice of oncology,* ed 4, Philadelphia, 1993, JB Lippincott.
11. Vande Woude S, Vande Woude GF: Principles of molecular cell biology of cancer: introduction to methods in molecular biology. In De Vita VT Jr, Hellman S, Rosenberg SA, editors: *Cancer: principles and practice of oncology,* ed 4, Philadelphia, 1993, JB Lippincott.

BIBLIOGRAPHY

Anthony CP, Kolthoff NJ: *Textbook of anatomy and physiology,* ed 9, St Louis, 1974, Mosby.
Boyd CM, Dalrymple GV: *Basic science principles of nuclear medicine,* St Louis, 1974, Mosby.
del Regato JA, Spjut HJ, Cox JD: *Ackerman and del Regato's cancer: diagnosis, treatment, and prognosis,* ed 6, St Louis, 1985, Mosby.
Kiemar V, Cotran RS, Robbins SL: *Basic pathology,* ed 5, Philadelphia, 1992, WB Saunders.

Principles of Surgical Oncology

Wesley English

Outline

Key terms

SCOPE OF SURGICAL ONCOLOGY

 "Surgical oncology emphasizes the application of surgical techniques in the diagnosis, staging, and treatment of neoplasms."[6] Through the years, general surgeons and surgical specialists (such as urologists; gynecologists; and ear, nose, and throat specialists) have performed cancer surgery. Having emerged in the last 20 years, surgical oncologists (surgeons who limit their practices to caring for cancer patients) are relative newcomers to the cancer care team. Although the number of surgical oncologists is increasing in the United States, community general surgeons and other surgical specialists still perform the great majority of cancer surgeries. Therefore in this chapter the term *surgical oncologist* is broad and includes all surgeons treating cancer.

Of the three standard treatments for cancer (surgery, radiation therapy, and chemotherapy), surgery was the first. Even today, more patients are cured of their cancers by surgery than by the other modalities of treatment.

According to the American Cancer Society, over 100 sites in the human body are capable of forming cancers. Each year, that organization publishes statistics on 24 of the most common cancer sites. This report is titled *Cancer Facts and Figures.*[1] Many of these cancers have similar behaviors. They spend a certain part of their natural histories in noninvasive forms. During this time, they are most curable by surgery. Cancers then invade surrounding tissues and spread to nearby lymph nodes called *regional lymph nodes,* or they may spread to more distant sites via the bloodstream. However, a modest number of malignancies exhibit specific behaviors. For example, basal cell carcinomas almost never spread to regional nodes but can continue to invade locally into surrounding tissues. **Sarcomas** rarely spread through the lymphatic channels but commonly metastasize to the lungs. Although certain general principles are followed in surgical oncology, the surgical oncologist must recognize situations in which the usual principles do not apply. The oncologist must consider each treatment case individually and take into account many factors before reaching a treatment plan.

Historical perspectives and evolution to present status

As explained in Chapter 5, cancer was not perceived in history as curable by surgery. This teaching was followed until about 1700, when Valsalva introduced the theory that a tumor begins in a localized form in the tissue of origin and is therefore curable by surgery as long as it is in this regional stage. Further application of this thinking led to the first modern cancer operation in 1881. This operation (a subtotal gastrectomy for cancer) was performed by Theodor Billroth, a Viennese surgical pioneer who attained great stature in surgical history.[6] By 1890 the principle of **en bloc resection** (still commonly used in treating breast, colon, gastric, and numerous other cancers) had been formulated by William Halsted, another surgical forefather at Johns Hopkins University (see Chapter 5) (Fig. 7-1).

Because little was known of modern concepts, radical procedures were applied to many cancers regardless of the size of the tumor, the apparent involvement or noninvolvement of regional nodes, and the lack of knowledge of tumor-host factors or other prognostic information. In fact, when the removal of entire organs with their regional nodes (e.g., radical mastectomies and radical hysterectomies [Fig. 7-2]) failed to cure some of the cancers, surgeons concluded that the operations were not radical enough and must not be removing all the cancer cells. Surgeons designed even more radical operations such as pelvic **exenterations** and super-radical mastectomies to give cancers even wider berth. When these extensive operations did not produce better treatment outcomes, surgeons realized that a better understanding of tumor biology was needed.

The present understanding of tumor biology includes the belief that the spread of a tumor through blood vessels probably occurs much earlier than previously thought. Tiny colonies of tumor cells known as *micrometastases* may already be present in the liver, lungs, brain, or bones in many patients by the time of the primary tumor's diagnosis (Fig. 7-3). Whether these micrometastases lead to clinically recognizable disease depends on complex tumor-host relationships, many of which are immune related. Therefore a trend in modern surgical oncology is the scaling down of

A
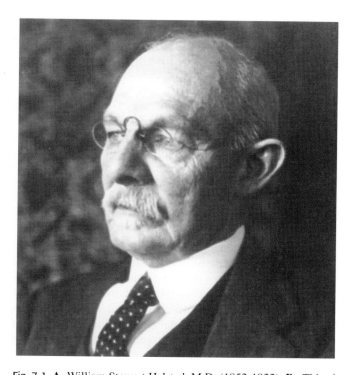

B
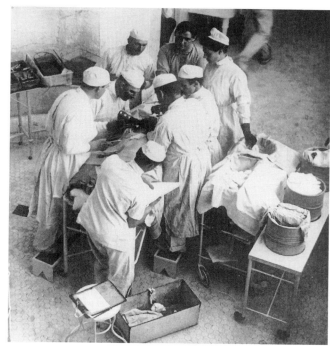

Fig. 7-1 **A,** William Stewart Halsted, M.D. (1852-1922). **B,** This photograph was taken of Dr. Halsted operating with a chisel and mallet on a patient who had osteomyelitis of the left femur. (Courtesy The Alan Mason Chesney Medical Archives of The Johns Hopkins Medical Institutions, Baltimore, Maryland.)

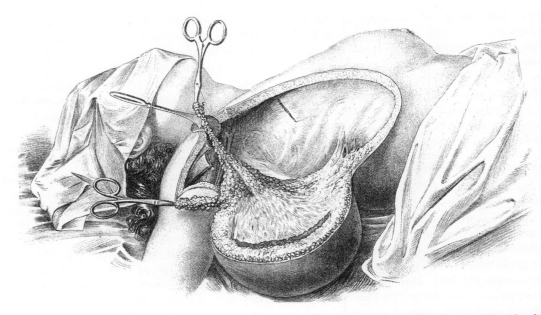

Fig. 7-2 A technique of a radical mastectomy at the end of the nineteenth century at Johns Hopkins. (Courtesy The Alan Mason Chesney Medical Archives of the Johns Hopkins Medical Institutions, Baltimore, Maryland.)

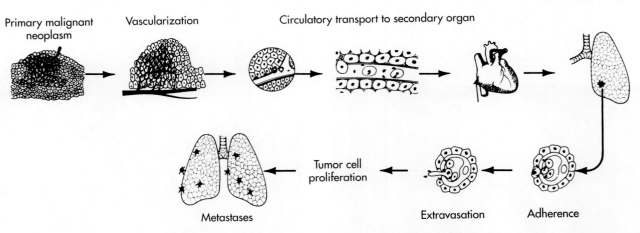

Fig. 7-3 A schematic representation of the process of lymphatic-hematogenic spread of tumor cells. (From Beare P, Meyers J: *Principles and practice of adult health nursing,* ed 1, St Louis, 1990, Mosby.)

some of the former radical and mutilating operations. Through the combination of smaller and less radical procedures with radiation therapy and chemotherapy, the goals of preserving function and reconstructing defects caused by the surgery are achieved.[5,7]

Surgical philosophy of cancer care and treatment

Surgery, like radiation therapy, is a locoregional treatment modality. If the tumor is spread from the primary site to distant organs such as the liver and lungs, surgery cannot remove all the tumor. Surgery can cure only cancers that are in a local or regional stage at the time of diagnosis. If cure is not possible, combinations of surgery, radiation therapy, and chemotherapy may provide relief **(palliation)** at least temporarily from symptoms caused by cancers. The well-trained surgical oncologist knows whether radical surgery is appropriate and can recognize special circumstances in which an aggressive surgical approach to a tumor is justified, when to some observers such an approach may be considered overtreatment. However, the surgical oncologist also functions as part of a cancer care team and recognizes the value of a team approach, known as **multidisciplinary care.**

THE ROLE OF SURGERY IN MULTIDISCIPLINARY CANCER CARE

A varying range of surgical options is available in the care of most cancers, depending on the stage in which the cancer is diagnosed. The options may range from a simple needle aspiration biopsy of a tumor requiring only a few minutes and causing minimal pain for the patient to a radical surgical procedure requiring 8 or more hours to perform and days to weeks for recovery. With some malignancies, surgery is the major treatment; with others, it may have only a diagnostic role.

As an example, a breast cancer with a 1.5-cm mass may be considered. The surgeon, working as part of a team with a radiation oncologist and medical oncologist, must choose from five or more types of biopsies. The most appropriate biopsy for the patient must take into consideration factors such as the age of the patient, location of the tumor, size of the breast, presence or absence of enlarged nodes in the axilla, and desire for breast preservation. The type of biopsy chosen for a patient with a 1.5-cm breast cancer might be completely different from that chosen for a cancer 6 cm in diameter.

After one of these types of biopsies confirms a diagnosis of breast cancer, decisions are made for a breast-conserving surgical procedure or total removal of the breast and regional lymph nodes. During planning discussions, patients must be fully informed and their wishes and concerns must be considered. In counseling the patient while making these decisions the surgeon frequently consults with the pathologist and offers consultation with a radiation oncologist and/or medical oncologist. When patients are under particular duress, nurse specialists and oncology social workers may be involved in supportive roles.

Recommendations given to the patient who has advanced stages of cancer are sometimes formulated in tumor conferences attended by the surgeon, radiation oncologist, medical oncologist, pathologist, specialized nurses, and others on the cancer care team. In such tumor conferences the ideal of multidisciplinary care is often best realized.

PRINCIPLES OF SURGICAL ONCOLOGY
Tissue diagnosis

Although the finding of a cancer in a specific organ suggests that the tumor began in that organ, some organs not only form cancers themselves, but also are common **metastatic** sites. The lungs, liver, bones, brain, ovaries, and adrenal glands are organs that can be affected by primary cancer, but they are also sites possibly involved by cancer from other organs. Because the biological behavior and response to treatment of many cancers differ, a tissue diagnosis obtained by a surgical procedure called a *biopsy,* is needed early in treatment planning to establish the exact tissue from which the cancer arose. In most situations in which tissue from the cancer can be examined under the microscope, the pathologist can identify the original site of the cancer based on the

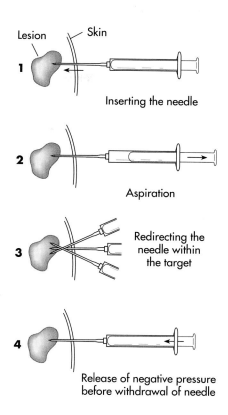

Fig. 7-4 The steps in aspiration of a palpable lesion. Step 3 indicates the way the needle should be redirected in the target, and step 4 emphasizes the importance of releasing the negative pressure before withdrawing the needle. (From Koss LG: Needle aspiration cytology of tumors at various body sites. In Silver CE et al: *Current problems in surgery,* vol 22, Chicago, 1985, Year Book Medical Publishers.)

appearance of the tissue. When identification by light microscope appearance is not apparent or obvious, special stains of the tissue can be used. In other situations, electron microscopy may be helpful. Only on rare occasions (such as an obvious relapse or confrontation of particular risks) does the treatment team choose to forego a biopsy. Various biopsies can be performed, including the following:

Needle aspiration biopsy. A needle with a fine diameter (usually from 18 to 22 gauge) is passed into the tumor with suction applied via an attached syringe (Fig. 7-4). A small specimen of tissue "juice" containing some floating cells from the tumor enters the barrel of the needle (not the syringe) and is then transferred to a microscope slide to make, in effect, a "Pap test."[4] A cytologist scans these slides for cancer cells. Although it can confirm the presence or absence of a cancer, this technique usually cannot identify the tissue source of the cancer. It is used frequently in investigating masses in the breast or neck that are suspicious for cancer.

Core-needle biopsy. A larger bore needle (14 or 16 gauge) is passed into the tumor to retrieve a core of tumor tis-

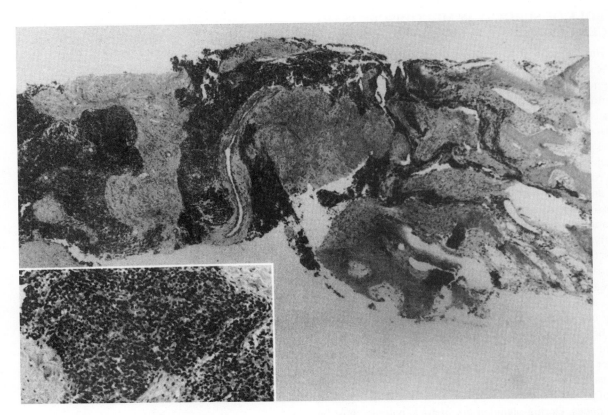

Fig. 7-5 An example of the tissue core obtained by needle biopsy of a Ewing's sarcoma as seen microscpically. The insert demonstrates good preservation of cells. (From del Regato JA, Spjut HJ, and Cox JD: *Ackerman and del Regato's cancer: diagnosis, treatment and prognosis,* ed 6, St Louis, 1985, Mosby.)

sue (Fig. 7-5) to imbed in paraffin and make microscope sections. An advantage is that the cells of the tumor can be seen in relation to neighboring cells so that the architecture of the tumor can be recognized. Architecture is an important feature in the identification of the tissue of origin.

Endoscopic biopsy. When tumors of the bronchial tree or gastrointestinal tract are seen through an endoscope, a flexible biopsy tool with a tip looking like tiny pincers can be passed through the scope to retrieve a fragment of tumor tissue to examine microscopically.

Incisional biopsy. Only a sample (sometimes referred to as a *wedge*) is removed from the primary tumor by incising into it (Fig. 7-6). The aim is to identify the tumor in a diagnostic way, and no attempt is made to remove the entire tumor. Incisional biopsies are often used on large tumors, locally advanced tumors, and tumors that are not removed surgically as an initial step. A punch biopsy is a type of incisional biopsy in which a tool resembling a leather punch is used to remove a small portion from the tumor.

Excisional biopsy The entire tumor is removed for purposes of the biopsy examination. The magnitude of the rim of normal tissue also excised with the tumor depends on the body site that is involved. For example, removing a large rim of normal tissue is common if a mass is in the skin and is suspected of being a **melanoma.** The orientation of the biopsy

incision should always anticipate large-scale surgery so that the incision may be easily included in a reexcision of the biopsy site.

Staging

A cancer may be diagnosed at almost any point in its natural history as it progresses from one cell to billions of cells. Systems have been devised to describe just where in this continuum the cancer is when it is discovered: early on one end of the scale, or late on the other end. These systems are called *staging systems.* Cancers were first described as *local* if diagnosed while still confined to their tissues of origin, *regional* if diagnosed after metastasis to regional lymph nodes, and *disseminated* if spread occurred beyond regional lymph nodes to other organs. Although these terms are still used today in oncology vocabulary, staging has become more precise.

Staging systems have been refined to better reflect certain characteristic behaviors of cancers in specific tissues. In 1932 Cuthbert Dukes proposed a staging system for malignancies of the colon and rectum based on the depth of the tumor's invasion into the wall of the intestine and whether lymph nodes were involved by spread of the tumor.[3] He used letters of the alphabet to indicate the state of the tumor's advancement. Stage A tumors were the least advanced, and stage C tumors penetrated the wall of the bowel. The staging

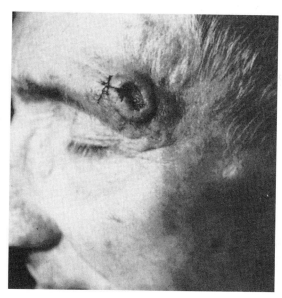

Fig. 7-6 In an incisional biopsy, a specimen is removed from the edge of the tumor. (From del Regato JA, Spjut HJ, and Cox JD: *Ackerman and del Regato's cancer: diagnosis, treatment and prognosis,* ed 6, St Louis, 1985, Mosby.)

systems tended to correlate with prognosis in that tumors in early stages proved to have higher cure rates.

With improvements in staging systems the American Joint Committee for Cancer Staging and End Results Reporting (AJCC) attempted to lend some uniformity to staging by developing and promoting the use of the TNM system.[2] In this system the letter T stands for tumor and is usually followed by a number from 1 to 4 indicating tumor size (1 for the smallest and 4 for the largest) (Fig. 7-7). The letter *N* stands for *nodes* and with numbers after the letter indicates whether local nodes contain no cancer (N_0) or are involved with metastatic cancer (N_1, N_2, etc.). The letter *M* stands for *metastases* and indicates no sign of metastatic spread at the time of diagnosis (M_0) or the presence of cancer in organs distant from the primary site (M_1). Many combinations of these letters and numbers are possible to describe accurately the many possible presentations of tumors. For example, a breast cancer that is 2.5 cm in diameter with metastatic cancer in three local lymph nodes but with no other sign of metastatic spread is described by the TNM system as T_2, N_1, M_0. By referring to a table provided by the AJCC for each cancer site, the TNM classification can be converted to a stage expressed in Roman numerals. In the breast system, T_2, N_1, M_0 is a stage II cancer.

By defining the stage at which a cancer is diagnosed, treatment may be planned appropriately and a prognosis may be forecast based on accumulated knowledge of the way a large group of patients with the same stage has fared after treatment. After being staged correctly, a cancer may be added to the pool of information on cancer treatment because investigators can compare the results of this cancer treatment with others of exactly the same stage that have been treated in the past. Part of the function of a cancer registry is to gather data on staged cancers and follow the cases over time to record the outcome of treatment. Most registries are linked to national data-gathering centers such as the National Cancer Institute and the American College of Surgeons Cancer Registry. These institutions are the source of cancer statistics.

Importance of the first procedure

The first operative procedure has the best chance of successfully effecting a curable cancer; therefore this procedure should be well planned, based on staging and executed expertly according to specific principles that are meant to minimize the danger of a recurrence. After recurring in an operative site, a cancer becomes increasingly difficult to eradicate surgically.

Resection with adequate margins

Operations that leave cancer cells in the tissue invite a recurrence of the cancer. A good policy during surgery to remove a cancer is to never actually see the cancer tissue being excised if possible. This policy is achieved by excising widely enough from the tumor that a grossly visible rim of normal tissue acts as a buffer zone between the cutting instrument and tumor. When free of cancer cells at all margins, this zone is referred to as a *clear margin of resection.* If the knife or another cutting instrument cuts through cancer tissue, cancer cells may be implanted in the site of excision (seeding) or some of the cancer is simply left behind in the host tissue. The surgeon's naked eye may not always recognize cancer at the surgical margin. Using a microscope, a pathologist examines the tissue to determine whether a clear margin of resection is present. The pattern of cancer invasion into surrounding tissues varies in different malignant sites so that some cancers need a wider margin of excision than others. The surgeon must be aware of these differences in the way cancers invade tissue planes.

Removal of regional lymph nodes

In many sites, regional lymph nodes are removed in one large block of tissue with the primary cancer whether they appear enlarged or not. This type of surgical approach is referred to as *en bloc resection.* As more information accumulates on the likelihood of nodal metastasis in certain sizes and depths of tumors, situations are being defined in which it may not help the patient to remove the regional lymph nodes. An example might be that in thin melanomas (those that are less than 0.7 mm thick and thus have not invaded into the dermis to any depth where they can invade the lymphatic channels), lymph node metastases are extremely uncommon. Likewise, with in-situ breast cancer in which the cancer has not invaded through the wall of the breast ducts, lymph node metastases are unlikely. In many surgical sites the major morbidity of the surgery is a result of the lymph node excision. Therefore if the involvement of lymph nodes by cancer spread appears

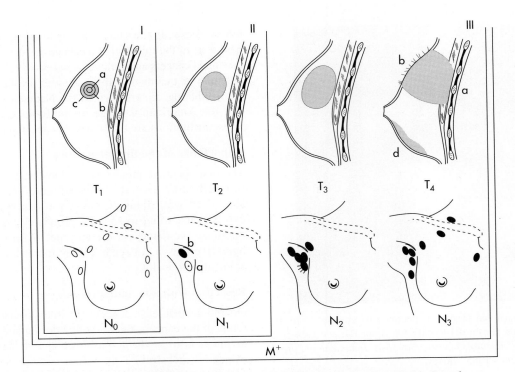

Fig. 7-7 A diagrammatic depiction of the breast cancer staging system. (From Rubin P et al: *Clinical oncology*, ed 7, Philadelphia, 1993, WB Saunders.)

unlikely, the surgery causes fewer side effects if the lymph nodes do not require removal.

Excision of slow-growing cancers

Cancers with long doubling times are best treated surgically. Even late metastases may be successfully excised if they occur after long disease-free intervals in which the patient was clinically free of cancer.

Palliation

Even if treatment for cure is impossible, tumor excision may simplify nursing care, relieve pain or obstruction of an organ, and control blood loss from a tumor. To palliate means to give treatment that makes symptoms less severe. An example of palliative excision is the removal of a cancer of the right colon even in the presence of known liver metastases. The surgeon knows that removing the colon cancer does not cure the patient, but doing so allows recovery from anemia and averts a possible bowel obstruction in future months.

Multidisciplinary approach

Combinations of surgery, radiation therapy, and chemotherapy may improve survival in certain malignancies and can reduce the magnitude of the surgical procedure required. By combining excision of a breast tumor with radiation therapy, breast-conserving treatment of breast cancer can provide the same chance for cure that can be provided by a modified radical mastectomy in properly selected cases. Combining radi-

ation therapy and chemotherapy in carcinomas of the anus can often provide excellent results in a disease that at one time was treated by surgical removal of the rectum and anus with creation of a permanent **colostomy.**

Procedures for pain relief

If cancer is advanced and causing considerable pain, the usual approaches of using oral or **parenteral** analgesic drugs may not relieve pain. In such situations, neurosurgical procedures are available to interrupt pain pathways. Rhizotomies (division of nerves and nerve trunks) and cordotomies (division of a portion of the spinal cord) are time-honored but now seldom-used techniques to alleviate severe pain. A more modern approach to such pain is the implantation of a delivery pump attached to a catheter placed in the epidural space. The pump infuses an analgesic into the space around the dura of the spinal cord, thus relieving pain and allowing the patient to continue to function.

Isolation perfusion. This procedure is used to deliver short-term (only a few hours), high-concentration chemotherapeutic agents directly into the circulation of a limb. Isolation perfusion is done by temporarily interrupting the arterial inflow and venous outflow of the extremity while pumping the agent into the artery by using a delivery system similar to a heart-lung machine. The usefulness of this procedure has been limited to only a few malignancies, notably to the treatment of malignant melanoma arising in an extremity.

Arterial infusion. A more commonly used practice for delivering cancer-treatment drugs to a specific site is arterial infusion. In this technique a fine plastic catheter is placed surgically or by percutaneous methods into an artery feeding an organ containing cancer. Hepatic tumors and metastases are sometimes treated this way.

Special procedures

Debulking. Debulking is a surgical procedure used to remove deposits of metastatic cancer. The aim of this procedure is to reduce the number of cancer cells to be treated by chemotherapy (often referred to as the *tumor burden*). Debulking is useful only when the tumor burden must be reduced and has particular application to the management of implants of ovarian cancer spread about the abdominal cavity.

Second-look operations. About 20 years ago the theory was advanced that the outcome of treatment could be favorably affected by reopening the abdomen at some interval after the primary resection of a colon cancer or ovarian cancer to search for possible recurrence of the tumor and remove it before it could become too advanced. Today, second-look operations are seldom performed because the practice has little effect on final outcome in the great majority of cancer patients.

Resection of isolated metastases. A benefit appears to exist in removing solitary brain and pulmonary metastases in patients who have sarcomas and colon cancer, provided a disease-free interval (a time in which the patient appeared free of metastatic disease) of over 1 year has taken place. In certain sarcomas metastatic to the lungs, multiple metastases may be resected with benefit.

Surgical endocrine ablation. Endocrine **ablation** refers to the removal of hormone-producing tissues such as ovaries, testes, and adrenal glands to halt the growth of cancers that seem to be stimulated to grow in the presence of hormones. This surgical technique applies most often in the treatment of metastatic breast and prostate cancers. Recently, hormone-blocking medications have been found to produce similar effects to surgical endocrine ablation. Therefore this type of cancer surgery is now done less frequently.

Laser destruction and cryosurgery. Primary tumors that are incurable because of metastatic disease or unre-sectable because of critical location may be largely destroyed by laser vaporization or application of an extremely cold probe (cryoablation). These techniques are useful because they may be carried out with the aid of a scope to approach the tumor. They are used to open airways (esophagi, or urethrae) obstructed by tumors.

The art of surgery

Any number of psychological factors are at play in each patient faced with a diagnosis of cancer. Fear, anger, bewilderment, and frustration are common emotions that surface during the cancer-treatment experience. The recognition of these emotions and even their anticipation can be vital to getting the patient through treatment without the development of handicapping emotional upheaval. Because in many cancer cases the surgeon is the first member of the multidisciplinary team to work with the patient, taking more than just a cold, scientific approach to cancer care can be extremely important. Patients must have feelings of hope and a sense that their concerns are being heard and addressed.

SUMMARY

Approximately 100 years have passed since the first bold attempts at a scientifically based surgical approach to the treatment of cancer. Exciting new discoveries about the role of genetics in cancer induction suggest that new approaches to cancer treatment are near and will reduce pain and suffering for cancer patients. Until a cancer cure is found, surgery will continue to play a major role in the diagnosis and management of a majority of cancers and will be used with radiation therapy and chemotherapy to reduce the extent of the surgery needed. Time-honored principles governing biopsy, staging, and resection with adequate margins will continue to have major importance in surgical cancer care and will be enhanced by new techniques of postoperative pain management, a team approach to cancer care, and ongoing emotional support of patients going through their cancer-treatment experiences. If treatment fails and the patient is dying of cancer, something can always be done, even if it is simply relieving pain and permitting death with dignity.

Review Questions

Fill in the Blank

1. _____ is a single word that may be used to describe the essence of multidisciplinary cancer care.
2. In the TNM staging system for cancers the letter *T* stands for _____ .
3. In staging terminology a cancer that has spread to nearby lymph nodes but not to other organs is referred to as _____ .

Multiple Choice

4. In making a tissue diagnosis of cancer a core needle biopsy has the advantage over a needle aspiration biopsy of showing which of the following?
   a. Tissue architecture
   b. Cell nuclei
   c. Golgi apparatus
5. Which of the following is a cancer treatment in which anitcancer drugs are pumped into an artery supplying the cancer?
   a. Isolation perfusion therapy
   b. Arterial infusion therapy
   c. Debulking

Questions to Ponder

1. What goal is accomplished by surgical removal of a colon malignancy that is already extensively metastatic to the liver?
2. What is the meaning of the term *en bloc resection*? Why is is considered an important concept in surgical cancer care?
3. Explain the meaning of a clear margin of resection.

REFERENCES

1. American Cancer Society: *Cancer facts and figures,* Atlanta, 1995, The Society.
2. American Joint Committee on Cancer: *Manual for staging of cancer,* Philadelphia, 1992, JB Lippincott.
3. Dukes CE: The classification of cancer of the rectum, *J Pathol Bacteriol* 35:323-332, 1932.
4. Koss LG: Needle aspiration cytology of tumors at various body sites. In Silver CE et al: *Current problems in surgery,* vol 22, Chicago, 1985, Year Book Medical Publishers.
5. Langmuir VK et al: Principles of surgical oncology. In Ruben P et al, editors: *Clinical oncology,* ed 7, Philadelphia, 1993, WB Saunders.
6. Pilch YH: *Surgical oncology,* New York, 1984, McGraw-Hill.
7. Rosenberg SA: Principles of surgical oncology. In DeVita VT et al, editors: *Cancer: principles and practice of oncology,* ed 4, Philadelphia, 1993, JB Lippincott.

8

Principles of
Medical Oncology

Shirley E. Otto

Outline

Key terms

Adjuvant
Cytotoxic
Informed consent
Metastasis
Mitosis
Palliation

Proliferation

Radiosensitizers
Randomized
Synergistic
Synthesis

About 1,300,000 people will be diagnosed as having cancer in 1996. More than half of these people received systemic chemotherapy because of disease recurrence, secondary therapy after a local treatment, and treatment of hematological disease. The primary focus of chemotherapy is to prevent cancer cells from multiplying, invading adjacent tissue, and developing **metastatsis.**

Chemotherapy is the use of **cytotoxic** drugs in the treatment of cancer. It is one of the three modalities (surgery and radiation therapy are the others) that provide cure, control, or **palliation.** Biotherapy and bone marrow transplants are also used in varied disease-treatment protocols. Chemotherapy is systemic, whereas surgery and radiation therapy are localized treatments. Chemotherapy may be used in the following five ways[4,5]:

1. **Adjuvant** therapy is a course of chemotherapy used with another treatment modality (surgery, radiation therapy, biotherapy, and bone marrow transplant) and aimed at treating micrometastases.
2. Neoadjuvant therapy is the administration of chemotherapy before surgery to reduce the tumor burden at the primary site, thus rendering efforts at local control more likely to be completely successful. Reducing the number of cancerous cells before surgery may reduce the chance of resistant clones developing.
3. Primary therapy is the treatment of patients who have localized cancer for which an alternative but less than completely effective treatment exists.

4. Induction chemotherapy is the drug therapy given as the primary treatment for patients who have cancer for which *no* alternative treatment exists.

5. Combination chemotherapy is the administration of two or more chemotherapeutic agents in the treatment of patients with cancer, therefore allowing each medication to enhance the action of the other or act in a **synergistic** manner.[10]

PRINCIPLES OF CHEMOTHERAPY
Cell generation cycle

The cell generation cycle is the sequence of events involved in the replication and distribution of deoxyribonucleic acid (DNA) to the daughter cells produced by cell division. All cells (nonmalignant and malignant) progress through the five phases of the cell cycle.[5, 19] These five phases are G_0, G_1, S, G_2, and M (Fig. 8-1).

The G_0 phase (postmitotic resting) encompasses the period of the cell cycle in which normal renewable tissue is not actively proliferating. In this phase, cells perform all functions except those related to **proliferation.** This category includes nondividing and resting cells. Normal cells in the G_0 phase are activated to reenter the reproductive cycle only by certain stimuli.

G_1 phase (growth or postmitotic-presynthesis) extends from the completion of the previous cell division to the beginning of chromosome replication. This is a period of decreased metabolic activity. Cells carry out their designated physiological functions by synthesizing proteins needed in the formation of ribonucleic acid (RNA). The G_1 phase is primarily a stage of readiness as the cells prepare for entry into the S phase.

In the S phase (**synthesis**), RNA is synethesized. This is essential for the synthesis of DNA, which is limited to this phase. Histones (the basic protein of chromatin) are also synthesized in the S phase. Cells are *most vulnerable* to damage during the S phase.

The G_2 phase (postsynthetic-premitotic) is one of relative hypoactivity as the cells await entry into the mitotic phase. This phase encompasses the interval from the termination of DNA synthesis to the beginning of cell division. Some additional protein synthesis, but mostly synthesis of structural proteins versus enzymes, occurs in G_2.

In the M phase (**mitosis**), cell division and mitosis occur. Protein synthesis continues but is drastically reduced. Duplication of DNA must be complete before cells enter the mitotic cycle. After mitosis the daughter cells return to the G_0 phase and stop dividing or, if a stimulus for cell division exists, enter the G_1 phase and begin the cell reproductive cycle again.

Cancer cells are able to complete the cell cycle quicker by decreasing the length of time in the G_1 phase. They are also much less likely than normal cells to enter or remain in the G_0 phase of the cell cycle; thus cancer cells divide continu-

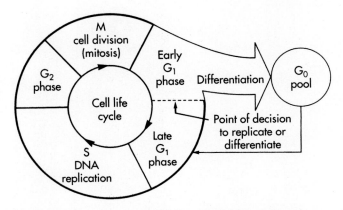

Fig. 8-1 Cell generation cycle. (From Otto SE: *Oncology nursing,* ed 2, St Louis, 1994, Mosby.)

ously. Chemotherapeutic drugs are most active against frequently dividing cells or in all phases of the cell cycle except G_0.[4,5,9]

Tumor growth

The regulatory mechanism controlling the growth of cancer cells differs from that of normal cells. Unlike normal cells, cancer cells grow via a pyramid effect; however, cancer cells grow at the same rate as the tissue from which they originated (e.g., breast cancer develops at the same rate of growth as normal breast tissue development).

The time required for a tumor to reach a certain size is called *doubling time.* Tumors undergo approximately 30 doublings from a single cell before they are clinically detected. Between the seventh and tenth doubling time a possibility exists for the tumor to shed cells. This process is called *micrometastasis.* Doubling time is more rapid during early stages of tumor growth than at later stages. This pattern of growth is called *Gompertz' function* (Fig. 8-2). The growth curve illustrates the initial exponential growth of cancer cells followed by the steady and progressive decrease in the growth fraction. This is due to a decrease in the fraction of proliferating cells and an increase in the rate of cell death.[4,5,19]

Cell-kill hypothesis

A single cancer cell is capable of multiplying and eventually killing the host. Every tumor cell must be killed in order to cure cancer. With each course of the drug therapy a dose of the chemotherapy drug kills only *a fraction, not all,* of the cancer cells (Fig. 8-3). Repeated courses of chemotherapy must be used in order to reduce the total number of cancer cells. This cardinal rule of chemotherapy (i.e., the inverse relationship between cell number and curability) was established by Skipper and his colleagues in the early 1960s.[4,5]

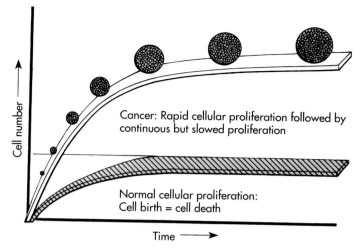

Fig. 8-2 Gompertz' function as viewed by growth curve. (From Otto SE: *Oncology nursing*, ed 2, St Louis, 1994, Mosby.)

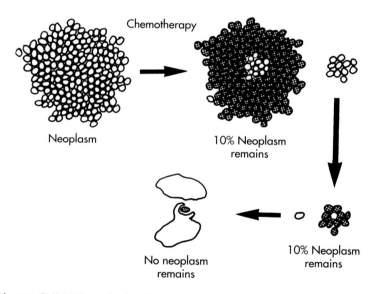

Fig. 8-3 Cell-kill hypothesis. (From Otto SE: *Oncology nursing*, ed 2, St Louis, 1994, Mosby.)

Drug classification

Chemotherapeutic drugs are classified according to their pharmacological action and interference with cellular reproduction. The basic groups and their potential actions are as follows[15,22]:

Cell-cycle phase specific drugs. These drugs are active on cells undergoing division in the cell cycle. Examples include antimetabolites, plant alkaloids, and miscellaneous agents such as asparaginase. These drugs are most effective against actively growing tumors that have a greater proportion of cells cycling through the phase in which the drug attacks

the cancer cell. Cell-cycle phase specific drugs are given in minimum concentration via continuous dosing methods.

Cell-cycle phase nonspecific drugs. These drugs are active on cells in a dividing or resting state. Examples include alkylating drugs, antitumor antibiotics, nitrosoureas, hormone and steroid drugs, and miscellaneous agents such as procarbazine. These drugs are active in all phases of the cell cycle and may be effective in large tumors with few active cells dividing at the time of administration. Drugs of this nature are often given as single bolus injections.

The function of most chemotherapy drugs is targeting of the cell's DNA in some manner. This action may result in direct interference with the DNA, inhibition of enzymes related to RNA or DNA synthesis or both, and destruction of the cells' necessary proteins.

A general description of each drug classification follows, and detailed information regarding specific drugs in each class can be found in Table 8-1.[11,15,22]

- *Alkylating agents* are cell-cycle phase nonspecific. They act primarily to form a molecular bond with the nucleic acids. This interferes with nucleic acid duplication, thus preventing mitosis. This category of drugs has similar phase activity to that observed in radiation therapy with two peaks of maximal lethal activity (one in the G_2 to M phase and one near the G_1-S phase boundary).
- *Antimetabolites* are cell-cycle phase specific. They exhibit action by blocking essential enzymes necessary for DNA synthesis or become incorporated into the DNA and RNA so that a false message is transmitted.
- *Antitumor antibiotics* are cell-cycle nonspecific. These drugs disrupt DNA transcription and inhibit DNA and RNA synthesis.

Table 8-1	Chemotherapeutic drug classification with side effects
Drugs	**Major side effects**
Alkylating agents	
Busulfan	Nausea and vomiting, diarrhea, pulmonary fibrosis, bone marrow suppression, impotence, amenorrhea, and skin hyperpigmentation
Carboplatin	Nausea and vomiting, bone marrow suppression, ototoxicity, neurotoxicity, and hyperuricemia
Chlorambucil	Myelosuppression and interstitial pneumonia-pulmonary fibrosis
Cisplatin	Neurotoxicity, myelosuppression, nephrotoxicity, nausea and vomiting, hypokalemia, and hypomagnesemia
Cyclophosphamide	Myelosuppression, anorexia, stomatitis, alopecia, gonadal suppression, nail hyperpigmentation, nausea and vomiting, diarrhea, and hemorrhagic cystitis
Dacarbazine	Nausea and vomiting, anorexia, vein irritation, alopecia, myelosuppression, facial flushing, and radiation recall
Hexamethylmelamine	Nausea and vomiting, diarrhea, abdominal cramps, alopecia, myelosuppression and neuropathy
Melphalan	Hypersensitivity, nausea, myelosuppression, amenorrhea, pulmonary infiltrates, and sterility
Nitrogen mustard	Nausea and vomiting, fever, chills, anorexia, vesication, gonadal suppression, myelosuppression, hyperpigmentation, and alopecia
Thiotepa	Nausea and vomiting, bone marrow suppression, mucositis, and gonadal dysfunction
Antimetabolites	
Cytarabine	Myelosuppression, diarrhea, nausea and vomiting, alopecia, rash, fever, conjunctivitis, neurotoxicity, hepatotoxicity, pulmonary edema, and skin desquamation of the palms and soles of the feet
Floxuridine	Nausea and vomiting, diarrhea, oral and gastrointestinal ulcers, bone marrow suppression, alopecia, and hepatotoxicity
Fludarabine	Chills, fever, hyperuricemia, nausea and vomiting, bone marrow suppression, neurotoxicity, and pulmonary toxicity
Fluorouracil (5-FU)	Oral and gastrointestinal ulcers, nausea and vomiting, diarrhea, alopecia, vein hyperpigmentation, and radiation recall
6-Mercaptopurine	Nausea and vomiting, anorexia, myelosuppression, diarrhea, hepatotoxicity, and hyperpigmentation
6-Thioguanine	Anorexia, stomatitis, rash, vein irritation, hepatotoxicity, myelosuppression, and nausea and vomiting
Antitumor antibiotics	
Bleomycin	Anaphylaxis, pneumonitis, pulmonary fibrosis, alopecia, stomatitis, anorexia, radiation recall, skin hyperpigmentation, fever, chills, and nausea and vomiting
Dactinomycin (actinomycin D)	Nausea and vomiting, stomatitis, vesication, alopecia, radiation recall, myelosuppression, and diarrhea
Daunorubicin	Myelosuppression, vesication, cardiotoxicity, stomatitis, radiation recall, nausea and vomiting, alopecia, and facial flushing
Doxorubicin	Myelosuppression, vesication, cardiotoxicity, stomatitis, alopecia, nausea and vomiting, radiation recall, and diarrhea
Idarubicin	Myelosuppression, alopecia, stomatitis, cardiotoxicity, nausea and vomiting, and vesication
Mithramycin	Myelosuppression, hepatotoxicity, hyperpigmentation, nausea and vomiting, facial flushing, and nephrotoxicity
Mitomycin	Myelosuppression, vesication, nausea and vomiting, alopecia, pulmonary fibrosis, hepatotoxicity, stomatitis, and hyperuricemia

- *Hormones* are cell-cycle phase nonspecific. These chemicals, secreted by the endocrine glands, alter the environment of the cell by affecting the cell membrane's permeability. By manipulating hormone levels, tumor growth can be suppressed. Corticosteroids provide an antiinflammatory effect on body tissues.
- *Nitrosoureas* are cell-cycle phase nonspecific. They have the ability to cross the blood-brain barrier. Their actions are similar to those of alkylating agents; DNA and RNA synthesis are inhibited.

- *Vinca plant alkaloids* are cell-cycle phase specific. They exert a cytotoxic effect by binding to microtubular proteins during metaphase, thus causing mitotic arrest. The cell loses its ability to divide and therefore dies.
- *Miscellaneous agents* may be cell-cycle phase specific, nonspecific, or both. These drugs act via a variety of mechanisms (inhibiting protein synthesis, interfering with DNA replication, and disrupting RNA processing).

Table 8-1	Chemotherapeutic drug classification with side effects—cont'd
Drugs	**Major side effects**
Hormonal agents	
Corticosteroids	
Dexamethasone	Nausea, suppression of immune function, weight gain, hyperglycemia, increased appetite, cataracts,
Hydrocortisone	impaired wound healing, menstrual irregularity, and interruption in sleep and rest patterns
Prednisone	
Solu-Cortef	
Antiandrogen	
Flutamide	Impotence and gynecomastia
Antiestrogen	
Tamoxifen	Nausea and vomiting, hot flashes, fluid retention, changes in menstrual pattern, increase in bone pain,
Zoladex	and hypercalcemia
Gonadotropin-releasing hormone	
Leuprolide	Impotence, decreased libido, increase in bone and tumor pain, genital atrophy, and gynecomastia
Nitrosoureas	
Carmustine	Nausea and vomiting, vein irritation, myelosuppression, stomatitis, nephrotoxicity, and pulmonary fibrosis
Lomustine	Nausea and vomiting, stomatitis, anorexia, myelosuppression, pulmonary fibrosis, and nephrotoxicity
Semustine	Myelosuppression, nausea and vomiting, hepatoxicity, nephrotoxicity, and pulmonary fibrosis
Streptozocin	Nausea and vomiting, fever, chills, nephrotoxicity, diarrhea, myelosuppression, and hypoglycemia
Plant alkaloid	
Etoposide	Nausea and vomiting, diarrhea, stomatitis, parotitis, anaphylaxis, hypotension, myelosuppression, radiation recall, hepatotoxicity, and alopecia
Taxol	Anaphylaxis, hypotension, nausea and vomiting, cardiotoxicity, myelosuppression, neurotoxicity, alopecia, stomatitis, and diarrhea
Teniposide	Nausea and vomiting, hypotension, anaphylaxis, myelosuppression, neuropathy, alopecia, and phlebitis
Vinblastine	Neurotoxicity, anorexia, myelosuppression, stomatitis, alopecia, gonadal suppression, peripheral neuropathy, and vesication
Vincristine	Neurotoxocity, constipation, myelosuppression, alopecia, vesication, peripheral neuropathy, and paralytic ileus
Vindesine	Nausea and vomiting, jaw pain, myelosuppression, paresthesia, alopecia, paralytic ileus, and stomatitis
Miscellaneous agents	
Asparaginase	Anaphylaxis, nausea and vomiting, fever, chills, myelosuppression, hyperglycemia, abdominal pain, diarrhea, pancreatitis, and anorexia
Hydroxyurea	Nausea and vomiting, alopecia, myelosuppression, allergic reactions, radiation recall, rash, azotemia, and dysuria
Pentostatin	Nausea and vomiting, rash, myelosuppression, vein irritation, nephrotoxicity, and hyperuricemia
Procarbazine	Nausea and vomiting; stomatitis; peripheral neuropathy; and severe gastrointestinal and central nervous system effects if taken with foods containing tyramine, alcohol, and monoamine oxidase inhibitor medications
Topotecan	Diarrhea, nausea and vomiting, myelosuppression, anorexia, and influenzalike symptoms

The following factors should be considered during drug selection:

1. Patient's eligibility for chemotherapy (confirmed diagnosis; bone marrow, nutritional, hepatic, and renal status; expectation of longevity; and history of chemotherapy and radiation therapy).
2. Cancer cell type (e.g., squamous cell, adenocarcinoma).
3. Rate of drug absorption (e.g., treatment interval and routes: oral, intraarterial, intraperitoneal).
4. Tumor location (many drugs do not cross the blood-brain barrier). The blood-brain barrier provides a protective mechanism that does not allow toxic agents to penetrate into this protective environment.
5. Tumor burden (larger tumors are generally less responsive to chemotherapy).
6. Tumor resistance to chemotherapy (tumor cells can mutate and produce variant cells distinct from the tumor stem cell of origin).[5,8]

Combination chemotherapy

Chemotherapeutic drugs are most frequently given in combinations to enhance their effect on the tumor cell kill. Consideration for drugs used in combination include verified effectiveness as a single agent, results in increased tumor cell kill, increased patient survival, presence of a synergistic action, varied toxicities, different mechanisms of action, and administration in repeated courses to minimize the immunosuppressive effects that might otherwise occur. Combination chemotherapy provides additional benefits not possible with single drug treatments. Such benefits include maximum cell kill in the range of toxicity tolerated by the host for each drug, a broader range of coverage of resistant cell lines in a heterogenous tumor population, and prevention or slowing of the development of new resistant lines.[6,9,12]

Because numerous cellular variants exist in a metastasis by the time it is detected, therapy for metastatic disease is often directed toward characteristics of the secondary rather than primary tumor. Combination chemotherapy rather than single, sequential therapy maximizes therapeutic response by addressing the diversity of cellular response (Table 8-2).

Interactions of chemotherapy and radiation therapy

Concomitant chemoradiotherapy is primarily aimed at overcoming mechanisms of radiation resistance at the locoregional tumor site. Multiple mechanisms of interaction have been proposed.[3,26,28-31]

Chemotherapy and radiation therapy can have activity against different tumor cell subpopulations; cells with intrinsic resistance against one treatment modality may be sensitive to the other. The early eradication of such resistant cells by the second treatment modality may prevent their subsequent proliferation.

Tumor cell repopulation after administration of radiation therapy is also an important mechanism of treatment failure.

Table 8-2	Combination chemotherapeutic regimens
Disease	**Drugs**
Acute lymphocytic leukemia (induction)	Asparaginase, vincristine, prednisone, and daunorubicin
Acute myelogenous leukemia (postinduction)	High-dose cytarabine, etoposide, and idarubicin
Brain	PLV—Procarbazine, lomustine, and vincristine
Breast	CAFVP—Cyclophosphamide, adriamycin, 5-FU, vinblastine, and prednisone CMF—Cyclophosphamide, methotrexate, and 5-FU FUVAC—5-FU, vinblastine, adriamycin, and cyclophosphamide
Colorectal Adjuvant Metastatic Hepatic metastases	 5-FU and levamisole 5-FU and leucovorin Floxuridine and mitomycin (intraarterial)
Ewing's sarcoma	CAV—Cyclophosphamide, adriamycin, vincrisitine, and dactinomycin
Hodgkin's	ABVD—Adriamycin, bleomycin, vinblastine, and dacarbazine MOPP—Nitrogen mustard, Oncovin, prednisone, and procarbazine
Kaposi's sarcoma	ABV—Adriamycin, bleomycin, and vincristine
Lung	ACE—Adriamycin, cyclophosphamide, and etoposide ICE—Ifosfamide, cyclophosphamide, and etoposide CAV—Cyclophosphamide, adriamycin, and vincristine CEP—Cyclophosphamide, etoposide, and cisplatin
Lymphoma	CHOP-BLEO—Cyclophosphamide, adriamycin, Oncovin, prednisone, and bleomycin PROMACE-CytaBOM—Prednisone, Oncovine, methotrexate, adriamycin, cyclophosphamide, etoposide, cytarabine, bleomycin, leucovorin, dexamethasone, and trimethoprim sulfa
Myeloma	VAD—Vincristine, adriamycin, and dexamethasone
Testicular	VBP—Vinblastine, bleomycin, and cisplatin VPV-VP-16—Etoposide, cisplatin, and vinblastine

Chemotherapy may be able to slow this process if drugs with activity against the specific tumor are available.

Tumor cell oxygenation and response to radiation therapy may be improved. Small masses may have better vasculation, thus allowing for improved delivery of chemotherapy to cancer cells.

Certain chemotherapeutic drugs decrease the ability of cancer cells to repair sublethal and potentially lethal radiation damage. This is thought to be an important mechanism of clinical radiation resistance (see Chapter 9). Various chemotherapeutic drugs have been studied in laboratory and clinical settings to characterize the interaction with radiation therapy (Table 8-3).

CONCOMITANT CHEMORADIOTHERAPEUTIC REGIMENS

The current approach of combination therapies is based on the premise that cytotoxic effects of chemotherapy interacts with local effects of radiation therapy and sensitizes cells to radiation cell kill. In addition to this, chemotherapy offers a systemic means of eradicating micrometastasis. The drug regimens usually contain agents that are known to have radiosensitizing properties. This approach has shown promise in the management of various cancer diseases (Table 8-4).[6,12,13,17]

Table 8-3 Chemotherapeutic and radiation therapeutic interactions

Drug	Cytotoxic effect
Bleomycin	Inhibits DNA synethsis; causes single-double strand breaks in DNA
Cisplatin	Alters DNA intrastrand cross-links; inhibits cellular repair after radiation
Cyclophosphamide	Inhibits DNA and RNA synthesis
Dactinomycin (actinomycin D)	Inhibits DNA and RNA synthesis; causes single-double strand breaks
Doxorubicin	Inhibits enzyme repair of replication-induced single strand breaks in DNA
5-FU	Inhibits synthesis of DNA by binding thymidylate synthase
Floxuridine	Decreases repair of radiation-induced, DNA double-strand breaks
Hydroxyurea	Inhibits repair of radiation-induced, single-strand breaks; selectively eradicates cells in the S phase
Methotrexate	Inhibits DNA synthesis
Mitomycin	Metabolites interact with DNA, leading to DNA interstrand cross-links
Nitrogen mustard	Inhibits DNA, RNA, and protein synthesis by single-strand breaks
Vinblastine and vincristine	Binds tubulin; poisons mitotic spindle, thus causing mitotic arrest

Table 8-4 Concomitant chemoradiotherapeutic regimens

Disease	Chemotherapy	Radiation therapy
Anus	5-FU 1000 mg/m2 96-hr infusion in weeks one and four; mitomycin C 10 mg first day of radiation therapy	4500 cGy in 4 to 5 weeks followed by a perineal boost of 1500 cGy
Bladder	5-FU 1000 mg/m2/day for 4 days in weeks one and three Cisplatin 25 mg/m2/day in weeks one and five	4000 to 6000 cGy in 5 weeks 4140 cGy in 4 to 5 weeks to whole pelvis +1000 cGy boost to bladder
Esophagus	5-FU 1000 mg/m2 infusion plus mitomycin 10 mg/m2 and/or cisplatin 75 mg/m2 bolus	3000 cGy in 3 weeks to 6000 cGy in 6 weeks
Head and neck	5-FU 1000 mg/m2 infusion plus mitomycin 10 mg/m2 and/or cisplatin 60 mg/m2 bolus	Hyperfractionated 125 cGy dose/twice daily; total dose of 6000 to 7200 cGy
Hodgkin's	Combination: nitrogen mustard, Oncovin, prednisone, procarbazine/Adriamycin, bleomycin, vinblastine, and dacarbazine	4000 to 4400 cGy over 4 weeks
Pancreas	Combination: 5-FU, mitomycin, and streptozocin infusion	4000 to 6000 cGy of split-course therapy
Rectal	Combination: 5-FU, lomustine, and mitomycin	4000 to 4700 cGy in 26 or 27 fractions
Non–small cell lung	Combination: cisplatin, carboplatin, etoposide, ifosfamide, and vincristine	Hyperfractionated 6000 cGy over 6 weeks

COMPLICATIONS OF COMBINED CHEMOTHERAPY AND RADIATION THERAPY

Safe and effective combination therapy requires cooperation and frequent interactions among the various specialists. Careful pretreatment planning is essential to maximize the chance of cure and minimize side effects. The various modalities can interact in many ways. For example, different sequences of radiation therapy and chemotherapy can lead to different side effects in patients who have head and neck cancer. Radiation recall (an increased redness and tenderness at the radiated skin site) occurs when certain chemotherapeutic drugs (e.g., dactinomycin, doxorubicin) are given with radiation therapy. Radiation therapy and chemotherapy can lower blood cell counts. This may lead to infection, bleeding, and fatigue. Additional side effects that may result in increased toxicity include stomatitis-mucositis, diarrhea, nausea and vomiting, cystitis, and xerostomia. Side effects and toxicity vary in severity according to the patient's response to the combination therapy. Acute treatment reactions not only may occur earlier in the treatment course, but also are more severe. Pertinent information related to the major systemic toxicities (cardiac, hepatic, hypersensitive, neurologic, pulmonary, and bone marrow suppression) has dose-limiting restrictions for many of the drugs. All the toxicities require astute observations and interventions by the health care team members (Table 8-5).[4,7,10,18,20,21,25,27]

Table 8-5	Complications: combination chemotherapy and radiation therapy
Drug	**Toxicity**
Bleomycin	Pulmonary fibrosis, rash, skin hyperpigmentaion, and radiation recall (dermatitis in previously irradiated areas)
Cyclophosphamide	Hemorrhagic cystitis, alopecia, and stomatitis
Cytarabine	Optic nerve, pulmonary edema, and skin desquamation on palms and soles of feet
Dactinomycin (actinomycin D)	Radiation recall, bone marrow suppression, and stomatitis
Daunorubicin	Bone marrow suppression, cardiotoxicity, alopecia, radiation recall, and stomatitis
Doxorubicin	Bone marrow suppression, cardiotoxicity, alopecia, radiation recall, and stomatitis
Etoposide	Bone marrow suppression, hepatotoxicity, alopecia, radiation recall, and mucositis
5-FU	Oral and gastrointestinal ulcerations, alopecia, and radiation recall
Hydroxyurea	Radiation recall and rash
Methotrexate	Pulmonary fibrosis, oral and gastrointestinal ulcerations, hepatotoxicity, and bone marrow suppression
Mitomycin	Bone marrow suppression, interstitial pneumonitis, alopecia, and stomatitis
Vindesine	Interstitial pneumonitis and local pulmonary fibrosis

RADIOSENSITIZERS

Chemical radiosensitizing compounds are used to increase lethal effects of radiation therapy. Nonhypoxic sensitizers such as iodoxyuridine (IUdR) incorporate into the DNA and increase the susceptibility of the cell to radiation damage. Hypoxic cell sensitizers such as metronidazole, misonidazole, and desmethymisonidazole increase oxygen to hypoxic cells and promote damage of the DNA, thus preventing cell repair. Certain chemotherapy agents such as carboplatin, cyclophosphamide, cisplatin, fluorouracil, and floxuridine are also used as **radiosensitizers** and given with radiation therapy. Radiosensitizers are commonly used with chemotherapy in the treatment of colorectal, cervical, glioblastoma, and head and neck cancers.[2,16,21,23,24,32]

CANCER CLINICAL TRIALS

Oncology as a medical and nursing speciality has grown rapidly over the past 25 years. The efforts of a nationwide network of physicians and nurses performing clinical trials resulted in improved surgical outcomes, new chemotherapeutic agents, less toxic radiation therapy, and the testing of numerous biological and growth hormones. Clinical trials for cancer patients focus on the development of new drugs and agents or combinations of therapies, improved prevention and detection methods, and psychological and physiological effects of cancer on patients.[14,19]

Clinical research on cancer is done primarily through the support and direction of the National Cancer Institute (NCI), which was established in 1937. In 1971 the National Cancer Act mandated the NCI to pursue basic cancer research and take responsibility for the organized application of research results to reduce the incidence, morbidity, and mortality of cancer.[17]

A comprehensive nationwide program designed to reach the public was needed to increase the efficacy of treatments, decrease toxicity, and improve the quality of life for cancer patients. To facilitate this, NCI-sponsored cooperative groups (e.g., brain tumor, leukemia, gynecological, pediatric, and radiation therapy), comprehensive cancer centers, and community clinical oncology programs conduct clinical trials.

The comprehensive cancer center program sponsored by the NCI designates national resources for research. Each center needs to have a multidisciplinary approach to cancer treatment and provide cancer resources for the community.

Community-based oncologists care for approximately 80% of cancer patients. The NCI developed the Community Clinical Oncology Program (CCOP) in 1984. CCOP institutions consist of community-based physicians linked to cooperative groups and cancer centers.[14,19]

Drug development

The NCI is the largest sponsor of studies using chemotherapeutic drugs. More than 100 such agents are currently in clinical testing. Pharmaceutical companies also develop new drugs. The drugs are identified and screened through stringent in vitro methods. Preclinical testing for drug toxicity is required after the formulation and resolution of production problems. The goals of toxicology studies are to predict organ system toxicity and the safest starting dose for clinical trials.[9,14]

Investigational new drug application

Before a drug can be studied in humans, its sponsor (the NCI or a pharmaceutical company) submits an Investigational New Drug Application to the Food and Drug Administration to request permission to evaluate the agent in human cancer. The developmental process for a new drug is lengthy (approximately 12 years) and costly ($50 to 70 million from screening to commercial availability).

Clinical trials

Clinical trials are carefully controlled experiments aimed at using the smallest number of subjects to determine with statistical confidence the effectiveness of treatments and simultaneously maintaining patient safety. Several steps must occur before a clinical trial is implemented. The first is the design and writing of the cancer treatment protocol; the second is the approval of regulatory boards. A protocol is best described as the following:

- A verbal plan that describes the study's methodology
- A written plan that communicates only the principal investigator's purpose in undertaking the study
- A written plan that clearly describes the way the clinical trial is conducted
- A verbal plan that provides the investigator's direction for the research study

An essential component of the protocol is the **informed consent.** The purpose of the informed consent is to maintain human dignity while conducting human research studies. The principle investigator is responsible for developing a protocol-specific informed consent. This informed consent must review the research study and identify all possible risk factors involved in the study. The informed consent must be written in language that is understandable to the patient. Signing an informed consent does not bind a patient to remain on the clinical trial; participation is voluntary. Patients may terminate their participation in the study at any time.[15,19]

An Institutional Review Board (IRB) must first approve federally funded and regulated clinical trials. The IRB is a multidisciplinary committee that includes physicians, nurses, scientists, lawyers, clergy, and people from the community. The purpose of this board is to act as the patient's advocate by reviewing all proposed clinical trials to ensure that the research design is scientifically sound. An IRB must approve a clinical trial before the trial can begin. The trial must then be reviewed annually until the study is completed.[6,17,28]

Clinical trials in humans have three phases (I, II, and III). The purpose of phase I is to determine the maximum tolerated dose (MTD) in humans, ascertain the most effective schedule of administration, and identify and quantify toxic effects in normal organ systems. Phase II is the evaluation of a new anticancer drug to determine whether the compound has objective antitumor activity in a variety of cancers. Attention is focused on the types of tumors that respond and the dose-response relationship. Phase III establishes the value of the new treatment relative to standard treatments by a **randomized** (e.g., a designated sample drawn from a population so that each member has an equal chance to be selected) or comparative study. Study methods that may be used to define this role are comparison of the new drug to the best standard drug; use of the new agent in a current, effective drug combination; and combined modality treatment versus the previous best single modality.

Many of the advances in the care of cancer patients can be attributed to successful clinical trials. A growing number of community hospitals and outpatient settings are becoming involved in the implementation of clinical trials. All health care professionals need to increase their understanding of the clinical trial process and recognize the importance of their contributions to the success of clincial trial research to promote the progressive advancement of cancer care options.[17,18,21]

SUMMARY

These are exciting times for all health care professionals involved in cancer care. New chemotherapeutic agents are being identified; technology is rapidly changing the world of diagnostics; and because of the combination of surgery, biotherapy, chemotherapy, and radiation therapy, disease-free intervals are significantly expanded.

Review Questions

Multiple Choice

1. What is the most common dose-limiting toxicity for chemotherapeutic drugs?
   a. Nerve toxicity
   b. Gastrointestinal toxicity
   c. Myelosuppression
   d. Respiratory capacity

2. The incidence of anaphylaxis after drug administration is common in all *except* which of the following?
   a. Asparaginase
   b. Bleomycin
   c. Vincristine
   d. Taxol

3. The factors considered in chemotherapeutic drug selection include which of the following?
   I. Cancer cell type (squamous-adenocarcinoma)
   II. Tumor location (brain-lung)
   III. Rate of drug absorption (route-treatment interval)
   IV. Tumor resistance to chemotherapy
      a. I and II only
      b. I and III only
      c. II, III, and IV only
      d. I, II, III, and IV

4. A phase II clinical trial is used to determine which of the following?
   a. The drug's promotion of anticancer activity
   b. The maximum-tolerated dose
   c. The new treatment in comparison with the current, conventional treatment
   d. None of the above

5. What chemotherapeutic drugs are used to increase the lethal effects of radiation therapy?
   a. Radiosensitizers
   b. Phase III drugs
   c. Phase IV drugs
   d. Proliferation drugs

6. Which of the following is *not* a possible side effect from chemotherapeutic drugs?
   a. Nausea and vomiting
   b. Cardiac toxicity
   c. Myelosuppression
   d. Alopecia
   e. None of the above

Fill in the Blank

7. Many cancer treatments work by modifying or interfering with DNA synthesis. In the _____ phase of the cell cycle, DNA synethesis occurs.

8. Cardiotoxicity is the dose-limiting factor for some of the antitumor antibiotics. Two key drugs are_____ and _____.

9. The administration of two or more chemotherapeutic drugs is known as _____ chemotherapy.

Questions to Ponder

1. Discuss the way chemotherapeutic treatments work by modifying or interfering with DNA synthesis.
2. Describe the components of the informed consent for a cancer research protocol.
3. Describe the factors that promote the success of chemotherapy.
4. Compare the similarities and differences among primary, neoadjuvant, induction, and combination chemotherapy.
5. Compare the difference between cell-cycle specific and nonspecific drugs used in chemotherapy.

REFERENCES

1. Boring CC et al: Cancer statistics, *CA Cancer J Clin* 44(1):7, 1994.
2. Bruner DW et al, editors: *Manual for radiation oncology nursing practice and education*, Pittsburgh, 1992, Oncology Nursing Society.
3. Bruner DW, McGinn-Byer M: Ostomy care considerations for patients before and after radiation therapy, *Progressions* 5(3):18, 1993.
4. Chabner BA: Anticancer drugs. In De Vita VT Jr, Hellman S, Rosenberg SA, editors: *Cancer: principles and practice of oncology*, ed 4, Phildelphia, 1993, JB Lippincott.
5. Devine SM, Vokes EE, Weichselbaum RR: Chemotherapeutic and biologic radiologic enhancement, *Curr Opin Oncol* 3(6):1087, 1991.
6. De Vita VT Jr: Principles of chemotherapy. In De Vita VT Jr, Hellman S, Rosenberg SA, editors: *Cancer: principles and practice of oncology*, ed 4, Phildelphia, 1993, JB Lippincott.
7. Dini D et al: Management of acute radiodermatitis, *Cancer Nurs* 16(5):366, 1993.
8. Ensminger WD: Regional chemotherapy, *Semin Oncol* 20(1):3, 1993.
9. Fields SM, Von Hoff DD: New anticancer agents, *Highlights on Antineoplastic Drugs* 10(2):16, 1992.
10. Finley RS: Drug interactions in the oncology patient, *Semin Oncol Nurs* 8(2):95, 1992.

11. Finley RS: Update on differentiating agent therapy in chemoprevention and cancer treatment, *Highlights on Antineoplastic Drugs* 11(4):76, 1993.

12. Green MR: Chemotherapy and radiation in the nonoperative management of stage III non-small-cell lung cancer: the right chemotherapy works in the right setting, *Important Adv Oncol* 8:25, 1993.

13. Harris JR, Recht A: How to combine adjuvant chemotherapy and radiation therapy, *Recent Results Cancer Res* 127:129, 1993.

14. Lake T, Jenkins J: Cancer chemotherapy: clinical trials, *Cancer Nurs* 16(6):486, 1993.

15. Levy W et al: Chemotherapy agents, part I, *Cancer Nurs* 16(4):321, 1993.

16. Looney WB, Hopkins HA: Rationale for different chemotherapeutic and radiation therapy strategies in cancer management, *Cancer* 67(6):1471, 1991.

17. Meehan JL, Johnson BJ: The neurotoxicity of antineoplastic agents, *Curr Issues Cancer Nurs Practice Updates* 1(8):1, 1992.

18. Murren JR, Buzaid AC: Chemotherapy and radiation for the treatment of non-small-cell lung cancer, *Clin Chest Med* 14(1):161, 1993.

19. Otto SE, editor: *Oncology nursing*, ed 2, St Louis, 1994, Mosby.

20. Patel NH, Koeller J: Cancer chemotherapy in the elderly, *Highlights on Antineoplastic Drugs* 11(4):58, 1993.

21. Perez CA, Brady LW, editors: *Principles and practice of radiation oncology*, ed 2, Phildephia, 1992, JB Lippincott.

22. Quint-Kasner S et al: Chemotherapy agents, part II, *Cancer Nurs* 16(5):398, 1993.

23. Robert NJ et al: Overall principles of cancer management chemotherapy. In Osteen RT, editor: *Cancer manual*, ed 8, Atlanta, 1990, American Cancer Society.

24. Rotman MZ: Chemoirradiation: a new initiative in cancer treatment, *Radiology* 184(2):319, 1992.

25. Servodidio CA, Abramson DH: Acute and long-term effects of radiation therapy to the eye in children, *Cancer Nurs* 16(5):371, 1993.

26. Tepper JE: Combined radiotherapy and chemotherapy in the treatment of gastrointestinal malignancies, *Semin Oncol* 19(4, suppl 11):96, 1992.

27. Thomas CR Jr, Taylor SG IV: Controversies in the modality management of head and neck cancer, *Hematology, Oncology Clin North America* 5(4):769, 1991.

28. Trimble EL et al: Neoadjuvant therapy in cancer treatment, *Cancer Suppl* 72(11):3515, 1993.

29. Vokes EE: Interactions of chemotherapy and radiation, *Semin Oncol* 20(1):70, 1993.

30. Walkenstein MD, McGinn-Byer M: Ostomy care for patients receiving chemotherapy or biological response modifers, *Progressions* 5(3):11, 1993.

31. Wood LS, Gulilo SM: IV vesicants: how to avoid extravasation, *AJN* 93(4):42, 1993.

32. Zietman AL, Shipley WU, Kaufman DS: The combination of cisplatin based chemotherapy and radiation in the treatment of muscel-invading transitional cell cancer of the bladder, *Int J Radiat Oncol* 27(1):161, 1993.

Overview of Radiobiology

Stephen M. Waldow

Outline

Key terms

INTERACTION OF RADIATION AND MATTER

 Since the discovery of x-rays by Roentgen in 1895, scientists and clinicians have investigated the interaction of **ionizing* radiations** and various target materials, including biological tissue. *Radiation biology*, or *radiobiology*, has evolved since Roentgen's time and can be defined as the study of the sequence of events following the absorption of energy from ionizing radiations, the efforts of the organism to compensate, and the damage to the organism that may be produced.[62]

In evaluating the response of a living cell to ionizing radiation, the following must be considered[62]:

1. Radiation may or may not interact with a cell.

---

*Ionization refers to the ejection of an electron from an atom, thus resulting in a charged particle or ion.

2. If an interaction occurs, damage may or may not be produced in the cell.
3. The initial energy deposition occurs extremely rapidly (much less than 1 second) and is nonselective or random in the cell.
4. Visible tissue changes after irradiation are not usually distinguishable from those caused by other traumas. (The only exception to this may be cataracts, which will be discussed later.)
5. Biological changes that occur after irradiation do so after some time has elapsed. The duration of this latent period is inversely related to the dose administered and can range from minutes to years.

Types of interactions

When radiation interacts with a cell, the ionizations are direct or indirect.[26] When a beam of charged particles (alpha particles, protons, or electrons) is incident on living tissue, direct ionization (the result of the incident particle itself) of a critical target (**deoxyribonucleic acid [DNA]**) is highly probable because of the relatively densely ionizing nature of most particulate radiations. This form of damage, in which a charged particle directly ionizes the critical target, is not modifiable by physical, chemical, or biological factors.

The other form of ionization is indirect because of the effects of specific secondary particles on the target. This mechanism predominates when the incident beam is composed of x-rays, gamma rays, or neutrons. These indirectly ionizing radiations give rise to fast (high energy), charged secondary particles that can then directly or indirectly cause ionizations in the critical target. Direct effects predominate when neutrons compose the primary beam because the secondary particles produced (protons, alpha particles, or heavy nuclear fragments) from the neutron's interaction with the nucleus of the atom may cause damage directly to the DNA or other important macromolecules (large molecules) in the cell.

The other possible interaction after indirect ionization is known as an *indirect effect*.[26] This occurs predominantly when x-rays or gamma rays compose the primary beam, thus producing fast electrons as the secondary particles that interact with the cellular medium, water (H_2O). Indirect effects involve a series of reactions known as **radiolysis** (splitting) of water. The initial event in radiolysis involves the ionization or ejection of an electron from a water molecule, thus producing a water ion (charged molecule):

$$H_2O \rightarrow H_2O^+ + e^-$$

The ejected electron (e^-), known as a *fast electron* because of its high energy, may now be absorbed by a second water molecule forming another water ion (H_2O^-):

$$e^- + H_2O \rightarrow H_2O^-$$

The pair of water ions produced are chemically unstable and tend to rapidly break down or dissociate into another ion

and a **free radical** (a highly reactive species with an unpaired valence [outer shell] electron):

$$H_2O^+ \rightarrow H^+ + OH^• \quad \text{and} \quad H_2O^- \rightarrow H^• + OH^-$$

The ion pair (H^+ and OH^-) may recombine, thus forming a normal water molecule with no net damage to the cell. The probability of recombination is high if the two ions are formed closely to each other. If these ions persist in the cell, they can react with and damage important macromolecules.

Free radicals may also recombine like the previous ion pair, thus forming a normal water molecule:

$$H^• + OH^• \rightarrow H_2O$$

Free radicals may also combine with other nearby free radicals, thus forming a new molecule like hydrogen peroxide that is toxic to the cell:

$$OH^• + OH^• \rightarrow H_2O_2 \text{ (hydrogen peroxide)}$$

Free radicals can participate in several other reactions involving normal cellular components, including DNA. Because the majority of the cell (80%) consists of water, the probability of damage by indirect effects is much greater than for direct effects with the use of indirectly ionizing radiations. Of the several reactions just presented for indirect effects, the predominant pathway that accounts for approximately two thirds of cellular damage involves the hydroxyl ($OH^•$) radical. As will be discussed later, indirect effects predominate with sparsely ionizing or low **linear energy transfer (LET)** radiations, and can be modified by physical, chemical, or biological factors.

Linear energy transfer and relative biological effectiveness

Depending on the composition of the incident beam of radiation, various secondary particles are produced in the cell. These secondary particles may directly or indirectly ionize the critical target. The physical properties of these secondary particles (mass and charge) give rise to a characteristic path of damage in the cell. Radiations can therefore be categorized by the rate at which energy is deposited by charged particles (incident or secondary) as they travel through matter. This is the LET of the radiation.[73] The LET is an average value calculated by dividing the energy deposited in kiloelectron volts (keV) by the distance traveled in micrometers (μm or 10^{-6} meters). Sparsely ionizing radiations such as x-rays and gamma rays are therefore classified as low LET because the secondary electrons produced are small particles that deposit their energy over great distances in tissue. Typical LET values for sparsely ionizing radiations may range from 0.3 to 3.0 keV/μm.[62] Densely ionizing radiations, which include charged particles such as protons and alpha particles, are classified as high LET because these particles are much bulkier in terms of mass than electrons and therefore deposit their energy over much smaller distances in the cell. Typical LET values may range from 30 to 100 keV/μm or greater, depending on the particle energy. Generally, a large, charged particle such as a proton or alpha particle does not penetrate nearly as far as a smaller, charged particle (electron) and not quite as far as an uncharged particle of equal mass (neutron). Neutrons usually have intermediate LET values (usually within 5 to 20 keV/μm). As the neutron's energy increases, its penetration in tissue also increases; therefore its LET decreases.

Knowing the LET of the radiation is important because the discovery was made early in the radiation therapy process that different LET radiations produce different degrees of the same biological response. In other words, equal doses of different LET radiations do not produce the same biological response. This is called the **relative biological effectiveness (RBE)** of the radiation.[26] The RBE relates the ability of radiations with different LETs delivered under the same conditions to produce the same biological effect. The equation for determining the RBE of a test radiation is as follows:

$$\text{RBE of test radiation} = \frac{\text{Dose from 250 - keV x-ray}}{\substack{\text{Dose from test radiation to produce} \\ \text{the same biological effect}}}$$

The test radiation referred to includes any type of radiation beam being used. The effectiveness of the beam is determined by a historical comparison with a 250-keV x-ray beam that was the primary radiation beam available in the early days of radiation therapy. For example, if 400 cGy of 250-keV x-rays and 200 cGy of neutrons both result in 50% cell kill, the RBE of the neutrons equals 2. This means that the neutrons are twice as effective as the x-rays. In general, as the LET of the radiation increases, so does its RBE.

Radiation effects on deoxyribonucleic acid

The key molecule in the nucleus of the cell for radiation damage is thought to be DNA. Damage to a key molecule may be lethal to a cell and has led to the development of a target theory for radiation damage. This theory states that when ionizing radiation interacts with or near a key molecule (DNA), the sensitive area is termed a *target*. An ionization event that occurs in the target is termed a *hit*. These terms are applied only under conditions in which radiation interacts with the target by direct effects. This theory does not account for damage to DNA that is the result of free radical-mediated pathways.

Regardless of whether DNA is damaged by direct or indirect effects caused by radiation, several types of damage can occur.[51] One form of damage involves the change in or loss of one or more of the four nitrogenous (nitrogen-containing) bases: adenine (A), thymine (T), cytosine (C), and guanine (G). A second form of damage may involve breakage of hydrogen bonds between the A-T and C-G base pairs, which function to keep the two DNA strands together. Bonds may also be broken between the components of the backbone of each DNA strand (i.e., between the deoxyribose sugar and phosphate groups connected to each base and known collec-

tively as a *nucleotide*). This may lead to intrastrand or interstrand cross-linking of DNA.

The consequences of these types of DNA damage vary. Loss or change of a base results in a new base sequence, which can cause minor or major effects on protein synthesis. A change in base sequence not rectified by the cell is an example of a mutation (change in the genetic material). Agents such as ionizing radiation that cause mutations are mutagenic. Single-strand breaks in the DNA backbone (common after irradiation with low LET radiations) may or may not be repaired. If they are not repaired, damage may occur. Single-strand breaks are more readily repaired than double-strand breaks, which are more apparent after exposure to high LET radiations. The production of multiple-strand breaks compared with single strand breaks correlates much more strongly with cell lethality. Radiation interaction with DNA does not always result in damage, and most of the damage can be and probably is repaired. Consequences of DNA damage in somatic (body) cells involve the irradiated organism or individual, whereas DNA damage in germ (reproductive) cells may also affect future generations.

Radiation effects on chromosomes

A review of the four phases of mitosis, which is a continuous process of organizing and arranging nuclear DNA during cell division, is helpful in understanding radiation effects on chromosomes. The box on p. 97 shows the major events of mitosis. Because DNA molecules form genes and thousands of genes compose a chromosome, studying genetic damage from ionizing radiation in terms of gross structural damage to chromosomes is often easiest.[17]

Early studies in this area often involved plant chromosomes because their small diploid number (number of chromosomes in each somatic cell) and large relative size facilitated study under the light microscope. The fact that radiation is an efficient breaker of chromosomes by indirect or direct pathways is now well documented. Gross structural changes in chromosomes are referred to as *aberrations*, *lesions*, or *anomalies*. A distinction also exists between chromosome and chromatid aberrations. A chromosome aberration occurs when radiation is administered to cells in the G_1 phase or before the cell replicates its DNA in the S phase (see the section on the cell cycle in Chapter 6). A chromosome aberration may involve both daughter cells after mitosis, because if the break is not repaired, it is replicated by the cell during the S phase. A chromatid aberration results when radiation is administered to cells in the G_2 phase or after they have completed DNA synthesis. This term applies to the arms (chromatids) of a replicated (duplicated) chromosome. In this situation, only one of the two daughter cells formed after cell division is affected if the damage is not repaired.

Structural changes induced in chromosomes by radiation include single breaks, multiple breaks, and a phenomenon known as *chromosome stickiness,* or *clumping.* Consequences

The Major Events of Mitosis

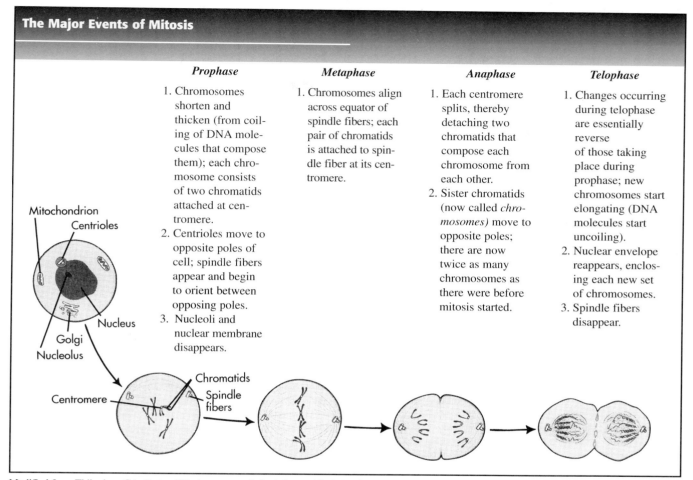

Prophase	Metaphase	Anaphase	Telophase
1. Chromosomes shorten and thicken (from coiling of DNA molecules that compose them); each chromosome consists of two chromatids attached at centromere. 2. Centrioles move to opposite poles of cell; spindle fibers appear and begin to orient between opposing poles. 3. Nucleoli and nuclear membrane disappears.	1. Chromosomes align across equator of spindle fibers; each pair of chromatids is attached to spindle fiber at its centromere.	1. Each centromere splits, thereby detaching two chromatids that compose each chromosome from each other. 2. Sister chromatids (now called *chromosomes*) move to opposite poles; there are now twice as many chromosomes as there were before mitosis started.	1. Changes occurring during telophase are essentially reverse of those taking place during prophase; new chromosomes start elongating (DNA molecules start uncoiling). 2. Nuclear envelope reappears, enclosing each new set of chromosomes. 3. Spindle fibers disappear.

Modified from Thibodeau GA, Patton KT: *Anatomy and physiology,* ed 3, St Louis, 1996, Mosby.

of these structural changes may include healing with no damage and loss or rearrangement of genetic material.

A single radiation-induced break in any part of a chromosome results in two chromosome fragments. One fragment contains the centromere (the place the mitotic spindle attaches during mitosis), and the other (known as the *acentric fragment*) does not.[62] The rejoining of these fragments, termed *restitution*, has a high probability of occurring because of their proximity.[17] Approximately 95% of all single breaks heal by restitution with the result being no damage to the cell.

If irradiation occurs in G_1 cells and restitution does not occur, both fragments are replicated during the S phase, thus resulting in four fragments (each with a broken end).[62] Two of these chromatids contain a centromere, whereas the other two do not. The two centromere-containing chromatids may now join, thus forming a dicentric fragment. The other two fragments may also join, thus forming an acentric fragment.

These structural aberrations become evident during the metaphase and anaphase stages of mitosis. Because the acentric fragment does not contain a centromere, the spindle fibers do not attach to it during the metaphase stage. Therefore the genetic material it contains probably will not be transmitted to either daughter cell. The dicentric fragment, however, has two centromeres and will therefore be attached to the mitotic spindle at two sites instead of one. Therefore this fragment is pulled simultaneously toward both poles of the cell. The fragment between the two centromeres therefore becomes stretched, thus giving rise to a characteristic anaphase bridge, which eventually tears by the end of the anaphase stage, thus resulting in an unequal transmission of genetic information to each daughter cell (Fig. 9-1).

A single break in one chromatid in two different chromosomes also produces four fragments. Two fragments contain a centromere and two do not.[62] Again, dicentric and acentric chromosomes may result by the joining of the broken fragments (Fig. 9-2, *A*). In addition, the acentric fragment from one broken chromosome may join to a centromere-containing fragment of the other broken chromosome, thus forming a new normal-appearing chromosome. This rearrangement is known as *translocation* (Fig. 9-2, *B*). Although translocation does not necessarily result in a loss of genetic information, the

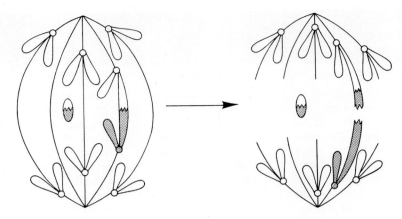

Fig. 9-1 The fate of the dicentric and acentric fragments during anaphase, thus leading to anaphase bridge formation. The dicentric fragment attaches to the mitotic spindle at each centomere and is pulled toward both poles of the cell *(left)* and ultimately breaks again *(right)*. The acentric fragment does not attach to the spindle, thus resulting in loss of genetic material to the new daughter cells. (From Travis EL: *Primer of medical radiobiology,* ed 2, St Louis, 1989, Mosby.)

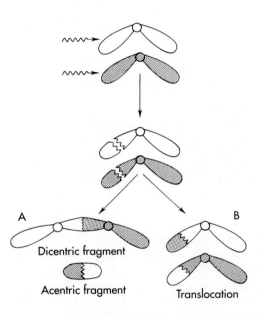

Fig. 9-2 Two different chromosomes *(top)* may sustain a single break in one arm *(center)* and result in formation of dicentric and acentric fragments *(A)*, or translocation of genetic material between the two *(B)*. In the latter process, two complete chromosomes are formed. However, the exchange of chromosome parts and therefore genetic information should be noted. (From Travis EL: *Primer of medical radiobiology,* ed 2, St Louis, 1989, Mosby.)

sequence of genes in the new translocated chromosome is different from the original sequence before radiation damage. The consequences of radiation-induced translocations can vary from no effects in somatic cells to malformed or nonviable offspring if these translocations occur in germ cells.

When high-LET radiation is administered to cells, a high probability exists of producing multiple breaks in the same chromosome because of the densely ionizing nature of the secondary particles involved. These multiple breaks can occur in the same chromatid or separately in each chromatid. When multiple breaks occur close together on the chromosome, repair is not as efficient as repair of single breaks. Repair of multiple breaks is more efficient if the breaks are sufficiently spaced from each other. The cell then handles each break independently as with the restitution of a single break. Because cell death after radiation exposure correlates strongly with the production of double breaks, the consequences of two breaks in a chromosome should be carefully considered.

A double break in one arm (chromatid) of a chromosome results in three fragments, each with a broken end.[62] Of these three, one fragment contains the centromere and the other two are acentric. The major consequences of a double break are known as *deletions* and *inversions* (Fig. 9-3). A deletion of genetic material results when the fragment between the breaks is lost and the joining of the remaining two fragments join (Fig. 9-3, *A*). The effect of a deletion varies depending on the amount and significance of the genetic information that was in the lost fragment. An inversion of genetic material results when the middle fragment with two broken ends turns around or inverts before rejoining the other two fragments (Fig. 9-3, *B*). Although no loss of genetic material occurs after an inversion, the DNA base sequences and therefore the gene sequence is altered. This affects the types and amounts of critical proteins synthesized by the cell and can certainly affect the long-term viability of the cell.

Because of the random absorption of ionizing radiation in the cell, a single break can be induced in each chromatid of the same chromosome, thus again producing three fragments. The fragment with two broken ends contains the centromere and the other two fragments are acentric. This may result in the formation of a ring chromosome and an acentric

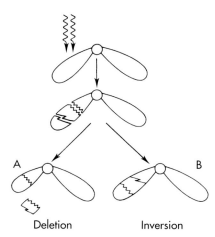

Fig. 9-3 Two breaks occurring in the same arm of a chromosome (*top* and *middle*) may result in deletion of the fragment between the breaks *(A)*, or inversion of the fragment, which is illustrated by the change in positions of the break lines *(B)*. (From Travis EL: *Primer of medical radiobiology,* ed 2, St Louis, 1989, Mosby.)

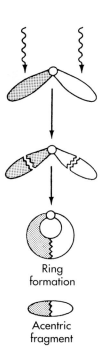

Fig. 9-4 One possible consequence of breaks in both arms of a chromosome by radiation is that the broken arms join to form a ring. The remaining fragments join but are left without a centromere (acentric fragment). (From Travis EL: *Primer of medical radiobiology,* ed 2, St Louis, 1989, Mosby.)

chromosome (Fig. 9-4).[62] The ring chromosome is replicated and transmitted to the daughter cells, whereas the acentric fragment and its genetic information is not passed on. If a replicated ring chromosome becomes tangled before the metaphase stage, unequal separation of each ring during the anaphase stage may result, so the daughter cells therefore do not inherit equal amounts of genetic information.

Several factors influence the type and extent of chromosome damage induced by ionizing radiations. The number of single breaks produced is directly proportional to the total dose of radiation administered. The frequency of single breaks, or simple aberrations, also increases as the LET of the radiation decreases. Therefore low-LET radiations such as x-rays and gamma rays produce more simple than complex (multiple break) aberrations. However, the production of single breaks is not influenced by the dose rate at which the radiation is administered.

The frequency of multiple breaks or complex aberrations is not directly related to the total dose but is proportional to the dose rate administered because at high dose rates, restitution of single breaks is less efficient. Therefore fewer break sites can be repaired, thus resulting in an increase in multiple breaks. The relationship between multiple breaks and LET is the opposite of that for single breaks (i.e., as the LET of the radiation increases, so does the probability of multiple break formation).

Radiation effects on other cell components

Although nuclear DNA is the critical target for radiation-induced cell damage, other structures in the cell are also damaged by ionizing radiations and contribute to cell damage and death. Among these cellular components is the plasma or cell membrane. Absorption of energy by the structural components of the plasma membrane (i.e., the phospholipid bilayer and proteins) can result in membrane damage and therefore changes in the permeability of the membrane with regard to the transport of substances in and out of the cell. Damage to the mitochondrial and lysosomal membranes in the cytoplasm can also result in drastic consequences to the cell. All cellular components (including vital proteins, enzymes, carbohydrates, and lipids) can undergo structural and functional changes after irradiation that can be deadly to the cell. Because the deposition of energy from secondary particles (electrons, protons, or alpha particles) is random in matter, any site in the cell can be at risk for damage from radiation exposure.

RADIOSENSITIVITY
Law of Bergonié and Tribondeau

In 1906 two scientists named Bergonié and Tribondeau performed experiments by using rodent testes to investigate reported clinical effects of radiation known at the time.[7] Testes were chosen as the model for the experiments because they contain cells differing in function and mitotic activity. These cell types ranged from immature, mitotically active spermatogonia to mature, nondividing spermatozoa (sperm).

The results of the animal experiments indicated that immature, dividing cells were damaged at lower radiation doses than mature, nondividing cells. This result led to the formation of the **law of Bergonié and Tribondeau,** which states that ionizing radiation is more effective against cells that (1) are actively mitotic, (2) are undifferentiated, and (3) have a long mitotic future. Bergonié and Tribondeau therefore defined radiosensitivity in terms of the mitotic activity and the level of differentiation. These two characteristics determined a cell's sensitivity to radiation. Therefore cells dividing more often are more radiosensitive than cells dividing less often or not all.

The level of maturity or differentiation of a cell refers to its level of functional and/or structural specialization. According to Bergonié and Tribondeau, cells that are undifferentiated (i.e., immature cells whose primary function is to divide and replace more mature cells lost from the population) are extremely radiosensitive. These cells are also known as *stem* or *precursor cells.* In the testes a spermatogonia is an example of a stem cell. A fully differentiated cell, known as an *end cell,* has a specialized structure or function, does not divide, and is radioresistant. Two examples of end cells are spermatozoa in the testes and erythrocytes in the circulating blood.

In 1925 Ancel and Vitemberger added to the findings of Bergonié and Tribondeau.[3] Ancel and Vitemberger proposed that the environmental conditions of a cell before, during, or after radiation treatment could influence the extent and appearance of radiation damage. Current knowledge indicates that the expression of radiation damage generally occurs when the cell is stressed, usually during reproduction. The sensitivity of a cell to radiation can also be modified. This change in sensitivity, known as *conditional sensitivity,* will be discussed later.

Cell populations

In 1968 Rubin and Casarett grouped mammalian cell populations into five basic categories based on radiation sensitivity[45] (Table 9-1). The endpoint chosen was radiation-induced cell death. The most radiosensitive of these groups is known as *vegetative intermitotic (VIM) cells.* VIM cells are rapidly dividing, undifferentiated cells with short life spans. Examples include basal cells, crypt cells, erythroblasts, and type A spermatogonia.

The second most radiosensitive group is known as *differentiating intermitotic (DIM) cells.* These cells are also actively mitotic but a little more differentiated than VIM cells. In fact, VIM cells such as type A spermatogonia divide and mature into DIM cells such as type B spermatogonia.

The third group of cells, known as *multipotential connective tissue cells,* is intermediate in radiosensitivity. These cells (such as endothelial cells of blood vessels and fibroblasts of connective tissue) divide irregularly and are more differentiated than VIM and DIM cells.

The fourth group, *reverting postmitotic (RPM) cells,* normally do not divide but are capable of doing so. RPM cells typically live longer and are more differentiated than the three previously discussed groups. These cells, including liver cells, are relatively radioresistant. Another example of an RPM cell is the mature lymphocyte. This cell, however, is very radiosensitive despite its characteristics and is therefore an exception to the law of Bergonié and Tribondeau.

The most radioresistant group of cells in the body are known as *fixed postmitotic (FPM) cells.* FPM cells are highly differentiated, do not divide, and may or may not be replaced when they die. Examples include certain nerve cells, muscle cells, erythrocytes, and spermatozoa.

Table 9-1	Classification of mammalian cells according to their characteristics and radiosensitivities		
Cell type	**Characteristics**	**Examples**	**Radiosensitivity**
VIM	Divide regularly and rapidly, are undifferentiated, and do not differentiate between divisions	Type A spermatogonia, erythroblasts, crypt cells, and basal cells	Extremely high
DIM	Actively divide, are more differentiated than VIMs, and differentiate between divisions	Intermediate spermatogonia and myelocytes	High
Vessels/connective tissue	Irregularly divide and are more differentiated than VIMs or DIMs	Endothelial cells and fibroblasts	Intermediate
RPM	Do not normally divide but retain capability of division and are variably differentiated	Parenchymal cells of liver and lymphocytes*	Low
FPM	Do not divide and are highly differentiated	Nerve cells, muscle cells, erythrocytes, and spermatozoa	Extremely low

From Travis EL: *Primer of medical radiobiology,* ed 2, St Louis, 1989, Mosby.
*Lymphocytes, although classified as relatively radioresistant by their characteristics, are extremely radiosensitive.

Tissue and organ sensitivity

Because radiosensitivities of specific cells in the body are now known, that information can be used to determine radiosensitivities of organized tissues and organs. Structurally, tissues and organs are composed of two compartments: the parenchyma and stroma. The parenchymal compartment contains characteristic cells of that tissue or organ. VIM, DIM, RPM, and FPM cells are examples of parenchymal cells. Regardless of the types of parenchymal cells in a tissue or organ, they also have a supporting stromal compartment.[62] The stroma consists of connective tissue and the vasculature and is generally considered intermediate in radiosensitivity, according to Rubin and Casarett.[45]

The radiosensitivity of a tissue or organ is a function of the most sensitive cell it contains.[45] For example, the testes and bone marrow are considered radiosensitive because of the presence of VIM stem cells in their parenchymal compartments. In these two organs, parenchymal cells are damaged at lower radiation doses than stromal cells (fibroblasts and endothelial cells). Radiation-induced sterility in males can occur after high doses because of destruction of immature spermatogonia cells that were destined to become mature spermatozoa.[70] A decrease in circulating erythrocytes in the blood after irradiation is due to destruction of the more sensitive stem cell (erythroblast) in the bone marrow.[60]

Tissues and organs that contain only RPM or FPM parenchymal cells are therefore more radioresistant. Examples include the liver, muscle, brain, and spinal cord. In this situation, stromal cells are damaged at lower doses than parenchymal cells. Blood vessels in these organs become damaged, thus decreasing blood flow and therefore the supply of oxygen and nutrients to the parenchymal cells. Therefore radiation-induced death of parenchymal cells in these organs is predominantly due to stromal damage. This form of indirect cell death is a significant mechanism of radiation damage in radioresistant tissues and organs.

CELLULAR RESPONSE TO RADIATION

Since the mid 1950s, when Puck and Marcus[42] first irradiated human cervical carcinoma cells in a Petri dish, the response of human, animal, and plant cells to radiation has been intensely studied. The response of cells after irradiation can now be placed into one of three categories: interphase death, division delay, or reproductive failure.

Interphase death

If irradiation of the cell during the G_1, S, or G_2 phase results in death, this mode of response is termed an *interphase death*.[62] This form of cell response can occur in nondividing cells (such as adult nerve cells) and rapidly dividing cells. In general, radiosensitive cells (VIM and DIM) succumb to an interphase death at lower radiation doses than radioresistant cells (RPM and FPM). The exception to this is the lympho-cyte, which is sensitive to interphase death at a dose as low as 50 cGy. In most cell types (except the lymphocyte), interphase death is not the primary mode of response to irradiation. The mechanism of interphase death is not clear but may involve damage to one or more biochemical pathways involved in cell metabolism.

Division delay

Another mode of cell response is known as *division delay*,[62] which after irradiation involves a disruption in the mitotic index (MI), the ratio of the number of mitotic cells to the total number of cells in the irradiated population. This results in cells in interphase at the time of irradiation to be delayed in the G_2 phase. This is known as *mitotic delay*.

The consequence of mitotic delay is a decrease in the MI for the population, which means that fewer cells than normal will enter mitosis and divide. Therefore fewer new daughter cells will be produced. The magnitude of this response to radiation is dose dependent; the higher the radiation dose, the longer the mitotic delay and therefore the greater the decrease in MI. If the dose is less than 1000 cGy, most cell lines recover and eventually proceed through mitosis. This results in a higher than normal number of cells dividing and is termed *mitotic overshoot*.

Canti and Spear first observed division delay in 1929 when they exposed chick fibroblasts in vitro to various doses of radiation.[11] The mechanism behind division delay is thought to involve the inhibition or delay of DNA and/or protein synthesis after irradiation. Apparently, cells attempt to repair radiation damage before mitosis by stopping in the G_2 phase to confirm that the DNA and proteins are intact. Any damage found is repaired during this phase of the cell cycle so that it does not disrupt cell division or possibly lead to cell death.

Reproductive failure

The third and most common endpoint for response of cells to radiation is **reproductive failure,**[42] which is defined as a decrease in the reproductive integrity or ability of a cell to undergo an indefinite number of divisions after irradiation. This effect on the reproductive capacity of cells can be traced to the extent of chromosome damage induced by the radiation dose.

Puck and Marcus[42] first quantified this effect in 1956 when they irradiated human cervical cancer cells (known as *HeLa cells*) in vitro and plotted the results (number of colonies formed) on a semilogarithmic graph. Their results, termed a *survival curve*, was a plot of the radiation dose administered on the x-axis versus the surviving fraction of cells on the y-axis (Fig. 9-5).

This survival curve is characteristic of the survival of cells exposed to low-LET radiations such as x-rays or gamma rays. A shoulder region or flattening of the curve occurs at doses below 150 cGy and indicates that cells must accumulate damage in multiple targets to be killed. Because this sur-

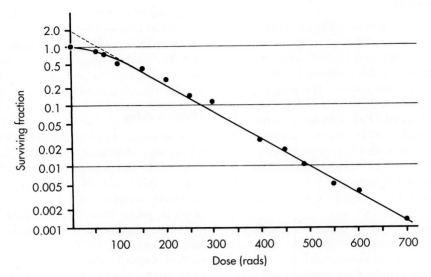

Fig. 9-5 The first survival curve using HeLa cells by Puck and Marcus. Below 150 cGy the curve exhibits a shoulder region and becomes exponential (straight) at higher doses. (From Puck TT, Marcus TI: Action of x-rays on mammalian cells, *J Exp Med* 103:653, 1956.)

Table 9-2	The exponential relationship between a radiation dose and surviving fraction		
Original cell number	Dose delivered (Gy)	Fraction of cells killed	Number of cells killed
100,000	5	50	50,000
50,000	5	50	25,000
25,000	5	50	12,500
12,500	5	50	6,250
6,250	5	50	3,125

From Travis EL: *Primer of medical radiobiology,* ed 2, St Louis, 1989, Mosby.

vival curve is graphed on a semilog plot, the linear portion of the curve (above a dose of 150 cGy) indicates that equal increases in dose causes equal decreases in the surviving fraction of cells (SF) but the absolute number of cells killed varies[62] (Table 9-2).

This exponential response of cells to radiation is due to the random probability of radiation interacting with critical targets in the cell. On irradiation of a cell population with n targets/cell (with n > 1), (1) some cells are lethally damaged (all targets are hit), (2) some cells are sublethally damaged (a few targets are hit), and (3) some cells are not damaged (no targets are hit). As the radiation dose increases, the probability of cellular targets being hit also increases.

Cell survival curves now exist for numerous cell lines exposed to various types of ionizing radiations. Three important parameters that allow interpretation of survival curves are the **extrapolation number (n)**, D_0 dose, and quasi-

threshold dose (D_q). A characteristic survival curve for cells exposed to x-rays is shown in Fig. 9-6.[10]

The n, originally known as the *target number*, is determined by extrapolating the linear portion of the curve back until it intersects the y-axis. In Fig. 9-6, the n equals 2, which theoretically means two critical targets are in the cell and must be inactivated. For mammalian cells exposed to x-rays the n ranges from 2 to 10. With the exception of simple, single-celled organisms such as bacteria (in which n probably equals 1), n is likely greater than or equal to 2 for complex cell types.

Another measure of cell response at low doses is the D_q. This parameter represents the dose at which survival becomes exponential. The D_q is a measure of the width of the shoulder region of the survival curve and is determined by drawing a horizontal line from an SF of 1 on the y-axis to the place it intersects the line extrapolated back from the linear portion of the curve for determination of n. The D_q is also a measure of the cell's ability to accumulate and repair sublethal damage.[6,19]

The third parameter, known as the D_0 *(or D_{37}) dose,* reduces the surviving fraction of cells by 63%. In other words, 37% of the cells survive. The D_0 equals the reciprocal of the slope of the curve's linear portion, and is a measure of the cells' radiosensitivity. Radiosensitive cells have a low D_0 whereas radioresistant cells have a high D_0. For mammalian cells the D_0 usually is between 100 to 220 cGy.[26]

Several equations describe the dose-response relationships expressed by survival curves.[10] The three survival-curve parameters are related by the equation $\log_e n = D_q/D_0$. The surviving fraction can be calculated as $SF = 1 - (1 - e^{-D/D_0})^n$. In

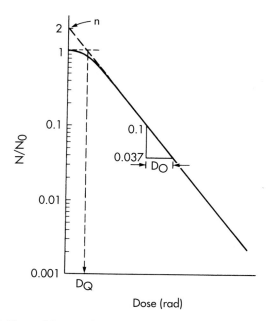

Fig. 9-6 The multitarget, single-hit model of cell survival characteristic of low-LET radiations (x-rays and gamma rays). The parameters n, D_o, and D_q should be noted. (From Bushong SC: *Radiologic science for technologists: physics, biology, and protection,* St Louis, 1993, Mosby.)

this equation, n is the extrapolation number and D is the total dose.[10] This equation accurately predicts the response of complex cell types, including most mammalian cells in which the number of targets is presumed to be greater than one. (This is known as the *multitarget, single-hit model.*)

Factors influencing response

As proposed by Ancel and Vitemberger in 1925, various external factors influence cellular response to radiation.[3] This change in response is termed *conditional sensitivity.* Three groups of factors (physical, chemical, and biological) can affect cellular radioresponse and therefore change the overall appearance of a cell line's survival curve and magnitude of the parameters n, D_q, and D_o.

Physical factors. The response of cells to high-LET radiation differs from that seen after exposure to low-LET radiation.[8] The response of five mammalian cell lines to 300-kV x-rays and 15-MeV neutrons is shown in Fig. 9-7. The shoulder region (D_q) is usually decreased or even absent after irradiation with high-LET radiations such as alpha particles and neutrons. In addition, survival curves tend to be steeper (the D_o is lower) after high-LET treatment. The effects of LET on biological response are due to differences in the density of energy deposition in the cell. Because DNA is thought to be the critical target in cells, the most efficient radiation with the highest RBE induces two strand breaks in the DNA molecule, thus leading to a high probability of cell death. This optimum LET is thought to be approximately

160 keV/μm. Therefore all radiations with LETs above or below the optimum level are less efficient (having a lower RBE) in terms of cell killing.

A second physical factor that influences cellular radioresponse is dose rate.[5] A dose-rate effect has been observed for reproductive failure, division delay, chromosome aberrations, and survival time after whole-body irradiation. Low dose rates are less efficient in producing damage than high dose rates. Survival curves generally shift to the right, thus becoming shallower (D_o increases), and the shoulder becomes indistinguishable at low dose rates (Fig. 9-8). This change in the appearance of the survival curve is explained by the cells' ability to repair sublethal damage from radiation treatment during and after exposure when given at a low enough dose rate. This dose-rate effect is significant with low-LET radiations such as x-rays and gamma rays but is not observed with high-LET radiations.

Chemical factors. Two major chemical factors influence cellular response to radiation. Certain chemicals that enhance response to radiation are known as **radiosensitizers**. Other chemicals, termed **radioprotectors**, have the opposite effect (i.e., they decrease the cellular response to radiation).

The most potent radiosensitizer to date is molecular oxygen. The oxygen effect has been observed in all organisms exposed to ionizing radiation.[72] Although the exact mechanism of the oxygen effect is unknown, the presence of oxygen may enhance the formation of free radicals and fix or make permanent radiation damage that is otherwise reversible. Oxygen must be present during the radiation exposure for sensitization to occur. The sensitizing effects of oxygen are most significant with low-LET radiations in which indirect effects caused by free radical formation predominate over direct effects.

Cell survival curves differ for oxic (normal oxygen level) versus hypoxic (reduced oxygen level) cell populations.[9] As the availability of oxygen decreases, cell response also decreases such that the survival curve shifts to the right because D_q and D_o increase. This effect is most pronounced with x-rays and gamma rays. The effects are less as the LET of the radiation increases (Fig. 9-9). The magnitude of the oxygen effect is termed the **oxygen enhancement ratio (OER)**.[26] The OER compares the response of cells with radiation in the presence and absence of oxygen. The equation for determining the OER for ionizing radiations is as follows:

$$OER = \frac{\text{Radiation dose under hypoxic/anoxic conditions}}{\substack{\text{Radiation dose under oxic conditions to produce} \\ \text{the same biological effect}}}$$

One common endpoint used for determination of the OER is the D_o. For example, if the D_o = 300 cGy under hypoxic conditions but is reduced to 100 cGy under oxic conditions, the OER for the radiation in the experiment is 300/100 = 3.0. For mammalian cells the OER for x-rays and gamma rays is

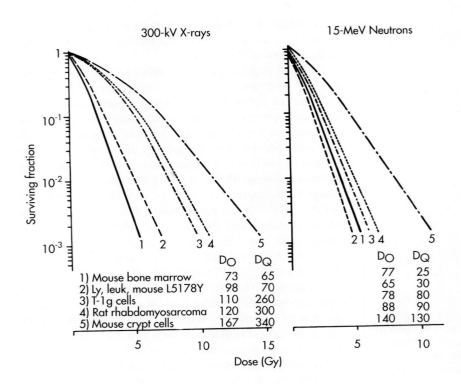

Fig. 9-7 Survival curves for various types of mammalian cells irradiated with 300-kV x-rays or 15-MeV neutrons. The wide variability in the shoulder (D_q) and slope (D_o) seen in the x-ray survival curves is reduced after neutron irradiation. The D_o and D_q values shown are expressed in cGy. (From Broerse JJ, Barendsen GW: Current topics, *Radiat Res Q* 8:305-350, 1973.)

300-kV X-rays

	D_O	D_Q
1) Mouse bone marrow	73	65
2) Ly, leuk, mouse L5178Y	98	70
3) T-1g cells	110	260
4) Rat rhabdomyosarcoma	120	300
5) Mouse crypt cells	167	340

15-MeV Neutrons

D_O	D_Q
77	25
65	30
78	80
88	90
140	130

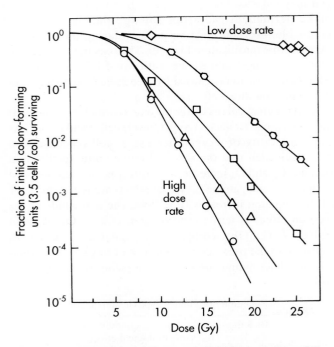

Fig. 9-8 Dose-response curves for an established mammalian cell line irradiated with a wide range of dose rates from a high of 1.07 Gy/min to a low of 0.0036 Gy/min. Reducing the dose rate makes the survival curve more shallow and causes the shoulder to eventually disappear. (From Bedford JS, Mitchell JB: Dose-rates effects in synchronous mammalian cells in culture, *Radiat Res* 54:316-327, 1973.)

generally 2.5 to 3.0. This means that hypoxic cells are 2.5 to 3.0 times more resistant than oxic cells to a dose of low-LET radiation. The oxygen effect is less significant with neutrons[24] (OER = 1.6) and may not be observable with high-LET radiations such as alpha particles (OER = 1.0).

Whereas oxygenation conditions are easily modifiable with cells in vitro, measurement of oxygen levels (known as *oxygen tension* or pO_2) are more difficult to determine and modify in vivo. In vivo oxygen tensions of 20 to 30 mmHg appear to render cells fully sensitive to low-LET radiations. The radiosensitivity of cells decreases as the pO_2 decreases, thus limiting the response of hypoxic cells in tumors treated with radiation.

Other compounds have also been tested as radiosensitizers. Most notable among these are halogenated pyrimidines and nitroimidazoles. Halogenated pyrimidines such as 5-bromodeoxyuridine and 5-iododeoxyuridine are analogs of the DNA base thymidine.[27] These agents act as nonhypoxic cell sensitizers and are taken up by cycling cells during DNA synthesis (S phase). If enough of these compounds are substituted for thymidine, the DNA of the cell becomes more susceptible to radiation by a factor approaching 2. The rationale for the clinical use of these compounds is based on the shorter cycle times observed for tumor cells versus their normal cell counterparts. This should result in preferential uptake by tumors.

Nitroimidazoles such as misonidazole are oxygen-mimicking agents[1] (i.e., they behave chemically like oxygen

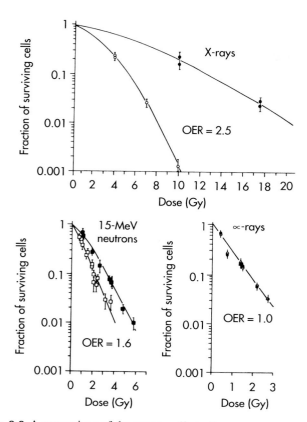

Fig. 9-9 A comparison of the oxygen effect after x-ray, neutron, or alpha-particle irradiation. The OER is highest after sparsely ionizing radiations (OER = 2.5), compared with densely ionizing radiations such as alpha particles (OER = 1.0). In the x-ray and neutron curves shown, the curve to the left represents the response of oxic cells and the curve to the right represents the hypoxic cell response. The oxic and hypoxic curves overlap when alpha particles are used. (From Broerse JJ, Barendsen GW, van Kersen GR: Survival of cultured human cells after irradiation with fast neutrons at different energies in hypoxic and oxygenated conditions, *Int J Radiat Biol* 13:559-572, 1967.)

in terms of indirect effects involving free radicals). In addition, nitroimidazoles may diffuse further than oxygen from blood vessels, thereby reaching radioresistant hypoxic cells in a tumor. These agents are classified as *hypoxic cell sensitizers.* The idea behind their use is to selectively increase the radiosensitivity of hypoxic tumor cells. This desired selective sensitization of tumors has not been achieved in the clinic. Two major reasons for this are that (1) neither of these sensitizing agents exclusively localizes in malignant tissue and (2) both of these agents cause side effects at therapeutic doses. New and improved sensitizing agents that localize in malignant tissues without toxic side effects are under development in the United States and England.

In some clinical situations, attempts have been made to protect normal tissues instead of sensitizing tumors to a dose of radiation. The agents used are known as *radiation protectors,* or *dose-modifying compounds.*[39] The most important group of protectors are sulfhydryls, agents that contain a free or potentially free sulfur (S) atom in their structure. Examples of sulfhydryls include cysteine, cysteamine, and WR-2721. Sulfhydryls act as free radical scavengers that compete with oxygen for free radicals formed after the radiolysis of water. If the sulfhydryl binds to the free radical before the oxygen does, the free radical can decay back to a harmless chemical species instead of causing damage to vital structures in the cell. The ability of a radioprotector to diminish the effects of a dose of radiation is called the *dose reduction factor (DRF).* The equation for determining the DRF is as follows[26]:

$$DRF = \frac{\text{Radiation dose with the radioprotector}}{\begin{array}{c}\text{Radiation dose without the radioprotector}\\\text{to produce an equal biological effect}\end{array}}$$

As with the oxygen effect, radioprotectors must be present during the irradiation. In practice, radioprotectors are administered at short time intervals (within 30 minutes) before radiation therapy. In general, this allows uptake by normal tissues so that they are protected without allowing enough time for significant tumor uptake. This therefore precludes protection of the tumor. If the radioprotector is effective, a DRF of 2.0 to 2.7 may be achieved, depending on the normal tissue that is involved. Similar to the oxygen effect, protection by sulfhydryls is much more significant against low-LET radiations that depend on free radical mechanisms, whereas little or no protection against high-LET radiations can be achieved. As with radiosensitizers, therapeutic doses of radioprotectors often cause side effects in patients. This has limited the widespread clinical use of radioprotectors.

Biological factors. Cellular response is also affected by two important biological factors: position in the cell cycle and ability to repair sublethal damage. Cellular radiosensitivity is dependent on the specific phase of the cell cycle containing the cells at the time of irradiation. (This is also referred to as *age response.*) In general, cells are most sensitive in the G_2 and M phases, of intermediate sensitivity in the G_1 phase, and most resistant in the S phase, especially during late S[53] (Fig. 9-10). This variation in response of cells should not be discounted because the D_0 for late S-phase cells may be as much as 2.5 times higher than for the same cells in the G_2 and M phases. During irradiation of asynchronous cells with low doses, the majority of survivors are expected to be S-phase cells.

In addition to the variation in sensitivity caused by position in the cell cycle, Elkind and Sutton-Gilbert showed in 1960 that cell survival increases if a dose of radiation is administered in fractions as a split dose instead of as a single dose (with the total dose remaining the same).[19] Elkind and Sutton-Gilbert showed that, depending on the time interval between each fraction, the survival curve parameters n, D_q,

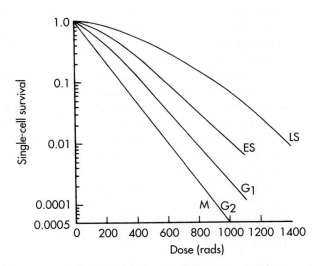

Fig. 9-10 The effect of cell-cycle position on survival of a synchronous population of cells. The M and G_2 phases are the most radiosensitive, whereas the early S period *(ES)* and late S period *(LS)* are the most resistant. (From Sinclair WK: Cyclic responses in mammalian cells in vitro, *Radiat Res* 33:620, 1968.)

and D_0 can remain the same as expected after a single-dose treatment. With low-LET radiations, Elkind and Sutton-Gilbert showed that the shoulder on the survival curve repeated after each fraction. This indicated that cells were repairing sublethal damage from the first fraction before exposure to the second fraction. This repair of sublethal damage after low-LET irradiation appears to be completed in most cell lines tested within several hours of each exposure depending on the dose/fraction. This repair of sublethal damage in normal tissues during fractionated radiation therapy in the clinic may account for the sparing of normal tissues relative to tumors. In addition, hypoxia reduces a cell's capacity to repair sublethal damage. This may partially account for the favorable tumor responses after fractionation compared with single-dose radiation therapy.

SYSTEMIC RESPONSE TO RADIATION
Response and healing

Response to ionizing radiation treatment refers to visible (detectable) structural and functional changes that a dose produces in a certain period. Response at all levels (whether in a cell, a tissue, an organ, a system, or the entire organism) is a function of the dose administered, the volume irradiated, and the time of observation after exposure. With the exception of cataracts of the ocular lens, radiation-induced changes are neither unique nor distinguishable from biological effects caused by other forms of trauma.

Structural or morphological response after irradiation is usually grouped into two phases: early or acute changes observed within 6 months of treatment and late or chronic

changes occurring more than 6 months later.[62] The appearance of late changes is a consequence of early changes that were irreversible and progressive. The probability of late changes occurring depends on the dose administered, the volume irradiated, and the healing ability of the irradiated structure (organ).

Organ healing can occur after radiation exposure by the process of regeneration or repair.[62] *Regeneration* refers to the replacement of damaged cells by the same cell type. Regeneration results in partial or total reversal of early radiation changes and is likely to occur in organs containing actively dividing VIM and DIM parenchymal cells. Examples include the skin, small intestine, and bone marrow. Regeneration is the desired healing process and can restore an organ to its preirradiated state.

Irreversible early changes, however, heal by the process of repair. *Repair* refers to the replacement of damaged cells by a different cell type, thus resulting in scar formation or fibrosis. Healing by repair does not restore an organ to its preirradiated state. Repair can occur in any organ and is more likely after high doses (1000 cGy or above) that destroy parenchymal cells, thus making regeneration impossible. Repair is the predominant healing process in radioresistant organs containing RPM and FPM parenchymal cells that do not divide or have lost the ability to do so.

Under conditions that produce massive and extensive damage to the organ, neither healing process may occur and tissue death or necrosis results. Therefore the type of healing if any that occurs is a function of the dose received and volume of the organ receiving it.

The other important factor that must be considered is the time after the treatment. In general, radiosensitive organs (e.g., skin) respond faster and more severely than radioresistant organs.[62] The reverse situation may hold true at a later time. For example, irradiation of skin and lung tissue with a dose of 2000 cGy induces severe early skin changes but minimal early lung changes (within 6 months). However, if the same tissues are examined 6 to 12 months after irradiation, minimal late changes are found in the skin but severe late changes are observed in the lung. This rate of response depends mostly on the cell cycle or generation times of the parenchymal cells in each organ. Because most cells die when attempting to divide after irradiation, cells with short cycle times show radiation damage sooner than cells with long cycle times. In comparing skin and lung parenchymal cells, cycle times are considerably shorter for parenchymal cells of the skin.

General organ changes

The most common early or acute changes after irradiation include inflammation, edema, and possible hemorrhaging in the exposed area. If doses are high enough, these early changes may progress to characteristic late or chronic changes, including fibrosis, atrophy, and ulceration. These late changes are not reversible and therefore permanent. The most severe late response is tissue necrosis or death. The sensitivity of the most radiosensitive organ of a system determines the general response of that system in the body.

Hematopoietic system

The hematopoietic system includes the bone marrow, circulating blood, lymph nodes, spleen, and thymus. This discussion is limited to radiation effects on the bone marrow and circulating blood.

Bone marrow contains parenchymal cells, including undifferentiated stem cells, circulating differentiated (end) cells, fat cells, and a connective-tissue stroma. Adults have two types of marrow: red and yellow. Red marrow supplies mature cells to the circulating blood and consists of numerous stem cells and fewer fat cells. Red marrow is present in the ribs, ends of the long bones, vertebrae, sternum, and skull bones. Yellow marrow consists primarily of fat cells, thus giving rise to the name *fatty marrow*. Because yellow marrow does not supply mature cells to the circulation, only red-marrow response to irradiation is presented.

The primary effect of radiation on bone marrow is a decrease in the number of stem cells.[60] Low doses (< 100 cGy) lead to a slight decrease in the stem cell count, but recovery should be complete in several weeks. Higher doses may cause a more severe, possibly permanent depletion of stem cells. In addition, an increase in the number of fat cells and connective tissue may also occur at higher doses. Stem cells in bone marrow are extremely radiosensitive, but each stem cell's response varies. The most radiosensitive stem cell is the erythroblast, which is the precursor to the erythrocyte, or red blood cell. Myelocytes (precursors to white blood cells) are next in sensitivity, and megakaryocytes (precursors to platelets) are the least sensitive of the three. Therefore after a dose of radiation, erythroblasts decrease first, then myelocytes, and finally megakaryocytes. Depending on the dose, recovery takes at least 1 week for erythroblasts and approximately 2 to 6 weeks for myelocytes and megakaryocytes.

In comparison with these stem cells, circulating blood cells (except lymphocytes) are relatively radioresistant. Radiation damage to bone marrow is eventually reflected in decreases in circulating blood cells. The order of decrease in end cells in the blood depends on the sensitivity and circulating life span of each stem cell. In addition, all cells in the circulation have finite life spans ranging from 24 hours for granulocytes to 120 days for erythrocytes. Therefore after radiation exposure, lymphocytes decrease first (minimum dose = 10 cGy), then neutrophils (minimum dose = 50 cGy), and finally platelets and erythrocytes (minimum dose > 50 cGy).[62] Decreases in the number of these cells in circulation can have serious consequences. Because neutrophils and lymphocytes are important components of the immune system, decreases in their levels can lead to infec-

tion. A decrease in platelets can result in hemorrhaging, and a decrease in erythrocytes leads to anemia. The extent and reversibility of these conditions is a function of the radiation dose received.

Skin

The radioresponse of human skin has been well documented since Roentgen's discovery of the x-ray in 1895.[38] As with all organs, skin response after irradiation is related to characteristics of its component cells. The outermost layer of cells, known as the *epidermis*, consists of mature, nondividing cells at the surface and immature, dividing cells at the base. Cells lost (sloughed off) from the surface are replaced by cells at the base, known as *basal cells*. The skin as a whole is considered radiosensitive because of characteristics of these basal cells. Early skin changes after moderate (100 to 1000 cGy) or high (> 1000 cGy) radiation doses include inflammation, erythema, and dry or moist desquamation. Erythema similar to that observed after overexposure to ultraviolet radiation (sunburn) is induced by a dose of 1000 cGy. Moderate doses allow healing in the epidermis by regeneration. Late changes after high doses include atrophy, fibrosis, increased or decreased levels of pigmentation, ulceration, necrosis, and possibly skin cancer years later.

Below the epidermis lies the dermis, which contains the vasculature and several accessory structures, including hair follicles and sebaceous and sweat glands. Because hair follicles are actively growing, they are radiosensitive. Moderate doses can result in temporary epilation (hair loss) and alopecia (balding), whereas doses in excess of 1000 cGy may result in permanent epilation. Although sebaceous and sweat glands are relatively radioresistant, high doses can result in glandular atrophy, fibrosis, and consequent loss of function.

Digestive system

The digestive system is composed of a closed tube lined by a mucous membrane from one end to the other. This tube, known as the *alimentary canal*, begins with the oral cavity (mouth) and includes the esophagus, stomach, duodenum and jejunum (small intestine), colon (large intestine), and rectum. (The liver, usually also considered part of the digestive system, will be considered separately.) The mucous membrane contains layers of cells (like the skin), some of which are undifferentiated and dividing (radiosensitive) and others that are differentiated and nondividing (radioresistant).

A common effect of moderate radiation doses is inflammation in the oral cavity (mucositis) and esophagus (esophagitis). This early change usually heals if the dose is below 1000 cGy. Higher doses may result in atrophy, ulceration, fibrosis, and esophageal stricture. The same late changes occur in the more radiosensitive stomach at lower doses.

The small intestine represents the most radiosensitive portion of the gastrointestinal tract.[69] The lining of the small intestine consists of fingerlike projections known as *villi*, which increase the surface area available to cells for absorption of digested materials. The cells of the villi are nondividing and slough off daily. They are replaced by cells from the crypts of Lieberkühn (crypt cells) located at the base. These crypt cells are rapidly dividing, undifferentiated stem cells and are therefore extremely radiosensitive. Radiation damage in the small intestine is the result of direct damage to crypt cells.

Radiation doses below 1000 cGy result in decreased mitotic activity of crypt cells followed by shortening of the villi. Regeneration of crypt cells gradually repopulates the villi again. Radiation doses above 1000 cGy induce much more pronounced effects (see the discussion on the gastrointestinal syndrome). Doses of this magnitude result in a shortening and eventual flattening of the villi because of a severe depopulation of crypt cells. Minimal recovery occurs under these conditions. The intestine may undergo denudation (villi are completely flat) with ulceration, hemorrhaging, fibrosis, and necrosis. These effects, when induced by a whole-body dose of 1000 cGy or more, invariably lead to death in 30 to 60 days. Radiation damage to the large intestine and rectum are similar after such high doses.

Reproductive system

Most tissues of the male reproductive system (except the testes) are radioresistant.[70] The testes contain radioresistant end cells (mature spermatozoa or sperm) and radiosensitive stem cells known as *immature spermatogonia*. The primary effect of irradiation of the testes is damage and depopulation of spermatogonia. This eventually leads to a depletion of mature sperm (known as *maturation depletion*). After exposure, temporary or permanent sterility may occur depending on the radiation dose. Sterility is ultimately due to the loss of immature spermatogonia and permanent after an acute dose of 500 to 600 cGy. A dose of 250 cGy may induce temporary sterility for a period of up to 12 months. An additional hazard of testicular irradiation is the production of chromosome aberrations in surviving germ (reproductive) cells capable of fertilization. This may result in the transmission of genetic abnormalities to subsequent generations.

In females the oocytes (eggs) are contained in saclike structures known as *follicles* in the ovaries. The size of these follicles determines their radiosensitivity. Small follicles are the most resistant, intermediate-sized follicles are the most sensitive, and large follicles have an intermediate sensitivity.[26] In females, germ cells do not constantly divide (as spermatogonia do in males). Therefore an oocyte is not replaced when it is released from a mature follicle (ovulation). After ovulation, fertilization or menstruation occurs. Moderate doses of radiation (below 300 cGy) to the ovaries usually result in temporary sterility soon after exposure. Doses above 600 cGy likely induce permanent sterility in most exposed females, although age is an important factor (young women are more resistant than older women). As in the male, genetic effects are a major concern in surviving, mature oocytes capable of fertilization.

Eye

The ocular lens contains actively dividing cells that may be damaged after radiation exposure to the orbital region (eyes).[26] Because no mechanism exists for removal of these damaged cells, the lens eventually becomes opaque as a result of a cataract's formation. Cataracts are rare in patients receiving doses up to 200 cGy, but the incidence is 100% with an acute dose of 700 cGy. The degree of visual impairment is minimal after 200 cGy but is progressive with increasing doses. Cataracts are classified as a nonstochastic, late effect of radiation. In other words, cataracts do not occur below an apparent threshold dose, and above this threshold the severity of the opacity increases with the dose.[26] The apparent threshold doses for cataracts are approximately 400 cGy (single dose) and 1200 cGy when fractionated. Eye shields should be used when possible to minimize the dose to the lens during therapeutic or diagnostic procedures. Radiation-induced cataracts do not become evident for many years (known as the *latent period*) after radiation exposure, and they typically progress in a different pattern than naturally occurring cataracts. Long-term follow-up of potential cataract patients is therefore required to document the occurrence and unique progression of this late effect of radiation.

Cardiovascular system

The extensive cardiovascular network is a common target of radiation-induced damage. Vessel occlusion may result from radiation damage to endothelial cells and lead to hemorrhaging and blood-clot formation (thrombosis). Small vessels tend to be more sensitive than larger vessels. If high enough doses are received, late changes in vessels (including petechial hemorrhages, telangiectasia, and vessel sclerosis) may result. The heart itself is considered to be relatively radioresistant.[62] Low-to-moderate doses of radiation do not usually result in obvious damage except for functional electrocardiographic changes, but high doses (4000 cGy or more) may result in pericarditis and even pancarditis.

Bone and cartilage

Mature bone and cartilage are radioresistant. However, growing bone and cartilage are moderately radiosensitive.[62] The parenchyma of growing bone and cartilage consists of resistant osteocytes and chondrocytes (nondividing, differentiated cells) and more sensitive osteoblasts and chondroblasts (rapidly dividing, undifferentiated cells). In addition, radiation injury to small blood vessels and bone marrow cells contributes to damage to growing bone.

High doses of radiation may produce permanent depopulation of proliferating stem cells in the bone and eventually lead to cessation of bone growth. Late changes after high doses include altered shapes and sizes of the bones irradiated and scoliosis. Radiation therapy for certain malignancies in children that involve irradiation of one or more bones in the treatment field may produce permanent bone changes. The incidence of radiation-induced bone abnormalities decreases with the decreasing dose and increasing age of the patient.

Liver

The liver is moderately sensitive to radiation treatment.[45] The parenchymal cells in the liver are RPM cells and are therefore relatively resistant. These cells normally do not divide but are capable of doing so. Because of the abundant vascular supply of the liver, damage to parenchymal cells is likely to be indirectly caused by vessel damage and the resulting decrease in oxygen and nutrient levels to these cells. After high doses, the liver may enlarge and fluid may accumulate in the abdominal cavity (referred to as *ascites*). Late changes in the liver, collectively known as *radiation hepatitis*, occur as a result of vascular sclerosis and consist primarily of fibrosis (cirrhosis) and possibly necrosis. Liver function eventually becomes impaired, thus resulting in liver failure and jaundice. Total doses of 3500 to 4500 cGy delivered in a standard, fractionated schedule to the majority of the liver can induce radiation hepatitis.[62] This effect is dependent on the volume of the liver irradiated because the tolerance of the liver (or any organ) increases as the volume irradiated decreases.

Respiratory system

The respiratory system includes the nose, pharynx, trachea, and lungs. This section concerns the response of lungs to radiation treatment. Lungs are late-responding organs of moderate radiosensitivity.[63] The primary early change after radiation is inflammation or radiation pneumonitis. Recovery usually occurs after moderate doses (below 1000 cGy). High doses above 1000 cGy to both lungs produce progressive reactions ranging from inflammation (early) to chronic fibrosis (late). Progressive fibrosis is likely in 50% of patients receiving 3000 cGy to both lungs. Higher doses are tolerable if only one lung is being treated.

Urinary system

The urinary system consists of the kidneys, ureters, urinary bladder, and urethra. The response of the kidneys to radiation is significant during irradiation of the abdominal cavity. Kidneys are also late responding and moderately radiosensitive to radiation (similar to lungs). As with the liver, radiation injury to parenchymal cells is primarily due to damage to the vascular stroma.[71] Radiation-induced changes in the kidney, termed *radiation nephritis*, range from edema (early) to atrophy, fibrosis, hypertension, and renal failure (late). Fractionated radiation therapy consisting of more than 2500 cGy over 5 weeks to the abdomen results in a high probabil-

ity of fatal radiation nephritis if the kidneys are not shielded.[62] As with the lungs, these early and late changes are diminished if only one or a portion of one kidney is involved.

Central nervous system

The central nervous system, consisting of the brain and spinal cord, is the most radioresistant system in the adult human.[45] Parenchymal cells are nondividing and fully differentiated and therefore nonresponsive to low radiation doses. The primary early change observed after high doses (1000 cGy or above) is inflammation (referred to as *myelitis* if occurring in the spinal cord). Late changes, including fibrosis and necrosis, are likely at doses in excess of 2000 cGy as a consequence of progressive vascular changes. Radiation necrosis in the brain is a common late effect after a total dose of 5000 cGy.[62] Spinal cord response varies depending on the total volume and part of the cord involved. The cervical and thoracic regions are more sensitive than the lumbar region. Radiation myelitis is commonly induced by doses of 4500 to 5000 cGy even if small volumes of the spinal cord are involved. Because the brain and spinal cord are often included in the treatment for a number of diseases, great care should be given to avoid unnecessary exposure to these structures.

TOTAL-BODY RESPONSE TO RADIATION

This section involves specific signs and symptoms induced by exposure of the entire body at one time to ionizing radiation. The total-body response to radiation is presented in terms of three radiation syndromes.[26] Characteristics of each syndrome are dependent on the dose received and exposure conditions. Three specific exposure conditions apply in dealing with radiation syndromes: (1) exposure must be acute (minutes); (2) total or nearly total-body exposure must occur; and (3) exposure must be from an external penetrating source rather than ingested, inhaled, or implanted radioactive sources.[62]

Radiation syndromes in animals

The primary effect of acute whole-body exposure to radiation is a dose-dependent, shortened life span in animals that is species specific. This effect on survival is expressed in terms of the **LD$_{50/30}$**, which is the lethal dose to 50% of the exposed population within 30 days. The LD$_{50/30}$ varies considerably among animal species. It ranges from 250 cGy for a pig to 3000 cGy for a salamanderlike amphibian known as a *newt*.[10] The 30-day period is used for small animals because radiation-induced death, if it occurs, usually does so within this time. Humans tend to respond more slowly (for better or worse) to total-body irradiation than lower animals. Therefore the critical period after exposure is usually 60 days instead of 30.[26]

The relationship between dose and survival time is rather straightforward: as the dose increases, the percentage and length of survival typically decreases.[10] If a total-body dose of 100 to 1000 cGy is received, death may occur as a result of damage to the hematopoietic system (bone marrow). This gives rise to the hematopoietic syndrome, the only one of the three radiation syndromes that may have survivors. With doses between 1000 and 10,000 cGy, death occurs primarily as a result of damage in the gastrointestinal tract (small intestine). This is known as the *gastrointestinal syndrome*. Doses above 10,000 cGy give rise to the cerebrovascular syndrome, which reflects damage to the central nervous system.

Animals exposed to these dose ranges of total-body radiation proceed through three stages of response.[62] The first stage of response (the prodromal stage or syndrome) is characterized by nausea, vomiting, and diarrhea. These symptoms last from minutes to days and then subside for a period (known as the *latent stage*), in which animals appear healthy because they have no obvious external symptoms. If a dose of less than 500 cGy is received, this latent stage may last several weeks. If a dose of 10,000 cGy or more is received, this stage may last only several hours or even less. The third and final stage, known as the *manifest illness stage*, marks a return of a variety of symptoms depending on the dose received. At doses indicative of the hematopoietic syndrome, fever and malaise are common. In the gastrointestinal syndrome, severe diarrhea, fever, dehydration, and electrolyte imbalance occur. After high doses indicative of the cerebrovascular syndrome, lethargy, tremors, convulsions, nervousness, watery diarrhea, and coma are observed. The duration of the manifest illness stage ranges from minutes to weeks depending on the dose and is followed by the recovery or death of the animal. Animals typically recover only from the effects of the hematopoietic syndrome, especially under conditions in which the dose is significantly less than the $LD_{50/30}$ for that species.

Radiation syndromes in humans

Although an abundance of animal data regarding the effects of total-body exposure to radiation exists, considerably less human data under the same conditions are available. However, human data are available from (1) industrial and laboratory accidents, (2) fallout from atomic bomb test sites, (3) therapeutic medical exposures, and (4) individuals exposed at Hiroshima and Nagasaki. As with lower animals, humans suffer the three radiation syndromes if the same exposure conditions are met.[26] Table 9-3 contains a summary of the acute radiation syndromes in humans after whole-body irradiation.

Hematopoietic syndrome. The hematopoietic syndrome in humans is induced by total-body doses of 100 to 1000 cGy.[26] The $LD_{50/60}$ for humans is estimated to be between 350 and 400 cGy but varies with age, health, and gender. Typically, females are more resistant than males, and the extremely young and old tend to be a little more sensitive than middle-aged persons. The prodromal stage or syndrome is observed within hours after exposure and is characterized by nausea and vomiting. The latent stage then occurs and lasts from a few days up to 3 weeks. Although the affected individual feels well at this time, bone marrow stem cells are dying. Peripheral blood cell counts decrease during the subsequent manifest illness stage at 3 to 5 weeks after exposure. Depression of all blood cell counts, termed *pancytopenia*, results in anemia (from a decreased number of erythrocytes), hemorrhaging (from a decreased number of platelets), and serious infection (from a decreased number of leukocytes).

Table 9-3	Summary of acute radiation syndromes in humans after whole-body irradiation				
Syndrome	Dose range	Time of death	Organ and system damaged	Signs and symptoms	Recovery time
Hematopoietic	100-1000 cGy*	3 weeks to 2 months	Bone marrow	Decreased number of stem cells in bone marrow, increased amount of fat in bone marrow, pancytopenia, anemia, hemorrhage, and infection	Dose dependent— 3 weeks to 6 months; some individuals do not survive
Gastrointestinal	1000-5000 cGy†	3 to 10 days	Small intestine	Denudation of villi in small intestine, neutropenia, infection, bone marrow depression, electrolyte imbalance, and watery diarrhea	None
Cerebrovascular	> 5000 cGy	< 3 days	Brain	Vasculitis, edema, and meningitis	None

Modified from Travis EL: *Primer of medical radiobiology*, ed 2, St Louis, 1989, Mosby.
R, Roentgen.
*$LD_{50/60}$ for humans in this dose range (450 cGy).
†LD_{100} for humans in this dose range (1000 cGy).

The probability of survival decreases with an increasing dose. The majority of individuals receiving doses less than 300 cGy survive and eventually recover over the next 3 to 6 months. As the dose increases, the survival time decreases. After 300 to 500 cGy, death may occur in 4 to 6 weeks. After 500 to 1000 cGy, death is likely within 2 weeks.[62] No record exists of human survival when the total body dose exceeds 1000 cGy.[26] The primary causes of death from the hematopoietic syndrome are infection and hemorrhaging after destruction of the bone marrow.

Gastrointestinal syndrome. If the total body dose is between 1000 and 10,000 cGy, the gastrointestinal syndrome is induced.[26] This syndrome may also be induced by a dose as low as 600 cGy and overlaps with the cerebrovascular syndrome above doses of 5000 cGy. The mean survival time for this syndrome is 3 to 10 days or up to 2 weeks with medical support and is largely independent of the actual dose received. The prodromal stage occurs within hours after exposure and is characterized by nausea, vomiting, diarrhea, and cramps. The latent stage then occurs 2 to 5 days after exposure. At 5 to 10 days after exposure, nausea, vomiting, diarrhea, and fever mark the manifest illness stage. Death occurs during the second week after exposure.

The gastrointestinal syndrome occurs as a result of damage to the gastrointestinal tract and bone marrow. As discussed previously, the small intestine is the most radiosensitive portion of the digestive system.[69] After exposure to doses in excess of 1000 cGy, severe depopulation of crypt cells leads to partial or complete denudation of the villi lining the lumen of the small intestine. Consequences of this damage include decreased absorption of materials across the intestinal wall, leakage of fluids into the lumen (thus resulting in dehydration), and overwhelming infection as bacteria gain access to the circulating blood. Significant changes in bone marrow also occur, highlighted by a severe decrease in circulating leukocytes. However, death occurs before the other peripheral blood cell counts significantly decrease. Despite attempts at regeneration of crypt cells in the small intestine, bone marrow damage likely leads to death as a result of the overwhelming infection, dehydration, and electrolyte imbalance.

Cerebrovascular syndrome. The third and final radiation syndrome is the cerebrovascular syndrome. This syndrome, which was formerly known as the *central nervous system syndrome*, occurs exclusively above 10,000 cGy but can overlap with the gastrointestinal syndrome because it can be induced by a dose as low as 5000 cGy.[26] Death after such high total-body doses occurs in several days or less. The prodromal stage lasts only minutes to several hours (depending on the dose) and is characterized by nervousness, confusion, severe nausea and vomiting, loss of consciousness, and a burning sensation in the skin. The latent period (if distinguishable) lasts only several hours or less. Within 5 to 6 hours after exposure, the manifest illness stage

begins and is characterized by watery diarrhea, convulsions, coma, and death.

The cause of death from the cerebrovascular syndrome is not completely known at this time. At autopsy, brain parenchymal cells appear almost completely normal despite the high dose. These parenchymal cells are extremely radioresistant fixed postmitotic cells, according to Rubin and Casarett.[45] Autopsy findings show extensive blood vessel (stromal) damage in the brain, thus resulting in vasculitis, meningitis, and edema in the cranial vault. The resulting increase in intracranial pressure is probably the major cause of death. In addition, peripheral blood counts and the villi of the small intestine do not exhibit significant changes in these individuals when examined at autopsy. This is due to the exposed person not living long enough for these effects to become evident.

Response of the embryo and fetus

Radiation exposure can also damage the developing embryo and fetus in utero. Generally, in utero radiation damage is manifested as lethal effects, congenital abnormalities present at birth, or late effects observed years later. These effects can be produced by (1) irradiation of the sperm or ovum before fertilization, thus resulting in inherited effects, or (2) exposure of the fetus to radiation, thus resulting in congenital defects. This section deals only with congenital abnormalities resulting from radiation exposure.

Stages of fetal development. The husband-and-wife research team of Russell and Russell divided fetal development into three stages: preimplantation, major organogenesis, and the fetal growth stage.[48] Extensive mouse studies have established that the effect induced by radiation depends not only on the radiation dose, but also on the time of the exposure's occurrence during gestation.[46] In humans the preimplantation stage occurs from conception (day 0) to 10 days after conception. During this time the fertilized ovum is actively dividing, thus forming a ball of highly undifferentiated cells.

The newly formed ball of cells, known as the *embryo*, then implants in the uterine wall and begins the major organogenesis stage (from day 10 to week 6). During this time, on specific gestational days, embryonic cells differentiate into the stem cells that eventually form each organ in the body. At the end of the sixth week the embryo is known as a *fetus* and enters the fetal growth stage, in which it continues to grow until birth. The central nervous system in the fetus differs from that in the adult because the neuroblasts (stem cells) of the fetus are still mitotically active and not fully differentiated. Therefore unlike that in the adult, the fetal central nervous system is responsive to radiation and can be damaged at relatively low doses.

Radiation effects on mice in utero. During preimplantation the mouse embryo is extremely radiosensitive. The major consequence of radiation exposure during this stage is prenatal death,[47,48] which can be induced by doses that are as low as 10 cGy. In most situations, surviving embryos develop normally during gestation, although a small percentage may exhibit exencephaly (brain formation outside the skull) at birth.

The incidence of prenatal deaths decreases, but the incidence of congenital abnormalities increases when irradiation occurs during major organogenesis.[47,48] Gross abnormalities have been observed in mouse embryos that were exposed to as little as 25 cGy during this stage. The highest frequency of congenital abnormalities takes place when exposure occurs during days 8 to 12 in the mouse (analogous to days 23 to 37 in human embryos).[62] For example, the exposure of mouse embryos on day 9 of gestation results in abnormalities of the ear and nose, whereas exposure on day 10 leads to abnormalities of the bone.

Radiation effects in mouse embryos irradiated during major organogenesis primarily involve the central nervous system and sensory organs (e.g., eyes). The most common central nervous system abnormalities in mice include microcephaly (underdevelopment of the brain) and hydrocephaly (water on the brain). Eye defects include microphthalmia, or small eyes. The musculoskeletal system is also radiosensitive during its development because stunted growth and abnormal limbs can be observed after radiation exposure. Whereas the incidence of prenatal deaths decreases during major organogenesis, the frequency of deaths at birth (neonatal death) peaks during this stage.

The incidence of prenatal and neonatal deaths and congenital abnormalities decrease if radiation exposure occurs during the fetal growth stage.[47,48] High radiation doses are required to induce lethal effects and gross abnormalities in mouse fetuses during this stage. Fetal exposure to radiation may result in late effects such as cancer and sterility later in the animal's life.[55]

Radiation effects on humans in utero. Radiation effects on human embryos have also been investigated with data sources that were described previously (atomic bomb survivors in Japan after World War II, fallout exposures, occupational exposures, and diagnostic or therapeutic exposures of pregnant women).[25,30] Despite the results of the animal studies just presented, a definitive cause-and-effect relationship between radiation and a specific abnormality is difficult to prove in human beings. Two major reasons account for this: (1) The background incidence of spontaneous congenital abnormalities is approximately 6%, and (2) radiation does not induce unique congenital abnormalities (excluding cataracts). Therefore implicating a certain radiation exposure as the sole cause of a specific congenital abnormality is difficult. The results of animal studies have been extrapolated to humans to allow predictions with regard to effects that might occur in irradiated human embryos and fetuses. However, the assumption should not be made that in utero effects in mice will be observed under the same conditions in human beings. Viable comparisons may indicate that the

mouse embryo is slightly more radioresistant than the human embryo. In addition, the mouse gestational period ends in 20 days versus 270 days or more in human beings. Therefore although the same developmental stages occur for the most part in mice and humans, they certainly occur much more rapidly in mice.[62] This should be taken into account during comparisons of animal and human radiation effects in utero.

Unfortunately, human data exist for radiation effects from in utero exposure. A report in 1930 by Murphy and Goldstein described congenital defects (microcephaly) attributed to radiation exposure in utero.[36] In one study of children born to 11 women who were pregnant and received high doses from the bomb dropped in Hiroshima, 7 of the 11 children (64%) had microcephaly and were mentally retarded.[41] In another study of 30 children who were irradiated in utero at Nagasaki, 17 (57%) were affected (7 fetal deaths, 6 neonatal deaths, and 4 surviving children who were mentally retarded).[37]

Dekaban in 1968 studied children born to women irradiated with a therapeutic dose of 250 cGy during various stages of gestation.[16] The results of this study indicated that exposure to the dose during the first 2 to 3 weeks of gestation produced a high frequency of prenatal death but few severe abnormalities in surviving children who were brought to term (similar to the mouse studies). Irradiation between 4 and 11 weeks correlated with severe central nervous system and skeletal abnormalities. The same dose (250 cGy) administered between the eleventh and sixteenth week frequently resulted in mental retardation and microcephaly, whereas irradiation after the twentieth week resulted in functional defects such as sterility.

In summary, although difficult to prove conclusively, the embryo and fetus are considered to be the most radiosensitive forms of animals and humans. Radiation, if it must be administered during a known pregnancy, should be delayed as much as possible because the fetus is more radioresistant than the embryo. As mentioned previously, the most radiosensitive period for induction of abnormalities in humans is between days 23 and 37. These effects usually involve the central nervous system and most commonly include microcephaly, mental retardation, sensory organ damage, and stunted growth. Skeletal changes (bone) appear to be most prevalent when radiation is administered between weeks 3 and 20.

LATE EFFECTS OF RADIATION

The previous section dealt with the total-body response to high doses of radiation, which usually results in lethality. Of equal and possibly even more concern is the biological response resulting from exposure to much lower doses of radiation. Because the latent period for an effect is inversely proportional to radiation dose, the biological response to low doses is not observable for extended periods, ranging from years to generations.[26] These effects are therefore known as *late effects* and are termed *somatic effects* if body cells are involved or *genetic effects* if reproductive (germ) cells are involved.

Somatic effects (carcinogenesis)

Historical background. The most important late somatic effect induced by radiation is carcinogenesis.[64,66] Radiation is therefore classified as a *carcinogen,* or *cancer-causing agent.* In 1902 (only 7 years after Roentgen's discovery of the x-ray) the first reported case of radiation-induced carcinoma appeared in the literature. By 1910 at least 100 cases of skin cancer were reported in radiologists and radiation oncologists who were unaware of the potential hazards of this new modality.

Carcinogenesis is considered to be an all-or-nothing event. This means that any dose, no matter how low, has some potential of inducing cancer. Cancer induction is therefore a nonthreshold event with the probability of an effect increasing as the dose increases. Carcinogenesis is therefore an example of a stochastic effect, in which every dose carries some magnitude of risk.[26]

Sufficient human data exist to implicate radiation as a cancer-causing agent. Most of the early data involve occupational exposures by radiation scientists, clinicians, and therapists who were chronically exposed to various radiation sources before the risks of such exposures were known. Ionizing radiation has been implicated as a cause of skin cancer, leukemia, osteosarcoma, lung cancer, breast cancer, and thyroid cancer.

Leukemia. Radiation was first implicated as a cause of leukemia in 1911. That study involved 11 cases of leukemia in occupationally exposed individuals.[62] Atomic bomb survivors in Hiroshima and Nagasaki had higher incidences of leukemia than the nonexposed population.[26] From 1935 to 1944, approximately 15,000 patients with ankylosing spondylitis in Great Britain received single or fractionated radiation treatment to their spines and pelvic regions, usually in the dose range of 100 to 2000 cGy.[13] An increased incidence of leukemia occurred in these patients, especially those irradiated with doses greater than 2000 cGy. Early radiologists in the United States who died between 1948 and 1961 had a much higher frequency of leukemia (300%) than the general population.[18,31] However, a similar study involving British radiologists showed no increased leukemia incidence in an early group (before 1921) compared with later groups who used some level of radiation safety.[12]

The latent period for leukemia induction by radiation is usually 4 to 7 years with peak incidence approximately 7 to 10 years after exposure. This period is much shorter than that observed for radiation-induced solid tumors, which have latent periods ranging from 20 to 30 years or longer.[26]

Radiation induction of leukemia is somewhat specific in that only certain types of leukemia show an increased incidence in irradiated individuals. For example, only acute and

chronic myeloid leukemia types are more prevalent in irradiated adults, whereas acute lymphocytic leukemia is more common in irradiated children.[14] Radiation exposure does not seem to affect the incidence of chronic lymphocytic leukemia. The available evidence suggests that leukemia induction is a nonthreshold (stochastic), linear response to radiation[62] (Fig. 9-11). However, other cancers induced by radiation may follow linear-quadratic rather than a linear relationship to radiation dose.[26]

Skin carcinoma. The first reported case of radiation-induced skin cancer (which occurred on the hand of a radiologist) was in 1902.[38] Because early x-ray machines were crude, radiologists placed their hands in the beam path to check its efficiency. This led to early skin changes (erythema) that were used to gauge the output of the beam, but skin tumors were observed years later in many of these individuals. Patients treated with radiation for several benign conditions such as acne and ringworm of the scalp also showed an increased incidence of skin cancer years later.[2] As a result of modern radiation safety procedures, skin cancers in radiation workers are no longer observed.

Osteosarcoma. The most striking example of radiation-induced osteosarcoma, or bone cancer, is the group of young female watch-dial painters who used radium to paint clock faces for a company in northern New Jersey from 1915 to 1930.[32] These workers regularly licked their brushes (which contained radium paint) to make the brush tip come to a point before painting the watch dials. This resulted in chronic ingestion of radium, which is a bone-seeking radioactive element.[23] Of the several hundred workers exposed this way,

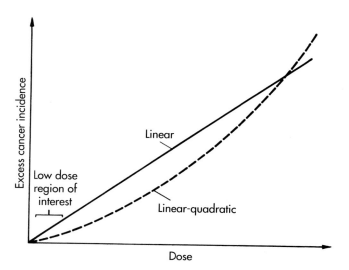

Fig. 9-11 A schematic of the linear and linear-quadratic models used to extrapolate the incidence of cancer from high-dose data down to low doses. Both models fit high-dose data well, but at low doses the estimated incidence depends on the model. (From: Travis EL: *Primer of medical radiobiology,* ed 2, St Louis, 1989, Mosby.)

approximately 40 cases of osteosarcoma were observed years later. The dose response for bone cancer in this group followed a linear-quadratic relationship that was dependent on the activities of the two radium isotopes (^{226}Ra and ^{228}Ra) contained in the paint.[44]

Lung carcinoma. German pitchblende miners in Germany more than 500 years ago suffered from a condition known as *mountain sickness*, which was later determined to be lung cancer.[26] Inhaling chronic amounts of radon gas in the air of the mines, these miners exposed their lungs to high-LET alpha particles that were emitted as the radon decayed. Uranium miners in the United States who were studied from 1950 to 1967 also had an increased incidence of lung cancer, most likely for the same reasons.[49] Radon gas and its decay products are now known to be significant contributors (200 mrem/yr) to annual background radiation levels and are the major risk factors for lung cancer in nonsmokers.

Thyroid carcinoma. Irradiation of enlarged thymuses in children before the 1930s over the dose range from 1200 to 6000 cGy was a popular treatment.[52,61] Unfortunately, a 100-fold increase in thyroid cancer was observed in these children. An increased incidence of thyroid cancer also occurred in individuals exposed as children from the bombs in Hiroshima and Nagasaki. Some of these individuals who developed thyroid cancer may have received doses as low as 100 cGy. Extensive follow-up is required in order to track the occurrence of these tumors because of their typical latent period of 10 to 20 years (which varies inversely with the dose that is received).

Breast carcinoma. Three major groups of irradiated women with increased incidences of breast cancer seem to implicate radiation as the causative agent[26]: (1) irradiated female survivors in Hiroshima and Nagasaki, Japan, (2) Canadian women in a Nova Scotia sanitorium who had tuberculosis and were subjected to numerous fluoroscopies, and (3) women treated for benign breast diseases such as postpartum mastitis. The best data that are available (with the Canadian study as the largest source) indicate that radiation induction of breast cancer most closely follows a linear dose-response relationship.[33]

Nonspecific life-shortening effects

Research studies have shown that animals chronically exposed to low doses of radiation die younger than nonexposed animals.[43] Autopsy examinations (known as *necropsies* in animals) revealed a decreased number of parenchymal cells and blood vessels and an increased amount of connective tissue in organs. These changes resembled those seen in older animals and have been referred to as *radiation-induced aging*.[15] The effect on life span in these animals indicated a nonthreshold, linear relationship with radiation dose. However, more recent studies indicate that the life-shortening effect in these animals was probably due to cancer induction at moderate doses and organ atrophy, cell killing, and

cell loss at high doses. Therefore the life-shortening result can be explained by the occurrence of specific rather than nonspecific effects. Most of the human data available support the statement that specific causes of radiation-induced life shortening are identifiable, although some exceptions to this probably exist.

Genetic effects

Somatic late effects can occur in an irradiated individual, and exposure of reproductive (germ) cells in that individual may affect future generations. As mentioned previously, ionizing radiation is a known mutagen (i.e., it can induce mutations in the genetic material [DNA/genes] found in the cell nucleus). Mutations (which are permanent, heritable [transmittable to subsequent generations], and generally detrimental) occur spontaneously in genes and DNA. The number of spontaneous mutations that occur in each generation of an organism is described as the *mutation frequency*, which can be increased by any mutagenic agent, including radiation.[28] If the mutation frequency in a generation is doubled by exposure to radiation, the radiation dose is then known as the *doubling dose*.[50] In humans the doubling dose is estimated to range from 50 to 250 rem (0.5 to 2.5 Sv) with an average figure given as 100 rem (1.0 Sv).[26]

The classic study that demonstrated the mutagenic potential of radiation was performed by H.J. Müller in 1927 and involved the use of the Drosophila melanogaster, or fruit fly.[35] Müller irradiated male and female fruit flies under a number of conditions and observed the mutation frequencies in the next several generations. The fruit fly was used as the model for these experiments because it has a number of easily identifiable mutations such as those involving its wing shape and eye and body color. In addition, large populations of fruit flies can be maintained and bred relatively quickly and easily.

The results of Müller's fruit fly experiments (which have not been contradicted by subsequent studies with mice) include the following[35]:

1. Radiation does not produce new or unique mutations but increases the frequency of spontaneous mutations in each generation.
2. Mutation frequency is linearly related to radiation dose.
3. Radiation induction of mutations has no clear threshold; it is a stochastic effect like carcinogenesis.

In addition to Müller's experiments, subsequent animal studies have indicated that high dose rates can cause more genetic damage than low dose rates, males are more sensitive than females at low doses and low dose rates to genetic effects, and not all mutations show the same susceptibility to induction by radiation.[26] The estimated doubling dose for humans is based on extrapolations from the numerous animal experiments.

RADIATION THERAPY
Goal of radiation therapy

The goal of radiation therapy for cancer is to eradicate the tumor while not destroying normal tissues in the treatment field. This is easier said than done because radiation interaction in matter is a nonspecific, random process that does not distinguish between malignant and normal tissues. Biological damage can be induced in tumor and normal tissues. Therefore the tolerance of the normal tissue in the treatment field limits the dose that can be administered to the tumor. Several methods have been attempted to deal with this limiting factor during treatment so that more effective tumor treatments can be given. Several of these methods will be discussed in this section.

General tumor characteristics

Parenchymal and stromal compartments. Like normal tissues, malignant tumors are composed of parenchymal and stromal compartments. A tumor parenchyma may contain up to four subpopulations or groups of cells.[62]

Cells belonging to group 1 are viable, actively mitotic (cycling) cells that are responsible for tumor growth. The percentage of group 1 cells in a tumor type usually varies from 30% to 50% and is termed the *growth fraction (GF)*.[34] The GF typically decreases as the size (volume) of the tumor increases.

Group 2 cells are typically viable but nondividing (not cycling). These cells, also known as G_0 *cells*, have retained the ability to reenter the cell cycle and divide if properly stimulated.

Groups 3 or 4 are composed of nonviable cells. Group 3 cells appear structurally intact, whereas group 4 cells do not. Group 3 and 4 cells therefore do not contribute to tumor growth.

The exact percentage of cells in each group varies with the size and type of tumor. In addition, each tumor contains a stromal compartment of blood vessels and connective tissue. In small, newly formed tumors the stroma may be entirely composed of normal host vessels, whereas large, older tumors contain a mix of normal and tumor vessels, or the supporting vasculature may be due to angiogenesis factors released by the tumor cells themselves. As will be discussed later, the tumor vasculature plays an important role in tumor growth and the oxygen effect.

Factors affecting tumor growth. The rate at which tumors grow depends on three major factors: (1) the division rate of proliferating parenchymal cells, (2) the percentage of these cells in the tumor (GF), and (3) the degree of cell loss from the tumor.[54] The division rate of group 1 cells in a tumor tends to be faster than the division rate for normal parenchymal cells from the same tissue.[29] For example, malignant skin cells cycle faster than normal skin cells. (Several other examples are shown in Table 9-4.) This might seem to imply that tumors have short doubling times (the time it takes to double in volume), but tumor doubling times

Table 9-4	Cell-cycle times for solid tumors and their normal cell counterparts		
Normal tissue	**Cell-cycle time (hr)**	**Tumors**	**Cell-cycle time (hr)**
Rat liver	21.5	Chemically induced hepatomas	14-16
Mouse skin	150	Epidermoid carcinomas	32
Mouse alveoli	64	Mammary tumors	33
Hamster cheek pouch epithelium	130-155	Chemically induced carcinomas	11
Rabbit epidermis	125-750	S-hope papilloma virus–induced papillomas	21
Mouse stomach epithelium	28-55	Squamous cell carcinomas	8-12
Human cervical epithelium	100-600	Squamous cell carcinomas	15

Modified from Hall EJ: *Radiobiology for the radiobiologist,* Philadelphia, ed 4, 1994, JB Lippincott.

in vivo are actually much longer than expected. The two major reasons for this are GF and cell loss. Although group 1 cells have short cycle times versus normal cells of the same origin, only an average of 30% to 50% of all cells in the tumor are included in this category.[34] In addition, of the new cells produced by mitosis at the end of each cycle, up to 90% may be lost from the primary tumor itself. This cell-loss factor (ϕ), which is manifested by metastases, cell death, and exfoliation (shedding of cells as in gastrointestinal tumors), is thought to be the most significant in vivo factor with regard to tumor growth.[54] A high cell-loss factor slows the growth of the primary tumor, but if cells are lost by metastasis, new tumors form in other sites in the body and limit the curative potential of any treatment, including radiation therapy.

The oxygen effect. Tumor growth is characteristically unorganized compared with that of normal cells. During their early growth stages, tumors begin to outgrow their vascular supply. This results in differing levels of oxygen availability (known as *oxygen tension*, or pO_2) for the tumor cells depending on their proximity to functioning blood vessels. This was first observed clinically in 1955 by Thomlinson and Gray, who examined human bronchial carcinoma specimens.[59] Thomlinson and Gray observed that the amount of necrotic (dead) tissue in the tumor was related to the size of the tumor itself. A tumor with a radius of less than 100 μm did not contain necrotic areas. A tumor with a radius of greater than 160 μm showed a necrotic area surrounded by a viable rim of cells approximately 100 to 180 μm thick.

Thomlinson and Gray concluded that tumor cells located more than 200 μm from the nearest blood vessels (capillaries) are anoxic (no oxygen available) and unable to proliferate. These cells then die, thus forming the necrotic area. Tumor cells closest to blood vessels, however, are well oxygenated (known as *oxic cells*), are actively dividing, and comprise the GF of the tumor. Between the oxic and anoxic cells are cells exposed to gradually decreasing oxygen tensions. These are known as *hypoxic cells*. Although hypoxic cells do not have normal levels of oxygen available to them, they are viable and capable of dividing. Data from animal tumors estimate that approximately 15% or more of the tumor-cell population may be hypoxic. This is known as the *hypoxic fraction* of the tumor.[65] Thomlinson and Gray's study estimated that the oxic, hypoxic, and anoxic populations in tumors were a result of the limited ability of oxygen to diffuse large distances in tissue. They estimated this diffusion distance of oxygen to be approximately 160 to 200 μm.[59] More recent studies indicate that a diffusion distance closer to 70 μm for oxygen may be more accurate.[26]

The vasculature network that forms in each growing tumor with factors such as division rate, GF, and cell loss ultimately gives rise to oxic, hypoxic, and anoxic cell populations in that tumor. The radioresponse of a tumor depends (among other factors) on these cell populations. Anoxic cells do not contribute to the GF and therefore do not affect clinical outcome. Cells that are fully oxygenated (oxic) are highly radiosensitive to low-LET radiations (see the previous discussion on OER). The third group (viable hypoxic cells) are resistant to low-LET radiations by a factor up to 2.5 to 3.0. The hypoxic fraction in each tumor is presumed to be responsible, at least in part, for tumor regrowth after radiation therapy. One of the reasons for the fractionation of a radiation dose is an attempt to increase the radioresponse of these hypoxic cells (see the discussion on reoxygenation).

Theory of dose-fractionation techniques

Modern radiation therapy treatments are given in daily fractions over an extended period (up to 6 or 8 weeks) so that a high total dose is given to the tumor while ideally sparing normal tissues.[40] This technique, known as **fractionation**, originated in 1927 and replaced a single, high-dose radiation treatment. The type of tumor and tolerance of the normal tissue in the treatment field determine the total dose, size and number of fractions, and treatment duration.

A fractionated dose of radiation is less efficient biologically than a single dose. Therefore higher total doses are necessary during fractionation to produce the same damage compared with a single dose. For example, a single dose of 1000 cGy causes more damage than two fractions of 500 cGy separated by 24 hours, although the total delivered dose remains the same.

A typical fractionation scheme may involve a daily fraction size of 180 to 200 cGy given 5 times a week for 6 weeks for a total of 30 fractions. This results in a total treatment dose ranging from 5400 to 6000 cGy (54 to 60 Gy). Depending on the tumor to be treated, the actual total dose may be higher or lower than this.

The biological effects on tissue from fractionated radiation therapy depend on the four Rs of radiation biology. These are repopulation, redistribution, repair, and reoxygenation.[68]

Repopulation. During protracted radiation therapy, surviving cells in the tumor and adjacent normal tissues may divide, thus repopulating these tissues partially or completely. Normal tissue repopulation is highly desirable and decreases the risk of late effects. Fractionated doses take advantage of normal tissue repopulation that occurs between fractions. This can result in the sparing of normal tissues in the treatment field.[68] In contrast, tumor repopulation is highly undesirable and contributes to tumor regrowth during or after treatment.

Redistribution. Irradiation of an asynchronous cell population (in which cells are distributed in all phases of the cell cycle) typically results in death to cells in the most sensitive phases (G_2 and M), whereas more resistant cells (especially in late S) survive. This process, known as *partial synchronization*, results in a redistribution or reassortment of surviving cells after irradiation.[67] The ideal clinical situation for radiation treatment exists when tumor cells have moved into a sensitive phase and normal cells have moved into a resistant phase. Theoretically, the timing of each radiation fraction can be based on the progression of cells into a sensitive or resistant phase. However, because this cannot be determined clinically, the partial synchronization of cell populations by radiation and other modalities (e.g., hydroxyurea) that may occur has not yet been successfully exploited.

Repair of sublethal damage. Repair of sublethal damage has occurred within hours of radiation exposure in normal and tumor cells in vitro.[16] Fractionated radiation treatment takes advantage of repair processes in normal tissues active between radiation fractions. This partially accounts for the sparing effect on normal tissues that fractionation can achieve. Repair of sublethal damage is oxygen dependent (i.e., cells require a certain amount of oxygen to efficiently carry out repair mechanisms). Because a proportion of tumor cells are thought to be hypoxic, tumors in general are presumed to be incapable of repairing sublethal radiation damage as efficiently as normal tissues.[5] Although demonstrated in animal models, this differential repair between tumors and normal tissues may not be clinically significant in human tumors.

Reoxygenation. The fourth R of radiobiology, unlike the other three, is presumed to apply only to tumors. This phenomenon, termed *reoxygenation*, is the process by which hypoxic cells gain access to oxygen and become radiosensitive between radiation fractions.

As discussed previously, the OER for x-rays and gamma rays is 2.5 to 3.0 when delivered as a single dose. However, the OER decreases during fractionation of x-rays and gamma rays. This implies that a proportion of hypoxic cells reoxygenate and therefore become more sensitive to the next fraction. Although the exact mechanisms of reoxygenation are not clear, clinical trials of fractionated radiation therapy seem to indicate that tumor response is improved compared with that from single-dose treatment. During fractionation, the initial dose fraction should kill a significant proportion of well-oxygenated (oxic), radiosensitive cells near blood vessels in the tumor. The effects on hypoxic, radioresistant cells is considerably less from the same dose fraction. Therefore immediately after exposure the percentage of hypoxic tumor cells increases significantly and may even reach 100% for a short time. Within 24 hours, hypoxic cells somehow gain access to oxygen. Because cells nearest the blood vessels are likely killed by the radiation fraction, oxygen may diffuse beyond these dead cells and reach a percentage of the hypoxic cells. Studies on animal tumors have demonstrated that the hypoxic fraction reestablishes itself in the tumor, usually within 24 hours of treatment.[58] In other words, if a tumor had a hypoxic fraction of 15% before treatment, it eventually reestablishes this percentage after reoxygenation is complete. The standard time interval of 24 hours between radiation fractions in human tumors was extrapolated from animal experiments. This time interval coincides with the range of reoxygenation rates in animal tumors and presumably occurs in human tumors. Because healthy normal tissues do not usually have hypoxic cells, the process of reoxygenation does not apply to these tissues.

Methods of improving tumor radioresponse. Reoxygenation does not rid the tumor of all hypoxic cells. If it did, fractionated treatments using low-LET radiations would be highly curative. Unfortunately, some tumors remain resistant to fractionated radiation therapy. This has given rise to a number of methods to overcome this persistent oxygen effect.

One early method involved the use of a chamber of hyperbaric (high-pressure) oxygen.[62] Patients were placed in sealed chambers containing pure oxygen at a pressure of 3 atmospheres. The rationale behind this was that the diffusion distance of oxygen would increase as a result of the high pressure used in the chamber so that it might reach the hypoxic areas in the tumor. However, this technique did not produce improved clinical results.

A related method involved the administration of perfluorochemicals (drugs that can carry oxygen) with 100% oxygen or carbogen (95% O_2/5% CO_2) breathing before and during radiation treatment.[62] The clinical results seemed to indicate improved response for several tumor types (most notably head and neck tumors), but the overall results were disappointing.

Radiosensitizers, radioprotectors, high-LET radiations, chemotherapy agents, and hyperthermia (heat) have all been used with varying degrees of success in terms of improved tumor response. However, each method is limited by biological or technical constraints.[26]

Concept of tolerance

Strandquist isoeffect curves. Although the preference of fractionated radiation treatments over high single doses is now established, the exact protocol for administration of fractionated doses continues to evolve. In 1944 Strandquist made the first attempt to establish a relationship between radiation dose and treatment time.[56] He developed plots of total dose (on a logarithmic scale) versus treatment duration (time in days on a linear scale) and called them *isoeffect curves* (Fig. 9-12). These isoeffect curves related the treatment schedule in terms of total dose and time with the clinical outcome, including early effects, late effects, and tumor cure. The use of isoeffect curves led to treatment schedules for fractionated radiation therapy that gave a high probability of tumor control without exceeding the tolerance of normal tissue. Also during this time the discovery was made that the tolerance of normal tissue is more dependent on the number and size of fractions than on the overall duration between the first and last fractions.

Tolerance and tolerance dose. Because the radiation dose applied to the tumor mass is limited by the tolerance of the normal tissue in the treatment field, identifing doses that can be used on normal tissues and factors affecting these doses is important. Tolerance doses have therefore been established for normal tissues in terms of the total dose delivered by a standard fractionation schedule that causes a minimal (5%) or maximal (50%) complication rate within 5 years (**$TD_{5/5}$** or **$TD_{50/5}$**, respectively). According to Travis, these normal tissue tolerance doses (NTTDs) range from 10 to 20 Gy for the gonads, bone marrow, and ocular lens to 75 Gy or more for muscle, bile ducts, ureters, and breast tissue.[62]

The NTTD is affected by two factors: the volume irradiated and fraction size. In terms of organ tolerance to radiation, the organ as a whole can tolerate higher radiation doses if the volume of the organ receiving that dose is small. As the volume of the organ affected by the treatment increases, the tolerance dose for the whole organ decreases. According to Rubin and Casarett, for example, the $TD_{50/5}$ for the heart is 55 Gy if 60% of the heart is irradiated. If only 25% of the heart is irradiated, the $TD_{50/5}$ increases to approximately 80 Gy.[45]

The other factor that affects the NTTD is the size of the daily radiation fraction used. In general, as the size of the

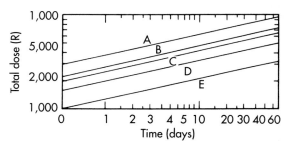

Fig. 9-12 Isoeffect curves from Strandquist's data that relate various treatment schedules to the following clinical results: *A*, skin necrosis; *B*, cure of skin cancer; *C*, moist desquamation; *D*, dry desquamation; *E*, skin erythema. (From Strandquist M: Studien über die kumulative Wirkung der Röntgenstrahlen bei Fraktionierung, *Acta Radiol [suppl]* 55:1-300, 1944.)

daily fraction increases, cell killing increases, and the cell's ability to repair sublethal damage decreases, thus resulting in a decrease in the radiation tolerance of normal tissues.

Nominal standard dose. In an attempt to design treatment schedules that result in optimal tumor response with acceptable normal tissue damage, Ellis in 1968 proposed the concept of nominal standard dose (NSD).[21] Ellis derived the following equation from the isoeffect curves of Strandquist that took into account several parameters of fractionated radiation therapy:

$$D = NSD \times T^{0.11} \times N^{0.24}$$

In the equation, D is the total dose, NSD is the nominal standard dose, T is the overall treatment time in days between the first and last fractions, and N is the number of fractions.[21] Ellis proposed the unit of rets (rad equivalent therapy) for NSD, and in many situations NSD = 1800 rets was considered the standard for comparison.[22] The NSD equation allowed radiation oncologists to enter their treatment data, calculate the NSD for their centers, and compare this with other centers. The limitations of this concept, however, include the following: (1) The equation is based on connective tissue response and therefore is not useful for late-responding normal tissues; and (2) the equation does not take into account the volume irradiated, which is critical to determining the tolerance of normal tissues. Although the NSD concept was popular in the 1970s, it is now useful for only an extremely limited number of clinical situations in radiation therapy.

Present status of radiation therapy

A number of treatment techniques combine the use of radiation therapy with other modalities. This is now the method of choice for many human malignancies. Because of the limited effect of low-LET radiations on hypoxic and S-phase tumor cells, the use of hyperthermia[4] and chemotherapeutic agents[26] with radiation has increased with improved clinical results for a number of tumor types. In addition, radiation fractionation techniques can be modified to deal with certain tumor types. For rapidly growing tumors of the head and neck, techniques known as *hyperfraction* and *accelerated treatment* have been used.[57] Hyperfraction involves administration of two fractions per day instead of the usual one, thus necessitating a decrease in the fraction size for each fraction so that normal tissue response is not significantly increased. Instead of a total of 30 to 40 fractions over 6 to 8 weeks, 60 to 80 fractions are given in a hyperfractionation scheme. Accelerated treatment also involves the use of multiple daily fractions. However, with accelerated treatment the entire dose is delivered in half the time (i.e., 3 to 4 weeks instead of 6 to 8 weeks) in an attempt to depopulate an aggressively growing tumor. In an accelerated treatment scheme the usual number of fractions given (30 to 40) remains the same. Again, care must be used so that normal tissue damage does not exceed acceptable levels. With the knowledge gained from clinical trials and preclinical experimentation, improvements in tumor responses and survival rates after radiation therapy continue to be realized.

Review Questions

Multiple Choice

1. What is the term describing certain chemicals or drugs that enhance the response of cells to radiation?
   a. Free radicals
   b. Radiosensitizers
   c. Radioprotectors
   d. Biological rescue factors
2. What is applied to the tolerance of normal tissue in which a tissue dose of radiation is associated with a 5% complication rate in 5 years?
   a. D_o
   b. D_q
   c. $TD_{5/5}$
   d. $TD_{50/5}$
3. Which of the following tissues is the least radiosensitive?
   a. Ovaries
   b. Ocular lens
   c. Small intestine
   d. Bone and cartilage
4. Which of the following is *not* one of the four Rs of radiation therapy?
   a. Reconfirmation
   b. Reoxygenation
   c. Redistribution
   d. Repopulation
5. Strandquist's isoeffect curves are related to which of the following?
   a. Oxygen enhancement
   b. Translocation of DNA
   c. Fractionation
   d. Radiation syndromes

Questions to Ponder

1. Discuss the interactions of radiation and matter (specifically, the indirect and direct effects on the cellular level).
2. Apply the concepts of LET and RBE as they relate to the treatment of malignant disease with ionizing radiation.
3. How does radiation sensitivity relate to the goals of radiation oncology in terms of tumor control and the sparing of normal tissue structures?

4. Relate the three graphic components of the cell survival curve (n, D_o, and D_q) to the administration of radiation treatments.
5. Briefly describe the three total-body responses to radiation.

REFERENCES

1. Adams GE et al: Electron-affinic sensitization. VII. A correlation between structures, one-electron reduction potentials, and the efficiencies of nitroimidazoles as hypoxic cell radiosensitizer, *Radiat Res* 67:9-20, 1976.
2. Albert RW et al: Follow-up studies of patients treated by x-ray epilation for tinea capitis, *Arch Environ Health* 17:899, 1968.
3. Ancel P, Vitemberger P: Sur la radiosensibilitie cellulaire, *C R Soc Biol* 92:517, 1925.
4. Arcangeli G et al: Tumor control and therapeutic gain with different schedules of combined radiotherapy and local external hyperthermia in human cancer, *Int J Radiat Oncol Biol Phys* 9:1125-1134, 1983.
5. Bedford JS, Mitchell JB: Dose-rate effects in synchronous mammalian cells in culture, *Radiat Res* 54:316-327, 1973.
6. Belli JA et al: Radiation response of mammalian tumor cells. I. Repair of sublethal damage in vivo, *J Natl Cancer Inst* 38:673, 1967.
7. Bergonié J, Tribondeau L: De quelques resultats de la radiothérapie et essai de fixation d'une technique rationelle, *C R Acad Sci (Paris)* 143:983, 1906.
8. Broerse JJ, Barendsen GW: Current topics, *Radiat Res Q* 8:305-350, 1973.
9. Broerse JJ, Barendsen GW, van Kersen GR: Survival of cultured human cells after irradiation with fast neutrons at different energies in hypoxic and oxygenated conditions, *Int J Radiat Biol* 13:559-572, 1967.
10. Bushong SC: *Radiologic science for technologists: physics, biology and protection,* ed 4, St Louis, 1988, Mosby.
11. Canti RG, Spear FG: The effect of gamma irradiation on cell division in tissue culture in vitro, part II, *Proc R Soc Lond B Biol Sci* 105:93, 1929.
12. Court-Brown WM, Doll R: Expectation of life and mortality from cancer among British radiologists, *Br Med J* 2(5090):181, 1958.
13. Court-Brown WM, Doll R: Mortality from cancer and other causes after radiotherapy from ankylosing spondylitis, *Br Med J* 2(5474):1327, 1965.
14. Court-Brown WM et al: The incidence of leukemia after the exposure to diagnostic radiation in utero, *Br Med J* 2(5212):1599, 1960.
15. Curtis HJ: *Radiation-induced aging in mice,* London, 1961, Butterworth.
16. Dekaban AS: Abnormalities in children exposed to x-irradiation during various stages of gestation: tentative timetable of radiation injury to the human fetus, *J Nucl Med* 9:471, 1968.
17. Dewey WC, Humphrey RM: Restitution of radiation-induced chromosomal damage in Chinese hamster cells related to the cell's life cycle, *Exp Cell Res* 35:262, 1964.
18. Dublin LI, Spiegelman M: Mortality of medical specialists, 1938-1942, *JAMA* 137:1519, 1948.
19. Elkind MM, Sutton-Gilbert H: Radiation response of mammalian cells grown in culture. I. Repair of x-ray damage in surviving Chinese hamster cells, *Radiat Res* 13:556, 1960.
20. Ellis F: Dose, time, and fractionation: a clinical hypothesis, *Clin Radiol* 20:1-7, 1969.
21. Ellis F: Dose, time, and fractionation in radiotherapy. In Ebert M, Howard A, editors: *Current topics in radiation research,* Amsterdam, 1968, North Holland Publishing.

22. Ellis F: Nominal standard dose and the ret, *Br J Radiol* 44:101-108, 1971.
23. Evans RD et al: Radiogenic tumors in the radium and mesothorium cases studied at MIT. In May CW et al, editors: *Delayed effects of bone-seeking radionuclides,* Salt Lake City, 1969, University of Utah Press.
24. Field SB: The relative biological effectiveness of fast neutrons for mammalian tissues, *Radiology* 93:915, 1969.
25. Griem ML et al: Analysis of the morbidity and mortality of children irradiated in fetal life, *Radiology* 88:347, 1967.
26. Hall EJ: *Radiobiology for the radiologist,* ed 4, Philadelphia, 1994, JB Lippincott.
27. Kinsella T et al: The use of halogenated thymidine analog as clinical radiosensitizers: rationale, current status, and future prospects—nonhypoxic cell sensitizers, *Int J Radiat Oncol Biol Phys* 10:1399-1406, 1984.
28. Krall JF: Estimation of spontaneous and radiation-induced mutation rates in man, *Eugenics Q* 3:201, 1956.
29. Lyskin AB, Mendelsohn ML: Comparison of cell cycle in induced carcinomas and their normal counterparts, *Cancer Res* 24:1131, 1964.
30. MacMahon B: Pre-natal x-ray exposure and childhood cancer, *J Natl Cancer Inst* 28:231, 1962.
31. March HC: Leukemia in radiologists in a 20-year period, *Am J Med Sci* 220:282, 1950.
32. Martland HS: Occurrence of malignancy in radioactive persons: general review of data gathered in study of radium dial painters, with special reference to occurrence of osteogenic sarcoma and interrelationship of certain blood diseases, *Am J Cancer* 15:2435, 1931.
33. McKenzie I: Breast cancer following multiple fluoroscopes, *Br J Cancer* 19:1, 1965.
34. Mendelsohn ML: The growth fraction: a new concept applied to tumors, *Science* 132:1496, 1960.
35. Müller HJ: On the relation between chromosome changes and gene mutations, *Brookhaven Symposium on Biology* 8:126, 1956.
36. Murphy DP, Goldstein L: Micromelia in a child irradiated in utero, *Surg Gynecol Obstet* 50:79, 1930.
37. Otake M, Schull WJ: In utero exposure to A-bomb radiation and mental retardation: a reassessment, *Br J Radiol* 57: 409-414, 1984.
38. Pack GT, Davis J: Radiation cancer of the skin, *Radiology* 84:436, 1965.
39. Patt HM,et al: Cysteine protection against x-irradiation, *Science* 110:213, 1949.
40. Peters LJ, Withers HR, Thames HD: Radiobiological considerations for multiple daily fractionation. In Kaercher KH, Kogelnik HD, Reinartz G, editors: *Progress in radio-oncology,* vol 2, New York, 1982, Raven Press.
41. Plummer C: Anomalies occurring in children exposed in utero to the atomic bomb at Hiroshima, *Pediatrics* 10:687, 1952.
42. Puck TT, Marcus TI: Action of x-rays on mammalian cells, *J Exp Med* 10:653, 1956.
43. Rotblat J, Lindop P: Long-term effects of a single whole body exposure of mice to ionizing radiation. II. Causes of death, *Proc R Soc Lond B Biol Sci* 154:350, 1961.

44. Rowland RE, Stehney AF, Lucas HF: Dose response relationships for radium-induced bone sarcomas, *Health Phys* 44:15-31, 1983.

45. Rubin P, Casarett GW: *Clinical radiation pathology,* vols 1 and 2, Philadelphia, 1968, WB Saunders.

46. Rugh R: X–ray-induced teratogenesis in the mouse and its possible significance to man, *Radiology* 99:433, 1971.

47. Russell LB, Montgomery CS: Radiation sensitivity differences with cell-division cycles during mouse cleavage, *Int J Radiat Biol* 10:151, 1966.

48. Russell LB, Russell WL: An analysis of the changing radiation response of the developing mouse embryo, *J Cell Physiol* 43(suppl 1):103, 1954.

49. Saccomanno G et al: Lung cancer of uranium miners on the Colorado plateau, *Health Phys* 10:1195, 1964.

50. Schull WL, Otake M, Neal JV: Genetic effects of the atomic bomb: a reappraisal, *Science* 213:1220-1227, 1981.

51. Simic MG, Grossman L, Upton AC, editors: *Mechanisms of DNA damage and repair,* New York, 1986, Plenum Press.

52. Simpson CL, Hempelmann LH: The association of tumors and roentgen-ray treatment of the thorax in infancy, *Cancer* 10(1):42, 1957.

53. Sinclair WK: Cyclic responses in mammalian cells in vitro, *Radiat Res* 33:620, 1968.

54. Steel GG: Cell loss as a factor in the growth rate of human tumors, *Eur J Cancer* 3:381-387, 1967.

55. Stewart A et al: A survey of childhood malignancies, *Br Med J* 1(5086):1495, 1958.

56. Strandquist M: Studien über die kumulative Wirkung der Röntgenstrahlen bei Fraktionierung, *Acta Radiol (suppl)* 55:1-300, 1944.

57. Thames HD et al: Accelerated fractionation vs hyperfractionation: rationale for several treatments per day, *Int J Radiat Oncol Biol Phys* 9:127-138, 1983.

58. Thomlinson RH: Effect of fractionated irradiation on the proportion of anoxic cells in an intact experimental tumor, *Br J Radiol* 39:158, 1966.

59. Thomlinson RH, Gray LH: The histological structure of some human lung cancers and the possible implications for radiotherapy, *Br J Cancer* 9:539, 1955.

60. Till JE, McCulloch EA: A direct measurement of the radiation sensitivity of normal mouse bone marrow cells, *Radiat Res* 14:213-222, 1961.

61. Toyooka ET et al: Neoplasms in children treated with x-rays for thymic enlargement. II. Tumor incidence as a function of radiation factors, *J Natl Cancer Inst* 31:1357, 1963.

62. Travis EL: *Primer of medical radiobiology,* ed 2, St Louis, 1989, Mosby.

63. Travis EL et al: Radiation pneumonitis and fibrosis in mouse lung assayed by respiratory frequency and histology, *Radiat Res* 84:133-143, 1980.

64. Upton AC: Radiation carcinogenesis. In *Methods of cancer research,* vol 4, New York, 1968, Academic Press.

65. Van Putten LM, Kahlman LF: Oxygenation status of transplantable tumor during fractionated radiotherapy, *J Natl Cancer Inst* 40:441, 1968.

66. Warren S: Radiation carcinogenesis, *Bull NY Acad Med* 46:131, 1970.

67. Withers HR: Cell cycle redistribution as a factor of multi-fraction irradiation, *Radiology* 114:199-202, 1975.

68. Withers HR: The 4 R's of radiotherapy. In *Advances in radiation biology,* vol 5, San Francisco, 1975, Academic Press.

69. Withers HR, Elkind MM: Microcolony survival assay for cells of mouse intestinal mucosa exposed to radiation, *Int J Radiat Biol* 17:261-267, 1970.

70. Withers HR et al: Radiation survival and regeneration characteristics of spermatogenic stem cells of mouse testis, *Radiat Res* 57:88-103, 1974.

71. Withers HR, Mason KA, Thames HD Jr: Late radiation response of kidney assayed by tubule cell survival, *Br J Radiol* 59:587-595, 1986.

72. Wright EA, Howard-Flanders P: The influence of oxygen on the radiosensitivity of mammalian tissues, *Acta Radiol (Stockholm)* 48:26, 1957.

73. Zirkle RE: Partial cell irradiation, *Adv Biol Med Phys* 5:103, 1957.

10

Detection and Diagnosis

Judith Bastin

Outline

Key terms

Asymptomatic
Baseline
Excisional biopsy

Incisional biopsy
Paraneoplastic syndrome
Reed-Sternberg (R-S) cells

The practice of medicine is "not merely the application of scientific principles to a particular biologic aberration. Its focus is on the patient whose welfare is its continuing purpose."[17] Medicine today is an art based on the biological, physical, and behavioral sciences. It is the accumulation of knowledge that has been developed through discovery, systematic scientific study, and research.

Physicians use their medical skills in interpersonal relationships, organization, knowledge, synthesis, and clinical judgment to benefit the patient. Interpersonal skills are extremely important during interaction with the patient and professional staff members. The presence or absence of appropriate skills can determine the physician's effectiveness in practicing medicine.

A patient seeks the services of a physician for consultation, physical examinations, medical treatment for a specific symptom or set of symptoms, and follow-ups for previously treated conditions. The acquisition of data based on the patient's chief complaints and medical, personal, and family histories is an important part of the patient-physician encounter. Additional patient information is obtained through results of current medical procedures and tests. Using the patient's database, the physician puts the pieces of the medical puzzle together to obtain a diagnosis and treatment that fits the patient.

The routine physical examination is necessary to help maintain good health and detect conditions or diseases early so that intervention is possible before the patient demonstrates signs or experiences symptoms. The actual physical examination (whether routine or a result of the patient experiencing signs or symptoms) is a methodical process that covers all the systems.

A *sign* is "an objective finding as perceived by an examiner." For example, the examining physician may notice signs such as a rash, feel a mass, or note the color of the patient's skin. A *symptom* is a "subjective indication of a disease or a change in condition as perceived by the patient."[9] For example, the patient may complain of pain, numbness, dysphagia, hematuria, dyspnea, difficulty in sleeping, or lack of appetite.

A patient experiencing symptoms is usually an indication that the condition or disease process is more advanced. A set of signs or symptoms that arise from a common cause is referred to as a *syndrome*. Many diseases share the same signs and symptoms. Grouping signs and symptoms into a syndrome with results of tests and medical procedures helps the physician eliminate some diseases and narrow the choices for a correct diagnosis. A fever, night sweats, fatigue, general weakness, and weight loss can be indicative of many types of conditions and disease processes. However, with an additional finding of painless lymphadenopathy the choices for a diagnosis become fewer. The physician decides to perform a biopsy on the lymph node, and the pathology report indicates the presence of **Reed-Sternberg (R-S) cells.** Because R-S cells are found in a variety of infectious, inflammatory, and neoplastic disorders, the physician can concentrate on these areas for possible diagnosis and rule out other possibilities such as Hodgkin's disease. A final diagnosis may not be possible until a more extensive work-up is done.

A *diagnosis* is defined as the identification of a disease or condition. A diagnosis can be subjective or objective. A subjective diagnosis is based on several factors. The patient's complaints and medical history are considered subjective. The physician's preliminary diagnosis with no hard evidence for support is also considered subjective. An objective diagnosis is based on results of current medical procedures and tests and observations of the physician and other medical personnel.

The process for obtaining an objective diagnosis begins with the interview and physical examination to help assess the patient's current status and determine necessary steps (if any) to take. During a physical examination the physician follows a methodical process that includes the acquisition of data through the interview process, a review of past medical records, a physical examination, a list of the patient's chief complaints, recommendations for further action, treatment recommendations, and follow-ups.

THE INTERVIEW AS A DIAGNOSTIC TOOL

The most powerful diagnostic tool of the physician is the interview. By this means, one learns the chronological events and symptoms of the patient's illness. Diagnostic hypotheses are generated and tested as the patient's history unfolds, resulting in the formulation of the most likely diagnoses at the completion of the interview.[17]

The physician must interview the patient to acquire accurate information. If the patient is too ill or handicapped to provide the information, the physician uses other sources such as family, friends, prior medical records, and other health care providers.

In the interview process the physician asks questions, and the patient provides answers. The physician determines the patient's chief complaints and current status and obtains the patient's medical and psychosocial history. The interview is also used in order to establish the physician-patient relationship and demonstrate to the patient a caring, empathetic attitude.

Physicians must interview patients in a variety of conditions and situations (e.g., emergency rooms, offices, and hospital rooms.) In an emergency situation the physician conducts a short interview and concentrates only on handling the immediate problem. A longer, in-depth interview is done later.

Allowing enough time for an interview is important. If the interview is rushed, the patient may feel that the physician is not empathetic. Not allowing enough time may limit the amount of information the physician is able to acquire.

Interviewing requires active listening, which calls for no distractions. Distractions should be kept to a minimum if not eliminated. Phone calls, interruptions by staff members, and loud noises can interfere with good communication. Taking excessive notes during the interview can be a distraction for the patient and should be avoided.

The physician listens to the patients' own words and concentrates on the way the patient speaks (e.g., the choice of and emphasis on words and phrases). Equally important are the words the patient chooses not to say or cannot say. The patient may have a limited vocabulary and be unable to find the right word to describe the symptom. The patient may lack the ability to communicate because of a stroke or mental deficit. A patient simply may not remember or may be afraid to describe all the symptoms because of the fear of a diagnosis.

For various reasons, patients may not give completely accurate statements. Fear of being judged by the physician or embarrassment may prevent young men and women from giving a complete history of their sexual activity. Patients may be reluctant to give much information to the physician for fear that it may affect their ability to get or retain a job. Patients with medical conditions such as the human immunodeficiency virus (HIV), acquired immunodeficiency syndrome (AIDS), and cancer may be discriminated against in the work place and by insurance companies. Some insurance companies may limit or charge more for the coverage of patients who engage in certain lifestyle activities such as smoking and drinking alcoholic beverages. Insurance companies may also limit coverage for preexisting conditions. Medical and life insurance companies may not insure patients diagnosed with certain diseases. Patients may not be hired or may lose their jobs after a diagnosis is made. Discrimination by employers against patients with HIV,

AIDS, or cancer is illegal, but in reality discrimination can be subtle and often difficult to prove.

The physician must select words that are clear and mean the same to the patient. The meaning of words is relative. A physician may ask, "What medications are you taking?" The response may be "None," although the patient is taking aspirin for pain and an antacid for indigestion. In the patient's mind, these are not medications because they were not prescribed. The physician may also ask, "Have you had any seizures?" to which the patient may respond, "No." In reality, however, the patient has experienced petit mal seizures. To the patient a seizure may mean a grand mal epileptic seizure.

Many factors can interfere with or facilitate the interview, such as the patient's physical senses and the ability to process and interpret information. The senses and ability to process and interpret information can be affected by age, inherited or acquired conditions, the disease process, treatment and medication, language, and environmental conditions such as dim lighting in a room. Factors that help to facilitate the interview include the interviewer's ability to put the patient at ease, ask clear and concise questions, and use terminology having the same meaning to the patient and interviewer.

The objective of the interview is to obtain as much accurate information as possible. During the interview the physician assesses the patient's ability to communicate, level of cognitive functioning, appearance, movement, and facial expressions. The physician also considers the reliability of the patient's responses. This requires skill in patient communication and observation, a technique that involves the use of verbal and nonverbal communication.

Verbal communication involves the manner, quality, and intonation of speech. Forms of nonverbal communication include personal appearance, facial expressions, posture, and manner of movement.

Observing nonverbal communication while the patient is talking can help the physician determine the real meaning of the patient's words. The patient may say one thing but really mean another. For example, the physician asks the patient, "Are you having any pain?" The patient says, "No". However, the patient's appearance, posture, and facial expressions contradict the verbal response. The patient sits slouched over, grimaces during movement, and moves slowly with great deliberation. These are all nonverbal signs of pain. These signs may be related to a medical problem other than pain or a psychological problem, or they simply have no significance. A slouched posture may indicate pain, low self-esteem, depression, or some other unexplained phenomenon. A grimace may be a psychological response to the question or physician, a sign of indigestion, or a facial tic. Slow, deliberate movement may mean unfamiliarity with the surroundings, discomfort, or distraction. A physician observing this type of nonverbal communication must probe further to rule out pain.

The physician and therapist must ask questions in such a way so as not to lead the patient but to get the patient to respond with as much information as possible. In other words, the patient should do most of the talking. This means that the physician should avoid using closed-ended questions, which are usually answered with "yes" or "no" responses. An example of a closed-ended question is, "Do you have pain?" The patient will likely respond, "yes" or "no." The physician must know several things about the patient's pain. Is the pain sharp or dull? Does it radiate from one area to another? Does the pain pulsate? What precipitates or alleviates the pain? Does the pain occur at a certain time of day? A closed-ended question will not obtain this information. Open-ended questions are usually better. Examples of open-ended questions and requests include the following: "Tell me about the pain you are having," "When do you notice it?" "How bad is your pain?" "What brings you here?" and "What kind of problems are you having?"

Responses of the interviewer can facilitate or hinder the interview process. A nonverbal response that may facilitate the interview is nodding the head. Silence can be extremely helpful because it can give patients more time to respond, think about their choice of words, and compose themselves. Touch (such as a pat on the shoulder or holding the patient's hand) is another response that can help facilitate communication. However, touch must be used with caution because it may be misinterpreted. These types of responses can help demonstrate the physician's empathy and understanding of the patient's responses. The physician must be extremely careful, however, to avoid nonverbal actions that may be misinterpreted by the patient. Not allowing enough time for the interview may give the impression of a lack of interest on the part of the interviewer. Facial responses as interpreted by the patient may mean the physician has found something serious.

Some of the verbal responses that can facilitate the interview are minimal responses, reflecting feelings, and seeking clarification (Table 10-1). Responses that may hinder the interview are the use of social clichés, imposition of the interviewer's own values, and devaluing or minimizing the patient's feelings or responses (Table 10-2).

Table 10-1	Examples of facilitating verbal responses
Type of response	**Examples**
Minimal	"I see." "I understand."
Reflecting feelings	"I see you are very angry." "It is very scary."
Clarifications	"How bad did it hurt?" "This only bothers you at night?"

Table 10-2	Examples of hindering verbal responses
Type of response	**Examples**
Social clichés	"You will feel better soon." "Don't worry; everything will be alright."
Imposing values	"You should not be having sex outside of marriage." "Someone your age should be more responsible."
Devaluing the patient's feelings or responses	"I wish I had a nickel for every time I heard this." "This is just part of the aging process."

Table 10-3	Information gathered during the medical history interview
Type of data	**Information obtained**
Demographic data	Age, race, gender, marital status, and current occupation
Chief complaints	Symptoms, current illness, and current condition
Medical history	Childhood illnesses, allergies, immunizations, injuries, prior hospitalizations, psychological problems, and medications
Family history	Illnesses, causes of death, genetic disorders, and mental disorders
Personal history	Occupation, lifestyle, and sexual activity and preferences

THE MEDICAL RECORD

The medical record documents the patient's past medical experience. The format of the medical record may differ from institution to institution and according to whether the person was an inpatient or outpatient seen in the clinic or emergency room.

"The hospital medical record is a legal public document, in that it is available to the medical staff, medical departments of the hospital, clinic, insurance companies, or by subpoena to a court of law."[17] Patients do not own their medical records, but they may review them on request and have copies released to other physicians. The medical record contains the medical history, results of laboratory tests and medical procedures, progress notes, copies of consent forms, and correspondence.

THE MEDICAL HISTORY

The format for taking a medical history may vary from physician to physician but should always be done in logical manner. Table 10-3 contains a summary of the type of information obtained during the interview.

The need for demographic data

Demographic data provide the physician with an overview of the patient, including information on the patient's age, gender, race, and possibly national origin. The reason for obtaining demographic data is that certain disease conditions are found to be more prevalent for groups according to age, gender, race, and national origin.

For example, although cancer occurs at any age, the incidence is higher among older persons. However, certain types of cancer occur more frequently in other age groups. Wilms' tumor (a cancer of the kidney) frequently affects children between 1 and 5 years and is rare in children over 8 years of age.[4]

Some types of cancer occur more frequently by gender. For example, men are affected twice as often as women by renal cancer, whereas the incidences of colon and rectal cancer are higher in women[1] (Fig. 10-1).

The incidence of cancer among races and nationalities varies. For example, the incidence of esophageal cancer is extremely high in the Bantu of Africa, China, Russia, Japan, Scotland, and the Caspian region of Iran.[4]

Determination of the chief complaints

When assessing the patient's chief complaints, the physician compiles a list of symptoms, known illnesses, and conditions. Listening to the patient's chief complaints helps determine necessary diagnostic decisions. This is important because certain symptoms, illnesses, or conditions may indicate the possibility of a predisposing factor, premalignant condition, **paraneoplastic syndrome,** or other risk factors.

A predisposing factor given the correct stimuli has the potential of becoming malignant. Leukoplakia, an example of a predisposing factor, is identified as a white patch or patches in the mucosa of the oral cavity and on the tongue.

A premalignant condition eventually becomes malignant if left untreated. Premalignant conditions usually are manifested as dysplasia or atypical hyperplasia. *Dysplasia* is the abnormal development of cells in size and shape. *Hyperplasia* is an abnormal increase in the number of new cells. Dysplasia and hyperplasia can be determined only by microscopic examination.

Some forms of cancer produce a paraneoplastic syndrome. *Paraneoplastic syndrome* is a term that describes certain metabolic disorders associated with cancer. These disorders indirectly result from the disease and are not caused by the spread of cancer to an organ or other tissues. The syndrome is a result of hormonal, hematological, neurological, and biochemical disturbances on the patient's physiology.

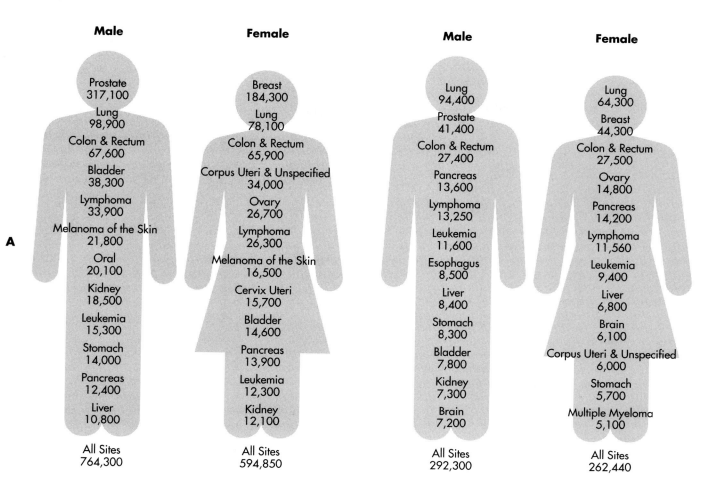

Male	Female	Male	Female
Prostate 317,100	Breast 184,300	Lung 94,400	Lung 64,300
Lung 98,900	Lung 78,100	Prostate 41,400	Breast 44,300
Colon & Rectum 67,600	Colon & Rectum 65,900	Colon & Rectum 27,400	Colon & Rectum 27,500
Bladder 38,300	Corpus Uteri & Unspecified 34,000	Pancreas 13,600	Ovary 14,800
Lymphoma 33,900	Ovary 26,700	Lymphoma 13,250	Pancreas 14,200
Melanoma of the Skin 21,800	Lymphoma 26,300	Leukemia 11,600	Lymphoma 11,560
Oral 20,100	Melanoma of the Skin 16,500	Esophagus 8,500	Leukemia 9,400
Kidney 18,500	Cervix Uteri 15,700	Liver 8,400	Liver 6,800
Leukemia 15,300	Bladder 14,600	Stomach 8,300	Brain 6,100
Stomach 14,000	Pancreas 13,900	Bladder 7,800	Corpus Uteri & Unspecified 6,000
Pancreas 12,400	Leukemia 12,300	Kidney 7,300	Stomach 5,700
Liver 10,800	Kidney 12,100	Brain 7,200	Multiple Myeloma 5,100
All Sites 764,300	All Sites 594,850	All Sites 292,300	All Sites 262,440

A   **B**

Fig. 10-1   Leading sites of new cancer cases and deaths, 1996 estimates. **A,** This illustration shows cancer cases by site and gender (excluding basal and squamous cell skin cancer and carcinoma in situ). **B,** This illustration shows cancer deaths by site and gender. (From The American Cancer Society: *Cancer facts and figures,* New York, 1996, The Society.)

Hypercalcemia and hypoglycemia are part of the paraneoplastic syndromes associated with hepatic cell carcinoma.[11] *Hypercalcemia* is an excessive amount of calcium in the blood. *Hypoglycemia* is a reduced amount of sugar in the blood. Thrombophlebitis and antidiuretic hormone excess are part of the paraneoplastic syndromes associated with lung cancer. *Thrombophlebitis* is the inflammation of a vein caused by the development or presence of a blood clot in the vein. Having any of these medical conditions does not necessarily mean that the individual has a malignant disease process. However, a patient who demonstrates several signs and symptoms of a particular syndrome needs to have a further work-up to rule out those possibilities.

Down syndrome is an example of a risk factor. Children born with Down syndrome (a genetic disease causing mongolism) have an increased risk of developing acute lymphoblastic leukemia (ALL) or acute myelogenous leukemia (AML).[4]

The importance of the medical history

The medical history gives a picture of the patient's prior medical problems and treatments. The determination of prior medical problems may establish risk factors for acquiring diseases in the future. For example, a patient who has a long history of indigestion and gastric reflux caused by a hiatal hernia may be at risk for ulcers or carcinoma of the esophagus.[11] A *gastric reflux* is the backward flow of contents of the stomach into the esophagus. A *hiatal hernia* is a congenital or acquired condition that is the result of movement of the stomach through the esophageal hiatus of the diaphragm into the thorax.

The medical history of immediate family members may determine additional risk factors. The immediate family consists of the parents, spouse, children, brothers, sisters, aunts, and uncles. The physician determines whether the parents are alive or deceased. If they are alive, the physician determines their ages and health status. If they are deceased, the physician needs to know the causes of death and the ages of the parents when they died. This is done to establish certain risk factors such as the acquisition of genetic disease and probability of developing medical conditions such as heart disease, arthritis, diabetes, and cancer.

Certain types of cancer appear to repeat in families. More than one sibling may develop leukemia. If the mother has breast cancer, the daughter is at a greater risk of developing the disease.[11]

The personal history encompasses the patient's lifestyle (past and present). The physician asks questions regarding dietary, exercise, alcohol, cigarette, and drug habits. The physician must also determine the patient's sexual activity frequency and preferences. Determining the patient's past occupations is also an important thing to do. For example, the patient may have been employed in an occupation that carried the risk of exposure to asbestos, disease, ionizing radiation, or other carcinogens.

THE PHYSICAL EXAMINATION

The physical examination, medical history, and test results help the physician detect variations in the normal state of the patient. The physical examination is an extremely organized, detailed exploration of the patient's anatomical regions. Performing a physical examination requires all the physician's senses and skills.

The following paragraphs list some examples of aspects in the physical examination and information the physician may be seeking. The information in this section is extremely general and far from comprehensive regarding all aspects of the physical examination. Inspection, palpation, percussion, and auscultation are the four classic techniques of the physical examination.

Inspection

Inspection is the use of sight to observe. A distinction must be made between seeing and observing. Something may be seen but not observed. For example, a person may see a group of people, but on observation of the group the person begins to make distinctions. The person may be able to say 10 people were the group and may observe differences in gender, race, age, appearance, and behavior.

The physician observes the color of the patient's skin, which may indicate signs of a disease condition. Many diseases and conditions affect skin coloration. The skin may be dark, pale, grey, flushed, jaundiced, or cyanotic. Dark skin may be natural or caused by irritation of another medical condition. Pale skin may be natural or caused by anemia. Flushed or reddened skin may be caused by hormones, infection, or burns. Jaundice, a yellow coloration of the skin, may be caused by obstruction of the bile ducts. Cyanosis, a blue coloration of the skin, may be caused by an excessive accumulation of reduced hemoglobin in the blood.

The physician looks for scarring or lesions such as warts, moles, ulcerations, tumors, and asymmetry on the surface of the skin. Scarring is an indication of prior medical procedures or injury. The presence of lesions or changes in warts and moles may be benign, a sign of malignant transformation, or cancer. Asymmetry may be an indication of edema, thrombosis, hematoma, injury, or an underlying tumor. *Edema* is a swelling of the tissue caused by the accumulation of excessive amounts of fluid. *Thrombosis* is the abnormal accumulation of blood factors in a blood vessel that causes a clot. A *hematoma* is the abnormal accumulation of blood in tissue from a blood vessel that has ruptured. An inspection may use the sense of smell to help in making a diagnosis. For example, the smell of the patient's breath, wound, urine, or sputum may indicate infection, ketoacidosis, or some other condition.

Palpation

Palpation is the use of touch to acquire information about the patient. The physician palpates the patient by using the tips of the fingers. Light palpation is used for a superficial examination. Heavy pressure may be necessary for deep-seated structures. Through palpation the physician tries to distinguish between hard and soft, rough and smooth, and warm and dry. Vibrations in the chest or abdomen can be felt through palpation. Palpation of an artery can help determine the pulse. Palpation is also used to determine whether pain is present. For example, the patient may not experience pain from an inflammatory process until pressure is applied or applied and released quickly.

Percussion

Percussion is different from palpation in that *percussion* is the act of striking or tapping the patient gently. The purpose of percussion is to determine pain in underlying tissue or cause vibrations. Making a fist and pounding it gently over the kidney area does not normally produce pain. However, if the patient has an underlying kidney infection, percussion may produce pain.

Another form of percussion is produced by placing the examiner's third finger of one hand flat on the surface of the patient over the lung or abdomen. With the third finger of the other hand the examiner gently raps the dorsal surface of the third finger that is resting on the patient. Depending on the location of the percussion, different sounds are produced. For example, if percussion is done over the lung (which is an air-filled cavity), the vibrations have a different sound than that of the abdominal cavity. Percussion over a normal lung produces a resonant sound, whereas percussion over the abdomen produces a distinctively duller sound. For the radiation therapist, percussion is helpful in determining the place the abdomen ends and the lung begins. The radiation therapist may have to take a simulation film that requires centering over the diaphragm.

Auscultation

With a stethoscope the physician performs *auscultation* by listening to the lungs, heart, arteries, stomach, and bowel sounds. Sounds in the lungs vary depending on the presence or absence of air and fluid. A pumping heart produces sounds that can be altered by changes or abnormalities of its structure and function. Listening to blood flowing through major arteries can tell the physician whether abnormalities such as atherosclerosis are present in the vessel. *Atherosclerosis* is the buildup of cholesterol and lipids on the inner surface of the blood vessel.

Vital signs

Vital signs are almost always taken during the physical examination. *Vital signs* include the temperature, pulse, respirations, and blood pressure of the patient. Vital signs can vary from patient to patient depending on the time of day and physical activity, condition, and age of the patient. Taking baseline values at various times to establish the patient's norm is important.

Temperatures are taken orally, rectally, in the ear, or in the axilla. Oral temperatures should not be taken on unreliable patients. This includes patients who are irrational, comatose, prone to convulsions, and young children. Patients in these categories should have rectal or ear temperatures taken. The rectal temperature is considered the most accurate. Devices most commonly used for taking temperatures are glass and electronic thermometers. Electronic thermometers give much quicker readings than glass thermometers. The electronic ear thermometer can be used on adults and children. Temperatures are measured in Fahrenheit (F) or Celsius (C), and some values are given in ranges. Textbooks may list slightly different values for normal and abnormal temperatures (Table 10-4).

Factors observed during the taking of a pulse are rate, rhythm, size, and tension. Rate indicates the number of beats per second. Rhythm is the pattern of beats. Size has to do with the size of the pulse wave and volume of blood felt during the ventricular contraction of the heart. Tension refers to the compressibility of the artery (e.g., soft or hard)[6] (Table 10-4).

Factors that are observed during the evaluation of respiration are rate, depth, rhythm, and character. *Rate* is the number of breaths that are taken in a minute. *Depth* refers to shallow or deep breathing. The deeper the breath, the greater the amount of air that is inhaled. *Rhythm* refers to the regularity of breathing (slow, normal, or rapid). *Character* refers to the type of breathing from normal to labored[6] (Table 10-4).

When taking a blood pressure, the systolic and diastolic pressures are noted. Systolic blood pressure represents the pressure in the blood vessels during the contraction of the heart and is the first sound heard through the stethoscope when taking a blood pressure. Diastolic pressure represents the pressure in the blood vessels during the relaxation phase of the heart after the contraction. The diastolic pressure is the last sound heard through the stethoscope when taking a blood pressure[6] (Table 10-4).

Table 10-4	Normal adult values for vital signs	
Vital signs	**Values**	
Temperature		
Oral	96.8° to 98.6° F	
	36° to 37° C	
Rectal	99.6° F	
Axillary	97.6° F	
Pulse	60 to 90 beats per minute	
Respirations	10 to 20 breaths per minute	
Blood pressure	$\dfrac{110 \text{ to } 140 \text{ mm Hg}}{60 \text{ to } 80 \text{ mm Hg}}$	

From Torres LS: *Basic medical techniques and patient care for radiologic technologists,* ed 4, Philadelphia, 1993, JB Lippincott.

SCREENING

Cancer prevention that takes place in the United States is grouped in three levels. The first level of cancer prevention is devoted to helping people maintain good health through education that encourages changes in lifestyle. Immunizations to prevent cancer, if they existed, would be encouraged. The second level of cancer prevention is concerned with the early detection of conditions and disease. Early detection makes intervening and perhaps improving the outcome for the patient possible. The third level is devoted to rehabilitation.

Cancer screening is part of the second level of health promotion.[1] Screening is the cornerstone of the diagnosis and management of the patient. It is done for large, **asymptomatic** populations at risk to detect deviations from the norm or signs of disease. Specific screening is performed for patients who are symptomatic, undergoing treatment, or being followed up. The determination to do mass screening is based on the results obtained, cost effectiveness, and risk to the patient.

Until the early 1960s the only routine screening that was available for asymptomatic patients included a chest x-ray, an electrocardiogram, a complete blood count (CBC), a blood chemistry test, a urinalysis, and a stool examination for occult blood. With the development of multichannel automated analyzers, many laboratory tests could be obtained for the same cost as that of the few tests that had been performed before. Later studies questioned the value of doing such a large number of tests. Many of the tests that were performed did not improve the outcome in asymptomatic outpatients.[17]

Most screening studies can be grouped into two major categories: laboratory studies and medical imaging. Hundreds of laboratory tests and medical imaging procedures exist today. Discretion must be exercised in selecting appropriate tests to be done, and studies are not performed unless logical reasons exist for doing so.

Cancer screening can be effective if a disease has a high incidence or prevalence in a population and the test has the ability to produce results having the appropriate sensitivity and specificity. *Incidence* is defined as the number of new cases of a disease over a period, and *prevalence* is defined as the total number of cases of a disease at a certain time. Screening may be set up to determine the incidence of new cancer cases over a period. Screening for the prevalence of cancer determines the number of cases at a certain time.[14]

In the United States, one of eight women develop breast cancer, and one in eight men develop prostate cancer.[3] Therefore a significant portion of the population benefits from mass medical screening. If the disease is caught early enough, morbidity and mortality rates may be reduced. Mass screening for breast cancer in China is not effective because the at-risk population is low. However, the reverse is true for cancer of the esophagus. The number of persons at risk for cancer of the esophagus is extremely high in certain regions of China. Whereas the population at risk for cancer of the esophagus is much lower in the United States, mass screening would not be beneficial in terms of outcome and cost effectiveness. In summary, the value of mass screening is determined by the number of the population at risk, cost of the studies, risks involved in the studies, and improvements in the morbidity and mortality rates.

Sensitivity, specificity, and predictive values

Other measures for determining the value of a study are the sensitivity, specificity, and predictive values. *Sensitivity* is defined as the ability of a test to give a true positive result when the disease is present. In other words, a person who tests positive for cancer from a high-sensitivity test probably has cancer. *Specificity* is defined as the ability of the test to obtain a true negative result. When the results of a high-specificity test are negative, that person probably does not have cancer.[10]

The ideal situation is for a test to yield a high sensitivity *and* high specificity. However, that is almost impossible. Because of the morbidity and mortality rates of cancer, the ability to detect cancer early in all individuals tested is important. High sensitivity is selected when the disease prevalence is low. A positive finding of cancer from a high-sensitivity test can be confirmed by subjecting the patient to a second test of high specificity. High specificity is selected when the disease prevalence is high. Determining the sensitivity and specificity of the test can affect its predictive value. The predictive value of a positive test increases with an increase in the sensitivity and specificity of the test. No single test should be relied on to establish a diagnosis of cancer.

COMMON SOURCES OF ERRORS

The sources of errors in medical studies are many. Any medical examination always has a margin of error in the results. The possibility of errors exist in the ordering of a study,

coordination of activities before the study, preparation of the patient, and performance of the procedure. Care must be taken in the ordering of the study and test, coordination of activities, and preparation of the patient[8] (Table 10-5).

The physician often asks radiation therapists to order certain tests. Request forms must be filled out completely and correctly. The individual filling out the form must know places to obtain the necessary information that must be recorded on the requisition. This information includes the patient's demographic data, symptoms, or diagnosis if available and the purpose of the test. Repeating a test because the requisition was not filled out properly or the patient was not prepared can put the patient at risk and may result in increased work hours and costs.

If the laboratory tests were done in the radiation therapy department, the radiation therapist may be responsible for labeling the specimens. The specimens must be labeled correctly according to institutional and departmental guidelines. Incorrect labeling may result in having to repeat tests. The worst case scenario is the wrong diagnosis for the wrong patient. In this situation, errors are compounded if they were not discovered in time because treatment may have been initiated based on results of the test.

Coordination of the patient's activities is important. Special consideration must be given to patients who are diabetic, have colostomies, or are infirm. Extra time may be necessary to accommodate these patients. Scheduling a battery of tests requires coordination so that the tests do not interfere with each other. For example, a glucose tolerance test takes place over 2 hours, at which time blood must be drawn. If the patient is not available when the blood is to be drawn, the results of the test are invalid. Some tests must be done before others because they may interfere with the next test. For example, an intravenous pyelogram should be done before x-ray contrast studies of the upper and lower gastrointestinal

Table 10-5	Actions that may alter test results
Person responsible	**Actions**
Caregiver	Incomplete or inaccurately filled-out requisitions
	Incomplete or inaccurate coordination of activities
	Incomplete or inaccurate patient instruction
	Incorrectly performed procedure
	Incorrect labeling of specimens
Patient	Incorrect interpretation of instructions
	Lack of cooperation
	Inability to follow instructions or noncompliance

(GI) systems. If the patient has an upper and lower GI study before the pyelogram, the contrast material left in the intestinal tract may obstruct the radiologist's view of the kidneys, ureters, and bladder. Improper coordination may result in the patient having to go through an uncomfortable preparation for the test again. (In the example just mentioned the preparation includes multiple enemas.) In addition, many of the tests are invasive, can be uncomfortable, and carry certain risks. Repeated radiographic procedures result in unnecessary exposure of the patient to ionizing radiation.[8]

The person ordering the test must have an understanding of the way it is done and elements of patient preparation. Certain examinations require specific preparation. Tests may require the patient to be nil per os (NPO), "nothing by mouth." Some tests require the patient to receive prior medication or contrast material. If this is true, the person ordering the test must determine whether the patient has any allergies.

A patient has a right to be informed about tests to be done and elements involved. Patients who are actively involved in their own care and informed are more likely to cooperate. Informed patients are more likely to be less apprehensive about medical procedures.

THE AMERICAN CANCER SOCIETY'S RECOMMENDATIONS FOR DETECTING CANCER

The American Cancer Society (ACS) strongly recommends mass screenings for colorectal, breast, cervical, prostate, and endometrial cancers. To date, results of mass screening for lung cancer have not proved beneficial in improving mortality rates. Getting people to stop smoking has the greatest effect on mortality statistics for lung cancer.[11]

Table 10-6 provides an excellent overview of recommendations for screening and detection by site and symptoms. New techniques for the diagnosis of prostate cancer (such as prostate-specific antigen [PSA] blood testing and ultrasound) are listed in Table 10-6. The ACS recommends that the PSA blood test be performed yearly for men over the age of 50. In addition, the ACS recommends prostatic ultrasounds for men who are at high risk. According to Rubin,[15] "the issue of screening asymptomatic men for prostate cancer with tests other than digital rectal examination is controversial." Rubin further states that although PSA and transrectal ultrasound used with the rectal examination increases the chances of making a diagnosis, the tests themselves are "associated with a high false positive rate and may identify a greater number of medically insignificant tumors."

Text continued on p. 134

Table 10-6	Screening and detection recommendations by cancer site*	
Cancer site	**Signs and symptoms**	**Screening, detection, and diagnostic tests**
Bladder	Painless hematuria in the absence of urinary frequency or difficulty voiding Frequent bladder irritability Bloody urine or urinary sediment >3-5 red cells per high-power field Marked urgency, dysuria, and frequency and a small volume of sterile urine Interstitial cystitis	Urine culture Urinary tract cytological study Washings of bladder Intravenous urography Pelvic CT Cytoscopical evaluation Biopsy
Breast	Painless lump or mass Unilateral serous nipple discharge Bloody discharge Dermatitis of nipple and areola Dimpling of skin in breast Nipple retraction Change in contour of breast Fixation of a mass to the pectoral fascia and chest wall Edema and erythema of breast skin Axillary adenopathy	Physical breast examination Mammography Ultrasound and thermography Percutaneous needle aspiration
Central nervous system	Increasing intracranial pressure resulting in headaches, vomiting, lethargy, edema, hemorrhage or infarction, and depression Contralateral homonymous hemianopsia Epileptic seizures	Neuroradiographic studies CT of brain with contrast material Carotid and vertebral arteriography MRI Analysis of cerebrospinal fluid Endocrine evaluation

*Childhood cancers not included.

Continued.

Table 10-6	Screening and detection recommendations by cancer site—cont'd	
Cancer site	**Signs and symptoms**	**Screening, detection, and diagnostic tests**
Colon and rectum	Change in bowel habits: obstruction and diarrhea Rectal bleeding Tenesmus Iron deficiency anemia	Fecal occult blood test Digital rectal examination Air contrast barium enema CT Cytoscopy Colonoscopy Flexible fiberoptic sigmoidoscopy

Esophagus	Subtle changes in digestive habits:
	    weight loss, malaise, and anorexia
	Dysphagia to solid foods followed by:
	    Dysphagia to liquids
	    Unexplained choking
	    Gastroesophageal reflux
		Careful physical examination
		Radiography (CT)
		Fluoroscopy and barium swallow
		Endoscopic examination (esophagoscopy with biopsy)
		Punch biopsies
		Brush biopsies
		Cytological studies of exfoliated cells

Extrahepatic bile duct	Jaundice followed by pruritus Anorexia and weight loss Fever Dyspepsia Nausea Vomiting	Physical examination (enlarged liver) Ultrasonography CT Endoscopic retrograde cholangiopancreatography Percutaneous transhepatic cholangiography by thin needle
Female genital tract Vulva Cervix Endometrium Ovary	 Pruritus valvae Postcoital spotting Postmenopausal bleeding (6 months after menopause) Enlarged abdomen Vague digestive disturbance	 Gynecological examination Inspection and palpation of superficial lymph nodes (supraclavicular, axillary and inguinal areas) Papanicolaou smear Bimanual palpation Fractional D and C Laparoscopy and laparotromy CT Cytological studies Directed biopsy

Gallbladder	Acute or chronic cholecystitis
	Abdominal pain
	Anorexia
	Weight loss
	Jaundice
	Nausea
	Vomiting
	Occasional fever
		Diagnostic x-ray studies
		Laboratory studies
		    Liver chemistry tests
		    Elevated alkaline phosphatase level
		Laparotomy

Head and neck Oral cavity Oropharynx	Red or white patch that persists Difficulty in chewing, swallowing, or moving tongue or jaws Firm unilateral lymph nodes in neck Swelling or ulcer that fails to heal Ipsilateral referred otalgia Indurated ulcer Dysphasia Local pain Pain on swallowing Referred otalgia	Careful examination of upper aerodigestive tract Individual indirect mirror examination Finger palpation Radiography Plain films CT Tomography Orthopantomography of mandible Barium swallow Laryngography

Table 10-6	Screening and detection recommendations by cancer site—cont'd	

Cancer site	Signs and symptoms	Screening, detection, and diagnostic tests
Head and neck—cont'd		
Hypopharnyx	Dysphasia Odynophagia Referred otalgia Neck mass	Chest x-ray studies Bone scan Arteriography Fiberoptic aerodigestive endoscopy
Larynx	Persistent hoarseness Pain Referred otalgia Dyspnea Stridor	Biopsy
Nasopharynx	Bloody nasal discharge Obstructed nostril Conductive deafness Neurological problems (atypical facial pain, diplopia, hoarseness, and Horner's syndrome) Neck mass	
Nose and sinuses	Bloody nasal discharge Nasal obstruction Facial pain Facial swelling Diplopia	
Parotic and submandibular glands	Painless local swelling Hemifacial paralysis	
Kidney	Pain Hematuria Palpable abdominal mass Weight loss Polycythemia Fever Erythrocytosis Hepatic dysfunction Seizures	Intravenous pyelography and arteriography Ultrasonography CT Urography and nephrotomography Radionuclide scan Aspiration Biopsy
Leukemia		
Acute leukemia	Viruslike syndrome with low-grade fever Anemia Fatigue Pallor Thrombocytopenia (oozing gums, epistaxis, petechiae, ecchymoses, menorrhagia, and excessive bleeding after tooth extraction) Infections of respiratory, dental, sinus, perirectal, and urinary tract with poor response to treatment Diffuse adenopathy Hepatosplenomegaly Bone pain Migratory joint pain accompanied by swelling and tenderness	Fundoscopic examination Laboratory findings of abnormal white blood cell count Peripheral blood smear Aspiration of bone marrow
Chronic myelogenous leukemia	Weight loss despite excellent appetite Low-grade fever Night sweats	Peripheral blood findings Reduced and absent leukocyte alkaline phosphatase (LAP) score

Continued.

Table 10-6	Screening and detection recommendations by cancer site—cont'd	
Cancer site	**Signs and symptoms**	**Screening, detection, and diagnostic tests**
Leukemia— cont'd Chronic myelogenous leukemia— cont'd	Fatiguability Splenomegaly (mild sensation of fullness or awareness of actual mass) Early satiety Peripheral leg edema Splenic pain referred to left shoulder Bone pain Bleeding problems Mucous membrane irritation Infection Pallor Adenopathy Hepatomegaly	Presence of Philadelphia chromosome (Phi) Hyperuricemia Hyperuricosuria
Chronic lymphocytic leukemia	Minimal diffuse adenopathy or splenomegaly Fatigue Malaise Occasional fever Infection Lymphadenopathy Night sweats Weight loss Uncomfortable neck masses Enlarged spleen Anemia Thrombocytopenia	Routine blood studies Bone marrow aspirations
Liver	Painful hepatomegaly Tender liver with nodular enlargement Splenomegaly Esophageal varices Ascites Jaundice GI bleeding Fever Edema	Tumor markers (e.g., AFP) Ultrasonography CT with contrast medium Liver scan Arteriography Portal venography Bone survey Chest radiography Needle biopsy
Lung	Change in pulmonary habits (cough, hoarseness, chest pain, rust-streaked or purulent sputum production, hemoptysis, and dyspnea) Recurrent pneumonitis Pleural effusion Shoulder and arm pain	Radiography Three-day sputum cytological study
Metastasis to brain	Paresthesias Headache Unsteadiness of gait	
Metastasis to liver	Neurological signs Weight loss Jaundice	
Metastasis to skeleton	Anorexia Bony pain Pathological fractures	

Table 10-6	Screening and detection recommendations by cancer site—cont'd	

Cancer site	Signs and symptoms	Screening, detection, and diagnostic tests
Lymphoma Hodgkin's disease	Adenopathy in supraclavicular or cervical area Fever Night sweats Weight loss	Physical examination CT of abdomen Radiography of chest Lymphagiography Laparotomy
Non-Hodgkin's lymphoma	Adenopathy Anemia	Laboratory findings of abnormal lymphocytes Leukemia composed of lymphoma cells Bone marrow aspiration Radiography of chest Bipedal lymphangiography Cytological examinations of any effusions Lung tomography Gallium and bone scans Radiographic examinations of gastrointestinal and urinary tract Liver biopsy Laparoscopy Laparotomy and splenectomy
Multiple myeloma	Anemia Back pain Painful skeletal lesions (osteolytic lesions) Proneness to pathological fractures that result in exacerbations of pain and skeletal instability Hypercalcemia (manifests in weakness, nausea, and altered mental status) Renal failure	Bone marrow examination Radiographic tests with contrast agents Laboratory studies Serum electrophoreses Erythrocyte sedimentation rate
Pancreas	Insidious onset of asthenia, anorexia, weight loss, gaseousness, and nausea Dull pain in epigastrium and back Jaundice Pruritus	CT with contrast medium Ultrasound Endoscopic retrograde cholangiopancreatography Thin-needle percutaneous biopsy
Prostate	Renal insufficiency and hematuria Weak or interrupted flow of urine Difficulty in starting and stopping urination Need to urinate frequently (especially at night) Painful, burning urination Blood in urine Bone pain Continuous pain in lower back, pelvis, or uppr thighs	Digital rectal examination Blood studies (serum acid phosphatase, alkaline acid phosphatase, prostate-specific antigen [PSA]) Radionuclide bone scan Conventional radiography Needle biopsy
Sarcoma of bone	Pain Presence of mass (initially painless) Functional deficit Pathological fracture	Physical examination Bone scan Chest CT Full lung planar tomography Biopsy
Skin and malignant melanoma	Loss of skin markings Variation in pigmentation Irregular hyperkeratotic areas Rough area that scabs over, rescabs, and fails to heal Persistent ulcer Any change in color, size, shape, elevation, surface, surrounding skin, sensation, and consistency	Complete cutaneous examinations Biopsy

Continued.

Table 10-6	Screening and detection recommendations by cancer site—cont'd	
Cancer site	**Signs and symptoms**	**Screening, detection, and diagnostic tests**

Soft-tissue sarcoma (tumors arising from supportive mesenchymal tissue other than bones)	Painless mass (especially in thigh area)
	Hard consistency of mass
	Peripheral neuralgia
	Paralysis
	Ischemia
	Bowel obstruction
	Weight loss
	Fever
	General malaise
	Episodic hypoglycemia
		Physical examination
		Radiographic studies
		  CT
		  Angiography
		Biopsy
		Radioisotope studies

Stomach	Complaints of indigestion and epigastric distress Loss of appetite Weight loss or anorexia Dysphagia Mass in abdomen Colonic obstruction Ulcer-type pain Iron deficiency anemia	Radiographic studies Endoscopic examination Gastroscopy with mucosal biopsies Abrasion balloon cytological study Flexible fiberoptic gastroscopy

Testis	Painless scrotal mass that does not illuminate
	Orchitis
	Infarction
	Feeling of heaviness
	Trauma at times
	Change in preexisting hydrocele
	Attack resembling epididymitis (it does not respond to medical treatment within 14 days)
	Spermatocele
	Hydrocele
	Fatigue
	Pallor (from anemia)
	Cough
	Hemoplysis
		Physical examination (palpation)
		Transillumination of intrascrotal lesions
		Abdominal examination
		Radiography of chest (abdominopelvic CT scanning)
		Hematological survey (RIA)
		  Chorionic gonadotropin levels
		  Alpha-feto protein levels
		  Lactic hydroglucose levels
		Lymphangiography

Thyroid	Mass in neck or cervical lymph node Existing goiter that may suddenly enlarge Hoarseness	Careful palpation of the thyroid gland Palpation of gland while patient swallows small quantities of water Indirect mirror laryngoscopy
Ureters	Hematuria Pain from obstruction	Urine examination Cytological study Excretory urography Cystoscopy Retrograde ureterography Pyelography

Modified from Baird SB, editor: *A cancer source book for nurses,* ed 6, New York, Boston, Atlanta, 1991, American Cancer Society.
CT, Computed tomography; *MRI,* magnetic resonance imaging.

LABORATORY STUDIES

Hundreds of laboratory studies are available today. Some studies are used to analyze the composition of the blood and bone marrow and rule out blood disorders. Blood studies are concerned with blood cells, whereas blood chemistry tests examine chemicals in the blood. Microbiological studies are helpful in detecting specific organisms that may be causing an infection. Urine studies are done to analyze the composition and concentration of the urine. These are helpful in detecting diseases and disorders of the kidney, urinary systems, and endocrine or metabolic disorders. Fecal studies are done to examine the waste products of digestion and metabolic disor-

Table 10-7	Normal ranges for complete blood count

Blood component	Range
White blood cells	3.90 to 10.80 thousand /mm^3
Red blood cells	3.90 to 5.40 million/mm^3
Hemoglobin	12.0 to 16.0 g/dl
Hematocrit	37.0% to 47.0%
Differential white blood cells (WBC)	
Neutrophils	42.0% to 72.0%
Lymphocytes	17.0% to 45.0%
Monocytes	3.0% to 10.0%
Eosinophils	0.0% to 12.0%
Basophils	0.0% to 2.0%
Platelets	150 to 425 thousand /mm^3

ders. These studies are useful in detecting GI diseases and disorders such as bleeding, obstruction, obstructive jaundice, and parasitic disease. Studies are also done to investigate the immune system. Immunological studies examine the antigen-antibody reactions. Serological tests are done to diagnose problems such as neoplastic disease, infectious disease, and allergic reactions.[5] Laboratory studies done to examine cells and tissue will be discussed in the following section.

Baseline values should always be obtained to observe any deviation. Table 10-7 contains normal ranges for a CBC. The values in this may vary from institution to institution depending on the methods used.

MEDICAL IMAGING

The physiology and anatomy of the body can be imaged in many ways, and the procedures used can be extremely simple or complex. Every procedure provides some element of risk to the patient. Noninvasive procedures provide extremely little risk to the patient. Most invasive procedures provide some risk, but the exact amount of acceptable risk depends on many factors. The physician and patient must discuss the risks.

Electrical imaging

Some medical imaging techniques use electrical impulses of the body to determine the ability of the heart, brain, and muscles to function. The electrocardiogram (ECG) demonstrates the electrical conductivity of the heart muscle. This aids in the detection and diagnosis of heart disease. During the examination, wave patterns representing the electrical pulse are drawn on special paper. The physician studies the wave patterns to check for any deviations. The electroencephalogram (EEG) records brain-wave activity. The EEG helps detect and diagnose seizure disorders, brain stem disorders, brain lesions, and states of consciousness. An electromyogram (EMG) measures the electrical conductivity of the

muscle, thus aiding in the detection and diagnosis of neuromuscular problems.

Nuclear medicine imaging

Nuclear imaging is achieved by the introduction of a radionuclide into the patient. A *radionuclide,* or *radiopharmaceutical,* is an isotope that undergoes radioactive decay. It is an unstable element that attempts to reach stability by emitting several types of ionizing radiation. The radionuclide may be injected, swallowed, or inhaled. After the introduction of the radionuclide into the patient, it follows a specific metabolic pathway in the body. Several minutes to several hours later an imaging device is placed outside the patient's body, and the resultant radiation from the radionuclide is measured and imaged. Hot spot and cold spot imaging are the two major types of imaging done in nuclear medicine. Hot spot imaging involves an increase in the concentration of the radionuclide in the area compared with normal tissue. Cold spot imaging is the opposite.

The two most common imaging devices are the gamma camera and rectilinear scanner. The gamma camera does not move and views the whole area of interest at one time. The rectilinear scanner starts at the top or bottom of the area of interest and then scans from side to side until the entire area of interest has been imaged. New imaging modalities in nuclear medicine include single photon emission computed tomography (SPECT) and positron emission tomography (PET). These modalities make possible the viewing of the organ's function and blood flow in addition to the image of its anatomy.[4]

Scans of the kidney, liver, thyroid gland, lung, brain, and bone are commonly used to detect cancer. Scans demonstrate the function, anatomy, and size of a particular organ. Bone scans are especially helpful in evaluating metastatic disease.

Routine radiographic studies

Routine radiographic studies consist of contrast and noncontrast types. The use of contrast media such as barium, Telepaque, Oragrafin, Cholografin, Hypaque and Conray helps to visualize anatomy that is radiolucent. If the anatomical structure is radiolucent, the x-rays are not absorbed by the structure and therefore cannot be demonstrated on a plain radiograph. For example, gas and fecal material in the colon may be visualized without contrast. However, to visualize the structure, position, filling, and movement of the colon, a barium-based contrast agent is necessary. For the esophagus to be visible, the patient must drink barium. Bone is radiopaque and can be demonstrated on a radiograph without the aid of contrast media.

Routine noncontrast studies consist of chest radiographs; films of the abdomen that include the kidneys, ureters, and bladder (KUB); and films of the sinuses, skull, spine, and other bones. Contrast studies include but are not limited to the intravenous pyelogram (IVP), upper and lower GI tract, and arteriograms.

Mammography

The ACS recommends a baseline mammogram for women between the ages of 35 and 40 and an annual or biennial mammogram to be determined by the physician for women between the ages of 40 and 50. For women 50 years and older the ACS recommends an annual mammogram. The self-breast examination (SBE) is strongly recommended by the ACS. Women who regularly engage in SBE often detect lesions before their physicians. Mammography can demonstrate lesions before they can be palpated. SBE has not been proved to improve survival rates. However, research has demonstrated that screening mammography can improve survival rates.[15]

Invasive radiographic studies

Angiography is the visualization of blood vessels by injecting contrast in the veins, arteries, or lymphatic system. During the procedure, stationary and moving pictures can be taken of the movement of the contrast media through the vessels. By this method the examiner can demonstrate abnormalities in the structure of veins, arteries, and lymphatic system.

Most routine radiographic studies give a two-dimensional (2-D) view of a three-dimensional (3-D) body. Images are superimposed on each other, and the depth of an object or anatomical structure cannot be determined. Multiple views in routine radiography are necessary to overcome this limitation.

Computed tomography

Seeing a complete 360-degree cross section of the body was not possible until 1972 with the development of the computerized axial tomographic (CT) scanning unit. Initially, the first CT scanners were head scanners. Later-generation scanners were able to demonstrate the whole body. CT scanners can demonstrate anatomical images in the transverse plane and the coronal plane.[7]

The CT scanner takes an x-ray image, digitizes it, and stores it in a computer. The computer can produce a high-resolution image.[16] Scanners that can produce a 3-D image are now available and being used for reconstructive surgery. Some of these units are found in radiation therapy departments and have great promise for 3-D treatment planning.

Routine radiographs can demonstrate differences between bone, air, and some degree of soft tissue. Because of the high-resolution capability of the CT scanner, radiologists can differentiate between bone, air, and soft tissue to a much higher degree than is possible with routine radiographs.[16] According to Levitt, Khan, and Potish,[13] "The CT has replaced upper gastrointestinal series and pancreatic angiography in the detection of pancreatic cancer."

Magnetic resonance imaging

Until the mid 1980s, magnetic resonance imaging (MRI) was called *nuclear magnetic resonance (NMR)*. The term *nuclear* was deleted because it was unpopular with the public. Unlike nuclear medicine and radiology, MRI does not use ionizing radiation. A major difference between the CT scanner and MRI is the ability of MRI scanners to obtain anatomical images in the sagittal plane. MRI units also have the ability to demonstrate soft tissue to a much greater degree than CT units. However, CT units can demonstrate bone better than MRI units.[7]

Ultrasonography

Ultrasonography is one of the least expensive imaging techniques. It is also quick and simple and usually causes only minimal patient discomfort. Ultrasound also differs from radiography in that its images are produced with high-frequency sound waves instead of ionizing radiation. Because of this, ultrasound has been used extensively in gynecological and prenatal imaging. Fetal weight, growth, and anatomy can be studied without exposure to ionizing radiation. Ovarian tumors are often difficult to image and detect, but with ultrasonography the ovary can be seen.

The ability of ultrasound to demonstrate soft tissue structures is helpful in demonstrating gallstones, kidney stones, and tumors. Ultrasound is the imaging modality of choice for demonstrating tumors of the prostate. With the digital color Doppler, embolism can be diagnosed and occlusion of an artery can be identified by studying the blood flow.

CANCER DIAGNOSIS

Histological evidence is vital in making a diagnosis of cancer. Tissue for diagnosis is obtained through scraping, needle aspiration, needle biopsy, **incisional biopsy,** and **excisional biopsy.**

Exfoliative cells can be found in all parts of the body. These are cells that have been scraped off deliberately or sloughed off naturally. They are found in the urine, sputum, feces, and mucus. Exfoliative cytological studies are extremely helpful in identifying neoplastic disease. The only problem with cytological studies is that individual cells are being viewed and the determination of cells as invasive or noninvasive is not possible.

Other methods of obtaining tissue are needle, incisional, and excisional biopsies. Needle biopsies and incisional biopsies can be done on an outpatient basis by using local anesthesia. Only small amounts of tissue can be obtained by needle and incisional biopsies. An excisional biopsy involves the removal of the entire tumor for diagnosis. This procedure provides for a more definitive diagnosis.[12]

When cancer is detected, determining the presence of metastatic disease is necessary. The use of a tumor marker may help detect widespread disease. A *tumor marker* is a substance manufactured and released by the tumor. Tumor markers "refer to a molecule that can be detected in serum, plasma, or other body fluids. . . . No tumor marker has been shown to have a specificity or sensitivity that is adequate for the screening detection of malignancies in the general population."[11] Tumor markers are useful in detecting metastatic disease and determining the effect of the treatment.

Studies are being done to develop tests that use clonal markers to detect cancer. This holds great promise, and these tests may be available in the near future.

STAGING SYSTEMS

After a histological diagnosis of cancer has been made, the cancer must be staged. Staging helps determine the extent of the disease. Treatment decisions are based on the histological diagnosis and extent of the disease. The natural growth for most cancers if untreated is that they extend beyond their original site by direct extension and then to the lymphatic system. They ultimately metastasize to distant sites. Staging systems are based on this concept.[2]

"Recommendations regarding staging of cancer by individual researchers, specialties, committees, and other groups have not been uniform."[2] The major groups who have been involved in staging and are working together to establish common terminology are the International Union Against Cancer (UICC), the International Federation of Gynecology and Obstetrics (FIGO), and the American Joint Committee for Cancer Staging and End Results Reporting (AJCC).[2]

The AJCC's general definitions of the TNM system are shown in Table 10-8 (subdivisions are not included). Another part of the staging system is the histological type and histological grade. *Histological type* refers to cell type, and *histological grade* refers to the differentiation of the cell. For example, the histological type may be squamous cell carcinoma, and the histological grade indicates the closeness of the cell's resemblance to a normal squamous cell. See the box for the histopathologic grades.

Another aspect of the staging system is the use of stage 0 through stage IV.* Stage 0 usually indicates carcinoma in situ. Stage I and II indicates the smallness of the tumor and/or involvement of early local and regional nodes with no distant metastases. Stage III indicates that the tumor is more extensive locally and may have regional node involvement. Stage IV indicates locally advanced tumors with invasion beyond the regional nodes to other areas. The categorizations of stage 0 through IV are often grouped with the TNM system of staging. For example, stage 0, Tis, N_0, M_0 indicates an extremely localized early disease, whereas stage II, T_2, N_0, M_0 indicates a more advanced disease. Stage IV, any T, any N, and M_1 indicates an extremely late advanced disease.

SUMMARY

As stated earlier in this chapter, medicine is the accumulation of knowledge that has been developed through discovery, systematic scientific study, and research. These processes help detect, diagnose, treat, and manage disease. After a diagnosis of cancer is made and the extent of the disease has been determined, appropriate treatment can be initiated.

*The definitions of these stages may vary according to the site and type of cancer.

Table 10-8	TNM clinical classification

TNM classification	Description
Primary tumor (T)	
TX	Primary tumor not assessable
T_O	No evidence of primary tumor
Tis	Carcinoma in situ
T_1, T_2, T_3, T_4	Increasing size and/or local extent of the primary tumor
Regional lymph nodes (N)	
NX	Regional lymph nodes not assessable
N_O	No regional lymph node metastasis
N_1, N_2, N_3	Increasing involvement of regional lymph nodes
Distant metastasis (M)	
MX	Presence of distant metastasis not assessable
M_O	No distant metastasis
M_1	Distant metastasis

From Beahrs OH, et al, editors: *American Joint Committee on Cancer manual for staging of cancer*, ed 4, Philadelphia, 1992, JB Lippincott.

Histopathologic grade (G)	
GX	Grade not assessable
G_1	Well differentiated
G_2	Moderately differentiated
G_3	Poorly differentiated
G_4	Undifferentiated

Review Questions

Multiple Choice

1. The presence of the Reed-Sternberg cell is necessary to make which of the following diagnoses?
   a. Adenocarcinoma of the breast
   b. Anaplastic carcinoma of the thyroid
   c. Hodgkin's disease
   d. Non-Hodgkin's lymphoma
2. What are the factors that must be observed when taking the pulse?

I. Rate	IV. Character
II. Rhythm	V. Tension
III. Size	

   a. I and II
   b. I, II, III, and V
   c. III and IV
   d. I, II, IV, and V
3. What are the factors that must be observed for respirations?

I. Rate	IV. Rhythm
II. Depth	V. Tension
III. Character	

   a. I, II, III, and IV
   b. III, IV, and V
   c. I and II
   d. IV and V

4. Which of the following statements is *not* true?
   a. Ultrasonography uses high-frequency sound waves.
   b. CT scans have a higher resolution than radiographs.
   c. Electroencephalograms use ionizing radiation.
   d. Most invasive procedures provide some risk to the patient.
5. What is the normal adult range for blood pressure?
   a. 110 to 140 mm Hg over 60 to 80 mm Hg
   b. 130 to 160 mm Hg over 90 to 99 mm Hg
   c. 90 to 100 mm Hg over 60 to 80 mm Hg
   d. 115 to 150 mm Hg over 60 to 90 mm Hg

Questions to Ponder

1. Describe the difference between an objective and subjective diagnosis.
2. Discuss the importance of the interview in helping to make a diagnosis.
3. Describe the factors that may interfere with an interview.
4. Describe the way to facilitate the interview process.
5. Describe nonverbal communication and give examples.
6. Discuss the way the radiation therapist can avoid making errors when ordering a test or procedure for a patient.
7. Identify measures used to determine the value of a study.
8. Describe the TNM staging system.
9. Describe the signs and symptoms for the following cancer sites: breast, prostate, lung, and colon.
10. Describe the screening, detection, and diagnostic tests for the following cancer sites: breast, prostate, lung, and colon.

REFERENCES

1. Baird SB, editor: *A cancer source book for nurses,* ed 6, New York, Boston, Atlanta, 1991, The American Cancer Society.
2. Beahrs OH et al, editors: *Manual staging of cancer,* ed 4, Philadelphia, 1992, JB Lippincott.
3. *Cancer facts and figures,* Atlanta, 1996, The American Cancer Society.
4. Casciato DA, Lowitz BB: *Manual of clinical oncology,* ed 2, Boston, 1991, Little, Brown.
5. DeGowins RL: *Diagnostic examination,* ed 6, New York, 1994, McGraw-Hill.
6. Du Gas BW: *Introduction to patient care: a comprehensive approach to nursing,* ed. 4, Philadelphia, 1983, WB Saunders.
7. Eisenberg RL: *Radiology: an illustrated history,* St Louis, 1992, Mosby.
8. Fischbach F: *A manual of laboratory diagnostic tests,* ed 3, Philadelphia, 1988, JB Lippincott.
9. Glanze WD, editor: *Mosby's medical and nursing dictionary,* ed 2, St Louis, 1986, Mosby.
10. Henry JB: *Clinical diagnosis & management by laboratory methods,* ed 18, Philadelphia, 1991, WB Saunders.
11. Holleb AI, Fink DJ, Murphy GP, editors: *American cancer society textbook of clinical oncology,* Atlanta, 1991, American Cancer Society.
12. Hossfeld DK et al, editors: *Manual of clinical oncology,* ed 5, Berlin, 1990, UICC International Union Against Cancer, Springer-Verlag.
13. Levitt SH, Khan FM, Potish RA, editors: *Levitt and Tapley's technological basis of radiation therapy: practical clinical applications,* ed 2, Philadelphia, 1992, Lea & Febiger.
14. Lewis SM, Collier IC: *Medical-surgical nursing,* New York, 1983, McGraw-Hill.
15. Rubin P: *Clinical oncology: a multidisciplinary approach for physicians and students,* ed 7, Philadelphia, 1993, WB Saunders.
16. Sochurek H: *Medicine's new vision,* Easton, Penn, 1988, Mack Publishing.
17. Wyngaarden JB, Smith LH, editors: *Cecil textbook of medicine,* Philadelphia, 1985, WB Saunders.

BIBLIOGRAPHY

Bates B: *A guide to physical examination,* Philadelphia, 1979, JB Lippincott.

Calabreis P, Schein PS: *Medical oncology,* ed 2, New York, 1993, McGraw-Hill.

The health professional and cancer prevention and detection, Atlanta, 1988, American Cancer Society.

Lyons AS, Petrucelli RJ: *Medicine: an illustrated history,* New York, 1978, Harry N Abrams.

Morton RF, Hebel JR, McCarter RJ: *A study guide to epidemiology and biostatistics,* ed 3, Gaithersburg, Md, 1989, Aspen Publishers.

Roses DF et al: *The diagnosis and management of common skin cancers,* Atlanta, 1989, American Cancer Society.

Segre E: *From x-rays to quarks: modern physicists and their discoveries,* New York, 1980, WH Freeman.

Sherman JL, Fields SK: *Guide to patient evaluation,* ed 3, Garden City, New York, 1978, Medical Examination Publishing Co.

The staging of cancer, Atlanta, 1989, American Cancer Society.

Stryker A: *Clinical oncology for students of radiation therapy technology,* St Louis, 1992, Warren H Green.

Tannock F, Hill P: *The basic science of oncology,* ed 2, New York, 1992, McGraw-Hill.

Torres LS: *Basic medical techniques and patient care for radiologic technologists,* ed 4, Philadelphia, 1993, JB Lippincott.

Principles of Radiation Therapy

Orientation to Radiation Oncology

Phyllis Thompson

Outline

Key terms

Accreditation
Certification
Cognitive

Curriculum
Licensure
Scope of practice

HISTORY OF RADIATION THERAPY

 Winston Churchill once stated, "The farther backward you can look, the farther forward you are likely to see." This narrative on the history of radiation oncology should be viewed as prescriptive for the future. Certain periods of history were relatively stagnant, whereas other periods had ongoing and remarkable progress.

The nineteenth century

Wilhelm Conrad Roentgen is credited with the discovery of x-rays. However, the stage for this discovery was set by other pioneers and discoverers. Nonetheless, on November 8, 1895, Roentgen observed a fluorescence in crystals of a bottle of barium platinocyanide located near a cathode tube in his laboratory. He passed the invisible light through his wife Anna's hand, and hence the first image using the rays was produced. Because Roentgen was not aware of this phenomenon, he called these invisible and unknown rays *x-rays*.

Diagnostic applications of rays developed rapidly, and within a month the therapeutic use evolved. One of the first uses for therapeutic treatment is credited to E.H. Grubbe for his treatment of breast carcinoma. The treatment of nasopharyngeal cancer, stomach cancers, ulcerating breast lesions, and various skin conditions followed.

Meanwhile, a French physicist by the name of Antoine Henri Becquerel reported his first communication on the emission of rays from uranium. This second discovery became known as Becquerel rays. Becquerel's discovery prompted Madam Marie Curie, a Polish scientist, to investigate these rays for her doctoral thesis. With her husband

Pierre, she discovered and reported radioactivity of polonium in July of 1898 and radium in December of 1898. These two discoveries—Roentgen for x-rays and Bacquerel and the Curies for radioactivity—formed the foundation for the treatment of malignant disease with radiation.

The twentieth century

The early 1900s realized the treatment of a variety of diseases with both types of radiation. Nicholas Senn and William Pusey treated leukemia, whereas Albert Friedlaender treated enlarged thymus. Throughout the remainder of the first half of the twentieth century, progress in radiation oncology advanced rapidly, lulled only by the effects of World Wars I and II. By the end of the second World War, interest was piqued. The 1920s and 1930s realized the building of the first x-ray beam unit by General Electric. External beam radiation therapy was successfully developed during this time. Most treatments were carried out with energies of 250 kVp or less. Treatment results were published, and in 1937 Robert Jemison Van de Graaff built the first electrostatic generator. These successes ushered in the use of higher penetrating beams. Also significant in the 1930s was a system of measuring radiation developed by Edith Quimby, thus making possible the comparison of treatment doses from patient to patient.

Significant growth and development occurred in the latter half of the twentieth century. In 1941 Donald A. Kerst built the betatron and thus created a radiation beam that produced electrons and photons for treatment. Postwar research efforts provided for additional use of this type of equipment. In 1950 cobalt 60 (used as a radium substitute) units were used for the first time in Regina, Saskatchewan. High-voltage sources such as electrostatic generators and linear accelerators became readily available for electron and x-radiation treatments.

Until the 1950s, physicians and nurses administered most radiation treatments. As the equipment and treatments became more successful, x-ray personnel performed these duties and became operators of the equipment. Sophisticated methods of treatment offered improved treatment results, thereby creating a demand for more specialized and educated persons to administer radiation treatments to patients. In 1962 two schools of radiation therapy technology were opened, and in 1967 the first educational standards for radiation therapy schools were established. Graduates of these schools were called *radiation therapy technologists.* In 1964 the first examination to establish credentialing in radiation therapy technology was given. Since 1960 the profession and education of radiation therapists has developed to include a diverse and complex set of numerable responsibilities. Growth of radiation oncology has paralleled the growth and expansion of the duties of the radiation therapist. As computers, simulators, and complex treatment equipment evolved, so did the demand for highly educated professional radiation therapists.

HEALTH SCIENCE PROFESSIONS
Medical profession

The term *medical profession* usually refers to the physician as a medical doctor (MD). A *physician* is a person who has successfully completed a prescribed course of studies in medicine and has acquired prerequisite qualifications for licensure in the practice of medicine. This profession is perhaps one of the oldest, dating back to prehistoric and primitive times. From the primitive healers of ancient Egypt, India, China, and Greece to modern times, healing rituals have been a part of everyday life. Hippocrates established himself as the father of medicine. His habits of observing and studying the patient (not the disease) and evaluating and assisting nature revolutionized medicine from the ancient past into a documentable, objective science. Born in 460 BC, Hippocrates' writings advised not only the physical aspects of disease, but also mental illness, anxiety, and depression. He also introduced ethical aspects of medicine.

Today, the practice of medicine is extremely complex. Since the middle of the nineteenth century, progress, discoveries, and advances in technology have been in a continuing state of evolution and change. The role of the physician has adapted and grown into new and more increased areas of specialization.

Nursing profession

Nursing is probably one of the first health professions. The first nurses were home caregivers, whereas the modern nurse fulfills a multitude of roles in the health care delivery system. Nursing is a diverse career in that it offers several career paths for persons in the profession.

Nurses are primarily employed in clinical settings. However, today their roles include administration, pharmacy, government, insurance, military, and public health. Historically, their roles have been assisting physicians. However, a modern day nurse can take health histories, perform physical examinations, provide information on health awareness and disease prevention, and (in some situations) prescribe and deliver treatments. The extent of nursing varies from simple patient care tasks to the most expert, professional techniques necessary in acute life-threatening situations. The role of the nurse is constantly changing as a result of the growth of biomedical knowledge; changes in the patterns of the demand for health services; and the evolution of professional relationships among nurses, physicians, and other health care professionals.

A variety of clinical specializations exist in nursing. For example, nurses may specialize in areas such as pediatrics, anesthesia, obstetrics, and gynecology. Of particular interest in radiation oncology is the nurse who specializes in medical oncology. Oncologic nurses care primarily for cancer patients by rendering physical and psychosocial support, providing acute nursing care, and administering chemotherapeutic drugs.

Health profession

Supportive services. A variety of supportive services provide assistance for patients undergoing radiation therapy. Individuals such as dietitians sometimes have direct contact with patients, whereas others such as medical record administrators and technicians, medical secretaries, and biomedical engineers rarely see patients. The dietitian's education and expertise are focused in the area of nutrition. This person has the ability to apply information to the regulation of diet in sick and healthy patients.

Dietitians work primarily in six areas: administrative, community, consultant, research, teaching, and clinical. The administrative dietitian is responsible for program planning and resource education, whereas the community dietitian specializes in community dietetics preparation and nutritional needs assessment for individuals and groups. The consultant dietitian has expertise in administration and clinical dietetics and provides advice for services in nutritional care to hospitals, retirement centers, and extended-care facilities. The research dietitian has advanced preparation in dietetics and research techniques. The teaching dietitian has advanced preparation in dietetics and conducts and evaluates educational programs for dietetics, medical, dental, and other students. The clinical dietitian (sometimes called a *therapeutic dietitian*) plans diets and supervises meal services to patients in hospitals, nursing homes, and clinics. This health professional probably interacts more directly with patients undergoing radiation therapy treatments than other dietitians. Oncology patients often have difficulty swallowing, eating, and maintaining good nutritional balance. The clinical dietitian serves as a consultant to these patients by counseling them and their families in the principles of nutrition. Clinical dietitians first confer with the radiation oncologist and other members of the health care team, and then the patient is evaluated, a nutritional care plan is developed, and patients are advised accordingly.

Another member of the support network for the radiation oncology patient is the individual involved in the health information sector. Health information specialists include medical record administrators (MRAs) and medical record technicians (MRTs). The MRA is responsible for the management of health information systems consistent with professional standards and the medical administrative, ethical, and legal requirements in the health care industry. Primarily, the MRA directs the activities of the medical records department. This includes planning; organizing the department; and preparing, monitoring, and analyzing the medical records of all patients. This forms the link between the increasing volume of medical data and the latest information-handling systems. The MRA is assisted by the MRT, who primarily maintains the information systems that include patient records. Both health professionals make significant contributions to oncology in that they serve as the backbone workers of the tumor registry.

Public health services. Public health provides protection and promotes community health through organized community effort. This community approach includes services that other health professionals provide and the particular focus of the public health sector. Public health officials aim to conserve human and fiscal resources by attacking the causes and spread of disease, educating citizens, and attempting to ensure health and medical services.

Several health professions are involved in public health services. Probably first and foremost is the epidemiologist. Epidemiology defines and explains the interrelationship of factors that determine disease, causation, frequency, and distribution. Public health officials aim to reduce the incidence and prevalence of disease, accidents, addictions, and environmental pollution. Their work is of particular interest to cancer patients, because it has often assisted with the prevention and control of disease. For example, epidemiological studies of smokers have made significant, notable progress in proving that nicotine is a contributing factor in lung cancer. The work of public health officials has also provided considerable attention in dietary concerns related to cancer. Epidemiologists investigate many facets of internal and external environments (i.e., diets, smoking, alcohol consumption, work surroundings and hazards, genetics, family composition, and the use of medical care and related services to provide valuable life-saving information).

Epidemiologists are assisted by biostatisticians, who apply statistical processes and methods to analyze biological data. For example, the work of biostatisticians with vital statistics provides information regarding births, deaths, and certain illnesses. This information can be of great value in cancer research activities.

Another health professional in the public health sector is the environmental health specialist. This individual is employed in a wide range of activities related to noise pollution, accident prevention, product safety, air-quality management, and radiation control. This work affects the general health of people today and is becoming more noticeable. Most environmental health specialists are employed in federal, state, and local environmental protection agencies. Public awareness and concern for environmental issues and their effect on health and safety are becoming significant in everyday life. Of particular concern to radiation oncology are the effects of the environment with regard to carcinogens, radiation workers, and the safety of the work environment.

Finally, public health administrators make a significant contribution to public health service. Public health administrators hold positions in all branches of public health, from the direction of health departments to the administration of special nutrition, population planning, public health nursing, alcoholism, and drug abuse programs. These administrators also work in insurance companies and health-planning agencies in government and private policy analysis.

Dental services. As the primary provider of dental services the dentist deals with the care of teeth and associated structures of the oral cavity. Dentists are concerned with the prevention, diagnosis, and treatment of the teeth and gums. Many dental specialists center their attention and expertise to specific areas. For example, the orthodontist deals with the prevention and treatment of irregularities of the teeth, the oral surgeon performs surgical procedures on the teeth, the periodontist deals with the diagnosis and treatment of diseases that invade the oral cavity, and the prosthodonist specializes in the mechanics of making and fitting artificial teeth. The prosthodonist is the type of dentist probably encountered most by radiation oncology patients when they undergo radiation to the head and neck area. Radiation of the head and neck area often necessitates the removal of teeth by the oral surgeon, and posttreatment of the patient is done by the prosthodontist, who replaces the natural teeth with fixed or removal devices.

Dentists are also useful agents in the detection of cancer. Dentists are often the first to observe and report precancerous conditions during patients' routine office visits. In addition, dentists often provide support before, during, and after treatment for patients with head and neck disease.

The dental hygienist is an assistant to the dentist. This health professional cleans teeth and provides counsel and education to the public. The dental hygienist works with patients to improve and protect their dental health. This is particularly important to cancer patients undergoing radiation treatments. The general counseling and educational advice of dental hygienists can offer cancer patients the emotional and physical support they need to maintain good oral dental hygiene.

Dental assistants also provide support and work with the dentist. They make patients comfortable, prepare them for treatments, and assist the dentist with instruments and materials. Dental assistants also make casts of teeth and mouths from impressions used to make dentures. Additionally, they may manage the office, make appointments, and handle billing procedures.

Pharmacy services. Pharmacy, the practice of compounding and dispensing medicine, dates to ancient times in the primitive medicine man. The practice of *pharmacology,* as it is known today, involves not only the preparation and dispensing of drugs, but also the education of patients. The pharmacist is the health professional licensed to prepare and dispense drugs. This health professional may specialize in several different areas in the health care setting. The most common is in the area of community pharmacy. The community pharmacist dispenses medicines and health supplies, provides health and drug information to consumers, and acts as an advisor to physicians and patients with regard to the science of drugs and their composition, contraindications, availability, and activity.

Another area of specialization for the pharmacist is in the hospital setting. In many institutions the hospital pharmacist's duties parallel those of the community pharmacist. However, in large medical centers the responsibilities of hospital pharmacists become more specialized and involved. Preparation of special fluids for intravenous administration, service on various hospital committees, and involvement with the drug therapy of patients are some of the additional tasks hospital pharmacists may perform.

Cancer patients are not usually directly involved with the hospital pharmacist. However, the pharmacist certainly provides services in terms of the various medications administered, especially for patients undergoing chemotherapy.

Laboratory services. Laboratory services are provided to cancer patients by several health professionals, including pathologists, medical technologists, cytotechnologists, histotechnologists, laboratory technicians, and assistants. These health professionals provide services primarily in the clinical setting and offer invaluable services to cancer patients, mostly through the diagnosis of malignant disease.

The pathologist is a doctor of medicine who specializes in diagnosing morbid changes in tissues removed during surgical procedures and postpartum examinations. Pathologists study the characteristics, causes, and progression of diseases; are actively involved in laboratory tests; and perform autopsies. Their expertise isolates, defines, and categorizes the specific tumor-size staging and provides the basis for the patient's prognosis.

The pathologist works with other health professionals to accomplish these tasks. The medical technologist is one of these individuals. Medical technologists perform tests with pathologists in detecting, diagnosing, and treating many diseases. For example, medical technologists develop data on blood, tissue, and body fluids by using a variety of precision instruments. The medical technologist often supervises the medical laboratory technician, who performs many of the routine tasks and procedures in the clinical laboratory. Histotechnologists also provide valuable services in the clinical laboratory. The histotechnologist prepares sections of body tissue for examination by the pathologist.

Another individual in the clinical laboratory setting is the cytotechnologist, who works with the pathologist to detect changes in body cells that may be important in the early diagnosis of cancer and other diseases. This is done primarily with the microscope to screen slide preparations of body cells for abnormalities in structure that indicate a benign or malignant condition.

Rehabilitation services. Rehabilitation involves processes of treatment and education that lead the disabled individual to attain maximal function, a sense of well-being, and a personally satisfying level of independence. Combined efforts of the individual; family; friends; medical, nursing, and allied health personnel; and community services make rehabilitation possible. The restoration of an ill or injured patient to self-sufficiency or gainful employment at its highest attainable skill in the shortest possible time is a goal in rehabilitation.

Rehabilitation can be the role of a number of health professionals. These health professionals work individually or sometimes with one another to achieve goals of rehabilitation. Rehabilitation experts can assist cancer patients, especially those undergoing radiation therapy, to return to the state and quality of life to which they are accustomed. Some of the health professionals who offer and assist in the rehabilitative process are physical therapists, occupational therapists, and prosthesists.

The physical therapist is legally responsible for planning, conducting, and evaluating a physical therapy program for a patient. Physical therapists examine, evaluate, and treat patients by using therapeutic procedures that include exercise and the use of artificial devices to improve the patient's quality of life. A patient is referred to a physical therapist by a physician. The physical therapist then evaluates the patient's condition and (after assessment is completed) plans a program of treatment that may include exercise, ultrasound waves, hydrotherapy, and infrared lamps. The physical therapist assists the cancer patient most often when surgery has rendered an area of the body immobile, amputation occurs, the use of artificial limbs requires instruction, and daily exercise patterns may benefit the overall recovery. Physical therapists often work with physical therapy assistants, who administer selected treatments and assist the physical therapist in patient-education activities and other daily routines.

The occupational therapist evaluates the self-care, work, play-time and leisure-time tasks, and performance skills of well and disabled clients. Occupational therapists then plan and implement programs. These programs can be social and interpersonal activities designed to restore, develop, and maintain the client's ability to accomplish everyday routines. The occupational therapist evaluates the psychosocial and physical needs of the patient, develops a treatment plan, and then determines activities and procedures necessary to facilitate an effective treatment. The occupational therapist is assisted by the occupational therapist assistant, an individual who (under the supervision of the occupational therapist) carries out the treatment, thereby restoring and developing the client's life-skill care and work and leisure skills.

A prosthesist is a specialist and maker of artificial limbs and dentures. The prosthesist writes specifications for, makes, fits, and repairs braces, appliances, and artificial limbs on prescription of a physician. The prosthesist assistant aids the prosthesist in caring for the patient by making casts, taking measurements and model specifications, and fitting supportive appliances or artificial limbs. Many cancer patients are referred to the prosthesist after surgery and before, during, and after treatment of radiation therapy to accommodate various treatment preparations and occurrences.

Other types of rehabilitative services that assist patients in adapting probably deal more with emotional, spiritual, and psychological considerations. These services include art, dance, and music therapy. Therapists in these areas apply the principles in art, dance, and music to the rehabilitation of physically and mentally handicapped patients. A music therapist can create an environment conducive to treatment, and art and dance therapists assist patients with creative adaptations to their disease.

Psychiatric services. Psychiatry deals with the diagnosis, treatment, and prevention of mental illness. The psychiatrist is a physician with specialized training in the diagnosis and treatment of mental and emotional disorders with medication, counseling, and psychotherapy. The psychiatrist also provides general supervision to other health professionals of the mental health care team, including psychologists, social workers, and psychiatric nurses.

Mental health services are provided in a variety of health care settings: hospitals, clinics, schools and universities, prisons, and private practice. Cancer patients may visit a psychiatrist, psychologist, or psychiatric nurse when they are experiencing unusual stress or related illnesses from their life-threatening disease. However, the medical social worker is more likely to interact with the cancer patient during the course of the radiation therapy. The medical social worker is trained to identify and understand emotional and social factors associated with the treatment of cancer patients. This person also helps resolve problems that interfere with the everyday life and treatment of cancer patients. For example, many times problems exist in the patient-treatment accommodations. The medical social worker recognizes these problems and offers counseling or refers critical life-threatening situations to a psychiatrist. The medical social worker also assists patients in dealing with psychosocial problems associated with their families. More important, medical social workers often help patients deal with situations and problematic circumstances associated with the treatment of their disease. For example, the medical social worker can make arrangements for transportation of the patient to treatment, support services in the home, and assist with other situations in making disease-coping mechanisms easier.

Medical specialty services. As stated earlier, the practice of medicine dates back to ancient times. Interest in and devotion to the art of healing and relieving pain has been ongoing since history has been recorded. Modern medicine is relatively new and can be traced to the late nineteenth century. Physicians in those times did not enjoy the respect, rank, and notoriety given to medical doctors today and were often associated with quackery and faith healers. The technological developments in the twentieth century effected monumental changes in the practice of medicine and established a legitimacy and standard of care in the United States that is admired throughout the world.

The physician is educated to diagnose and treat human disease. In the past, physicians were commonly called *general practitioners*. Specializations were available, but most physicians were general practitioners and provided generalized care. In the middle of the twentieth century an increase in specialization occurred, so many types of specialization are available today. However, a trend is growing toward generalized and family practice as a result of the escalating health care costs associated with specialized medicine today.

The number of specialties and subspecialties in medicine is large. All specialties have one commonality: The physician must complete medical school and a residency. The time involved in the preparation for each specialty varies. Certifying boards exist, and physicians must meet the criteria for individual certification.

Physicians practicing ophthamology and otolaryngology are referred to as *ophthamologists* and *otolaryngologists,* respectively. The ophthamologist specializes in the treatment of eye disorders and diseases, and the otolaryngologist specializes in the treatment of diseases of the head and neck. These specialists often refer patients to radiation oncology for assessment and treatment.

Pediatricians specialize in the treatment of children's diseases from birth to adolescence. The pediatrician provides preventive and ongoing care. Pediatrics encompasses several subspecialties, such as neonatology (the study of the newborn), pediatric cardiology, and pediatric hematology. During special and routine examinations, pediatricians may detect malignant conditions and provide referrals to surgeons or radiation oncologists for treatments.

Other physicians who specialize and make referrals to radiation oncologists include gynecologists, who study and treat the female reproductive system; urologists, who study and treat the urinary tract in both sexes; neurologists, who study and treat the nervous system; and pulmonologists and chest physicians, who study and treat diseases of the lung and chest. Dermatologists also study and specialize in the treatment of skin diseases and frequently refer patients with skin cancers for radiation treatment.

The surgeon specializes in surgery. This branch of medicine deals with manual and operative procedures for correcting deformities and defects (such as cancer), repairing injuries, and diagnosing and curing certain diseases. Radical surgery involves extensive excision or removal of a part of a diseased tissue or adjoining areas of lymphatic drainage in an attempt to obtain complete cure. The surgeon assesses the patient, determines whether surgery is necessary, and then performs the operation and supervises the preoperative and postoperative care of the patient. Numerous subspecialties exist that require additional certification (e.g., orthopedic, gynecological, thoracic, and plastic surgery). Because surgery is one of the primary cancer treatments, cancer patients interact often with surgeons.

The anesthesiologist specializes in the administration of local and general anesthesia for the preparation and performance of surgical procedures. Drugs and gas are used to render patients unconscious for surgical procedures. The anesthesiologist monitors the patient during and after surgery.

Internal medicine comprises another branch of medicine. Internists treat diseases of the internal organs with nonsurgical methods. Family practice is still a comprehensive method of patient care that focuses on the family unit. Physicians practicing in this area are responsible for health care that is not limited by the patient's age, gender, particular body organ, body system, or disease entity.

Preventive medicine is a specialty that includes public health and occupational medicine and encompasses mental and physical disease. Preventative effort has three levels, each of which affects the diagnosis and treatment of the cancer patient. The first level is concerned with preventing the occurrence of disease and includes general promotion of health and specific protection such as immunization. The second level involves early diagnosis and speedy treatment to reduce the severity and duration of disease. The third level is concerned with limiting the degree of disability and promoting rehabilitation of chronic disease.

Oncological services. Surgeons, medical oncologists, and radiation oncologists provide the major care for cancer patients. The surgeon specializes in manual and operative procedures for the correction of deformities and defects, repair of injuries, and diagnosis and cure of certain diseases. The surgeon's role in the cure and treatment of cancer involves mainly two procedures: conservative surgery (removal of as much as possible of a diseased part or structure) and radical surgery (extensive excision to remove diseased tissue or adjoining areas of lymphatic drainage in an attempt to obtain a complete cure).

The medical oncologist deals with the diagnosis and treatment of cancer from the medical aspect. This physician treats cancer patients by using chemotherapeutic drugs. Patients are treated usually as outpatients. However, sometimes extensive courses of chemotherapy are given to individuals as inpatients. The prescription and application of chemotherapy can be extremely complicated, and care is taken to ensure that the correct combination and dosage are given. These powerful drugs can kill if not properly prescribed and administered. A registered nurse who specializes in oncology often assists the medical oncologist. This area of specialization requires advanced certification and involves advanced levels of nursing care.

The radiation oncologist specializes in the treatment of cancer patients through the use of ionizing radiation. This physician assesses the patient's condition, prescribes the radiation treatment, and is responsible for the treatment and posttreatment care and follow-up. The radiation oncologist is a member of a team of specialists that includes the radiation therapist, radiation physicist, and dosimetrist. Others who may assist include nurses, dietitians, and social workers. Together, this team of caregivers provides the radiation dosage to the cancer patient to cure the disease, extend life, or make life more comfortable. The radiation oncologist has specialized training in radiation oncology and is board certified. The radiation therapist is a health professional educated to deliver a prescribed, planned course of radiation therapy to the cancer patient. The radiation therapist's duties include the administration of the radiation treatment, care and emotional support during treatment, observation of the patient's clinical progress, and education of the patient regarding treatments.

The medical physicist has worked with the radiation oncologist since the early days of radiation therapy. Medical physicists are responsible for many of the advances in technology and the movement into the modern age of radiation oncology. In small radiation oncology departments the medical physicist may be a part of the department. However, in large research institutions, departments exist that are dedicated solely to medical physics. The medial physicist in the radiation therapy department has primarily two responsibilities. One responsibility is relevant to the calibration of the radiation-producing equipment, and the other is focused on clinical dosimetry (the planning of the radiation treatment). The medical physicist is responsible for the daily calibration-dosage measurements; maintenance, calibration, and installation of new equipment; research; and the overall quality-assurance mechanisms used in the department. In clinical dosimetry the medical dosimetrist assists the medical physicist. Together, they plan the course of treatment for the cancer patient, computer applications relevant to the treatment, quality-assurance mechanisms regarding dose distribution, and evaluation and research of treatment results.

Radiologic services. Radiology is concerned with radiant energies, including x-rays, radioactive isotopes, and ionizing and nonionizing radiation, and the application of these radiant energies to the prevention, diagnosis, and treatment of disease. The radiologist uses these radiant energies for the diagnosis and treatment of disease. Radiologic services generally involve three main areas: radiation therapy, diagnostic radiology, and nuclear medicine.

Because of the rapid technological advances occurring in the past 25 years, diagnostic radiology has many areas of specialization. Some of these areas are general radiology, mammography, computed tomography (CT), magnetic resonance imaging (MRI), interventional radiology, and diagnostic medical sonography.

Most radiologists are involved in the practice of general radiology, which includes common x-ray examinations such as those prescribed for injury and the detection of common illnesses. Examinations with chest and skeletal x-rays are probably most common. Many times, contrast material is used to visualize selected body organs. The radiologist interprets the x-ray films and provides the referring physician with a report, thus rendering a diagnosis. To the untrained eye an x-ray study shows extremely little; yet to the radiologist the shadowing imaging reveals important information related to a patient's condition.

Some radiologists specialize in mammography (the x-ray study of breast tissue). Mammography is probably one of the most effective means of diagnosing breast cancer. Radiologists who specialize in mammography are trained to notice any abnormalities in the mammogram (an x-ray study of the breast).

Radiologists who specialize in CT are involved in the computer's application to medical imaging. CT images show organs of interest at selected levels of the body. These images are produced by rotating the x-ray around the patient. X-rays passing through the body are detected by an array of sensors, and the information from these sensors is computer processed and then displayed as an image on a video screen. The radiologist interprets these images and reports findings. CT can image internal organs and separate overlapping structures. It has become the diagnostic tool of choice in a variety of situations and has replaced a number of more painful radiologic procedures.

Radiologists who specialize in MRI practice in one of the newest areas for radiology specialization. MRI is similar to CT in that body sections are visualized. However, the source of energy for MRI is a large magnet rather than x-rays. The magnet produces a magnetic field up to 8000 times stronger than that of the earth. The magnetic field circles the patient, and an image is produced through interactions with the human body cell nuclei, radio frequencies, and the magnet. This data is computer processed, and an extremely detailed image of human anatomy is produced. MRI uses no ionizing radiation, presents no apparent risk to patients, and is replacing many painful and risky examinations.

Radiologists specializing in interventional radiology are involved with the treatment rather than the initial diagnoses of disease. These specialists use narrow tubes called *catheters* to treat conditions such as artery blockage by inserting the catheter into the blood vessel and threading it to the point of the blockage. A tiny balloon at the end of the catheter is then inflated, thereby breaking open the blockage and returning the normal blood flow. Because it is initiated from outside the body, this procedure offers an alternative to surgery and eliminates or shortens hospital stays.

Diagnostic medical sonography involves the use of reflected sound echoes to gather sonographic data necessary to reach diagnostic decisions. It includes general sonography, cardiac sonography, and various subspecialties. Sound waves are produced by a transducer that is placed in contact with the skin. The transducer also receives the sound echoes, an image is produced on a video screen, and the image is frequently recorded as it is being made. The radiologist then interprets the image.

Nuclear medicine is concerned with the diagnostic, therapeutic, and investigative use of radioactive substances called *radionuclides* or *radiopharmaceuticals*. Normally, a separate hospital department is dedicated to this specialty. However, nuclear medicine may often be practiced in areas such as pathology, radiology, and internal medicine. The radionuclides are administrated inside (in vivo) and outside (in vitro) the body for diagnostic and therapeutic purposes. Nuclear medicine studies visualize and document the function of organs rather than structures. A patient is injected with a radioactive chemical and scanned with a gamma camera that detects the radioactivity. The chemicals are specially formulated to be collected temporarily in parts of the body to be studied. For example, when spreading to bone, tumors may stimulate abnormal bone production. This abnormality causes more of the chemical (radionuclide) to collect in this region. The gamma camera visualizes the spread of the tumor because of the increased energy absorbed by the abnormal bone.

RADIATION THERAPIST PROFESSION
Accreditation

The radiation therapist's main duty is to provide long-term radiation treatments and emotional support to cancer patients. Radiation therapy requires independent judgment and the ability to provide the best possible care to patients. To become a radiation therapist an individual must graduate from an accredited program and pass a national certification examination. Programs in radiation therapy are available in practically every state and vary in length from 1 to 4 years depending on the student's educational background. Typically, the 1-year program admits radiologic technologists already certified in radiography. A 2-year program admits high school graduates and awards a certificate or associate degree, whereas the 4-year program also admits individuals with high school degrees and awards a baccalaureate degree. The professional organization for radiation therapists, the American Society of Radiologic Technologists (ASRT), has mandated that by the year 2000, a baccalaureate degree be required for entry to the profession.

Regardless of the type of program, it must be accredited. **Accreditation** is a process of voluntary, external peer review in which a nongovernmental agency grants public recognition to an institution or specialized program of study that meets current, established qualifications and educational standards as determined through initial and subsequent periodic evaluations. The purpose of accreditation is to provide a professional judgment of the quality of the educational institution or program and encourage its continued improvement. Accreditation is also assurance of acceptable educational quality. Accredited programs are required to meet national standards established by radiologic science professionals and communities of interest.

The process of accreditation is also meant to protect students from inadequate programs and provide assurance of quality health care to the public. The accrediting agency recognized by the U.S. Department of Education for radiation therapy is the Joint Review Committee on Education in Radiologic Technology (JRCERT).

The JRCERT interacts with nearly 800 institutions sponsoring radiography and radiation therapy educational programs. Through processes and procedures, documentation related to program compliance with the educational standards is collected and assessed. The JRCERT identifies a peer evaluator to conduct a site visit of the educational program. The function of the site visitor is to collect information from a variety of program interests such as institutional administrators, program officials, and students and to validate documentation that the institution of the program may have submitted. The JRCERT is governed by a board of directors composed of nine members, three physicians appointed by the American College of Radiology (ACR), five technologists appointed by the ASRT and the American Association of Educators in Radiologic Sciences, and one public member selected by the JRCERT from a pool of nominees.

After graduating from an accredited program, the student is eligible to apply to take a national certification examination. The American Registry of Radiologic Technologists (ARRT) administers this examination.

Certification

Certification is a process by which a governmental or nongovernmental agency or association grants an individual who has met predetermined qualifications the authority to use a specified title. Individuals passing the ARRT examination are certified and may then use the title *radiologic technologist* or RT (T), ARRT after their names. The *(T)* signifies certification in radiation therapy. A card is also issued with the name of the individual and the expiration date. The card and certification expires yearly and must be renewed annually by paying a fee. In January 1997, to renew the registration process, the radiation therapist will have to document proof of continuing education (12 hours per year) or be reexamined.

The purpose of the ARRT is to examine and certify eligible candidates for entry to the profession. The examination is given 3 times per year (March, July, and October), usually in a location near the candidate's home. A board of trustees composed of nine members administers the examination. The ACR appoints four members, and the ASRT appoints five members. Most hospitals hire only radiation therapists with ARRT certification, and nearly half the states require radiation therapists be licensed to practice. Certification by the ARRT is accepted by these states with licensure laws for licensing purposes.

Licensure is a process by which an agency or government grants permission to an individual to work in a specific occupation after finding the individual has attained the minimal degree of competency necessary to ensure that the health and safety of the public is well protected. Licensure is probably the most restrictive form of occupational regulation. It prevents individuals from engaging in activities covered in their scope of practice without permission from a government agency.

The ARRT also certifies other professions in radiologic technology, including the following: radiographer, RT (R); nuclear medicine technologist, RT (N); mammographer, RT (M); cardiovascular interventional technologist, RT (CV); computed tomographer, RT (CT); and magnetic resonance imager, RT (MR). Fig. 11-1 demonstrates the various certifications.

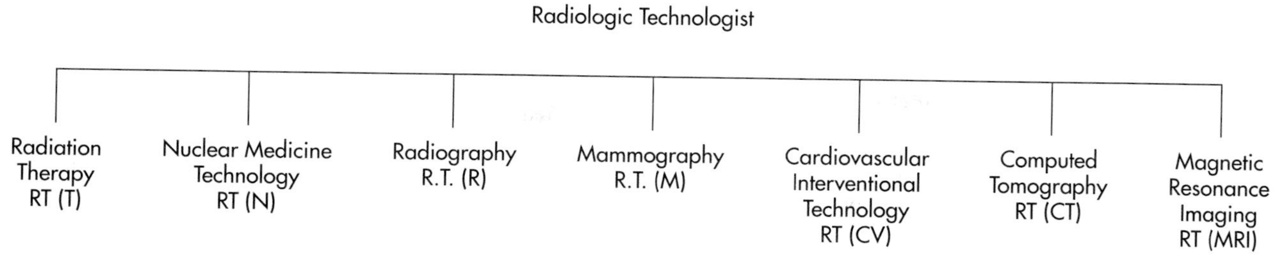

Radiologic Technologist

Fig. 11-1 Certifications available to the radiologic technologist.

Scope of practice document

The scope of practice document defines the role and responsibilities of radiation therapists in the contemporary practice of radiation therapy (see the box in Chapter 4). Accredited educational programs for radiation therapists encompass the cognitive, psychomotor, and affective elements fundamental to the scope of practice definition. The assumed and assigned role and responsibilities have developed over time and are consistent with contemporary clinical practice. Variations in local, state, or federal statutes or regulations supersede the specifics that are contained in the scope of practice document.

Code of ethics

The ASRT has adopted a code of ethics for radiation therapists (see the box in Chapter 4). This code sets forth a system of moral principles and standards governing the conduct of the therapist.

Career mobility

Graduate radiation therapists usually begin their careers as staff radiation therapists in hospitals or cancer centers. After a reasonable period, some radiation therapists feel a need for the opportunity to move laterally or advance in the profession. This is an individual decision based on the radiation therapist's personality, motivation, and ability to seek new pursuits. A radiation therapist's attitude toward professional development is an important factor in career mobility, whether the individual's goal is a lateral or upward move. Continuing education also plays a role. Usually, some advanced education, knowledge, and even change in attitude may be necessary to achieve personal goals.

After deciding to seek alternative employment, radiation therapists may consider several areas. Dosimetry is one of the most common career pathways chosen by radiation therapists. Dosimetrists are members of the treatment-planning team who plan the radiation treatments for patients and calculate the radiation dosage. Dosimetrists must be familiar with the physical and geometrical characteristics of radiation equipment and radioactive sources. Some hospitals teach radiation therapists to become dosimetrists on site. However, educational programs that are specifically

designed to educate dosimetrists are available. The profession of dosimetry is relatively young. As the professional growth and development of the specialty develops, attending approved schools rather than on-the-job training will become more important. Lists of dosimetry programs may be obtained from the American Association of Medical Dosimetrists (AAMD).

Another area in the clinical setting is quality management. The radiation therapist assigned to quality management is responsible for the overall effectiveness and precision of the department's treatment-delivery system. Interest in public safety and awareness of radiation dangers are extremely important. *Quality improvement* in radiation oncology is defined as planned and systemic actions that ensure the radiation therapy facility consistently delivers high-quality care in the treatment of patients, thereby leading to the best outcome assessment with the fewest number of side effects. All identified problems should be discussed and recorded with appropriate follow-up action plans initialed. Quality-management actions include quality-control techniques and quality-assurance procedures. *Quality control* refers to procedures and techniques used to monitor or test and maintain components of the radiation therapy quality-assurance program. Quality-control techniques are directly concerned with equipment and its use in patient treatment-delivery services. Accreditation standards overseen by the Joint Commission on Accreditation of Healthcare Organizations (JCAHO) require that each department meet specific criteria for accreditation. The radiation therapist involved in quality management is responsible for performing and overseeing activities related to the assurance of the most accurate treatment for the cancer patient.

Another area in radiation therapy departments is hyperthermia (the application of radiation treatments along with heat administered to patients). More opportunities exist in large departments with high treatment volumes and research activities.

Experienced radiation therapists are prime candidates for managing and administering the daily routine of the radiation oncology department. As the radiation oncology department grows to greater degrees of sophistication, so does the amount of experience and knowledge needed to manage the department. Ideally, the radiation oncology department manager should be a radiation therapist with clinical experience who has additional education in the area of human resources and management. The radiation oncology department manager is responsible for the planning, personnel management, budget preparation, state and federal regulations, and a variety of other tasks. A radiation therapist can gain the necessary knowledge for a career in management by enrolling in a health services administration program or traditional business administration program. Both of these options may be pursued at the baccalaureate or graduate level. The graduate degree is obviously the better route to pursue.

Another career option for the radiation therapist is in the area of education. If a radiation therapist is employed in a radiation oncology department that is a clinical education center of a radiation therapy program, the opportunity to be involved is excellent. After qualifying for the appointment of clinical instructor, the radiation therapist can provide clinical instruction in the clinical setting to students enrolled in the program. Clinical instructors are responsible for the student's achievement in the clinical portion of the radiation therapy program. Clinical instructors evaluate and report student clinical performance. Other educational opportunities are the positions of clinical supervisor and clinical coordinator. The clinical supervisor oversees the general education of students in the clinical setting, whereas the clinical coordinator is responsible for coordinating clinical and didactic programs as assigned by the program director. The position of program director is another area of education and requires the attainment of a degree (a master's is preferred). The program director is responsible for the organization, administration, periodic review, continued development, and general effectiveness of the radiation therapy program. The program director must demonstrate proficiency in instruction, **curriculum** design, program planning, and counseling.

In addition, positions are available in state and federal agencies that oversee radiation activities. Normally, a baccalaureate or graduate degree is required for these positions. Also, extensive clinical experience is usually required. Positions are available in commercial areas such as sales representative and application specialist. Both of these positions require advanced clinical and technical experience, and advanced education is preferred. The position of sales representative usually requires a baccalaureate degree with a marketing and business focus. Clinical and technical experience is useful because the sales representative must interact with the administrator and radiation oncologist regarding equipment purchases. An outgoing personality, good communication skills, and confidence in oneself and the product is essential. In contrast, the application specialist deals with the radiation therapist and radiation oncologist regarding equipment use. The application specialist must be knowledgeable about the function and feasibility of the equipment and must provide in-service training and orientation to clients.

PROFESSIONAL ORGANIZATIONS
Radiologic-technology related

The ASRT is the national professional organization representing radiation therapists, radiographers, other medical imaging specialists, and sonographers. The organization was founded in 1920 and has grown to a membership of over 40,000. The purposes of the Society are to advance the profession of radiation and imaging specialties, maintain high standards of education, enhance the quality of patient care, and further the welfare and social economics of radiologic technologists.

A board of directors and house of delegates composed of representatives from state affiliate societies, modality delegates, and chapter delegates govern the Society. The house of delegates meets once a year to conduct business affairs of the Society. Although the ASRT is involved in main facets of the health care delivery system, the Society's main focus is on continuing education. Through the ASRT Educational Foundation, which was founded in 1984, the ASRT provides high-quality continuing education and continuing educational materials to members and nonmembers. Also, the ASRT appoints representatives to the national certifying agency (the ARRT) and the national radiologic technology accreditation agencies (the JRCERT, the Joint Review Committee on Education in Nuclear Medicine [JRCENM], and the AAMD).

Individual states affiliate with the ASRT. Each state and several cities have professional organizations for radiologic technologists. Some state organizations have radiation therapist subgroups. The ASRT publishes two journals, *Radiologic Technology* and *Radiation Therapist,* and a monthly publication in which radiation therapists can find the current happenings and progress in the profession.

Two professional educational groups are specific to educators in radiologic technology: the Association of Educators in Radiologic Sciences (AERS) and the Association of Collegiate Educators in Radiologic Technology (ACERT). The AERS was founded in 1967 by a small group of radiologic technologists serving as educators and researchers in university radiology departments. The goals of the AERS are to foster the exchange of educational concepts, stimulation of interests in academic advancement and teaching, advancement of the profession by encouraging members to disseminate their work through publication, and attitudes that strive for a standard of excellence in the delivery of radiologic health care services. Today, the AERS is a nationally recognized organization of professionals that promotes advancement in education in the radiologic sciences. The ACERT is also an organization national in scope. The main purpose of the ACERT is to improve educational programs in the collegiate setting. Both organizations provide publications that provide educators with insight and information for the exchange of ideas.

Another group associated with the radiologic sciences is the American Radiologic Nurses Association (ARNA). The purposes of the ARNA are to promote health and wellness by defining the functions and educational criteria of radiology nurses; assess, record, and evaluate radiologic nursing standards; facilitate efficient networking among radiology nurses, allied health professionals, hospitals, and other health care agencies related to nursing; and stimulate and promote research in professional publications related to radiologic nursing.

One organization that is worldwide in scope is the International Society of Radiographers and Radiologic Technicians (ISRRT). The ISRRT is an international, nongovernmental organization with official relations with the World Health Organization. The chief purpose and aim of the ISRRT is to promote and encourage improved standards of education in radiography, radiation therapy, and allied subjects. The policy and decision-making body of this society is the counsel that is composed of one representative from each member country. A board of management is responsible for the activities of the Society within the guidelines established by the counsel. The ASRT is a member of the ISRRT.

Professional organizations also exist that are related to management activities in the radiologic sciences. The Society for Radiation Oncology Administrators (SROA) is a national organization for radiation oncology managers whose objectives are to improve the administration of the business and nonmedical management aspects of radiation oncology and the practice for radiation oncology as a cost-effective form of health care delivery, provide a forum for dialogue between members on matters of professional interest, disseminate information to members of the Society, and generally promote the field of radiation oncology administration. Another organization for radiologic science managers is the American Healthcare Radiology Administrators (AHRA). The AHRA was founded in 1973 and is an educational association organized to promote the highest level of management practice and administration of radiologic sciences. The AHRA is built on a strong foundation of active and regional local groups. Five regions offer programs and coordinate meetings that deal with topics of special interest to regional members. Membership in the AHRA constitutes membership with the region determined by the member's place of employment.

Physician related

The American Medical Association (AMA) is probably the nation's largest medical organization. Founded in 1847, the AMA's initial primary purpose was raising medical education standards and establishing a code of ethics. The AMA is a voluntary membership organization composed of physician members and is the patient's advocate, physician's voice, and standard for the medical profession. The Association is governed by a house of delegates that includes representatives

from every aspect of health care. The AMA maintains a high level of contact and lobbying activities with local, state, and federal governments.

The ACR is the principal organization serving radiologists with programs that focus on the practice of radiology and delivery of comprehensive radiologic health services. These programs in medical sciences, education, and practice management serve the public interest and interest of the medical community in which radiologists serve in diagnostic and therapeutic roles. The purposes of the ACR are to advance the science of radiology, improve radiologic services to the patient, study economic aspects of radiology, and encourage improved and continuing education for radiologists and other allied professional fields. Since 1969 the ACR has represented the interests of the specialty on matters of legislation and regulatory significance. For more than 15 years the ACR, through research efforts by its Philadelphia office, has contributed significantly to America's war on cancer. The ACR has enhanced the role of radiation oncology and cancer care.

The American Society of Therapeutic Radiology and Oncology (ASTRO) is the national professional organization for radiation oncologists. Other professionals such as medical physicists and radiation biologists may also be members. Founded in 1958, the Society's purposes are to extend the benefits of radiation therapy to patients who have cancer or other disorders, advance its scientific bases, and provide education and professional fellowship for its members. The organization publishes the *International Journal of Radiation Oncology, Biology, and Physics.*

Another physician-related organization is the American Radium Society (ARS), founded in 1916. The ARS is an organization of physicians and other scientists with common interests in cancer therapy. Members include radiation oncologists, surgeons, gynecologists, medical oncologists, radiologists, and physicists. The objectives of the Society are to promote the study of cancer in all its aspects, encourage a liaison among the various medical specialties concerned with the treatment of cancer, and continue the scientific study of the treatment of the cancer patient.

Another society is the Counsel of Affiliated Regional Radiation Oncology Studies (CARROS), which was founded in 1978. The Counsel, through its network of 30 constituent organizations, provides a mechanism for the exchange and dissemination of information pertaining to the clinical practice of radiation oncology at the national level. A board of representatives consisting of one representative from each constituent organization governs the affairs of the Counsel.

Medical-physics related

The AAMD was founded in 1976. Its membership consists primarily of medical dosimetrists, and its purposes are to promote the proper application of medical radiation dosimetry, clarify and strengthen the position of dosimetrists in the radiation therapy community, establish guidelines for the training and continuing education of dosimetrists, and develop direct lines of communication among dosimetrists. The AAMD publishes a quarterly journal, *Medical Dosimetry*. Radiation therapists find this journal of interest for reading and research.

Medical physicists also have a national professional organization, the American Association of Physicists in Medicine (AAPM). The AAPM was founded in 1958, and its purposes are to promote the application of physics in medicine and biology, encourage interests and training in medical physics, and prepare and disseminate technical information in this and other related fields. The scientific activities of the AAPM primarily involve radiologic physics of ionizing radiation such as dosimetry, physics of radiologic diagnosis, therapy, and radiation safety. However, an increasing emphasis exists on the physics of nonionizing techniques for the diagnosis and treatment of disease. The Association publishes a bimonthly journal *(Medical Physics)* and newsletters covering developments in the profession.

INTRODUCTION TO RADIATION ONCOLOGY

Radiation oncology, broadly defined, is the treatment of malignant disease (usually cancer) with ionizing radiation. Other conditions such as benign disease may also be treated. However, this is not as common. The primary three methods of treatment with radiation are external beam, interstitial implants, and intracavitary implants. Other methods such as contact therapy, intraoperative, stereotactic, and hyperthermia are practiced. However, not all radiation oncology centers have these capabilities.

External beam treatment

Cobalt machines were the mainstay of radiation oncology departments in the 1960s. These units, sometimes called *teletherapy units (tele* is Greek for "at a distance"), consisted of a large machine with cobalt 60 housed in the head of the treatment unit. The unit, although bulky, is diverse in its treatment scope because patients can be treated in a rotational or fixed-beam arrangement. The cobalt 60 radioactive source is located in the head of the machine and is shielded for protection. The radiation therapist prepares the patient for treatment and then activates the unit from a control panel located outside the treatment room. When the beam is activated, the cobalt source is brought out to an opening in the protective housing. Thus, the treatment beam is emitted. Collimators that can be set for varying lengths and widths control the beam size. Because cobalt 60 is a decaying isotope source, it must be replaced about every 5 years.

Linear accelerators are high-energy units that operate at extremely high voltages. This megavoltage unit (*mega* is Greek for "great") uses basically the same principle as x-ray units for the production of the treatment beam. Electrons from an electron gun are accelerated at speeds approaching the speed of light. If the beam produced is an x-ray beam, the electron is directed toward a target and x-rays are produced. If the desired beam is an electron beam, the target can be bypassed and the electron beam is directed toward scattering foils such as lead. Linear accelerators (linacs) are generally categorized into three levels of treatment capabilities: low-energy, high-energy, and dual-mode units. A low-energy unit normally operates at 4 to 6 MV, whereas the high-energy linac operates at 18 to 20 MV. The dual-mode linacs usually operate at 15 to 25 MV and provide an x-ray and electron beam for patient treatment. Linear accelerators are the most popular treatment units used today.

Interstitial and intracavitary treatment

Implant therapy (brachytherapy) is a method of radiation treatment using sealed radioactive sources placed at short distances from the patient's tumor. These radioactive sources can be best described as interstitial or intracavitary. The interstitial method is the placement of a sealed radioactive source directly into the tumor, such as the tongue. The intracavitary method is the placement of sealed radioactive sources in a body cavity close to the tumor, such as the cervix. In both instances, these radioactive sources can be permanent or removable. Sources come in different forms (e.g., needles, tubes, and seeds). Radioactive substitutes also vary and include cesium, gold, tantalum, and iridium. Radiation therapists often assist in the preparation of materials to be used for implant therapy.

Other methods of treatment

In addition to the conventional methods of radiation therapy previously mentioned, additional methods of treatment exist. Contact therapy is one of those methods. Simply defined, *contact therapy* is the placement of radioactive sources directly on the tumor. The source is usually embedded in a mold (plaque) and left on the tumor for a specified period. Intraoperative radiation therapy (IORT) and total-body irradiation (TBI) are two newer methods of treatment. IORT delivers the radiation dosage directly to the tumor during surgery. This technique is used in tumors that are deeply situated in the body where surrounding radiosensitive organs can be moved out of the treatment area. Therefore a larger single dose can be delivered directly to the tumor with the aim of destroying the tumor and any residual disease. It is a costly, time-consuming procedure because of the necessity of combining the operating room's sterile-technique situation with the high-energy equipment in a shielded room needed for radiation protection. This technique is used in selected cases. In contrast, TBI focuses on irradiation of the entire body rather than a specific site. This technique is also used for only specific diseases. Patients preparing for bone marrow transplants are probably the most common candidates for TBI. Doses higher than those that cause death from bone marrow depletion can be given because bone marrow is replaced during the transplant.

Hyperthermia is another method of treatment. The basic principle of hyperthermia is that heat sometimes causes regression in tumors. A special unit is needed to perform the heating procedure on the patient. Then the patient is treated with conventional radiation therapy. Stereotactic radiosurgery is a treatment technique that was introduced in the early 1950s. Stereotaxis (a method dealing with precise location in an area of the brain) is essential in this neurological procedure. The tumor is located, and stereotactic radio-

surgery delivers a high dose to a small volume of disease through customized arcing of the treatment unit. Stereotaxis is often performed on outpatients and is a time-consuming process involving the placement of a surgical frame, tumor location, treatment plan, and treatment delivery.

Other radiation therapy treatment modalities include neutron and proton therapy and the use of heavy ions and pions. These treatment modalities are used primarily in specialized radiation oncology centers and not in average departments.

Review Questions

Multiple Choice

1. Radiation therapists have opportunities to advance in the profession in which of the following areas?
   a. Education
   b. Management
   c. Dosimetry
   d. All of the above
2. The ARRT is the organization that provides radiation therapists with which of the following?
   a. Licensure
   b. Accreditation
   c. Certification
   d. All of the above
3. The JRCERT is the organization that provides which of the following?
   a. Licenses to radiation therapists
   b. Accreditation to radiation therapists
   c. Accreditation to educational programs
   d. Certification to educational programs
4. The ASRT provides which of the following?
   a. Membership in a professional organization
   b. Opportunities for licensure in the profession
   c. Opportunities for accreditation activities for professionals
   d. Membership in a licensure organization
5. Allied health professionals who provide rehabilitation services to cancer patients include which of the following?
   a. Medical record administrators
   b. Dental hygienists
   c. Physical therapists
   d. Dietitians
6. Allied health professionals who provide laboratory services to cancer patients include which of the following?
   a. Cytotechnologists
   b. Medical technologists
   c. Histotechnologists
   d. All of the above

7. A prothesist is an allied health professional who does which of the following?
   a. Provides dietary information to cancer patients
   b. Provides cancer patient information to the tumor registry
   c. Provides artificial limbs for cancer patients
   d. Provides social service information to cancer patients
8. The radiation therapist's scope of practice does which of the following?
   a. Provides radiation therapists with direction and counseling to assist in patient treatments
   b. Provides radiation therapists with ethical consideration regarding the treatment of cancer patients
   c. Provides radiation therapists with insight and awareness of the psychosocial aspects of treatment of cancer patients
   d. Provides radiation therapists with direction regarding professional responsibilities in providing quality care to cancer patients
9. Methods of radiation treatments for cancer patients include which of the following?
   a. External beam treatments
   b. Brachytherapy treatments
   c. Interstitial treatments
   d. All of the above
10. A newer method of treatment with radiation is which of the following?
    a. Brachytherapy treatment
    b. Hyperthermia treatment
    c. Contact therapy treatment
    d. All of the above

Questions to Ponder

1. Describe the rationale for and application of the radiation therapist's code of ethics in the daily performance of duties.
2. Trace the history of the radiation therapist profession and relate the levels of performance of the radiation therapist's role.
3. Describe rehabilitative services provided to cancer patients.
4. Who are the professionals involved in treating cancer patients? What role and function do they serve?
5. Describe radiologic services and the individuals involved.
6. Compare and contrast certification and licensure.
7. Analyze the benefits of accreditation.
8. Describe the career opportunities available for radiation therapists.
9. Briefly describe the three primary methods of radiation treatment.
10. Identify the professional organization for radiation therapists and state reasons for holding membership.

BIBLIOGRAPHY

Allied health education directory, ed 21, Chicago, 1993, American Medical Association.

American College of Radiology: *Organizations in radiology,* Reston, Va, 1991, The College.

American College of Radiology: *Radiology: an inside look,* Reston, Va, 1993, The College.

American Medical Association: *Physicians dedicated to the health of America,* Chicago, 1994, The Association.

American Registry of Radiologic Technologists: *Educators handbook,* Minneapolis, 1987, The Registry.

American Society of Radiologic Technologists: *Code of ethics for the radiation therapist,* Albuquerque, 1994, The Society.

American Society of Radiologic Technologists: *Scope of practice for the radiation therapist,* Albuquerque, 1994, The Society.

Boyles MV, Morgan KM, McCauley: *The health professions,* Philadelphia, 1992, WB Saunders.

Grigg ERN: *Trail of the invisible light,* Springfield, Ill, 1965, Charles C Thomas.

Gurley L, Calloway W: *Introduction to radiologic technology,* ed 3, St Louis, 1992, Mosby.

Joint Review Committee on Education in Radiologic Technology: *Essentials and guidelines of an accredited educational program for tradiation therapists,* Chicago, 1994, The Committee.

Joint Review Committee on Education in Radiologic Technology: *Handbook for educational programs,* Chicago, 1991, The Committee.

Miller-Alan P: *Introduction to the health professions,* Belmont, Calif, 1984, Wadsworth.

12

Radiographic Imaging

Dennis T. Leaver
Alan C. Miller

Outline

Key terms

Radiographic imaging plays a critical role in helping the cancer patient. In radiation therapy it provides a way to view the interior of the human body. The x-rays used in this process can penetrate matter and create an image on film. This information helps members of the cancer-management team achieve an important goal in radiation oncology: to maximize the radiation dose to the diseased tissue (cancer cells) and minimize the dose to the surrounding normal tissue.

In this chapter, several concepts are introduced, including the history of x-rays, their production, the design of the tube from which they are produced, their interaction with matter, and the art of creating high-quality radiographic images.

HISTORICAL OVERVIEW

Approximately 100 years ago in November of 1895, a little-known German physicist tinkered in his laboratory at the University of Würzburg, Germany, with a fancy piece of glassware known as a *Hittorf-Crookes tube*. In communicating to his friend Theodor Boveri in early December 1895, Wilhelm Conrad Roentgen said, "I have discovered something interesting, but I do not know if my observations are correct."[10] After energizing his tube in the darkened laboratory, Roentgen noticed a strange green light emanating from a nearby piece of cardboard coated with phosphorescent material. This was hardly momentous because phosphorescence was a well-known event. However, when he passed a heavy piece of paper between the end of the tube and the cardboard coated with barium platinocyanide, the glow persisted. At that moment the scientist realized his newly found

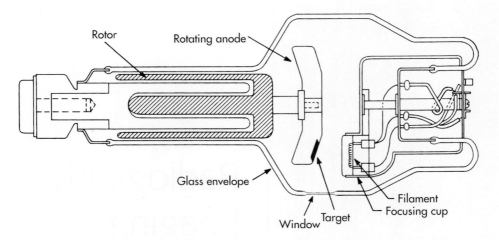

Fig. 12-1 Diagram of a rotating-anode x-ray tube illustrating the fundamental parts. (From Bushong S: *Radiologic science for technologists: physics, biology, and protection,* ed 5, St Louis, 1993, Mosby.)

rays could pass through matter. He appropriately named them *x-rays*.

The essential elements of x-ray production have not changed in the intervening 100 years. However, x-rays have changed regarding their application in medicine. Modern x-ray tubes (Fig. 12-1) still require a source of electrons (the cathode), a current capable of liberating them from their tungsten filament home, a target toward which they can be directed (the anode), and the extremely high voltage necessary to persuade this reluctant electron cloud to flow at the velocity required to produce x-rays.

RADIOGRAPHIC IMAGING CONCEPTS

Radiographic imaging has rapidly expanded its role in diagnosing disease over the last half of the twentieth century. X-rays have a variety of diagnostic and therapeutic purposes, and because of that, many modalities such as diagnostic radiology, nuclear medicine, mammography, cardiovascular imaging, and computed tomography (CT) scanning exist to aid the physician in the precise diagnosis of disease.

Several types of x-rays are used therapeutically in radiation oncolgy and its treatment of malignant disease. In the 40 to 300 kVp range, x-rays are used for two purposes. The first purpose is the treatment of skin cancers and other superficial tumors (most other tumors are treated with gamma rays and much higher energy x-rays above 1 million volts). The second purpose is the planning of a patient's treatment on the simulator. Simulation provides geometries similar to those found on treatment machines. This is done with x-ray equipment in the 50- to 120-kVp range. Diagnostic-quality images displayed on a radiograph or television monitor allow part of the cancer-management team to evaluate the geometry of the actual treatment. One of the

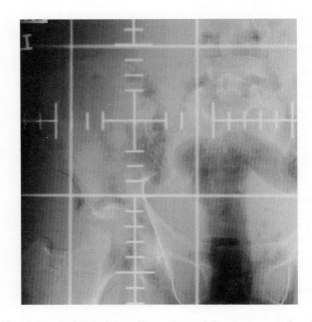

Fig. 12-2 A simulation radiograph used for treatment-planning purposes. Note the field-defining wires outlining the tumor and a small volume of normal tissue.

radiation therapy department's essential functions is to ensure that all definitive and many palliative treatments are planned with meticulous detail to optimize the treatment's outcome (see the box on p. 159).[2] The radiographic imaging capabilities of the simulator allow the outlining of the tumor and a small volume of surrounding tissue to be documented and stored on a radiograph (Fig. 12-2).

The major components of an imaging system on a radiation therapy simulator are an x-ray tube and a fluoroscope. Although these two components can be found hard at work in

"Radiation oncology assumes a significant role in the medical management and treatment of patients with cancer. Fifty to sixty (50-60%) of all cancer patients will be treated with radiation therapy as an integral component of their care. Optimal use of radiation therapy requires detailed attention to personnel, equipment, patient and personnel safety, education and quality assurance." The American College of Radiology (ACR) recommends that "all patients should have ready access to therapeutic equipment for the optimal management of their disease. If the equipment is not in place in the facility, it should be readily available for any patient who might benefit from it." Regular maintenance and repair of equipment is also recommended as part of the *ACR Standards for Radiation Oncology.*

Treatment units, simulation equipment, and ancillary supporting equipment are an integral part of the *ACR Standards for Radiation Oncology.* This equipment should specifically include the following items:

1. Supervoltage radiation therapy equipment for external beam therapy. This must be an x-ray generator of 1 million volts or more or cobalt 60 teletherapy unit. If the cobalt 60 unit is the only megavoltage unit, it must have a treatment distance of 80 cm or more.
2. Electron beam therapy equipment or low-energy x-ray equipment for treatment of skin lesions or superficially placed lesions.
3. Appropriate brachytherapy equipment for intracavity and interstitial treatment (or arrangements in place for referral to appropriate facilities).
4. Access to or presence of computerized dosimetry equipment capable of providing external beam isodose curves and brachytherapy isodose curves.
5. Simulation equipment.
6. Physical measurement equipment to calibrate all equipment.
7. Special field-shaping equipment.
8. Access to appropriate supporting facilities, including diagnostic laboratories and imaging facilities.

Modified from the American College of Radiology: *ACR standards for radiation oncology,* Reston, Va, 1990, ACR Publications Department.
*The standards of the ACR are not rules. Instead they attempt to define principles of practice that should generally produce high-quality patient care. Additional standards, which are not included here, are outlined by the *ACR Standards for Radiation Oncology* in areas of personnel (blue book), patient and personnel safety, education, and quality assurance.

most diagnostic radiology departments, their purpose is somewhat different in radiation oncology. X-ray tubes in diagnostic radiology settings and those on radiation therapy simulators are essentially the same devices. Both can produce the same mysterious rays Roentgen found interesting in 1895.

X-RAY TUBE

The electrical production of x-rays is possible only under special conditions, including a source of electrons, an appropriate target material, a high voltage, and a vacuum.[4] The production of x-rays occurs inside the tube because of high-speed electrons colliding with a metal object called the *anode.* The components of the tube, the **cathode** and **anode**, are enclosed in a glass envelope and protective housing.

Cathode

The *cathode* is one of the electrodes found in the x-ray tube and represents the negative side of the tube. It consists of two parts: the filament and focusing cup. As a first step in x-ray production, the primary function of the cathode is to produce electrons and focus the electron stream toward the metal anode.

Filament. The filament is a small coil of wire made of thoriated tungsten, which has an extremely high melting point ($3380°$ C) (Fig. 12-3). The coil of wire is a smaller version of that inside a light bulb or toaster. A current, which heats the filament, is passed through the small coil of wire where electrons boil off and are emitted from the filament.

Most modern x-ray tubes have dual filaments, thus permitting the selection of a large or small source of electrons. The length and width of the filament control the ability of the x-ray tube to produce fine imaging detail. Most modern x-ray machines are equipped with a rotating anode tube having 0.6-mm (small) and 1.0-mm (large) focal spots. Other x-ray machines having focal spots as small as 0.1 mm and as large as 2.0 mm are also commercially available.[6] Using a small focal spot allows the radiation therapist to radiographically display fine detail. This is especially important in imaging the field-defining wires used to localize the treatment area during the simulation process.

Focusing cup. The selection of a small or large focal spot is associated with the small and large filaments, which are embedded in a small oval depression in the cathode assembly called a *focusing cup.* The negative charge of the focusing cup helps direct electrons toward the anode in a straighter, less divergent path.

Anode

The *anode* is the positive side of the x-ray tube. It receives electrons from the cathode as a target, dissipates the great amount of heat as a result of x-ray production, and serves as the path for the flow of high voltage. Aspects of the anode assembly include the composition of the anode, the target, and the line-focus principle.

Composition. The anode is a circular disc composed of many different metals, each designed to contribute to the effectiveness of x-ray production (Fig. 12-4). The rotating tungsten disc serves as the target and can range up to 13 cm in diameter. Rhenium-alloyed tungsten serves as the target focal-track material because of its ability as a thermal conductor and the source of x-ray photons. The rotor, which

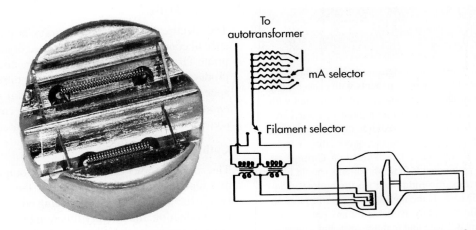

Fig. 12-3   The dual-filament cathode in a focusing cup allows the selection of a small or large focal spot. (From Bushong S: *Radiologic science for technologists: physics, biology, and protection,* ed 5, St Louis, 1993, Mosby.)

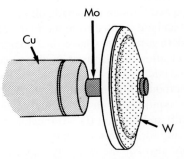

Fig. 12-4   Composition of a rotating anode. (From Bushong S: *Radiologic science for technologists: physics, biology, and protection,* ed 5, St Louis, 1993, Mosby.)

allows most anodes to reach 3400 revolutions per minute, is an excellent device to help dispel the great amounts of heat created.

Target. Electrons from the cathode strike the portion of the anode called the *target,* or *focal spot.* This is the point at which x-ray photons are produced and begin to fan out in a divergent path. Divergence of the x-rays from their focal spot is similar to the sun's divergent rays seen on a partly sunny day. As the rays get closer to the earth, they fan out more from their source, which is 93 million miles away.

Line-focus principle. The **focal spot** is the section of the target at which radiation is produced. With the use of a small focal spot, more detail is seen on the simulation radiograph. Simultaneously, however, more heat is created by bombarding a smaller area of the target. To overcome the disadvantage of creating more heat and still maintain radiographic detail, the target is angled as shown in Fig. 12-5. In this way a larger geometrical area can be heated while a small focal spot is maintained. Fig. 12-5 displays the line-focus princi-

ple. The actual focal-spot size of the target is larger than the effective focal-spot size. Most x-ray tubes have a target angle from 7 to 20 degrees.[6,12]

Glass envelope

The cathode and anode are in a vacuum in the x-ray tube. The removal of air from the glass envelope or x-ray tube permits the uninterrupted flow of electrons from the cathode to the anode. The efficiency of the tube is increased because no air molecules are floating around inside the x-ray tube to collide with the accelerated electrons. The tube may measure from 20 to 30 cm in length and be as large as 15 cm in diameter at the central portion.

Protective housing

To control unwanted radiation leakage and electrical shock, the x-ray tube is mounted inside the protective housing. Lead lining in the protective housing helps prevent radiation leakage during an exposure. A special oil fills the space between the protective housing and glass envelope to insulate the high-voltage potential and provide additional cooling capacity.

Recommendations for extending tube life

Proper care and use by the radiation therapist can extend the life of the x-ray tube, the cost of which may range up to $16,000. Several practical steps may extend the life of the x-ray tube (see the box on p. 161). The manufacturer's warm-up procedure should be followed to prevent excessive heat load on a cold anode; otherwise, serious damage can occur. Many systems have a digital display (measured in percent) of the heat capacity created on the tube after an exposure. This is a helpful tool in monitoring the heat units created. The rotor switch should not be held before an exposure. Most x-ray systems do not permit an exposure until the rotor has reached its full revolutions per minute. When the rotor

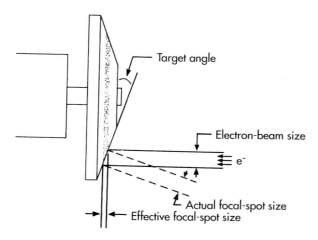

Fig. 12-5 By angling the target of the rotating anode (thus taking advantage of the line-focus principle), a larger geometric area can be heated while a small focal spot is maintained. (From Bushong S: *Radiologic science for technologists: physics, biology, and protection*, ed 5, St Louis, 1993, Mosby.)

Recommendations for Extending X-Ray Tube Life

1. Follow the manufacturer's warm-up procedure to prevent heat damage to the anode.
2. Monitor the heat units created during repeated exposures.
3. Avoid holding the rotor switch before an exposure. Double-press switches should be completely depressed in one motion, and dual switches should have the exposure switch pressed first, and then the rotor switch.[4]
4. Use low mA (filament current) values whenever possible.
5. Avoid multiple exposures near the tube limit.

switch is depressed, thermionic emission of the electrons from the filament occurs and continues until an exposure is made. Any delay in exposure causes unnecessary wear on the filament and decreases the tube life. The use of a low mA (filament current) values during an x-ray exposure decreases filament evaporation, thus extending tube life. Finally, making multiple exposures near the tube limit should be avoided; otherwise, unnecessary heat stress on the anode may occur and cause serious damage.

X-RAY PRODUCTION

The essentials of x-ray generation are remarkably simple. They willingly follow the orderly progression of rules in the physical sciences. X-rays are just one of the many forms of electromagnetic energy organized according to wavelength on the electromagnetic spectrum (Fig. 12-6). Initially, x-rays may appear to have little in common with their spectral

cousins: radio and microwaves, visible light, cosmic radiation, and a host of other energy forms. However, all these radiant energies share certain properties. They all travel at the speed of light (3×10^{10} cm per second); they all take the form of a wave, each with its own characteristic undulating pattern expressed as *wavelength* (the distance between the crests in the wave) and *frequency* (the number of complete wave cycles per second); and they all consist of photons, which are minute bundles of pure energy having no mass and no electrical charge. The concept of something made up of nothing may be difficult to appreciate because humans tend to think in terms of objects or things, even at the atomic level. However, photons (or quanta) exist and constantly roam around us at the speed of light.

Understanding the unique relationship that exists between photon wavelength and frequency is essential to understanding the dramatically different behaviors observed in various forms of electromagnetic radiation. For example, microwave television signals can transmit sound and image information across great distances, but they cannot readily pass through matter without being deflected. In contrast, x-rays are quite capable of penetrating matter and altering its atomic structure through a process called *ionization* (the ejection of orbital electrons). Because the velocity of all radiant energy forms is constant, the differing properties of radiant energy can be attributed only to variations in their wavelength and frequency.

X-ray radiations and gamma radiations are located at the high end of the spectrum and possess extremely short wavelengths. The relationship between wavelength and frequency is an inverse proportion (i.e., as wavelength decreases, frequency increases). In 1900 the German physicist Max Planck showed through his quantum theory that frequency and energy are directly proportional. Despite their constant velocities, different forms of electromagnetic radiation may have widely varying energies (from the low end of the spectrum [radio waves] to the high end [X-ray radiations, gamma radiations, and cosmic radiations]). As the wavelength decreases and frequency increases, so does the associated quantum energy.

X-rays are the classical form of artificially produced electromagnetic radiation. Unlike most spectral radiant energies, no spontaneous equivalent for x-rays exists in nature. They are purely a human-produced phenomenon. As described earlier in this chapter, producing x-rays is quite simple and requires only a source of electrons, a target at which to direct the electron stream, a high-vacuum glass tube, and a source of electricity of sufficient voltage.

Thermionic emission

In an oversimplification, x-rays are produced when a stream of electrons liberated from the cathode is directed across the tube vacuum at extremely high speeds to interact with the anode. These cathode electrons are freed from the tungsten filament atoms in a process called **thermionic emission.**

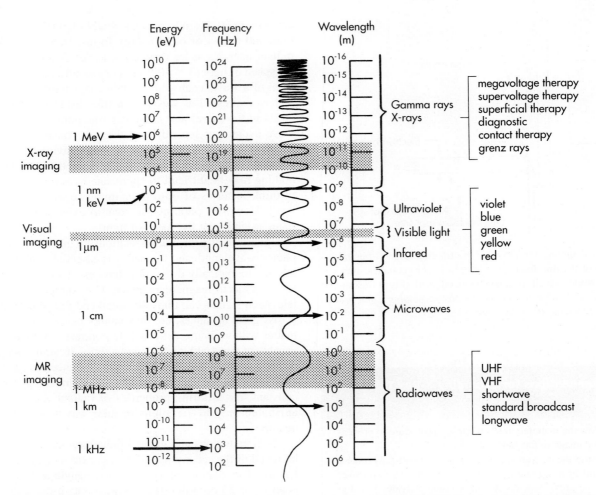

Fig. 12-6 The electromagnetic spectrum demonstrates specific values of energy, frequency, and wavelength for some regions of the spectrum. (From Bushong S: *Radiologic science for technologists: physics, biology, and protection,* ed 5, St Louis, 1993, Mosby.)

This elaborate-sounding term makes perfect sense if broken down into its root forms (*thermal* refers to heat, *ions* are charged particles, and *emission* is release).

The process of liberating electrons through the application of heat is quite similar to that seen in an ordinary light bulb. An electrical current is applied to the filament, which because of its resistance, begins to glow. As the current increases, the filament reaches the white-hot state necessary for outer-shell electrons to leave their orbits. This is known as *incandescence,* and the resulting electrons are called *thermions.* Thermionic emission begins when the filament circuit (usually the first stage in a two-stage exposure switch) is energized.

The process is silent, but in all modern rotating-anode x-ray tubes, filament heating is accompanied by the sound of the anode spinning. This statement may seem unnecessary to make for individuals already familiar with the essentials of x-ray generation, but it is worth repeating that during this initial stage of exposure the operator has activated nothing more

than an extremely expensive light bulb. No x-rays are produced; yet significant deterioration occurs in the tube, thus possibly shortening its life greatly. This is no small matter to individuals responsible for the economic health of the imaging or therapy department. Not only is the filament literally being boiled away, but the anode bearings are also subjected to wear. These factors are two of the major causes of tube failure.

Potential difference

The electron cloud or space charge produced from the filament hovers in the vicinity of the cathode indefinitely unless something is done to encourage it to move. The motivating force comes the moment the exposure switch is depressed. High voltage, typically on the order of 70,000 to 120,000 v (70 to 120 kVp), is applied to create a high potential difference between the negative and positive anodes. According to the basic laws of electrodynamics, this causes the negatively charged electrons to be strongly repelled from the cathode

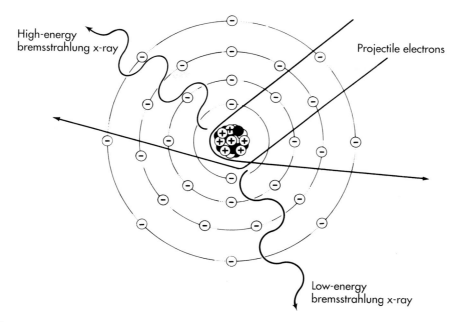

High-energy bremsstrahlung x-ray

Projectile electrons

Low-energy bremsstrahlung x-ray

Fig. 12-7 The bremsstrahlung interaction. (From Bushong S: *Radiologic science for technologists: physics, biology, and protection,* ed 5, St Louis, 1993, Mosby.)

and drawn at extreme speeds toward the attracting force of the positively charged anode. In modern three-phase radiographic equipment, the velocity of this electron stream can approach the speed of light.

Target interaction

X-rays are produced when the kinetic energy of the moving electron stream is given up as it enters the nuclear field of the anode. As noted earlier in the discussion of x-ray tube design, the anode (or target) is composed of materials selected for their high atomic number and high melting point. The former factor largely determines the energy efficiency of x-ray production resulting from interactions that take place in the tube. The latter minimizes the potential for damage from the intense heat those interactions produce. Over 99% of the electrical energy applied to the tube is converted to heat, and only a tiny fraction (about 0.6% at diagnostic energy levels) becomes x-rays.

The principal interaction in x-ray production results in the output of **bremsstrahlung** (German for "breaking") radiation (Fig. 12-7). Bremsstrahlung accounts for approximately 75% to 80% of the tube's output and is produced by the sudden deceleration of the high-speed electron as it is deflected around the nucleus of the tungsten atom. The therapist should remember that electrons have mass and moving electrons possess kinetic energy. When any moving object is abruptly slowed, the surplus energy must be given off. The greater the angle of deflection around the nucleus, the more pronounced the degree of deceleration and the more energy

released. A somewhat remote analogy may be found in an automobile rounding a bend in the road. As the automobile slows, some energy is converted to heat through friction with the brakes and tires. This same vehicle suddenly negotiating a sharp curve may have to slow almost to a stop, thereby giving off most or all its kinetic energy. In the target atoms of the anode the kinetic energy of the decelerating electron is given off as a bundle of pure energy, or an x-ray photon.

A second, lesser interaction also contributes to the production of x-rays. **Characteristic radiation** is created by the direct interaction of cathode electrons with inner-shell electrons of the target material. Some electrons may collide with tungsten orbital electrons that have sufficient energy to overcome their binding energy and eject them from orbit. This process is called *ionization* (Fig. 12-8). When an inner-shell electron is ejected from orbit, other electrons (generally from adjacent shells) move in to fill the hole left. The energy of x-rays produced in this manner is dependent on the binding energy of the target atom's electrons. As the atomic number of an element increases, so does the energy level of each shell. This is the rationale for using materials of high atomic number (such as tungsten) in the targets of x-ray tubes. Binding energy drops with each successive electron orbit away from the nucleus. Outer-shell, or valence, electrons have an extremely low binding energy and are easily ejected from orbit. Therefore ionization events in the O or P shell of the tungsten atom do not produce characteristic x-ray photons of sufficient energy to be useful. Tungsten K-shell electrons, however, have a binding energy of 69.5 keV.

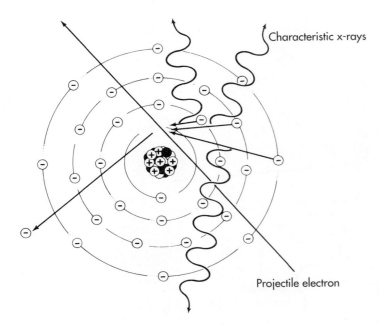

Fig. 12-8 The characteristic interaction. (From Bushong S: *Radiologic science for technologists: physics, biology, and protection,* ed 5, St Louis, 1993, Mosby.)

When a K-shell electron is ejected from orbit and replaced with a tungsten L-shell electron, a surplus energy of 57.4 keV is released in the form of a characteristic x-ray photon.[3] Energies of this magnitude are well within the useful range for diagnostic x-rays.

Physical relationships in x-ray production

A basic premise of physics is that matter can be neither created nor destroyed; it can only change its state. Thanks to the efforts of Albert Einstein, matter's conversion to energy is now known. Einstein, the undeniable father of modern nuclear physics, proved mathematically the theoretical relationship between the kinetic energy of moving matter and the production of light quanta (photons). In his historic theory of relativity, Einstein demonstrated that matter accelerated to a sufficient velocity can become pure energy.

On a more practical level (applied to the production of x-rays) the velocity of the cathode stream is determined by the energy supplied in volts; as the voltage increases, so does the energy available for conversion into x-ray photons. As may be expected, high-energy photons pass through matter more readily than low-energy photons. The ability of the photon stream to pass through matter such as human body tissues is critical to the production of a useful image on a radiograph. This ability is generally called *penetration.* A radiation beam of high energy penetrates structures with greater ease than a weak, low-voltage beam. Although this may appear obvious, the theory behind it is of great importance in diagnostic radiography and radiation therapy.

As the potential difference (voltage) is increased across the x-ray tube vacuum, the velocity of the cathode electron stream is increased. The greater the speed of the moving matter, the greater the resultant energy of the photon stream produced by target interactions. As noted earlier, when mass is slowed or stopped, its energy must be given up in some form. In this situation, mass is converted to heat and photons. Increasing voltage (kVp) increases photon energy.

This energy is commonly termed *beam quality.* A beam of radiation produced by using high kVp is a high-quality beam (i.e., it contains a large percentage of highly penetrating, extremely energetic photons). However, quality addresses only half of the x-ray beam equation. The number of photons in the beam must be considered, and the way quality and quantity may interrelate in radiographic image production must be examined.

From an extremely early age, children are taught a simple mathematical premise: if five oranges are given to a friend, the friend will have five oranges (quantity). Explaining that three of the oranges are nice and juicy (high quality) and the other two are rather dry and useless (low quality) is more difficult. Such is the relationship between x-ray tube current and x-ray production. The relationship is purely a question of the number of photons in the stream. Most students in radiation therapy find the concept of quantity easier to accept than issues involving the conversion of matter to energy.

Thankfully, the relationship between the number of cathode electrons released during thermionic emission and the production of x-ray photons is simple; they occur in direct proportion. As the operator of the radiation therapy simulation equipment increases tube current, a predictable increase in the number of electrons released occurs. The relationship between current (expressed in mAs) and the quantity of electrons liberated is a direct proportion. The relationship has no bearing on beam energy, penetrating ability, or any other variable necessarily useful. For example, it may be simply a question of producing 10-to-the-billionth-power photons for a certain mAs. If the mAs is doubled, 20-to-the-billionth power photons are produced. The fact that many of these photons will not have sufficient energy to contribute to any useful radiographic image (the dry oranges) is irrelevant, but an important correlation exists among energy, quantity, and image production.

X-RAY INTERACTIONS WITH MATTER
Overview

The ability of an x-ray beam to produce a latent radiographic image on film depends on certain key properties characteristic of extremely short-wavelength, high-frequency forms of radiant energy.[3,7,15] X-rays travel in straight lines and diverge from a point of origin. (This is critical in understanding the geometrical principals discussed in the previous section.) X-rays are capable of causing certain substances to fluoresce, ionizing materials through which they pass, and

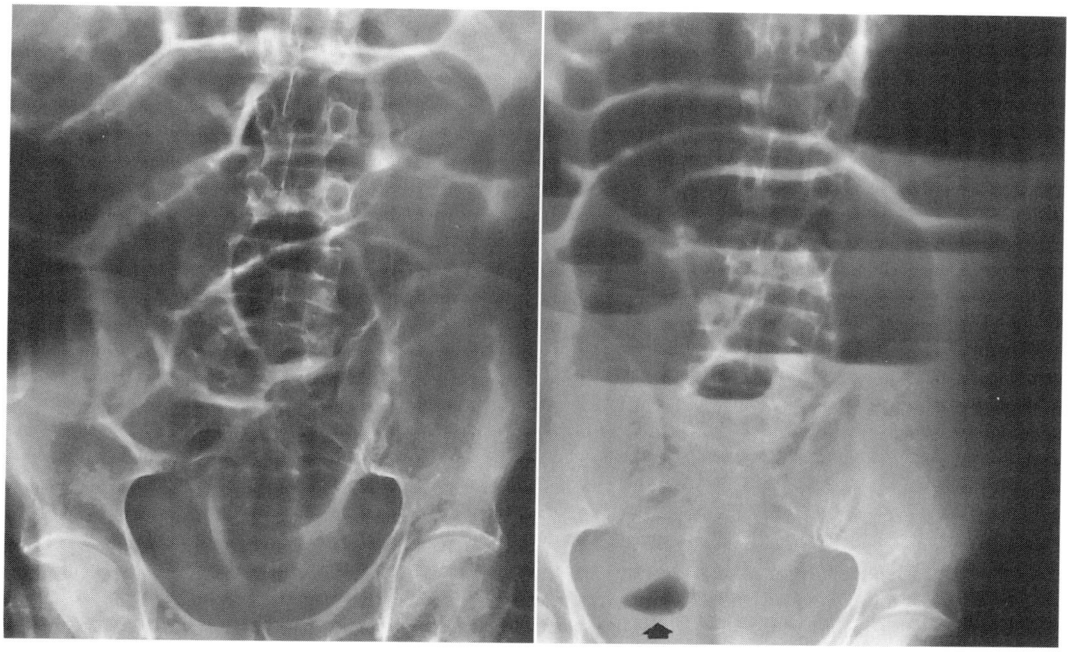

Fig. 12-9 These radiographs of the abdomen demonstrate an obstruction of the small bowel. Large amounts of gas (shown as dark areas on the radiograph) are seen on supine (**A**) and upright (**B**) abdominal films. Note the small amount of gas in the colon. Bone (whiter areas) and other soft-tissue structures are also demonstrated in both radiographs. (From Eisenberg RL, Dennis CA: *Comprehensive radiologic pathology,* St Louis, 1990, Mosby.)

causing chemical and biological changes in tissue. These properties are the basis of x-ray interactions with matter.

As it passes through matter, the x-ray beam undergoes a gradual reduction in the number of photons or exposure rate. This process is termed *absorption* or, more correctly, **attenuation.** Photons in the original or primary beam may also be scattered (i.e., they may change direction as they collide with atoms in their path). In the human body the rate of beam attenuation and degree of scattering is determined by tissue thickness, density, and effective atomic number. The net effect is a wide variation in the quantity of photons actually reaching the film. The nature of the tissues through which the beam must pass controls which photons strike and where they strike.

The human body is not a homogenous structure. It consists of varying quantities of air, fat, water, muscle, and bone, each with their own absorption properties. A radiograph of the abdomen (Fig. 12-9) provides an ideal demonstration of these differential absorption characteristics. Denser structures and those of higher-average atomic numbers appear as lighter areas on the radiograph because of their higher rates of attenuation. Air (as a result of its extremely low density) and fat (as a result of its relatively low atomic number) appear as dark areas, whereas bone (which is dense and has a high atomic number [z]) appears as a light shadow on the film. This range in differential absorption makes the viewing of anatomical detail possible. From a practical standpoint, the goal of the radition therapist is to select technical factors (appropriate kVp and mAs) that maximize the rate of differential absorption and increase the visibility of detail in the image.

Interactions in the diagnostic range

For an appreciation of the importance of differential absorption, some understanding of x-ray photons at the subatomic level is important. In the diagnostic energy range, three interactions occur. Photons may be absorbed photoelectrically or undergo Coherent (unmodified) or **Compton scattering** during an interaction. In general, a scattered photon is a bad photon. It rarely contributes to a useful image on the film, and therapists go to great lengths to minimize its detrimental effect. Technical factors are selected in an attempt to maximize differential absorption through photoelectric effect, minimize Compton scattering, and keep patient exposure within reasonable limits.

Unfortunately, the predominant interaction in the diagnostic energy range is the Compton effect (Fig. 12-10). Compton scattering is produced when an x-ray photon interacts with an outer-shell orbital electron with sufficient energy to eject it from orbit and alter its own path. The classic analogy is seen in the game of billiards, in which the cue ball collides with another ball and both fly off in different directions. In Compton scattering the freed electron likely travels only an extremely short distance before attaching itself to another atom. At high kVp settings the scattered photon may have

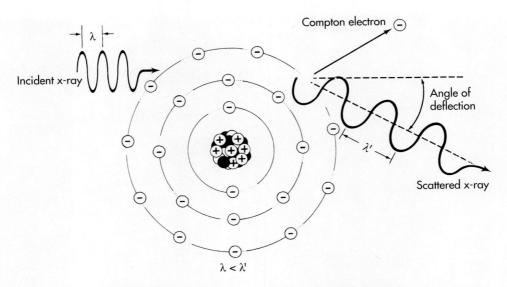

Fig. 12-10 The Compton effect is produced when an x-ray photon interacts with an outer-shell orbital electron. The photon must posses sufficient energy to eject it from orbit and alter its own path. (From Bushong S: *Radiologic science for technologists: physics, biology, and protection,* ed 5, St Louis, 1993, Mosby.)

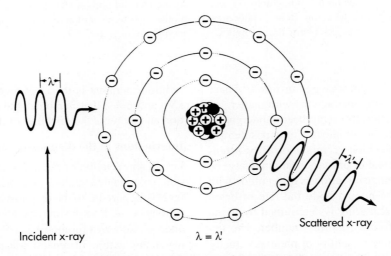

Fig. 12-11 Unmodified scattering is an interaction between extremely low energy (generally below 10 keV) and is of little importance in radiation therapy. (From Bushong S: *Radiologic science for technologists: physics, biology, and protection,* ed 5, St Louis, 1993, Mosby.)

enough energy remaining to interact with another atom (thus producing more scatter) or even exit the body part completely. If the photon reaches the film, it strikes it at random, thus producing unwanted density because its path no longer corresponds accurately to the portion of anatomy through which it passed. In any situation, the scattered photon is a bad photon and detrimental to image quality.

Unmodified scattering (Fig. 12-11) is of relatively little importance to diagnostic imaging. This scattering occurs at low energy levels (generally below 10 keV), and the resultant scattered photons do not have sufficient energy remain-

ing to be emitted from the part. Coherent scattering (also called *Thomson* or *unmodified scattering*) results in a change in the incident photon's direction but no change in energy. In this interaction, not enough energy exists to eject an electron from its orbit.

As noted earlier, the only interaction with the capacity to produce a useful image on the film is **photoelectric effect.** This interaction, sometimes described as *true absorption,* occurs when the incident photon penetrates deep into the atom and ejects an inner-shell electron from orbit (Fig. 12-12). Orbital electrons close to the nucleus have higher bind-

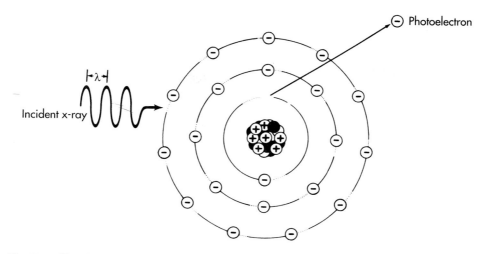

Fig. 12-12 The photoelectric effect, sometimes described as *true absorption*, occurs when the incident photon penetrates deep into the atom and ejects an inner-shell electron from orbit. (From Bushong S: *Radiologic science for technologists: physics, biology, and protection,* ed 5, St Louis, 1993, Mosby.)

ing energies, and all the photon's energy is required to remove them from orbit. Because a photon is nothing more than a bundle of pure energy, it ceases to exist or is absorbed in the process if all its energy is given up. The energy is transferred to the electron, now termed a *photoelectron,* with a kinetic energy equal to the original energy of the incident photon. This photoelectron has sufficient energy to undergo a variety of other interactions that are beyond the scope of this chapter.

An atom is ionized when it loses or gains an electron. Ionization is an unstable atomic state, and the ionized atom seeks to stabilize itself by filling the hole left in its inner electron shell. This effort sets off a chain reaction that can lead to as many as six different ionizing events, each with its own subsequent release of pure energy (a new photon). In practice, most of these events possess insufficient energy to be of any radiographic significance. However, atoms of high atomic number with K-shell binding energies of 20 or 30 keV can easily produce secondary or characteristic photons energetic enough to reach the film or undergo additional ionizing events.

The human body is composed primarily of carbon, hydrogen, and oxygen atoms, and none of these materials has sufficiently high k-energies to produce secondary photons of any magnitude. For this reason, most photoelectric interactions in tissue result simply in absorption with no appreciable secondary effect. This is desirable because to clearly define anatomical structures of differing densities and atomic number on the radiograph, their relative variation in absorption rates, however slight, must be used to the fullest imaging advantage.

Normal human anatomy provides a predictable variation in tissue densities. For example, kidneys can be seen in a plain radiograph of the abdomen not because of their density

difference compared with the greater surrounding tissue, but because they are outlined by a thin band of fat called the *adipose capsule*. Contrast materials such as iodine, barium, and other agents of high atomic number may be used to enhance the visibility of structures with similar composition that would otherwise remain unseen. Advanced imaging modalities such as CT scanning and magnetic resonance imaging (MRI) have done much to overcome this limitation in conventional diagnostic radiography.

Imaging pathology

Any diseased state in the body can dramatically alter the body's absorption characteristics. In many situations the changes that accompany pathology can actually improve radiographic demonstration. This phenomenon is of obvious value in diagnostic radiography and can also prove useful in radiation therapy treatment planning. After all, localizing disease that is not visible radiographically is difficult.

Tissue changes that occur in pathology are often characterized as *additive* or *destructive* (Fig. 12-13). Additive pathologies are those with increased tissue density and therefore appear as light regions on the radiograph. (The opposite is true with the reverse image on the television monitor during fluoroscopy, in which densities such as bone and tumor appear darker). The majority of nonmalignant disease entities are additive. They include edema, Paget's disease, atelectasis, abscesses, pleural effusions, and several other common illnesses. Hilar masses commonly associated with lung tumors are universally additive, and any large, fluid-filled mass also appears as an additive pathology. Necrotic areas in a tumor are generally destructive in appearance (typical of astrocytoma), but the band of actively mitotic, highly vascularized malignant tissue that surrounds this dead mass is often seen as additive in density.

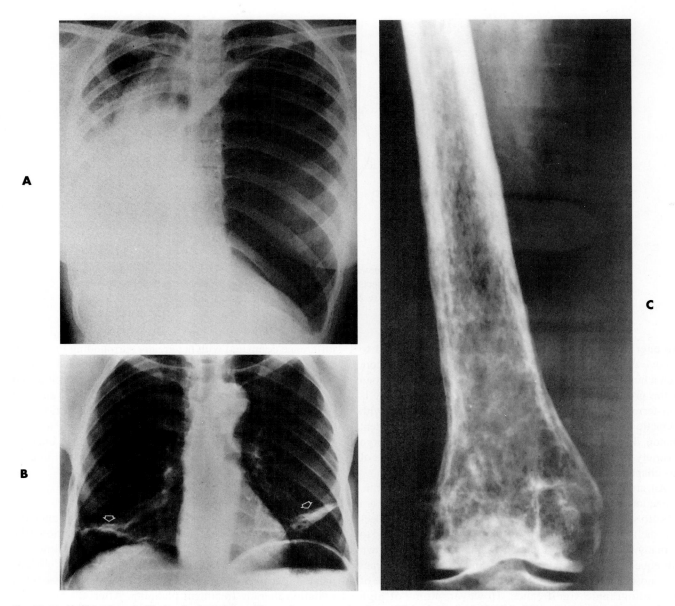

Fig. 12-13 A, This pleural effusion in the left hemithorax is an example of an additive pathology. **B,** This illustration demonstrates atelectasis in the lower portion of both lungs (another example of an additive pathology [an opacity on the radiograph]). **C,** A Ewing's sarcoma has destroyed part of the distal femur. (From Eisenberg RL, Dennis CA: *Comprehensive radiologic pathology,* St Louis, 1990, Mosby.)

Unfortunately, definite rules for malignant disease imaging do not exist because several tumors can cause increased tissue density. Certain cancers follow predictable patterns that can reliably guide the radiation oncologist and radiation therapist in their efforts to localize the lesion. Most patients with multiple myeloma or any osteolytic metastatic disease have a destructive pathological disease. Metastases from breast and prostate cancer can sometimes be seen as pathologically additive or destructive in the radiographic image when they are present in bone. Certain sarcomas and other soft-tissue tumors frequently differentiate poorly from surrounding tissues and are best localized by palpation and visual observation, although they can be seen radiographically through the use of low-kVp techniques.

The individual nature of healthy and diseased body tissues makes generalizations on levels of absorption difficult and possibly unwise. Far more important is the radiation therapist's understanding that dense structures absorb more photons photoelectrically and produce more Compton scattering. Conversely, tissues that are thin, less dense, and aged result in dramatically decreased attenuation and thus produce a disproportionately darker image on the film.

FUNDAMENTALS OF IMAGING
Introduction to concepts of contrast and density

The function of voltage (kVp) and current (mAs) in radiographic imaging involves the way more energetic photons (controlled by kVp) affect the film and the reason greater or lesser quantities of photons (controlled by mAs) make the film darker or lighter.[8,9] The explanation to these subjects focus on the two most important concepts in radiographic imaging: radiographic density and contrast.

Density. **Radiographic density** is defined as the degree of darkening on the film. This is not to be confused with *tissue density*, which refers to the compactness of molecules in the atomic structure of different body parts. Radiographic density is a relatively simple concept to grasp because it is easy to visualize. A radiograph of high density is dark, and a radiograph of low density is light. The rules governing radiographic density are equally straightforward. When more photons reach the film, density increases; when fewer photons reach the film, density decreases.

Many authors suggest that the principal factor governing radiographic density is mAs (i.e., mAs equals the tube current in milliamperes multiplied by the time of exposure). Although mAs largely determines the quantity of photons in the primary beam, giving mAs an enormous amount of credit in the regulation of density is inaccurate because numerous other factors may have equal or greater effect. For example, source-film distance (SFD), kVp, and grid ratio are important factors. However, mAs has a clear and predictable role in radiographic density. When all other factors remain the same, the relationship between mAs and density is a direct proportion (i.e., as mAs is doubled, so is the resulting density on the film). This makes mAs an extremely useful tool in the control of density and one that therapists find easy to use. By virtue of its convenience, this tool is also subject to abuse because as mAs is doubled to increase density, so is the dose of radiation exposure to the patient.

In addition, kVp may be used to change radiographic density. A far smaller increase in kVp is needed to significantly affect the film than is required by using mAs. When all other factors remain the same, a kVp increase of only 15% doubles the radiographic density. To put this in perspective, a scenario in which the therapist is involved in a prostate localization procedure may be considered. In the anteroposterior (AP) projection the therapist selects an mAs of 50 at 74 kVp. The resulting radiograph has insufficient density (too light) and must be repeated. The therapist may then use 100 mAs and 74 kVp or 50 mAs and 85 kVp to make the correction; either combination produces the same new radiographic density. One choice may be preferable to the other, and several variables yet to be discussed will determine the more desirable combination.

When mAs is used to control density, the only direct effects are on density and patient dose. However, extremely high mAs exposures, particularly those made by using the small focal spot, can shorten tube life dramatically. In contrast, when kVp is used to adjust density, a change in radio-

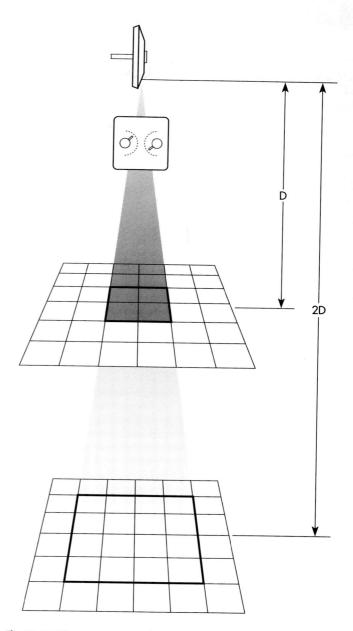

Fig. 12-14 The inverse square law means as distance *(D)* is doubled. A quantity of radiation is spread over an area 4 times as great, therefore reducing the intensity of the beam in any area to one fourth its original value. (Courtesy Eastman Kodak, Rochester, New York.)

graphic contrast also occurs, and this may not always be desirable.

Another major extrinsic factor influencing density is *distance,* which refers to the gap between the focal spot of the x-ray tube and the recording medium or film. The terminology used to describe this gap varies with the equipment in use and its application. SFD, focal-film distance (FFD), and source-image receptor distance (SID) refer to the same idea.

Distance can have a profound effect on radiographic density (Fig. 12-14), and although distance is a critical factor in

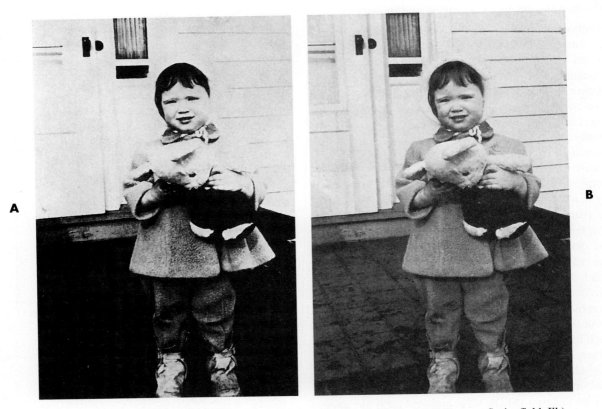

Fig. 12-15 Two photographs represent the variation in contrast. (Courtesy Charles C Thomas, Springfield, Ill.)

diagnostic radiography when the radiographer may have to negotiate a variety of distance changes, it is less important to the radiation therapist who generally works with one or two fixed distances. Still, some discussion on the effect of distance is important, not only for its relationship to radiographic density, but also because of its vital influence on occupational exposure. The relationship between distance and density follows the **inverse square law,** which states that the intensity of the beam of radiation is inversely proportional to the square of the distance. Put more simply, when distance is doubled, the quantity of radiation reaching the image receptor (or occupationally exposed personnel working with brachytherapy sources) is reduced to one fourth. From a practical standpoint, a film with a satisfactory radiographic density using 100 mAs at 80 cm SFD requires 400 mAs to produce the same density at 160 cm.

The inverse square law works because of the property of x-rays stating that they travel in straight lines and diverge from a point of origin. As distance is doubled, a quantity of radiation is spread over an area 4 times as great, therefore reducing the intensity of the beam in an area to one fourth its original value.

Contrast. Perhaps no element of radiographic imaging is more important or more misunderstood than contrast. **Radiographic contrast** is the element of imaging that provides visual evidence of the all-important differential absorp-

tion rates of various body tissues. Radiographic contrast has been described as the tonal range of densities from black to white or the number of shades of grey in the radiograph. Neither of these definitions (nor any of the others that have appeared in print over the years) provides an adequate description of the significance of contrast in defining information on the film.

When most homes had black and white television sets, describing the effect of contrast on a visible image was easier. With these old sets, contrast could be arbitrarily increased or decreased by the twist of a knob. Today, a similar demonstration can be conducted through black and white photographs.

The dramatic variation in the pair of photographs in Fig. 12-15 is clear. Initially, the image of the child on the left may be described as underexposed based on the obvious loss of optical information. However, both of these pictures exhibit identical overall density. However, they differ in that the photograph on the left is a high-contrast image, whereas the picture on the right demonstrates low contrast, or the greater number of grey shades needed to clearly define important details. The high-contrast image all but eliminates any definition of the child's hat, the surface on which she stands, the structure of the door behind her, and the bunny she is holding. The same ability to precisely define or destroy visible information exists

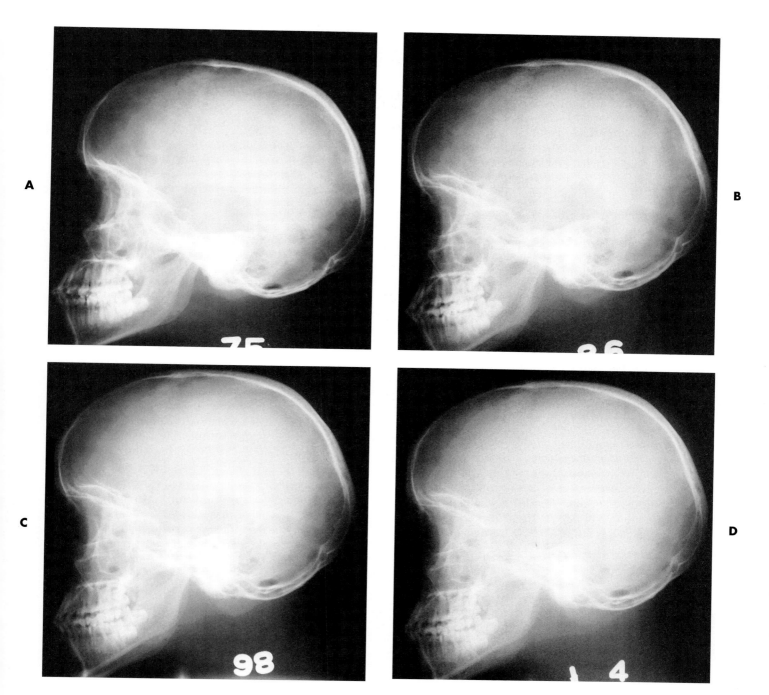

Fig. 12-16 In this series of four radiographs, density remains constant. A 15% increase in kVp (**A,** 75 kVp; **B,** 86 kVp; **C,** 98 kVp; and **D,** 114 kVp) and reduction in mAs demonstrates visible changes in contrast. Note the loss of detail from image **A** to image **D,** especially near the sella turcica. In **D** the contrast is low because of the overpenetration of the subject anatomy and increased production of scatter radiation.

in the medical imaging field and is the responsibility of the radiation therapist's correct application of technique.

The skull radiographs shown in Fig. 12-16 also exhibit identical densities. However, even to the casual observer, the difference in visible information is readily apparent. Fig. 12-16, *A* demonstrates clearly defined borders that may be

pleasing to the eye, but it lacks detailed anatomical information. Fig. 12-16, *D* is the opposite; the contrast is too low, and information is lost as a result of the overpenetration of the subject anatomy and increased production of scattered radiation. The other two images (Fig. 12-16, *B* and *C*) may represent optimal contrast. **Optimal contrast** results when technical factors (primarily kVp) are selected that maximize the rate of differential absorption between body parts of varying tissue density and effective atomic number. Optimal kVp ranges exist for all body parts. The most important factor in determining optimal kVp is part thickness, but numerous other elements such as grid ratio and field size may also influence the selection (Table 12-1).

Generally, any time the thickness of the body part exceeds 10 to 12 cm, a radiographic grid should be used. All tissues of the foot, hand, lower leg, forearm, and elbow can be adequately demonstrated without the use of a grid. In many situations the knee and upper arm may also be examined by using only screen-type radiographic techniques. Beyond this, a grid should be used to absorb the scattered radiation emitted from the thicker body parts and to allow the use of beam energies needed to maximize differential absorption between similar tissues. Chest and rib radiography may be an exception to this guideline, but only under specific circumstances. In general, even these procedures should be performed with a grid using high kVp ranges.

The ability of the radiation therapist to exercise control over contrast and density in an effective manner is not something that is readily learned from books. Medical imaging is certainly a visual science, and no amount of text will take the place of experience. Persons operating imaging equipment who wish to fully exercise their skills must understand the physics of radiographic imaging and then use all the tools available to them to produce quality radiographs. The temptation is great for persons to consider only easy and predictable options, such as mAs in the control of density. Disregarding the enormous flexibility available through varying kVp, use of a grid, field size, and other factors discussed throughout this chapter is easy, but doing so deprives the true professional of the right to practice medical imaging as an art and a science.

RECORDING MEDIA

One of the primary purposes of diagnostic-quality x-rays used in radiation oncology (as opposed to extremely high-energy x-rays used in the treatment of cancer) is to transfer information from the simulator's x-ray beam to a member of the radiation oncology team by using special recording media. The most common method of receiving and storing this information is with x-ray film. The construction and characteristics of x-ray film and photographic film are quite similar in that both are sensitive to light and radiation. However, x-ray film has a spectral response different from that of photographic film. In addition to conventional recording media (processing film), modern imaging technology has developed many other radiographic image receptors such as fluoroscopic screens, image intensifiers, computer-linked detectors, scintillation and piezoelectric crystals, and selenium plates.[4] More recently, effort has been invested in developing and perfecting an imaging technology without the use of film.[12] The conventional recording media (film, screens, and cassettes) used in capturing an x-ray image are discussed in this section.

Film

Construction. X-ray film has three major components: base, emulsion, and protective coating. The base is a rigid, transparent plastic onto which the emulsion is coated (Fig. 12-17). An x-ray film base must be flexible enough to maintain its size and shape during processing (immersion in a chemical solution) and handling, yet strong enough to withstand repeated viewing on a radiographic illuminator. To help reduce eye strain during viewing of the radiographic image, a blue dye is added to the film during manufacturing. Before the film base is coated with the emulsion that contains the photosensitive crystals, a thin adhesive layer is applied to the base.

The emulsion is composed of gelatin and photosensitive silver halide crystals (Fig. 12-18). The photosensitive crystals are suspended in the gelatin in much the same way as fruit is suspended in Jell-O during the preparation of a gelatin mold. The emulsion is spread onto the x-ray film in an

Table 12-1	Factors influencing contrast and density*		
Factor	**Change**	**Result**
Kilovoltage peak	Increase kVp	Decrease contrast
Part thickness	Increase thickness	Decrease contrast
Field size	Increase field size	Decrease contrast
Tissue density	Increase density	Decrease contrast
Grid ratio	Increase ratio	Increase contrast
Grid frequency	Increase frequency	Decrease contrast
Processing chemical temperature	Increase temperature	Decrease contrast
OFD	Increase OFD	Increase contrast

*Note that the change in contrast results when a single factor is modified alone and without compensation of other factors. Multiple concurrent changes can produce varying effects.
OFD, Object-film distance.

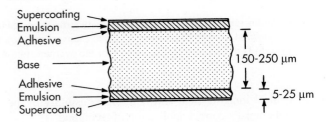

Fig. 12-17 A cross-sectional view of x-ray film. The base is a rigid, transparent plastic onto which the emulsion is coated. (From Bushong S: *Radiologic science for technologists: physics, biology, and protection,* ed 5, St Louis, 1993, Mosby.)

extremely thin, even coating. The silver halide crystals must be evenly distributed over the surface of the film so that one area of the film is not more photosensitive than another. The gelatin also allows the water and other chemicals to reach the silver halide crystals during the film processing.

About 95% of the photosensitive crystals are composed of silver bromide; the remainder consists of silver iodide. These crystals are the light-sensitive portion of the emulsion that allows it to interact with x-ray and light photons. These interactions are responsible primarily for the formation of the radiographic image on the film. To protect the image, a durable coating is applied to the emulsion to reduce the chance of damage from scratches, abrasions, and skin oils from handling.

Latent image formation. The remnant radiation (the amount of radiation leaving a patient after an x-ray exposure) that reaches the film's emulsion is responsible primarily for creating the latent image. The latent image is the image on the x-ray film that is not visible until the film is processed. The latent image exists on the film as an unseen change in the silver halide crystal's atomic structure. After processing, the invisible latent image becomes a manifest image, which contains a visible range of densities from black to white. The amount of radiation reaching the film after interaction with the patient greatly influences the degree of blackening on the film. This amount is proportional to the density and thickness of the anatomical part x-rayed. Denser and thicker parts of the body absorb more radiation and therefore allow less remnant radiation to reach the film. In many situations the x-ray photons and light photons are responsible for interacting with the atomic structure of the silver halide crystals. The affected silver halide crystals indirectly make up the image. Although much is still unknown about critical mechanisms that control the formation of the latent image, the theory of sensitivity specks and their essential involvement in the image-formation process (proposed by Gurney and Mott in 1938) remains almost unchallenged.[4]

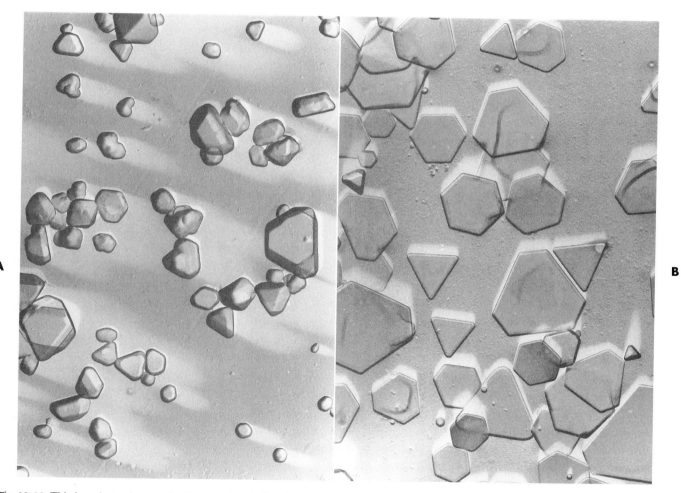

Fig. 12-18 This is a photomicrograph of conventional silver halide crystals (**A**) and newer technology, tabular grain silver halide crystals (**B**), which result in the coverage of a larger surface area. (Courtesy Eastman Kodak Company.)

Types of film used in radiation therapy. Mainly two types of film are used in radiation therapy. Intensifying screen film is primarily used in the simulation process, and direct-exposure film is used to check the patient's position before, during, or after treatment. This type of film, used to verify the patient's treatment position, is called *port film.*

Screen-type film, designed for use with intensifying screens, is available in a variety of speeds (sensitivity of the silver halide crystals). The speed of the film is also related to the thickness of the emulsion layer and number and size of the crystals in that layer. Most of the photons reaching the emulsion are light photons from the intensifying screens, which sandwich the film inside the cassette (Fig. 12-19). Emulsion is coated on both sides of screen-type film (double-emulsion film) to take advantage of the light generated from each of the intensifying screens mounted inside the cassette. This is especially important in diagnostic radiography, in which the dose to the patient is kept as low as reasonably possible. The patient generally receives a lower radiation dose when two intensifying screens help produce the image versus a single screen. If screen-type film were used with a direct-exposure technique (without screens), it would require 3 to 4 times the exposure than nonscreen film used in direct exposure.[19]

Some radiation oncology departments do use screen-type film without intensifying screens to verify the patient's position under treatment (also called port film). Thin sheets of lead and/or copper are mounted in the cassette in place of the intensifying screens. If screen-type film were used with intensifying screens for treatment verification, only a small amount of the high-energy radiation would interact with the emulsion and a poor image would result. The use of lead and copper screens in place of the intensifying screens produces a better, more acceptable image. Budget considerations make this port-filming technique more desirable than the technique with direct-exposure film.

Direct-exposure film, which produces an acceptable image without intensifying screens, is more expensive. Remnant radiation exiting from the patient during treatment verification interacts more directly with the emulsion to produce the image. True direct-exposure film (used for industrial radiography) has a single, thicker emulsion and requires a special, longer processing. Two types of direct-exposure film available are used for port filming. This type of direct-exposure film is developed through a conventional 90-second processor. With a shorter processing time than industrial direct-exposure film, X-OMAT TL@ and X-OMAT V @ direct-exposure films are convenient and efficient in radiation therapy portal imaging. However, the two direct-exposure films have different applications.

X-OMAT TL@ film. This type of direct-exposure film can be used with two short exposures of about 3 to 10 cGy (or equivalent monitor units) to verify the patient's position before or after a treatment. Individually packaged X-OMAT TL@ film comes in light-tight paper wrappers (unlike screen film that comes in boxes of 100 and needs a darkroom for

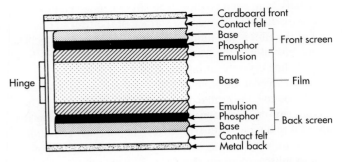

Fig. 12-19 A cross-sectional view of a cassette used for simulation purposes. (From Bushong S: *Radiologic science for technologists: physics, biology, and protection,* ed 5, St Louis, 1993, Mosby.)

storage and loading). The individual film package is positioned directly under a patient or placed inside a portal-imaging (therapy) cassette between the lead and/or copper screens. A double-exposure technique, in which one exposure area is larger than the other, verifies the treatment site in relationship to the surrounding anatomical area. This double-exposure technique is useful in identifying the patient's position because additional surrounding anatomical landmarks (outside the treatment area) become visible.

X-OMAT V@ film. This direct-exposure film (except for being 12 times slower) is similar to the X-OMAT TL@ film. This film also comes in individual light-tight packaging and can be placed directly underneath the patient. The density on the film results from a single, longer exposure. Usually, the film is left in place during the entire length of the treatment. This technique visualizes only the treatment area on the port film.

Film characteristics. Important characteristics of x-ray film are speed, contrast, and latitude. **Sensitometry,** which is the measurement of the film's response to exposure and processing, provides a mechanism to analyze these characteristics within the normal exposure range of the film. Sensitometric evaluation of the film may also be part of a quality-assurance program designed to monitor the simulator's exposure system and performance of the processing unit.

The **film speed** affects the degree of blackening (density) produced on the film for a certain amount of exposure. The thickness of the emulsion layer and size and shape of the silver halide crystals determine the speed of the film. For example, if two films with different speed are given similar exposures, one film would have less measured density. Several reasons may account for this. A film with large silver halide crystals produces a greater area of darkening than one with smaller crystals, given the same exposure. Similarly, a thicker emulsion layer provides more crystals in an area, thus producing more film density than a film with a thinner emulsion layer.

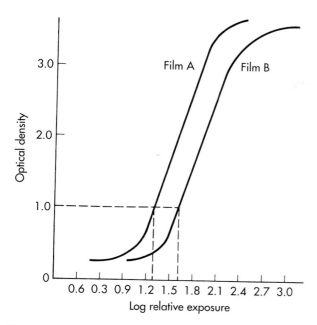

Fig. 12-20 A characteristic curve shows the speed of a film. Film speed is the reciprocal of the exposure in roentgens, needed to produce a density of 1.0. Notice that film A is faster than film B. (From Bushong S: *Radiologic science for technologists: physics, biology, and protection,* ed 5, St Louis, 1993, Mosby.)

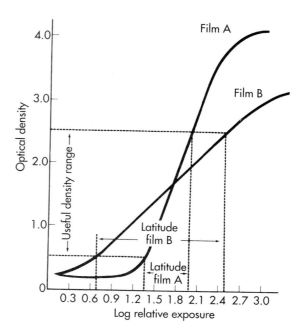

Fig. 12-21 A comparison of two characteristic curves showing a difference in latitude. Relative exposure ranges are indicated for film A and film B. (From Bushong S: *Radiologic science for technologists: physics, biology, and protection,* ed 5, St Louis, 1993, Mosby.)

The speed of two films can be compared through a graphic relationship called a *sensitometric, characteristic,* or *H & D curve* (Fig. 12-20). Hurter and Driffield are two British photographers who in 1890 first described the relationship between exposure and density. This graph represents the measured density on a processed film compared with exposure. A special device called a **densitometer** measures the degree of blackening on the film. The readings from the densitometer, plotted on logarithmic graph paper, correlate to the characteristics of the film. Logarithmic paper keeps the graph to a reasonable size. Density increases with exposure quite sharply along the straight line portion of the graph for film *A* in Fig. 12-20 and less sharply for film *B*. Film *A* is faster than film *B*. Both curves are sigmoidal (i.e., they have a toe and shoulder portion and are not just straight lines). A characteristic, or H & D, curve also graphically expresses film contrast and latitude.

Another important characteristic of x-ray film is *contrast,* which is the ability of the film to record differences in density. Film emulsion manufactured to produce high contrast (mammography) or low contrast (a longer scale of greys) is designed to have its own unique response to exposure factors (kVp, mAs, distance). Low-contrast film provides more film latitude and is therefore more forgiving of errors in the selection of technical factors, whereas high-contrast film provides better image detail.[5]

Latitude is the range of radiographic exposures that produce densities in the diagnostically useful range (Fig. 12-21).

Film *A* has a narrow latitude, whereas film *B* has a wider latitude and responds to an extended range of exposures. Film *B* is a more forgiving film because it allows a sizable variation in exposures while still displaying densities in the diagnostically useful range. An inversely proportional relationship exists between contrast and latitude. When contrast increases, latitude decreases. In other words, high-contrast film has narrow latitude and low-contrast film has wide latitude.

Storage and handling of film. Several factors such as light, radiation, heat and humidity, shelf life, and proper handling influence the safe storage and handling of x-ray film. Most x-ray film must be stored and handled in the dark. A darkroom with an appropriate safelight (a special orange-red light that permits low-level illumination without fogging the film) is an essential component. A darkroom is needed not only for processing exposed simulation and port films, but also for safely storing and handling the film. The unexposed film should be stored in a lightproof, lead-lined storage bin for added protection from light and radiation sources.

X-ray film is also sensitive to the effects of heat and humidity. Storage temperature should not exceed 68° F (20° C). Professional photographers know the benefits of refrigerating film, thus increasing its shelf life. Ideally, x-ray film should also be refrigerated. However, this is not always practical. Low humidity (below 30%) can cause unwanted static-discharge artifacts on the film, and high humidity (above 60%) may cause condensation or water spots on the radiograph.

The shelf life of x-ray film is determined by the expiration date stamped on each box of 100 sheets, much the same way a gallon of milk is stamped with an expiration date. Old film can cause a loss of speed and contrast as a result of an increase in fog (unwanted density on the film) from excessive heat, humidity, and background radiation. The fog on a film may reach a level at which it interferes with the quality of the radiographic image. Rotating film according to the expiration date reduces problems associated with old film.

Proper handling of x-ray film is also important in maintaining a high image quality. Boxes of film stored on end and not stacked flat prevent the film from warping and sticking together. Care must be taken when cardboard inserts and paper interleaves are removed from around the film or when a new box of film is opened. Rough handling and quick movements, even with the proper humidity, can cause unwanted film abrasions from unnecessary pressure and static-discharge artifacts.

Film identification. All port films and simulation radiographs should be identified with the patient's name, date, institution at which the exposure was made, identification number, and additional treatment-related information. This can be accomplished in several ways. Most cassettes have a small rectangular space in one corner reserved for patient identification. A lead blocker prevents radiation from reaching this rectangular area during the exposure. Then patient information, usually included on a small index card (flash card), can be added to the film through a special daylight identification and cassette system. Information can also be added in the darkroom with a special flash-card device after the film is removed from the cassette but before the film is processed. China markers (wax pencils) frequently used in radiation oncology provide a method of adding critical treatment-related information on the film after processing. All the information on the film becomes part of the patient's medical record.

Intensifying screens

Intensifying screens convert the invisible energy of an x-ray beam into visible light energy. About 99% of the latent image on the x-ray film is formed because of this visible light created by intensifying screens. The process of using intensifying screens with film is especially important in diagnostic radiology, where imaging detail and limiting the dose to the patient is more critical. Less exposure is required with film and screen systems than with direct-exposure film. These screens are commonly used in pairs to take full advantage of the double-coated emulsion on the film.

Construction. Intensifying screens are usually constructed of four distinct layers (Fig. 12-22). A typical screen, designed to emit visible light when struck by x-rays, has a base, reflective layer, phosphor layer, and protective coating. The base is made of cardboard or a thin sheet of plastic and must be flexible and rigid. A thin reflective layer is added between the base and active phosphor layer of the intensifying screen. This reflective layer increases the efficiency of the screen by redirecting light photons toward the center of the cassette where the x-ray film is sandwiched between two screens. A protective coating safeguards the phosphor layer from harmful scratches and abrasions.

Luminescence. The phosphor layer is the key to the conversion power of the intensifying screen. This layer has the ability to absorb the energy of an x-ray photon and emitting light photons. When Röntgen discovered x-rays in his laboratory, he observed light photons that were emitted (luminescence) from a piece of cardboard coated with a phosphor called *barium plantinocyanide*. Materials other than intensifying screens excited by x-rays can be caused to luminesce. For example, materials such as a watch dial, lightning bug, or glow light also glow in the dark or luminesce when stimulated. The two types of luminescence are called *fluorescence* and *phosphorescence*. If light is emitted only during the stimulation of the phosphor, the action is known as *fluorescence*. If light continues to be emitted from the phosphor after the stimulation stops, this is called *phosphorescence*, an undesirable quality of intensifying screens. An instantaneous emission of light from an intensifying screen (fluorescence) can be displayed by exposing an opened cassette in a darkened room. In contrast, a delayed emission of light (phosphores-

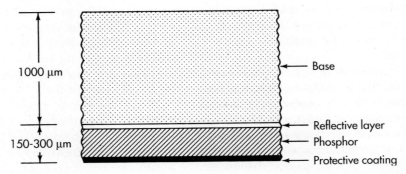

Fig. 12-22 The four layers of an intensifying screen are shown in this cross-sectional view. (From Bushong S: *Radiologic science for technologists: physics, biology, and protection,* ed 5, St Louis, 1993, Mosby.)

cence) occurs when the screens continue to glow after the exposure has ended. In each situation the phosphor produces light photons when stimulated with x-ray photons.

Over the years, several materials have been used as phosphors. Some of the older materials such as barium platinocyanide, zinc sulfide, barium lead sulfate, and calcium tungstate have a lower conversion factor. The newer, rare earth screens such as gadolinium, lanthanum, and yttrium have a more efficient x–ray-to-light conversion factor. The conversion factor for rare earth screens averages about 15% to 20% compared with 5% for calcium tungstate screens.[14] Table 12-2 summarizes some of the intensifying screens used in radiographic imaging.

Screens used in radiation therapy. Three types of screens are used in radiation therapy: intensifying, lead, and copper screens. Intensifying screens, which are necessary in the production of diagnostic-quality radiographs, are used on the treatment-planning simulator. In contrast, lead and copper screens are primarily used in portal imaging.

Intensifying screens used today on the treatment-planning simulator are probably the rare earth type, but some older calcium tungstate screens may still be found in use. Unlike the lead and copper screens used to check the patient's treatment, the calcium tungstate and rare earth type screens convert low-energy x-rays into visible light.

Lead and copper screens are used primarily for port filming on high-energy radiation therapy equipment. They do not convert x-ray photons to light photons. The image quality of a port film is considerably poor compared with that of a chest x-ray or simulator film. However, the film must be good

enough to determine field boundaries of the treatment area in relationship to anatomical or bony landmarks. Taking regular port films is good clinical practice and provides legal documentation of the patient's actual treatment area.

The thin metal screens can be used with screen-type or direct-exposure film (Fig. 12-23). The lead and copper screens used in port filming can be mounted in a screen-type cassette with the intensifying screens removed or secured to a cardboard film holder. The screens can range in thickness from 0.1 to 0.5 mm for lead and up to 3 mm for copper.[13] The thin metal sheets act as an intensifying screen by ejecting electrons from the screen through photon interaction, thus providing an image on the film that represents the variation of beam intensity transmitted through the patient.[1] The ejected electrons from the screen do not have far to travel before reaching the film. High-energy photons used in port filming cause electrons produced further in the patient to travel greater distances to the film emulsion. This adds to geometrical blurring of the image. The copper screen absorbs some of these unwanted electrons and at the same time produces some of its own. Good screen-film contact is important to avoid poor image quality. Intensifying screens are used in the diagnostic photon range to produce simulation radiographs, whereas lead and copper screens are used in the megavoltage photon range to produce port films.

Cassettes and film holders

The **cassette** provides the light-tight conditions necessary for x-ray film and intensifying screens to work properly. The cassette, which opens like a book, is made of material with a low atomic number such as cardboard, plastic, and carbon fiber. Because of its low atomic number and strength, carbon fiber is also used as table-top material for the radiation therapy simulator and CT couches. The x-ray film is loaded between the front and back intensifying screens, which are mounted inside the sturdy cassette (Fig. 12-19). Pressure pads, usually made of felt or a spongelike material, are mounted between each intensifying screen and the cassette cover. This design helps maintain good film-screen contact when the cassette is closed and loaded with film. The location of the lead blocker in one corner of the cassette provides space on the film for patient-identification purposes.

Phosphor	Primary emission color	Type
Barium lead sulfate	Violet or ultraviolet	Older
Calcium tungstate	Violet	Older
Barium fluorochloride	Blue	Older
Gadolinium oxysulfide	Green	Rare earth
Lanthanum oxybromide	Blue	Rare earth
Yttrium oxysulfide	Blue	Rare earth

Table 12-2 Intensifying screen phosphors used in radiographic imaging

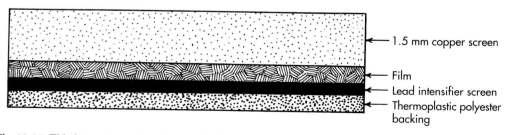

Fig. 12-23 This is a cross-sectional view of a therapy cassette with a 1.5-mm copper screen and lead-intensifying screen with the use of a thermoplastic polyester backing.

The back of the cassette is designed differently than the front of the cassette. Lead or other metal backing prevents unwanted scatter radiation from returning to the simulator film after it has exited the cassette. This type of backscatter radiation can cause unnecessary fog and reduce image contrast.

Cleaning. The proper cleaning of cassettes and intensifying screens is important to total image quality. Dust, dirt, and other such materials inside the cassette can interfere with image quality by preventing light photons produced by the screens from reaching the film. Special antistatic cleaning agents, which reduce static electricity that can discharge and expose the film, are commercially available to clean intensifying screens. Mild soap and water can be used to clean the screens and cassette if the water does not contain high levels of minerals, which may leave unwanted stains and deposits.

The use of film, screens, and cassettes as conventional recording media in radiation therapy serves as a convenient, relatively inexpensive method of recording important patient information. Simulation and port films are legal documents considered part of the patient's medical record. Proper understanding of the tools used in creating these legal documents is essential to producing good-quality port films and high-quality simulation radiographs. Until an imaging technology without the use of film is perfected and widely available, close attention needs to be given to the principles of conventional recording media.

PROCESSING

In the era of modern, high-speed automatic film processing, the challenges of darkroom chemistry and manual developing are easily forgotten. Gone are the days of hand tanks and cumbersome metal film hangers. Gone is the task of dipping and agitating the film in a five-step process that can take almost 2 hours to produce a completely developed, fixed, and dried radiograph. Gone is the arduous duty of the shift person who would begin each Monday morning at 6:30 AM with the noxious mess of mixing several caustic and unforgiving powdered chemicals with precise amounts of water. Gone are the little trays strategically located below each viewbox to catch the dripping solutions from films that required the urgent attention of the radiologist.

In diagnostic radiology, much of this rugged heritage still remains in daily terminology. Wet readings are still mentioned despite the fact that partially processed radiographs dripping from the wash water have not been delivered to the physician in 25 years. Occasionally, a requisition ordering a "flat plate of the abdomen" is still seen although glass plates have not been used as a film-base material since the advent of cellulose nitrate x-ray film over 70 years ago.

Despite advances brought on by automation in the darkroom, some rudimentary understanding of film processing should remain a part of the future therapist's curriculum. The standard textbook definition of radiographic *film processing* describes the procedure as the conversion of the latent image to a visible image.[3,4,17] The visible image must also be reasonably well preserved for storage.

Developer

The latent image is created when the remnant radiation reaching the intensifying screens of the cassette is converted to light. The light exposes the film in a pattern that precisely corresponds to the intensity of the remaining radiation beam after it passes through anatomy. Without delving too deeply into the chemistry involved, when the exposed film is placed in a developer solution, a reducing agent converts the light-sensitive silver halide crystals in the emulsion to black metallic silver. Unexposed crystals are chemically restrained from involvement in this process. In manual film development the hazy, milky image taking shape on the film is visible even under the dim illumination of the safelight. However, if the film is exposed to white light at this time, the unfixed image is destroyed.

Fixer

The function of the fixer is to remove the unexposed silver halide from the film. (The silver washed off the film in this process is quite valuable, thus leading to the use of silver-recovery systems in most darkrooms.) The fixer also preserves the image by hardening the emulsion and neutralizing any developer remaining on the film. The film is then placed in a bath of running water to remove residual chemicals. In manual processing the entire cycle from development through washing and drying can take up to 2 hours.

Automatic processing

Fortunately, modern diagnostic and simulation radiographic film development relies on a totally automated process requiring virtually no direct intervention from the therapist. The individual simply enters a darkened cubicle, removes the exposed film from the cassette, and places the film on a tray from which it is drawn into the complex inner reaches of the processor with its whirring rollers, various chemical baths, and heated blower system. About 90 seconds later, the completely processed and preserved image emerges, ready for viewing, analysis, and (ultimately) archival storage.

The diagram of a modern film processor (Fig. 12-24) is deceiving in its simplicity. Only a chain of rollers (the film-transport system) meandering through a row of three tanks is seen. However, this apparently simple processor took several major corporations nearly a generation to design and perfect.

The discussion on the construction of x-ray film in the previous section should be recalled. Film consists of a polyester plastic base coated with a gelatinous layer impregnated with light-sensitive compounds. For the chemicals involved in the development and fixing of the latent image to work effectively, the gelatin must absorb water, which serves as the chemical solvent. This is appropriately termed *gel swell*.

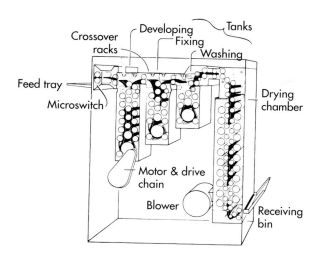

Fig. 12-24 A diagram of a modern film processor demonstrating the major components. (From Bushong S: *Radiologic science for technologists: physics, biology, and protection*, ed 5, St Louis, 1993, Mosby.)

In the days of manual processing, gel swell was of no significance because the increase in the thickness of the film was only a few microns. However, with the advent of primitive automatic processors, gel swell became the most important obstacle to a successful design. As it entered the water-based developer solution, the film promptly swelled sufficiently to become irretrievably lodged between the narrow gap of the rollers. Increasing roller separation proved ineffective because as the film passed to the fixer tank, it contracted so that it sat motionlessly between the now excessive roller play.

Automatic processing required the development of an entirely new set of chemicals, compounds that would limit gel swell and still provide adequate chemical penetration of the emulsion. The new chemicals also had to resist the increased oxidation that takes place at the higher processing temperatures necessary in rapid automatic equipment.

Troubleshooting

Modern film processors are usually remarkably reliable. However, having some limited troubleshooting skills for rare malfunctioning occasions is useful. In general, the condition of the film exiting the processor gives a good indication of the problem.

When the film feels sticky or greasy, probable causes include the following:

1. The fixer solution is exhausted.
2. The flow in the wash water is inadequate. (Check for plugged filters.)
3. The developer solution is contaminated.

In departments in which the demand placed on the processor is relatively low (including many therapy ser-

vices, operating room darkrooms, and small medical office practices), developer exhaustion is a common problem. This is caused by insufficient replenishment of solutions. Each time a film is fed into the processor, a microswitch is tripped, thus activating the replenisher pumps for the fixer and developer. Low-volume periods prevent fresh solutions from being pumped regularly into the tanks. This may not be obvious because the deterioration of the chemicals is relatively gradual. The therapist simply finds necessity in making increases in exposure factors to compensate for the loss of film density. This leads to excessive patient dose and general poor technique.

Film fogging can also be a problem. Fog results in an overall greying of the image and loss of contrast. Although fog can have many causes, the leading ones include the following:

1. The safelights are too bright. The bulbs may be of too high a wattage, or the safelights may be located too close to the work area.
2. The darkroom technique is poor. (Limit the time the film is exposed to the safelight.)
3. The film is stored too long or at excessive temperatures.
4. The film is exposed to ionizing radiation.
5. The chemical temperatures are too high.

One of the most common problems is related not to the automatic processor at all, but to the humidity conditions in the darkroom. Excessively dry air (below about 50% relative humidity) may cause a buildup of static electricity. When this static electricity is discharged on the film, the result is dramatic black artifacts that resemble lightening bolts or Christmas trees.

A strict program of preventive maintenance and quality control can eliminate almost all processor problems. Although it is not a common practice in some departments, sensitometric evaluation of the processor should be conducted regularly. This relatively simple and economic testing regimen detects problems before they become serious and substantially improves the technical proficiency of simulation and port-film radiography.

APPLICATION IN RADIATION ONCOLOGY

Producing quality radiographs is not an easy task. Many components should be considered, such as geometrical factors, control of unwanted scatter radiation, and problems associated with contrast and density on the radiograph. An understanding of the many factors affecting the production of good-quality simulation radiographs and port films is essential. In this section, a practical-application approach to these issues is explored.

Geometrical factors

Some principles in photography apply to radiography. Both areas require a certain intensity of light or x-ray energy and proper exposure time to create an image on the film. A recorded image is possible in both situations because x-ray and visible-light photons travel in straight, divergent lines. This principle of divergence, in which photons move in straight but different directions from a common point (focal spot), contributes greatly to the magnification and distortion seen on simulation radiographs and port films. Three geometrical factors are important in radiation oncology: magnification, distortion, and proper selection of focal-spot size.

Magnification. All images on a radiograph or port film appear larger than they are in reality. This condition is known as *magnification*. The images on the film represent objects in the path of the beam. These objects can be located closer to the common point source (e.g., objects on or near the block tray) or nearer to the film (anatomy in the patient). Fig. 12-25 illustrates the principle of divergence, in which more tissue is exposed at the level of the lumbar vertebrae *(B)* than at the skin surface *(A)*. The degree of magnification depends on several factors, all of which have to do with the geometrical arrangement of the x-ray target, the patient (object), and the radiographic film on which the image is displayed.[17]

Magnification can be measured and expressed as a factor. Magnification on a film is directly proportional to the distance of the object from the target or source and is dependent on the distance of the object from the film. The magnification factor is defined as follows:

$$\text{Magnification factor} = \frac{\text{Image size}}{\text{Object size}}$$

Example: If an object in the patient, such as the maximum width of a vertebral body, measures 5.3 cm and its image on the simulator film measures 7.5 cm, what is the magnification factor?

Answer:

$$\text{Magnification factor} = \frac{7.5 \text{ cm}}{5.3 \text{ cm}} = 1.415$$

Another method of determining the magnification factor is using the geometrical relationship between similar triangles. Two triangles are similar if the corresponding angles are equal and corresponding sides are proportional. Fig. 12-25 illustrates a typical divergent x-ray beam used on the simulator. In many radiation therapy imaging procedures, determining the size of an object (especially in a patient) is not possible. In these situations the magnification factor can be calculated by using the ratio of SFD and source-object distance (SOD):

$$\text{Magnification factor} = \frac{\text{SFD}}{\text{SOD}}$$

Example: A radiograph taken at 140 cm SFD during a simulation procedure produces an image measuring 6.5 cm on the radiograph. The distance from the target (source) to the object is 100 cm. What is the magnification factor?

Answer:

$$\text{Magnification factor} = \frac{140 \text{ cm}}{100 \text{ cm}} = 1.4$$

Magnification, expressed as a factor or ratio, is inherent in the production of all simulation radiographs and port films. This is due in part to limitations of the simulation and treatment equipment used in radiation oncology. A greater degree of magnification is tolerated in radiation oncology than in diagnostic radiology, in which loss of radiographic detail from magnification is more critical to image quality. The radiation therapist should posses an understanding of the practical applications of magnification and demonstrate the ability to measure its effects in the clinical setting.

Distortion. Distortion is a change in the size, shape, or appearance of the structures being examined. Magnification is a good example of size distortion. More magnification occurs with large SODs. Conversely, the greater the SFD, the less the magnification of the object on the image. For minimal distortion, the distance and angulation of the x-ray beam in relationship to the anatomical part (object) and image receptor must be given special attention.

Shape distortion is the misrepresentation by unequal magnification of the actual shape of the structure being examined.[4] This occurs when the object plane or part examined is not parallel with the image plane. If these two planes are parallel, only size distortion occurs, and that distortion is directly proportional to the SOD and SFD. Because of unequal magnification, shape distortion can be the result of the following two factors:

1. The angulation of the x-ray beam is in relationship to the part examined.
2. The object and image planes are not parallel in common anatomical projections such as AP, posteroanterior (PA), and lateral.

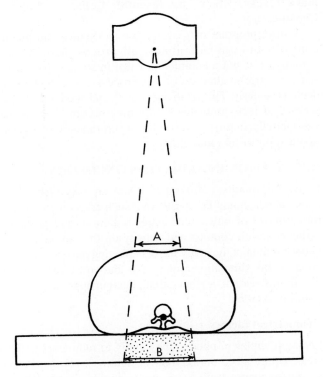

Fig. 12-25 Divergence of an x-ray beam. More tissue is exposed as the beam exits the patient than at the anterior skin surface.

In radiation therapy treatment planning, angling the beam to avoid treating sensitive normal tissue structures is frequently necessary. When this occurs, a certain amount of shape distortion is observed on the image. No formula exists (as it does in magnification) to assess the amount of shape distortion. Instead, the assessment is based on the radiation therapist's understanding of normal radiographic anatomy in certain situations. Fig. 12-26, *A* illustrates a common radiographic projection (AP), in which the object and image planes are closely parallel. Fig. 12-26, *B* illustrates shape distortion of a vertebral body when the simulator beam is angled 25 degrees. Greater shape distortion of an image is illustrated in Fig. 12-26, *C*, in which the beam is angled 40 degrees from the vertical. The distortion that occurs in the thoracic vertebrae should be noted. In this situation the objective in treatment planning may be to treat a lung mass while avoiding the spine (a sensitive critical structure).

Shape distortion can also occur when the object and image planes are not parallel. For example, in the pelvic region the obturator foramina are normally of equal size when radiographed in the anterior or posterior projection. If

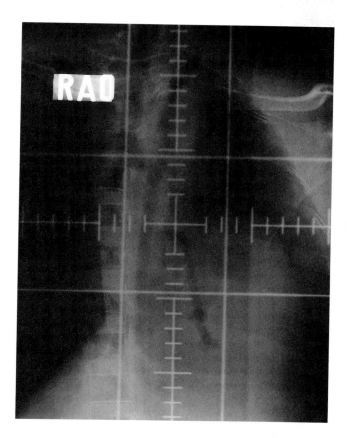

B

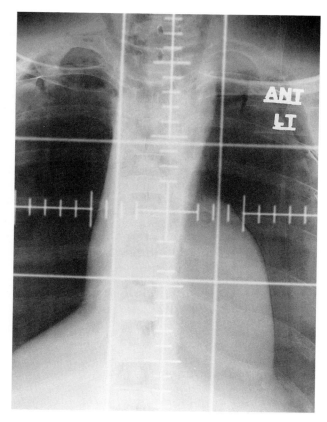

A

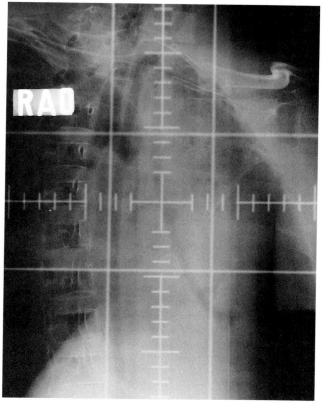

C

Fig. 12-26 These three radiographs illustrate the normal anatomy of a thoracic vertebral body in the AP projection **(A),** distorted anatomy with a 25-degree angulation of the beam **(B),** and distorted anatomy with a 40-degree angulation of the beam **(C).**

the pelvic bones are rotated slightly, shape distortion can be detected in the image, especially in the shape of the obturator foramina openings. Fig. 12-27 compares the amount of shape distortion as a result of unequal magnification when the object (the pelvis) and image planes are not parallel.

For reduction of the effects of distortion, the distances used for a specific procedure and angulation of the x-ray beam deserve particular attention. Otherwise, a misrepresentation of the size and shape of the anatomical part occurs. This misrepresentation, classified as *size* or *shape distortion,* can affect radiographic image quality. Other factors such as the selection of the focal-spot size can also contribute to distortion on the radiographic image.

Focal-spot selection. Focal-spot size and the line-focus principle (Fig. 12-5) influence radiographic image quality.[18] X-rays are not emitted from a common point source but from a measurable area on the anode, which is commonly referred to as a *spot* or *common point.* Thus, the focal spot (which can measure from 0.1 to 2.0 mm) is not a true point source, but a square or rectangular area of x-ray production.

The *penumbra* is the area of unsharpness or fuzziness at the edge of the beam. This is a result of photons emanating from various locations on the target area and intersecting the object at different angles. Penumbra is undesirable, but a certain amount of it is unavoidable because of the geometry of image formation. Three situations can contribute to unwanted penumbra: large focal spot, large object-film distance (OFD), and short SFD.

The *umbra* (Fig. 12-28, *A*) is the central, sharper portion of the image influenced by the size of the focal spot. The penumbra surrounds the umbra, or area of greater detail. Fig.

12-28, *B* illustrates the penumbra as a result of the selection of a large focal spot or mA station to produce a radiograph. Penumbra increases and image sharpness decreases as the focal spot becomes larger. Fig. 12-28, *C* and *D* illustrate the effect of small and large OFDs on image size and resolution. A large OFD increases penumbra and reduces image detail. Fig. 12-28, *E* and *F* illustrate the effect SFD has on penumbra. As SFD decreases, penumbra increases and resolution decreases.

Using a small focal spot in radiation therapy reduces the effects of penumbra, especially on the field-defining wires located in the collimator head of the simulator gantry. The large OFDs created by the field-defining wires located in the collimator head is unavoidable. Therefore to reduce the effects of penumbra, a small focal spot should be selected when possible. Any unsharpness or fuzziness of the field-defining wires on the radiographic image adds to the uncertainty of the treatment field outlined on the patient's skin. The difference in the width of the field-defining wires on the simulator radiographs should be noted in Fig. 12-29. The exposure factors for each radiograph used the same mAs and kVp. However, Fig. 12-29, *B* shows the use made of a large focal spot. An unnecessary amount of penumbra produced on the field-defining wires with the large focal spot can compromise the precision and accuracy demanded in radiation therapy.

Magnification, distortion, and the focal-spot size are controllable factors that affect radiographic image quality. A knowledge of these geometrical factors and an understanding of their application is necessary to produce quality radiographs. Other factors such as the control of scatter radiation can also improve radiographic image quality.

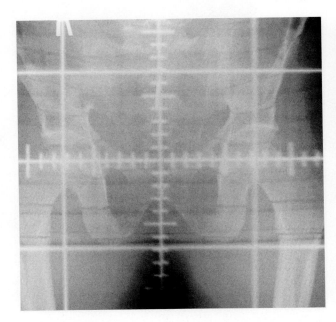

A

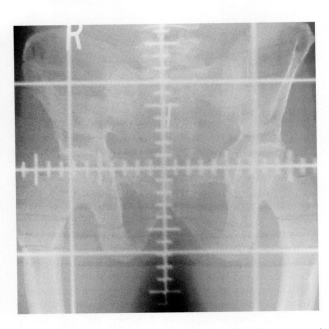

B

Fig. 12-27 These two radiographs compare an AP projection of the pelvis (**A**) and shape distortion of the obturator foramina as a result of unequal magnification when the image and object plane are not parallel (**B**). One obturator foramen appears smaller than the other because of rotation of the pelvis.

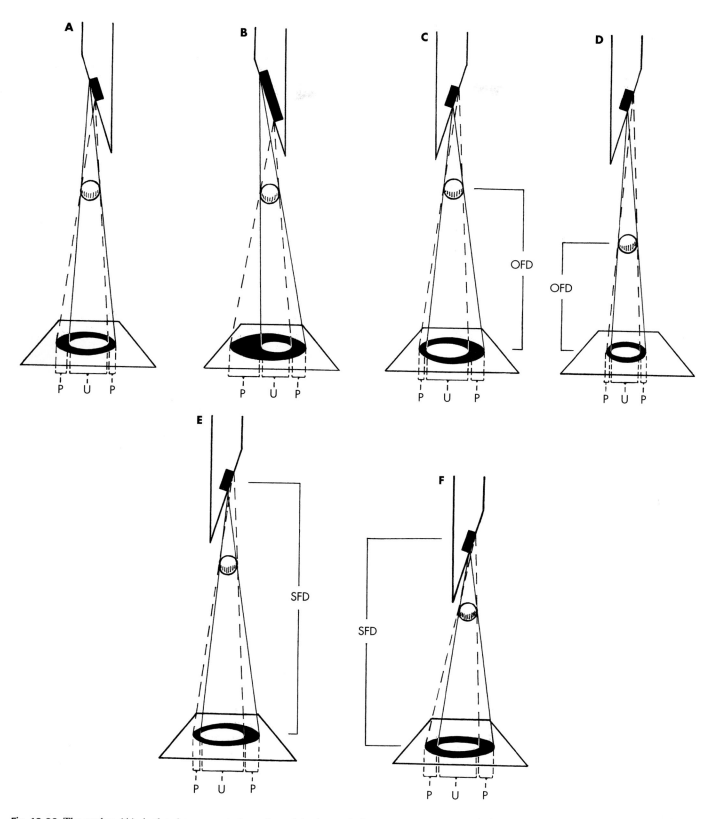

Fig. 12-28 The umbra **(A)** is the sharper central portion of the image influenced by the size of the focal spot. The penumbra surrounds the umbra, or area of greater detail. **B** illustrates the penumbra as a result of selecting a large focal spot or mA station to produce a radiograph **(B)**. Penumbra increases and image sharpness decreases as the focal spot becomes larger. **C** and **D** illustrate the effect of small and large OFDs on image size and resolution. A large OFD increases penumbra and reduces image detail. **E** and **F** illustrate the effect SFD has on penumbra. As SFD decreases, penumbra increases and resolution decreases. (From Carlton RR, McKenna-Adler AM: *Principles of radiographic imaging,* Albany, NY 1992, Delmar Publishing.)

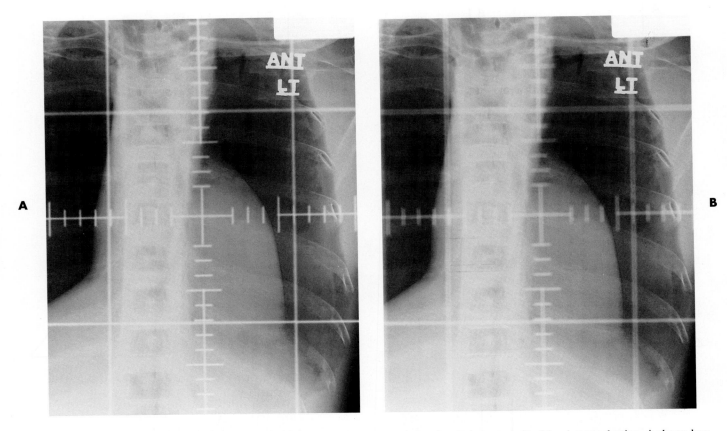

Fig. 12-29   Penumbra, demonstrated on the field-defining wires of a simulation radiograph, as a result of focal-spot selection. **A** shows less penumbra as a result of a smaller focal-spot selection than in **B.**

Control of scatter radiation

During an exposure, some x-rays are absorbed photoelectrically, and others pass through the patient to reach the film. This is partially a result of the kilovoltage. If more photons pass through the patient, the radiographic image has a greater density. The opposite is true if fewer photons reach the film and more photons are absorbed in the body; radiographic density decreases. A considerable amount of the radiographic density on the film is due to scatter radiation, in which photons arrive at the film after bouncing off matter rather haphazardly. However, the density on the film from scatter photons does not directly correlate to the anatomical structures of interest. Instead, the unwanted scatter radiation decreases contrast and reduces image quality.

Reducing scatter or secondary radiation, which is created during a Compton interaction, is essential to improving image quality. Scatter photons are produced when an incoming primary photon interacts with an outer-shell electron and is forced to change direction. Sometimes that scattered photon never reaches the film or image receptor. Other times it does. When it reaches the film, scatter radiation reduces contrast by causing additional density on the film and fogging

the image. The radiation therapist can create a better image by restricting the amount of scatter radiation reaching the film. Collimating the x-ray beam and using a grid reduces the effects of unwanted scatter radiation.

Less scatter radiation is produced by restricting the beam through careful collimation of the x-ray shutter blades. If fewer primary photons are emitted from the collimator head, fewer scatter photons are created. Collimating the primary x-ray beam is the first line of defense in controlling unwanted secondary radiation. A grid absorbs scatter photons as a second line of defense. The grid, which acts like a filter by absorbing some photons, is placed between the film and patient. On some simulator models, the grid is built into the cassette holder. Other models require the manual positioning of a grid in the cassette holder before exposure.

Several other factors influence image quality. The following four primary factors influence the amount of scatter radiation reaching the film: kilovoltage, irradiated material, lead shutter size, and use of a grid. If scatter radiation is to be controlled, understanding the influences of its production is important.

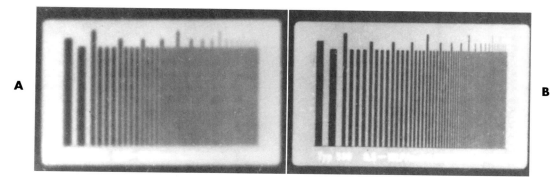

Fig. 12-30 Small field sizes are particularly important in fluoroscopy. These spot films of a test pattern embedded in the middle of 20 cm of tissue-equivalent material were taken with full-field exposure and the x-ray beam restricted to the area of the pattern: full-field exposure (**A**) and beam restricted to the area of the pattern (**B**). The radiograph in **B** is clearer because the smaller field size resulted in less scatter radiation. (From Bushong S: *Radiologic science for technologists: physics, biology, and protection,* ed 5, St Louis, 1993, Mosby.)

Kilovoltage. As x-ray energy increases, the penetrating ability of the beam increases. With extremely large patients, increasing the kVp considerably to penetrate the part being radiographed is sometimes necessary. When kVp increases, the amount of scatter radiation also increases and contrast decreases. More scatter radiation results with higher kVp because the percentage of x-rays undergoing Compton interactions also increases. For example, if the normal technical factors are not sufficient to penetrate an AP thorax, the radiation therapist can choose to increase kVp or mAs to compensate. An increase in mAs results in a higher radiation dose to the patient for that particular exposure, and a compensation in kVp increases the percentage of photons undergoing Compton interactions. Kilovoltage in the range of 60 to 90 kVp is appropriate for most examinations. Small increases in kVp of 10% to 15% or a larger increase in mAs may be all that is needed to sufficiently penetrate the anatomical part. In other situations, evidence of proper collimation on the radiograph and the use of a grid can help decrease the number of scatter photons.

Irradiated material. Large patients absorb and scatter more radiation than smaller patients. Not only does the amount of tissue irradiated influence the production of scatter, but the density of the tissue irradiated also affects the quantity of scatter. As the volume of tissue irradiated and atomic number of the material irradiated increases, the amount of scatter increases. The atomic number of the material irradiated affects the amount of scatter radiation produced because the x-ray photons have a greater chance of interacting with an electron in a material with a higher density. For example, more scatter occurs in the pelvis, which has more bone (higher atomic number), than in the thorax, which has more air (lower atomic number.) The patient's thickness and the lead shutter field size greatly influence the volume of tissue irradiated. Larger patients and larger shutter openings produce more scatter.

Shutter field size. Unlike the patient's thickness, the lead shutter (diaphragm) field size and kilovoltage are under the control of the radiation therapist. As the lead shutter field size increases, the amount of scatter radiation increases because more radiation is available to interact with the patient. To improve image quality, radiographic evidence of collimation on the film or image intensifier (fluoroscopy) of the lead shutters is important. Restricting the beam through collimation reduces the quantity of primary photons available to produce scatter radiation. The restriction of the lead shutter opening to improve image quality is critical during fluoroscopy (Fig. 12-30). When the beam size is not limited to the area under fluoroscopic examination, increased amounts of scatter reduce contrast and image quality, especially with large patient thicknesses.

Grids. A **grid** is a device placed between the patient and image receptor to absorb scatter radiation. The construction of a grid (including the materials, grid ratio, and grid type) is important to understanding the purpose of a grid. The primary purpose of a grid is to reduce scatter and improve contrast. A grid is recommended when the part thickness is greater than 10 cm.

A familiar term used in discussing the construction of a grid is *grid ratio,* which is the ratio of the height of the lead strips to the interspace material between them (Fig. 12-31). Grid ratios can range from 5:1 with an 85% scatter reduction to 16:1, which may absorb up to 97% of the scatter radiation. Thin foil lead strips are spaced between a radiolucent material such as plastic or aluminum and then bonded together in an aluminum or a carbon fiber casing.[11] The lead strips absorb stray scatter photons, and the radiolucent material allows primary photons to pass through the grid. Grid ratio affects the amount of radiation reaching the film by determining the maximum angle of the scattered photon allowed through the grid without being absorbed by the lead strips (Fig. 12-32).

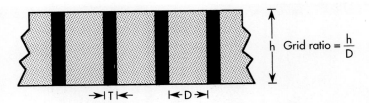

Fig. 12-31 *Grid ratio* is the ratio of the height of the lead strips to the distance between them. (From Bushong S: *Radiologic science for technologists: physics, biology, and protection,* ed 5, St Louis, 1993, Mosby.)

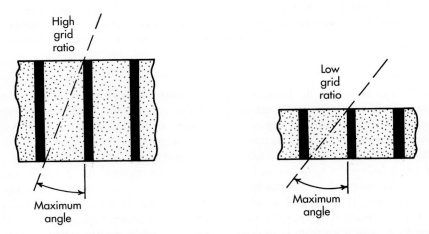

Fig. 12-32 The maximum angle of a scatter photon that can pass through a grid is a result of the height of the lead strips and their closeness.

When a grid is used for a simulation procedure, an increase in technical factors is necessary to compensate for the increased amount of absorption. An 8:1 parallel grid is commonly used in radiation therapy. A parallel grid is manufactured with the lead strips and interspace material parallel. Unlike parallel grids, focused grids have lead strips designed to coincide with the divergence of the x-ray beam. The lead strips in a focused grid extend along the same line as the divergence of the x-ray beam and are limited in use to a range of distances. The increase in technical factors necessary when using a grid is dependent on many factors such as the thickness of the patient, kVp used, grid ratio, and type of grid used.

SUMMARY

Radiographic imaging is a complex process. The application of knowledge and understanding concerning the construction of the x-ray tube, the production of x-rays, their interaction with matter, and the creation of high-quality images is fundamental for the precision and accuracy necessary in radiation therapy technology. Until conventional recording media are replaced or significantly augmented with a technology without film, the role of the radiation therapist in the art and science of radiographic imaging remains critical. X-ray film is still an important method of receiving and storing meaningful treatment-related information. Whether computer technology or conventional x-ray film is used, the goal of maximizing the radiation dose to the tumor and minimizing the dose to the surrounding normal tissue remains the same. The simulator and other diagnostic imaging equipment are essential tools in realizing this goal in radiation oncology. Correctly applying the principles and practice in radiographic imaging can only improve patient outcomes.

Review Questions

Multiple Choice

1. Which of the following additive or destructive conditions affect the radiographic image?
   - I. Hilar mass
   - II. Pnemonectomy
   - III. Edema
   - IV. Multiple myeloma
   - V. Atrophy
     - a. I, II, and III
     - b. II, III, and IV
     - c. II, IV, and V
     - d. V only
     - e. I, II, III, IV, and V

2. What is the positive side of the x-ray tube?
   - a. Filament
   - b. Anode
   - c. Cathode
   - d. Electrostatic triode

3. Which of the following are considered x-ray interactions occurring with matter?
   - I. Bremsstrahlung x-rays
   - II. Compton scattering
   - III. Photoelectric absorption
   - IV. Rectification
     - a. I and II
     - b. II and III
     - c. II, III, and IV
     - d. I, III, and IV

4. An AP radiograph of the pelvis taken at 100 mAs and 67 kVp has too much contrast but enough density. What should the new mAs be if the kVp is increased to 77?
   - a. 25 mAs
   - b. 50 mAs
   - c. 200 mAs
   - d. 400 mAs

5. Which of the following is *not* a method of reducing or controlling scatter radiation?
   - a. Using grids
   - b. Increasing kVp while reducing mAs
   - c. Using the diaphragms to collimate the beam
   - d. Decreasing kVp while increasing mAs

6. If a radiograph taken at 120 cm SFD produces an image measuring 3.5 cm on the radiograph through the use of a 90 cm SOD, what is the magnification factor?
   - a. 0.75
   - b. 1.33
   - c. 2.63
   - d. 4.66

7. *Sensitometry* is the measurement of the film's response to exposure and processing. What is used to demonstrate this response?
   - a. H & D curve
   - b. Characteristic curve
   - c. Inverse square law
   - d. Both a and b

Questions to Ponder

1 Discuss the way x-rays are used in radiation therapy. Are they different from those used in diagnostic radiology? Explain.

2 Discuss the conditions necessary for the production of x-rays.

3. Compare and contrast bremsstrahlung and characteristic target interactions.

4. Describe the two interactions in matter that have the most effect in the diagnostic imaging range.

5. How and why is scatter radiation controlled?

REFERENCES

1. Bentel CG, Nelson CE, Noell KT: *Treatment planning and dose calculation in radiation oncology,* ed 4, New York, 1989, Pergamon Press.
2. Bomford CK et al: Treatment simulators, *Br J Rad Suppl* 23:4-32, 1989.
3. Bushong SC: *Radiologic science for technologists: physics, biology, and protection,* ed 5, St Louis, 1993, Mosby.
4. Carlton RR, McKenna-Adler A: *Principles of radiographic imaging,* Albany, NY, 1992, Delmar Publishing.
5. Chow MF: The effect of a film's sensitivity to its speed, contrast, and latitude, *Can J Med Radiat Technol* 19(4):147, 1988.
6. Cullinan AM, Cullinan JE: *Producing quality radiographs,* ed 2, Philadelphia, 1994, JB Lippincott.
7. DeVos DC: *Basic principles of radiographic exposure,* Philadelphia, 1990, Lea & Febiger.
8. Fuchs AW: Relationship of tissue thickness to kilovoltage, *Radiol Technol* 19(6):287, 1948.
9. Fuchs AW: The rationale of radiographic exposure, *Radiol Technol,* 22(2):62, 1950.
10. Glasser O: *Dr W.C. Roentgen,* ed 2, Springfield, Ill, 1972, Charles C. Thomas.
11. Hufton AP et al: Low attenuation material for table tops, cassettes and grids: a review, *Radiography* 53(607):17, 1987.
12. Karzmark CJ, Nunan CS, Tanabe E: *Medical electron accelerators,* Princeton, NJ, 1993, McGraw-Hill.
13. Khan FM: *The physics of radiation therapy,* ed 2, Baltimore, 1994, Williams & Wilkins.

14. Kodera Y, Kunio D, Hwang-Ping C: Absolute speeds of screen-film systems and their absorbed-energy constants, *Radiology* 161:229-239, 1984.

15. Malott JC, Fodor J III: *The art and science of medical radiography,* ed 7, St Louis, 1993, Mosby.

16. Nation Council on Radiation Protection and Measurements: *Medical x-ray, electron beam, and gamma-ray protection of energies up to 50 MeV (equipment design performance and use),* NCRP Rep 102, Bethesda, Md, 1989, The Council.

17. Selman J: *The fundamentals of x-ray and radium physics,* ed 8, Springfield, Ill, 1994, Charles C Thomas.

18. Stears JG et al: Radiologic exchange: resolution according to focal spot size, *Radiol Technol* 60(5):429-430, 1989.

19. Taylor J: *Imaging in radiotherapy,* Kent, England, 1988, Croom Helm.

13

Linear Accelerator

Edward Aribisala
Dennis T. Leaver

Outline

Key terms

Many types of equipment, including the linear accelerator, are useful in the treatment of cancer. Various treatment machines are available to produce x-rays, electrons, and other particles such as neutrons, protons, and heavy nuclei. These machines may range in energy from 10 keV to 50 MeV.[16] In this chapter, x-ray and electron production as it relates to the linear accelerator are discussed.

The term **linear accelerator** means that charged particles travel in straight lines as they gain energy from an alternating electromagnetic field. The linear accelerator is distinguished from other types of particle accelerators such as the cyclotron, in which the particles travel in a spiral pattern, and the betatron, in which the particles travel in a circular pattern.[16]

In the linear accelerator, x-rays and electrons are generated and used to treat a variety of tumors. The accelerator structure, which resembles a length of pipe, is the basic element of the linear accelerator. The accelerator structure allows electrons produced from a hot cathode to gain energy until they exit the far end of the pipe.[16] Understanding the proper use of this equipment is significant to the radiation therapist because it is one of the essential tools enabling the radiation therapist to deliver a prescribed dose of radiation.

Aspects of the linear accelerator that are discussed in this chapter include a history of the electron accelerator, its basic design features, and a description of the major components. An explanation of the key components in a linear accelerator provides a basic overview of its operation. These components include the klystron, waveguide, circulator, water-cooling system, electron gun, accelerator structure, bending magnet, flattening filter, scattering foil, and other accessories.

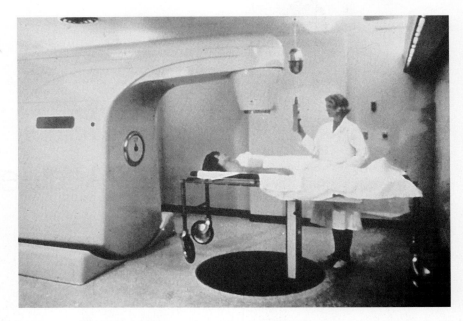

Fig. 13-1 The first 100-cm SAD fully isocentric medical linear accelerator manufactured in the United States in 1961 by Varian Associates. (Courtesy Varian Associates, Palo Alto, California.)

HISTORY

The first 100-cm source-axis-distance (SAD), fully isocentric linear accelerator was manufactured in the United States and installed in 1961 (Fig. 13-1). In many areas of the United States, the cobalt 60 unit was the most common treatment unit in the 1970s and 1980s (see Chapter 5). Over the last 2 decades, a gradual shift to the use of the linear accelerator has taken place. This is due primarily to advantages of the linear accelerator over cobalt 60. With the linear accelerator, higher energy beams can be generated with greater skin sparing, field edges are more sharply defined with less penumbra, and personnel receive less exposure to radiation leakage.

DEVELOPMENT

The development of the linear accelerator has its roots in the United States and England. In these countries, many men and women have contributed significantly to the research and development of the linear accelerator. Its development can be traced to the work of several key individuals.

In the 1930s William Hansen was a young instructor at Stanford University in Palo Alto, California. The physics department at Stanford University was conducting research in atomic physics in which the goal was to extract about 1 MeV of electron energy from a generator.

Meanwhile, David Sloan was working with his team on a new invention of his called a **cyclotron.** *Cyclo* describes the circular pathway, and *tron* refers to the place of occurrence. The cyclotron process involves heavy charged particles such as deuterons, positrons, and protons accelerating by an oscillating electric field through a circular or spiral path. A large magnet keeps these heavy particles in a pretuned pathway. At the time, this was a singularly pursued research project at Berkeley.

Microwave power

The **klystron** (Fig. 13-2) proved invaluable in the development of and is an important component in the high-energy linear accelerator. The klystron is a form of radiowave amplifier and multiplies the amount of introduced radiowaves greatly.

The British group of D.D. Fry at Telecommunication Research Establishment in Great Malvern, England, was at this time inventing the magnetron, a device similar to the klystron in its ability to generate microwave power.[11] A major difference between the klystron and magnetron is that a klystron is a linear-beam microwave amplifier requiring an external oscillator or radiofrequency (RF) source (driver), whereas the magnetron is an oscillator *and* amplifier.

Medical application

In the late 1940s the chief radiologist of Stanford's x-ray department, Dr. Henry Kaplan, became fascinated by the linear accelerator project. As a result of the medical application proposed by Ed Ginzton, Kaplan invited Dr. Ginzton to lunch in 1951 to discuss his theory. Medical application of the lin-

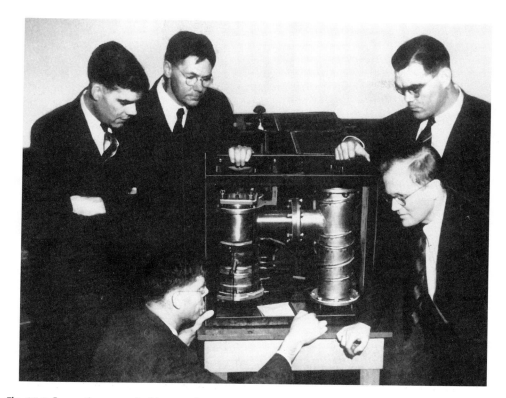

Fig. 13-2 Inspecting an early klystron that proved invaluable in high-energy linear accelerator development are (clockwise from lower left) Russel and Siguard Varian, Professor David Webster, William Hansen, and John Woodyard. (Courtesy Varian Associates, Palo Alto, California.)

ear accelerator could have a tremendous effect on the fields of radiation therapy and atomic physics. In addition, a working 1-MV linear accelerator was installed in 1948 at the Fermi Institute in Chicago. The mile-long waveguide, which ran under University Boulevard at the University of Chicago, provided photon and electron beams.[20] Work had also begun in England, but the Stanford University project proved most practical, partly because of the support of President Eisenhower in 1959 and subsequent funding by the U.S. Congress in 1961.

In 1948 the British Ministry of Health brought together the three main groups in England who were working on the linear accelerator project: the Medical Research Council (Dr. L.H. Gray et al.), the Atomic Energy Research Establishment (D.W. Fry), and the Metropolitan Vickers Electric Company (later Associate Electrical Industries) (C.W. Miller et al.). The resulting linear accelerator was installed at Hammersmith Hospital in London in June 1952. The first treatment was delivered on August 19, 1953, with an 8-MV photon beam. Another 4-MV linear accelerator was installed at Newcastle General Hospital (August 1953) and Christie Hospital in Manchester, England (October 1954). The first single gantry unit (Fig. 13-3) could be rotated over an arc of 120 degrees by lowering part of the treatment room floor.[16]

The linear accelerator was introduced in England and the United States in the 1950s. In England a 2-megawatt magnetron and 3-m stationary accelerator were used to produce an output of 100 cGy/min with the 8-MV machine.[11,16] This was a major achievement, even by today's standards. In the United States a linear accelerator was first clinically used at Stanford University Hospital in January 1956 to treat a child suffering from retinoblastoma. The patient was still disease-free 32 years later.[11]

A joint venture between the British industrial work and the Stanford University group under the direction of C.S. Nunan produced the first **ergonomic*** linear accelerator (a 6-MV, isocentric linear accelerator with the ability to rotate 360 degrees around a patient lying supine on the treatment couch).

---

*Ergonomics is the science that attempts to adapt a situation involving certain tasks or procedures to suit the worker. With a large, heavy piece of equipment such as a linear accelerator, ergonomics attempts to assist in delivering a prescribed dose of radiation therapy with the least exertion of energy by the operator and little inconvenience to the patient.

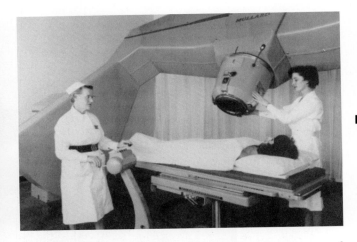

Fig. 13-3 A, The first single gantry unit installed at Christie Hospital in Manchester, England, in October 1954. It could rotate over an arc of 120 degrees by lowering part of the treatment floor. **B,** The first clinical linear accelerator manufactured by Mullard (later purchased by Philips Medical Systems) in the United Kingdom, circa 1953. (**A,** courtesy Christie Hospital, Manchester; **B,** courtesy Philips Medical Systems, Shelton, Connecticut.)

LINEAR ACCELERATOR COMPONENTS

A typical linear accelerator (Fig. 13-4) consists of a drive stand, gantry, patient-support assembly (PSA) (treatment couch), and console electronic cabinet. Some linear accelerators may also have a modulator cabinet, which contains components that distribute and monitor primary electrical power and high-voltage pulses to the magnetron or klystron. Each of the components is critical to the total function and operation of the linear accelerator.

U. S. distribution

A linear accelerator, unlike a cobalt 60 unit, produces a high-energy x-ray or electron beam to treat the cancer patient. Linear accelerators are growing in popularity in the United States. In 1994 a total of 2733 megavoltage treatment units were in the United States. This is a 17% increase since 1990. Of the 2733 treatment units, 2418 (88%) were linear accelerators or betatrons, and 315 (12%) were cobalt 60 units.[21] In 1990 the Patterns of Care group of the American College of Radiology (ACR) reported that 2336 megavoltage treatment machines were in the United States. Linear accelerators or betatrons comprised 79% of the megavoltage treatment units, and cobalt 60 units comprised 21%.[22] To serve a world population of 5 billion with the same incidence of cancer and the same average patient load per machine would in the United States in 1990 require about 20 times as many machines.[16] Table 13-1 shows the distribution of radiation therapy treatment machines in hospitals and freestanding clinics throughout the United States in 1986, 1990, and 1994.

The evolution of the linear accelerator is discussed in this section with reference to three types of linear accelerators: the early linear accelerators (1953 to 1961); second-generation, 360-degree rotational units (1962 to 1982); and new computer-driven, third-generation treatment machines.

Table 13-1	Distribution of radiation therapy treatment machines in radiation oncology facilities in the United States between 1986 and 1994		
Equipment type	**1986**	**1990**	**1994**
LINAC/betatron	1262	1847	2418
Cobalt	647	489	315
TOTAL	1909	2336	2733

Modified from Owen JB, Coia LR, Hanks GE: Recent patterns of growth in radiation therapy facilities in the United States: a pattern of care study report, *Int J Radiat Oncol Biol Phys* 24:983-986, 1993; Owen JB: Personal communication, July 1995.
LINAC, Linear accelerator.

Early accelerators

The early linear accelerators were extremely large and bulky compared with today's design features. In 1952 the first linear accelerator was installed at Hammersmith Hospital in London and had an 8-MeV x-ray beam and limited gantry motion. Several other linear accelerators with improved design features were also installed in England in the early to mid 1950s. As mentioned previously, the Stanford University linear accelerator in the United States treated its first patient in 1956. Since then, several manufacturers have designed and built linear accelerators for clinical purposes.

Second-generation accelerators

Second-generation linear accelerators can be referred to as the older *360-degree rotational units,* which are less sophisticated than their modern offspring. These isocentric units, some of which are still operational today, allow treatment to a patient from any gantry angle. They offered an improvement in accuracy and dose delivery over the extremely early

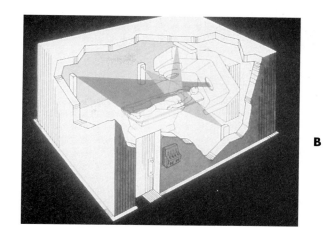

Drive stand

Gantry

A

B

Patient support assembly (treatment couch)

Fig. 13-4 **A,** The major components of a linear accelerator are a drive stand, gantry, PSA (treatment couch), control console (not shown), and modulator cabinet (also not shown). **B,** Two side lasers with an overhead laser combine to provide a patient-positioning system commonly used in radiation therapy. (**A,** courtesy Robert Morton and Medical Physics Publishing Corporation, Madison, Wis; **B,** courtesy Gammex, Inc, Middleton, Wis.)

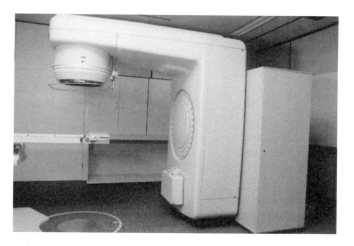

A

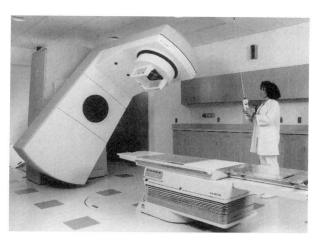

B

Fig. 13-5 Philips 75/5 linear accelerator gantry and stand (**A**). Siemans Mevatron illustrates gantry, stand, and PSA (**B**). (**A** and **B,** courtesy Philips Medical Systems, Shelton, Connecticut.)

models, primarily because of their 360-degree rotational ability around an isocenter.

If two linear-accelerator models built between 1962 and 1982 were compared, many more similarities than differences would be observed, regardless of the manufacturer. Fig. 13-5 illustrates two linear accelerators produced by different manufacturers. The similarities in design are related to their major features, such as gantry, treatment couch (PSA), and control console.

Second-generation linear accelerators are like some older cars on the road today. They may have more bumps, dents, and high mileage. They may work well at times but usually require a considerable amount of maintenance. An older car

has the same basic components as a newer one, such as an engine, transmission, and operator's panel (with fewer knobs and buttons), to accomplish the task. A third-generation linear accelerator is like the newer car of today. The newer car is equipped with many of the basic components of the older, less-sophisticated automobile but has added features such as aerodynamic design, antilock brakes, and computer-integrated components.

Third-generation accelerators

In general, third-generation accelerators have improved accelerator-guide, magnet systems, and beam-modifying systems to provide wide ranges of beam energy, dose rate,

Table 13-2	Improvements in medical linear accelerator technology from the 1950s to 1990s		
Item (accelerator guide type)	**Early** (traveling wave)	**Modern** (standing guide)	**Result** (doubled guide efficiency)
MV per meter of guide (shunt impedance, megohms/meter)	4 (13-47)	12-18 (86-112)	Shorter guide; simpler, more compact machine; and 360-degree gantry rotation
Bending magnet	Nonachromatic	Achromatic	Stable treatment
X-ray field size	Modest	Large	Full mantle at isocenter
X-ray dose rate (centigray per minute)	100-200	250-500	Short exposure, even with wedge filters
X-ray energies, MeV (number of modes)	4-6 (1)	4-24 (2)	Optimal for thin and thick sections of the patient
Electron energies	None or low	Low to high	Full useful penetration
Isodose distributions and their stability	Fair	Excellent	Protection of normal tissue and dose precision
Microwave tube life	Months	Years	Machine up-time and lower cost
Cleanliness	Oil pumps	Ion pumps and brazed guide	Freedom from arcing High-energy gradients
Electronics	Tubes and relays	Solid state modulator	Reliability and ease of service

From Karzmark CJ, Nunan CS, Tanabe E: *Medical electron accelerators*, New York, 1993, McGraw-Hill.

field size, and operating modes with improved beam characteristics. These accelerators are highly reliable and have compact design features.[16] Table 13-2 describes improvements in the technology of medical linear accelerators from the first- to third-generation treatment units.

Third-generation, computer-driven linear accelerators are available with a wide variety of options, which may include dual photon energies, multileaf collimation, a choice of several electron energies, and electronic portal verification systems. Because of the advances in three-dimensional treatment planning, some new linear accelerators provide additional features. Before some of these newer features are discussed, a basic understanding of components and design features of a linear accelerator are necessary.

DESIGN FEATURES

In the treatment room the major components of a linear accelerator can be divided into three specific areas: drive stand, gantry, and treatment couch (PSA) (Fig. 13-4, *A*). A typical treatment room is designed with thick concrete or lead walls for shielding purposes. In this space the gantry is mounted to the stand, which is secured to the floor. The treatment unit is positioned in a way that permits 360-degree rotation of the gantry. A treatment couch is mounted on a rotational axis around the isocenter. This permits the positioning of a patient lying supine or prone on the treatment couch. One ceiling and two side lasers project small dots or lines onto predetermined marks (established during the simulation process) on the patient (Fig. 13-4, *B*). Sometimes a fourth midsagittal laser is mounted opposite the drive stand, high on the wall in a way that directs a continuous line along the sagittal axis of the patient. This laser may be used to position the patient's midsagittal plane along the long axis of the

treatment couch. One or more closed-circuit television cameras may be mounted on the wall of the treatment room to enable the radiation therapist to monitor the patient during treatment.

DRIVE STAND

The gantry rotates on a horizontal axis on bearings within the **drive stand,** which is firmly secured to the floor in the treatment room. The drive stand appears as a large, rectangular cabinet, at least as large as the gantry itself. As its name indicates, the drive stand is a stand containing the apparatus that drives the linear accelerator. The drive stand is usually open on both sides with swinging doors for easy access to gauges, valves, tanks, and buttons. Four major components are housed in the stand: the klystron, waveguide, circulator, and cooling system (Fig. 13-6).

The klystron, invented by the Varian brothers in 1937, provides the source of microwave power used to accelerate electrons.[16] This microwave power is directed into the circulator and out to the **waveguide,** much like a copper wire delivers electricity to an outlet in a home. However, the waveguide is usually a hollow, tubelike structure. A **circulator** is placed between the klystron, directs the RF energy into the waveguide, and prevents any reflected microwaves from returning to the klystron. The circulator acts much like the valves found in human veins and the lymphatic system, which are designed to prevent the backflow of blood and lymphatic fluid. The water-cooling system, which is actually a thermal-stability system, allows many components in the gantry and drive stand to operate at a constant temperature. Components cooled by circulating water include the accelerator structure, klystron, circulator, target, and other important assemblies and components.

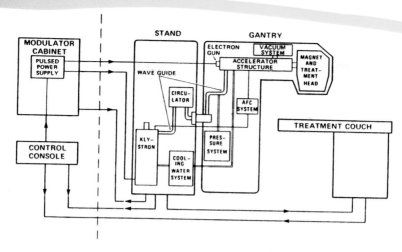

Fig. 13-6 A block diagram of a linear accelerator illustrating the major components, including the stand, gantry, PSA, modulator cabinet, and control console. (Courtesy Robert Morton and Medical Physics Publishing Corp, Madison, Wis.)

GANTRY

The **gantry** is responsible primarily for directing the photon (x-ray) or electron beam at a patient's tumor. It can accomplish this through a single-rotational or multiple-fixed fields positioned around a point called the *isocenter*. For isocentric-type treatment, this point is usually positioned in the patient's tumor. The three translations of the treatment couch (left/right, up/down, and in/out) move the patient in relationship to the isocenter, thus allowing for precise patient positioning (Fig. 13-7).

The controls to the gantry motions are located on a control pendant(s) or the dedicated keyboard outside the room at the console area. Digital readings are also displayed. Gantry angle, collimator rotation, and field size (defined by the X and Y collimators) are commonly displayed for easy reference at the throat of the gantry (Fig. 13-8).

The major components in the gantry are the electron gun, accelerator structure (guide), treatment head (Fig. 13-9), and optional beam stopper.

Electron gun

The **electron gun** is responsible for producing electrons and injecting them into the accelerator structure. Electron production in a diagnostic x-ray tube is quite similar to that in a linear accelerator.

Fig. 13-10 illustrates the design of a diode electron gun. The cathode is a spherically shaped structure made of a material with a high atomic number, such as tungsten. Tungsten is the element of choice because of the high temperatures required (between 800° and 1100° C). The anode, which carries a positive potential, is separated from the cathode to allow the focus electrode to direct the accelerated electrons through the beam hole in the anode.

Accelerator guide

The **accelerator guide,** sometimes called the *accelerator structure,* can be mounted in the gantry horizontally, as illustrated in Fig. 13-11 (high-energy machines) or vertically, as illustrated in Fig. 13-12 (low-energy machines). Microwave power (produced in the klystron) is transported to the accelerator structure, in which corrugations are used to slow up the waves (sometimes analogous to small jetties at a beach used to break up ocean waves). As a result, the crests of the microwave electric field are made approximately synchronous with the flowing bunches of electrons.[16,26] After the flowing electrons leave the accelerator structure, they are directed toward the target (for photon production) or scattering foil (for electron production) located in the treatment head. In the gantry, x-rays are produced or a treatment beam of electrons is shaped. Because x-rays are produced in the gantry of a linear accelerator, a discussion of their production is appropriate.

X-RAY PRODUCTION

X-ray production in a diagnostic tube serves as a review and provides the necessary background information for further discussion as it relates to x-ray production in a linear accelerator.

Diagnostic

A household electrical bulb has an evacuated glass bulb with a filament (a small, thin wire). When current is transported to the filament, electrical energy is converted to heat energy, thereby supplying illumination. Lack of evacuation in the bulb shortens the life span of such a filament as a result of oversaturation of electrons during the burn off.

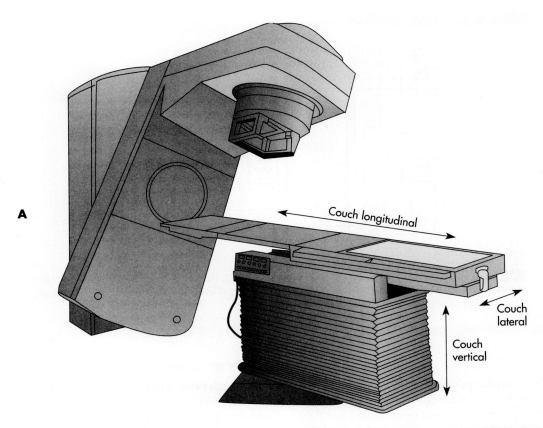

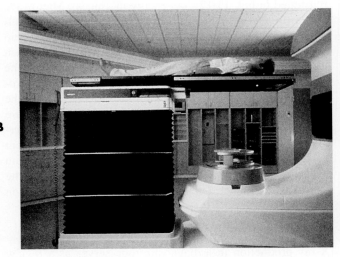

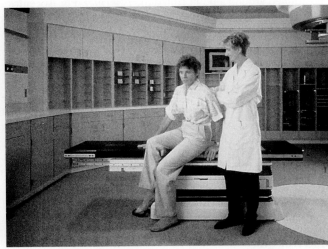

Fig. 13-7 Three translations of the treatment couch are shown: **A,** In/out, up/down, and left/right. **B,** Newer treatment couches extend higher for greater posterior treatment distances and **C,** travel lower to the floor for easy patient access. (**A,** courtesy Siemans Medical Systems, Concord, California; **B** and **C** courtesy Varian Associates, Palo Alto, California.)

In the same sense, a source of current is needed to produce x-rays. In a diagnostic x-ray tube the filament is situated at the cathode end of the tube in a focusing cup aimed at the positive terminal of the tube (anode). When applied, the current makes the filament glow (like in the light bulb) and electrons burn off. This process is called *thermionic emission* (see Chapter 12).

Tube voltage, when applied, speeds the stream of electrons toward the target at about the speed of light. The electron stream hits the target and is suddenly stopped, thus producing tremendous heat and a small amount of x-rays (about 1%). This phenomenon of x-ray production may be in the form of bremsstrahlung or characteristic radiation.

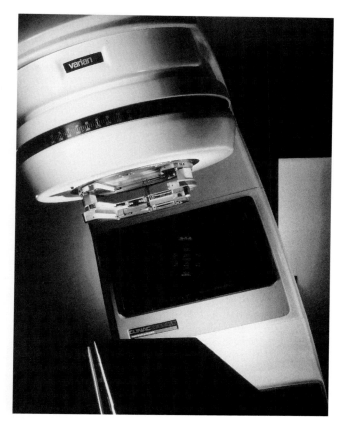

Fig. 13-8 Readout displays for collimator angle, gantry angle, and upper and lower jaws (X and Y collimator) are digitally displayed at the throat of the gantry. (Courtesy Varian Associates, Palo Alto, California.)

Linear accelerator

The production of x-rays in a linear accelerator has some similarities to x-ray production in a diagnostic tube. An illustration may be helpful in understanding x-ray production. Through the use of a battery at the cathode end to burn off electrons at its filament, a potential difference of 4 million V can be sent across the tube filtered by a thin metal window acting as the anode at the other end. The result is a stream of therapeutic electrons of 4 MeV. An anode (positive end of the tube) but no target is present in this schematic because the schematic's purpose is to produce only electrons. By adding a tungsten target to the same schematic with a constant alternating current of 4 million v of potential difference, the result is a 4-MV photon beam. X-ray production in a linear accelerator is similar.

In a linear accelerator the electron gun produces a stream of electrons, which are then injected into the accelerator structure. With the RF that is generated by the klystron, the electrons are accelerated to almost the speed of light. The stream of electrons can be used directly for electron therapy if a scattering foil is introduced or x-ray therapy if a tungsten-copper target is used.

A theoretical description on the way the electrons are brought up to speed can be described in two parts. First, the electromagnetic waves (RF) are traveling toward the exit port at the near end of the waveguide. Second, electrons surf along the electromagnetic waves. The waves push the electrons up to the desired speed. When the electrons crash into the target, the electron's mass is converted back to energy.[20]

Grid pulse. Two important factors in the acceleration of electrons toward the scattering foil or x-ray target are grid pulse and microwave power. The grid pulse is alternated with the RF pulse to maximize the acceleration of the electrons and therefore maximum beam current. The output dose rate is controlled by the variance of the grid pulse and RF pulse in a directly proportional manner. RF microwaves act as the highway of an electron, whereas the grid pulse is the driving force that pushes the electrons along to prevent gridlock on the linear accelerator highway. As it receives extremely high voltage pulses from the modulator, the klystron uses this energy to amplify the low-RF signals received from the RF driver.

The RF power pulse is also an important factor in a linear accelerator. The amplitude of the RF power pulse is maintained and tuned to a desired energy level by the waveguide and energy switch.

Microwave power. The klystron, or magnetron, has a single purpose. It is a specialized electron tube designed to provide amplified microwave for the electrons while in the accelerator structure. Microwave power, directed to the accelerator structure through the transmission waveguide, is produced in the magnetron or klystron. The magnetron is usually used for low-energy linear accelerators and the klystron for high-power accelerators. The magnetron is less expensive and lacks the stability of the klystron.

Circulator. The circulator is the link between the klystron and accelerating structure. It conveys microwave power to the accelerator structure and deflects reflected microwave power that could damage the klystron or magnetron. If any backup microwave power is not absorbed by the waterload attached to the circulator and the power escapes into the klystron or magnetron, damage can result.

Accelerator structure. From basic radiologic physics, *microwave* means "extremely small wavelengths." Because the length of waves is inversely proportional to its energy, energy is high. The microwave frequency needed for the linear accelerator is in the range of 3 million cycles per second. Amplification that occurs in the accelerator structure is in the closed-ended, precision-crafted copper cavities (Fig. 13-13). Here, the electrical power provides momentum to the low-level electron stream mixed with the microwaves. An alternating positive and negative electric charge accelerates the electrons toward the treatment head.

Velocity modulation. To increase the effectiveness of the electrons, velocity modulation is necessary. Because of the streaming of such electrons, early and late arrivals occur

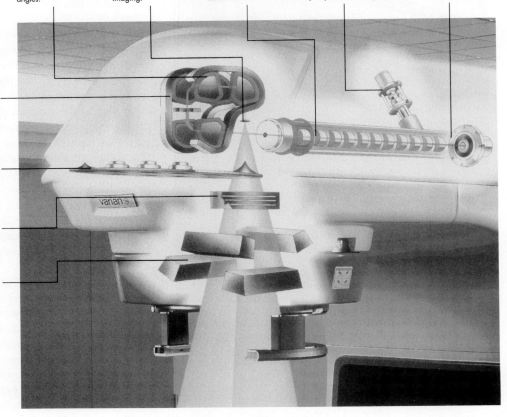

Steering System
Radial and transverse steering coils and a real-time feedback system ensure beam symmetry to within ±2% at all gantry angles.

Focal spot size
Even at maximum dose rate, the circular focal remains less than 3.0 mm, held constant by the achromatic bending magnet. Assures optimum image quality for portal imaging.

Standing Wave Accelerator Guide
Maintains optimal bunching for different acceleration conditions, providing high dose rates, stable dosimetry and low-stray radiation. Transport system minimizes power and electron source demands.

Energy Switch
Patented switch provides energies within the full therapeutic range, at consistently high, stable dose rates, even with low energy X-ray beams. Ensures optimum performance and spectral purity at both energies.

Gridded Electron Gun
Controls dose rate rapidly and accurately. Permits precise beam control for dynamic treatments since gun can be gated. Demountable, for cost-effective replacement.

Achromatic Dual-Plane Bending Magnet
Unique design with ±3% energy slits ensures exact replication of the input beam for every treatment. Clinac 2300C/D design enhancements allow wider range of beam energies.

10-Port Carousel with Scattering Foils/Flattening Filters
Extra ports allow future specialized beams to be developed. New electron scattering foils provide homogeneous electron beams at therapeutic depths.

Ion Chamber
Two independently sealed chambers, impervious to temperature and pressure changes, monitor beam dosimetry to within 2% for long-term consistency and stability.

Asymmetric Jaws
Four independent collimators provide flexible beam definition of symmetric or asymmetric fields.

Fig. 13-9 The major components of the gantry include the electron gun, accelerator guide, and treatment head, which includes components such as the bending magnet, beam-flattening filter, ion chamber, and upper-lower collimator jaws. (Courtesy Varian Associates Palo Alto, California.)

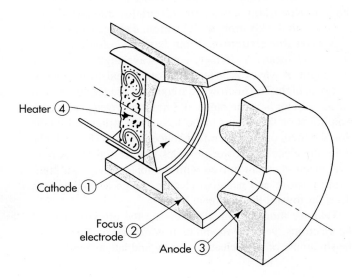

Heater ④
Cathode ①
Focus electrode ②
Anode ③

Fig. 13-10 Cross-sectional view of a diode electron gun demonstrating the cathode and anode. (From Karzmark CJ, Nunan CS, Tanabe E: *Medical electron accelerators*, New York, 1993, McGraw-Hill.)

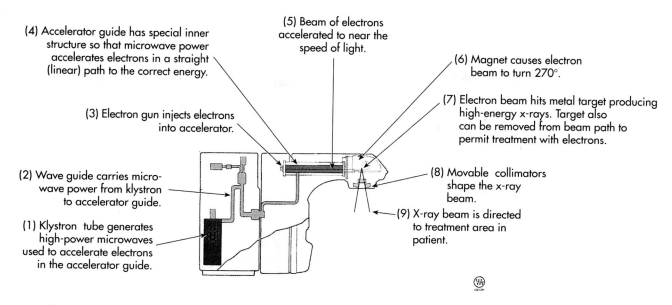

(4) Accelerator guide has special inner structure so that microwave power accelerates electrons in a straight (linear) path to the correct energy.

(5) Beam of electrons accelerated to near the speed of light.

(6) Magnet causes electron beam to turn 270°.

(7) Electron beam hits metal target producing high-energy x-rays. Target also can be removed from beam path to permit treatment with electrons.

(3) Electron gun injects electrons into accelerator.

(2) Wave guide carries micro-wave power from klystron to accelerator guide.

(1) Klystron tube generates high-power microwaves used to accelerate electrons in the accelerator guide.

(8) Movable collimators shape the x-ray beam.

(9) X-ray beam is directed to treatment area in patient.

Fig. 13-11 This high-energy radiation therapy treatment machine illustrates the horizontally mounted accelerator structure and 270-degree bending magnet. (Courtesy Varian Associates, Palo Alto, California.)

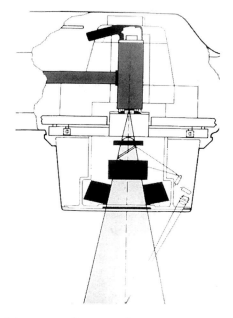

Fig. 13-12 A low-energy linear accelerator demonstrates the vertically mounted, straight-through beam design, which eliminates the need for complex beam-bending magnet systems. (Courtesy Varian Associates, Palo Alto, California.)

at crucial points of the cavity. Therefore the electrons are averaged together into an electron-cloud bunch in a process called *velocity modulation*.

This is similar to a group of students running a race. In the group a variety of running speeds is likely. Faster students who may have started later catch up with slower students by picking them up or nudging them along. In this way, all the students arrive as a team at the finish line. This means that slower students gain more speed from the nudging and faster students lose speed from helping to nudge the slower students, but the average speed is a gain for the group as a whole. A drift tube in a linear accelerator helps accomplish this task.

A drift tube acts like a synapse or link tunnel between the cavities and unit; electrons of different velocities are bunched together into more concrete electron bunches and parceled to the catcher or afferent cavity. In the catcher cavity, microwaves get highly amplified as a result of the effect of the kinetic energy of the bunched electrons. Excess electrons go to the anode or electron-beam collector end, where incidental electrons are converted to heat. Because of constant bombardment, some bremsstrahlung x-rays may result. For this reason the collector is usually lead-lined and the cold-water cooling system is used to draw the heat away from the system.

The length of the accelerator structure varies depending on the beam energy of the linear accelerator. The length may vary from 30 cm for a 4-MV unit to 1 m or more for high-energy units.[15,16] For high-energy linear accelerators, up to five cavities are sometimes used to accelerate the electron bunch enough to generate the desired microwave energy. The therapist should remember that as more cavities are used, higher energy is derived. After electrons leave the accelerator structure, they are directed toward the treatment head. The treatment head may contain various beam-shaping devices, radiation monitors, and possibly a bending magnet if a horizontal accelerator structure is used.

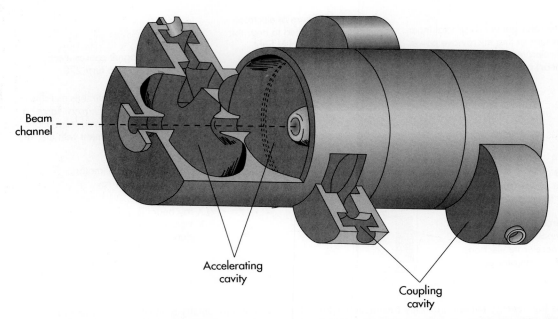

Beam channel

Accelerating cavity

Coupling cavity

Fig. 13-13 A cross-section of a standing-wave accelerator structure used in high-energy treatment units. (Courtesy Siemens Corporation, Concord, California.)

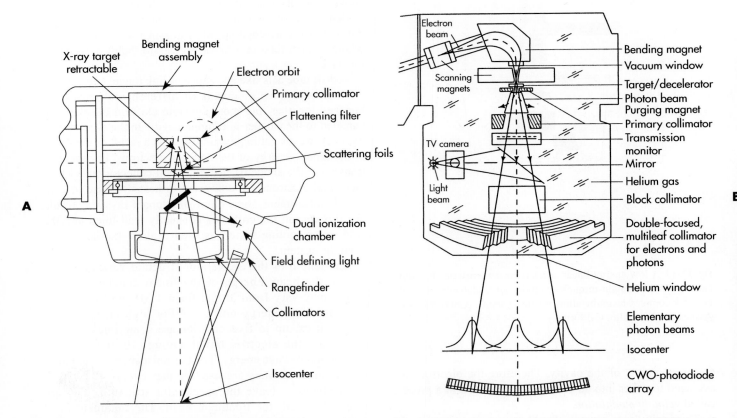

X-ray target retractable

Bending magnet assembly

Electron orbit

Primary collimator

Flattening filter

Scattering foils

Dual ionization chamber

Field defining light

Rangefinder

Collimators

Isocenter

A

Electron beam

Scanning magnets

TV camera

Light beam

Bending magnet

Vacuum window

Target/decelerator

Photon beam
Purging magnet

Primary collimator

Transmission monitor

Mirror

Helium gas

Block collimator

Double-focused, multileaf collimator for electrons and photons

Helium window

Elementary photon beams

Isocenter

CWO-photodiode array

B

Fig. 13-14 A, A cross section of the treatment head of a high-energy linear accelerator. **B,** A medical micotron. (**A,** courtesy CJ Karzmark and Varian Associates, Palo Alto, California; **B,** courtesy A Brahme and Scandinavian University Press, Stockholm.)

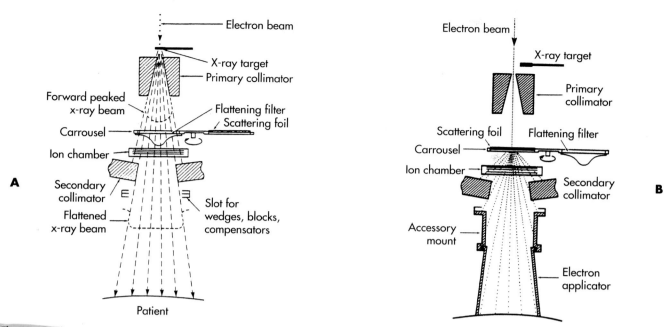

Fig. 13-15 The subsystem components with the treatment head of a high-energy linear accelerator. **A,** Note the beam subsystem is in the x-ray mode, indicated by the position of the flattening filter. **B,** The subsystem in the electron mode is indicated by the position of the scattering foil. (Courtesy Robert Morton and Medical Physics Publishing Corporation, Madison, Wis.)

TREATMENT HEAD

Several components designed to shape and monitor the treatment beam are located in the treatment head (Fig. 13-14). For x-ray therapy, these components may consist of a bending magnet, x-ray target, primary collimator, beam-flattening filter, ion chamber, secondary collimators, and one or more slots for wedges, blocks, and compensators.

The horizontal accelerator structure required for an 18-MV photon beam needs a **bending magnet** to direct the electrons vertically toward a supine patient for an anterior treatment (otherwise, the electrons would continue straight out, horizontally through the treatment head of the gantry). A magnet system may bend the electron group through a net angle of approximately 90 to 270 degrees and onto the x-ray target (or scattering foil for electron production).[16] The electrons then disappear and are transformed into x-rays. After emerging from the x-ray target, the x-rays produced are shaped by a primary collimator, which is designed to limit the maximum field size. A **beam-flattening filter** located on the carousel with the scattering foil (Fig. 13-15) shapes the x-ray beam in its cross-sectional dimension. An ion chamber monitors the beam for its symmetry in the right-left and inferior-superior direction. Secondary collimation is achieved through the manual or remote control by using the setting knobs at the collimator head or pendant to adjust the upper and lower collimator jaws. On new units, secondary collimation may also be set from the treatment console outside

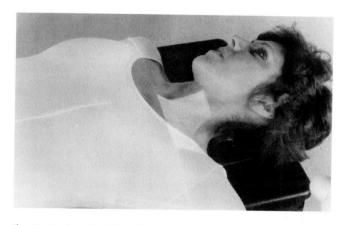

Fig. 13-16 A light field, directed from a quartz-iodine bulb in the treatment head, corresponds to the radiation field in this anterior supraclavicular field. (Courtesy Varian Associates, Palo Alto, California.)

the room. Additional beam-shaping and modifying devices such as a wedge, compensator, or custom shielding blocks can be placed in slots just below the secondary collimators.

In addition, a field light is located in the treatment head. Light from a quartz-iodine bulb outlines the dimensions of the radiation field as it appears on the patient (Fig. 13-16). This alignment of the radiation and light fields allows accurate positioning of the radiation field in relationship to skin marks or other reference points.

CONTROL CONSOLE

Because of similarities in the design features of many manufacturers, a single linear accelerator (the Varian 2300C) will be used to describe some of the additional components of a medical electron accelerator.

Monitoring and controlling of the linear accelerator occurs at the control console. Located outside the treatment room, the control console may take the form of a digital display, push-button panel or video display terminal (VDT) in which the machine status and patient-treatment information are incorporated into the computerized treatment unit.

Accelerator operational status is usually displayed at the control console. Certain states provide the operator with information regarding the accelerator's readiness to provide a treatment beam. These states include stand-by, preparatory, ready, beam-on, and complete or interlock.

Stand-by indicates that the machine is in a nap state in which the water, vacuum systems, and console electronic cabinet are still operational. From the stand-by mode the equipment can be operational in a short period. After the machine is brought out of stand-by, a delay of several minutes usually occurs before start up. The machine uses this time to self-test its circuitry. In addition, filament voltage is sent to the klystron and accelerator gun in preparation for use of the treatment beam.

Preparatory shows an operational status in which the equipment is programmable for a specific patient treatment. This may include setting the photon or electron energy monitor units, back-up timer, and other important patient parameters.

The *ready* state of the equipment allows the therapist to confirm the treatment parameters. All interlocks must be satisfied for the machine to allow the beam to be started. A lighted push-button or message on the VDT usually indicates the machine is in the ready state.

An indicator for the *beam-on* state (from a lighted push-button or message on the VDT) remains on throughout the patient's treatment until the prescribed dose is delivered.

Interlock displays can occur before or during a treatment. The interlock system is designed to protect the patient, staff members, and equipment from hazards. Patient-protection interlocks, including beam energy, beam symmetry, dose, and dose-rate monitoring, prevent radiation and mechanical hazards to the patient. For example, interlocks protect the patient against extremely high dose rates, especially if the treatment unit provides x-ray *and* electron beams. Because of the high electron-beam currents used for x-ray production, extremely high dose rates can result if the target or flattening filter do not intercept the beam. Machine interlocks protect the equipment from damage, which may include problems detected in the machine's high-voltage power supply, water-cooling system, or vacuum system.

Emergency off buttons, which can terminate irradiation and machine functions, are located on the control panel and at several other locations in the treatment room. These switches terminate all electrical power to the equipment and require a complete start-up procedure before the treatment machine can produce an electron or photon beam.

Besides displaying the operational mode of the treatment unit, the control console serves several other functions. It may provide a digital display for prescribed dose (monitor units), mechanical beam parameters such as collimator setting or gantry angle, and possibly up to 50 other status messages.[16] Overall, the treatment-control console provides a central location for controlling and operating the linear accelerator.

The control console on a Varian 2300C is usually divided into four main sections: mechanical motion keys, function keys, a cursor and numerical keypad, and beam-control sections. Mechanical motion keys allow the operator to move the gantry and collimator from the dedicated keyboard at the console area with the motion-enabling bar. The operator only needs to select the appropriate motion key, activate the enabling bar, and simultaneously depress the motion speed of *slow* or *fast* with the motion-control keys. Function keys are multipurpose keys coded to execute a logical series of commands depending on the screen window's mode of operation. In the cursor and numerical-keypad section, several functions are located. The set-up key is like an eraser in that it clears the screen and activates the opening screen, thus allowing the operator to initiate a new set of commands. *Enter* forwards commands to the computerized control system. Clear, set-up, and enter buttons and the numerical keypad with the directional keys allow numbers to be typed in cells and erased at the therapist's choice. These also make operation faster in terms of data entry into the control system or monitor screen.

TREATMENT COUCH

The **treatment couch** is sometimes referred to as the *PSA*. This is the area on which patients are positioned to receive their radiation treatment.

Several unique features of the PSA provide the tabletop with mobility. A standard feature allows the tabletop to move mechanically in a horizontal and lengthwise direction (Fig. 13-7, *A*). This movement must be smooth and accurate with the patient in the treatment position, thus allowing for precise and exact positioning of the isocenter during treatment positioning. Many tabletops support up to 140 kg (300 lbs) and range in width from 45 to 50 cm. If the couch width on the simulator is not similar to that of the treatment unit, reproducibility may become a problem, especially with large patients.

Unlike the tabletop on the simulator, patients may be positioned at either end of the treatment couch depending on the treatment plan (Fig. 13-17). At one end of the couch a rectangular or square segment of sturdy plastic or a frame with strings (similar to a tennis racket woven tightly together) can be located. After extended use, this racketlike section should be restrung to provide more patient support and reduce the amount of sag during treatment positioning. At the opposite end of the tabletop, some manufacturers have

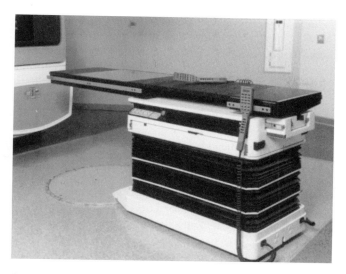

Fig. 13-17 This couchtop contains removable side-rail and center-spine sections for treating posterior and posterior oblique fields. The side-rail posterior support panel provides a 47 × 61 cm treatment window, and removable couch panels may be shifted over 30 cm to adjust to variances in patient size and tumor location. (Courtesy Varian Associates, Palo Alto, California.)

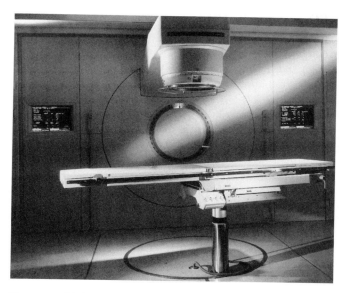

Fig. 13-18 Phillip's SL 75/5 Linear Accelerator with ram-type patient support. (Courtesy Philips Medical Systems, Shelton, Connecticut.)

developed removable inserts (two, three, or more segments located to the left or right of a sturdy metal support). Patient-positioning and support devices such as an arm board, breast board, and treatment chair may be attached at the sides or end of the tabletop.

In addition, a set of local controls may be located on the treatment couch. These can mimic those of the simulator unit as a pendant(s) (hand-held control) suspended from the ceiling or attached to the base of the treatment couch. In some models a portion of the local controls can be located on one or both sides of the treatment couch. In either situation the controls should allow access to the mechanical movements and optical features of the treatment unit.

Although PSA base support may differ, some treatment couches contain bellowlike curtain molding covering the motorized base that supports the horizontal tabletop. Other treatment couches (Fig. 13-18) may be mounted on a vertical column called a *ram*.

MODULATOR CABINET

This important component of the linear accelerator is usually located in the treatment room and is the noisiest part of the ensemble. In some systems the modulator cabinet contains three major components: the fan control, auxiliary power-distribution system, and primary power-distribution system. The fan-control switch automatically turns the fans off and on as the need arises for cooling the power distribution (auxiliary and primary) in the modulator cabinet. The auxiliary power-distribution panel contains the emergency off button that shuts off the power to the treatment unit.

In addition, located in the auxiliary power-distribution panel are fuse housings for the 360-Hz generator circuit board, contacts, and wiring in AC and DC circuits. The timer for the filament displays the amount of time since the last installation of the klystron, thyratron, and accelerator gun filament. Because these parts are made to last a long time as a result of their expensive cost, the timer monitors these components for warranty purposes.

Also on the panel is the high-voltage timer displaying the number of hours the beam is on. This is extremely useful for helping the service engineer determine the frequency the machine is in use. The timer provides information about when to schedule preventive maintenance on the machine.

The primary power-distribution panel is the third section of the modulator cabinet controls. It contains the major power route to the linear accelerator system. Several power circuit breakers are located in this section. The high-voltage power supply (HVPS) breaker is designed to protect the modulator HVPS by tripping a circuit breaker when the modulator has a current overload. Outside the room a high-volt circuit breaker (HVCB) interlock is displayed on the treatment console, and the switch on the modulator must be reset for the machine to produce a beam again. The pump breaker is designed to protect the power source to the water pump motor. With an excessive power surge to the motor, this breaker trips to avoid damage to the pump motor.

The modulator cabinet contains important components that control and regulate the linear accelerator. The fan control, auxiliary power-distribution system, and primary power-distribution system help provide this control.

APPLIED TECHNOLOGY

Computer-controlled accelerators include multimodality treatment units. Because of their increased flexibility in design and dose delivery, these accelerators have been used by more radiation treatment centers. Dual photon energies (ranging from a 6-MV low-energy x-ray beam to high-energy x-ray beams of 15 to 35 MV) provide the radiation oncologist with more options in treating a wide range of diseases. In addition, several electron energies ranging from 3 to 20 MeV are available to treat more superficial tumors. Table 13-3 categorizes linear accelerators based on energy, and Table 13-4 shows the type of beam preferred for certain tumor sites by radiation oncologists in the Philadelphia area.[16]

Multimodality treatment units offer several advantages. Because of their dual photon energies, they can provide backup for other treatment units that may experience downtime as a result of electrical, mechanical, or software problems. In addition, patients can be treated with multiple beam energies on the same treatment unit. Traditionally, a patient may have been moved to a second treatment unit for a boost or cone-down treatment.

New technologies

Numerous new technologies are allowing radiation oncologists and radiation therapists to increase radiation doses to various tumor sites. **Conformal therapy,** in which the field shape and beam angle change as the gantry moves around the patient, requires sophisticated computer-controlled equipment. Conformal therapy has certain advantages over other, more conventional forms of therapy (Fig. 13-19). If conformal therapy is not available, other new technologies

such as asymmetrical collimators, multileaf collimators (MLCs), dynamic wedge, electronic portal imaging, and linear-based stereotactic radiation therapy help increase the dose to the tumor and simultaneously spare as much normal tissue as possible.

Independent collimators, or dual asymmetrical jaws, allow increased flexibility in treatment planning. MLCs allow an increased number of treatment fields without the use of heavy cerrobend blocking. A dynamic wedge is used for computerized shaping of the treatment field (Fig. 13-20, *B*). Electronic portal imaging provides feedback on single-event set-up accuracy or observation of treatment in near realtime. Linear-based stereotactic radiation therapy may enhance dose delivery to specific tumor sites through radiosurgery.

Dual asymmetrical jaws provide a variety of options for treatment purposes. Traditionally, the upper and lower collimators, or jaws, moved symmetrically to define the width and length of a treatment field. However, for some treatments requiring abutting fields, independent motion of one or both

Table 13-3	Energy range of linear accelerators	
Energy range	**Features**	
Low	4 to 6 MV;	x-rays
Medium	8 to 12 MV;	x-rays and electrons
High	15 to 35 MV;	x-rays, electrons, and special features

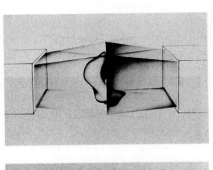
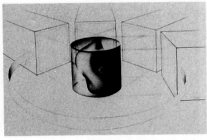
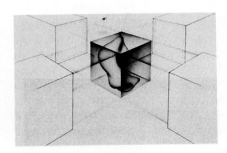
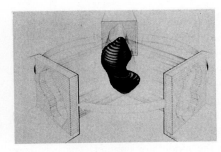

Fig. 13-19 Conformal therapy compared with conventional approaches. (Courtesy Dr. Alan Lichter, University of Michigan, Ann Arbor, Mich.)

Body area	Caseload (%)	Low X (%)	High X (%)	Electrons (%)
Table 13-4 Beam preference of radiation oncologists in the Philadelphia area for certain tumor sites				
Lung	22	35	43	13
Pelvis	20	—	—	—
Prostate	—	17	70	4
Cervix	—	4	78	4
Head and neck	7	83	0	57
Breast (intact)	7	96	0	52
Abdomen	5	—	—	—
Pancreas	—	0	87	15
Brain primary	4	74	9	9
Chest wall	3	52	0	57
Trachea and esophagus	2	78	61	0
Nodes	3	—	—	—
Bone mets	18	—	—	—
Brain CNS mets	3	—	—	—
Other	6	—	—	—
	—	71*	23*	12 (boost)* 6 (alone)*

Modified from Karzmark CJ, Nunan CS, Tanabe E: *Medical electron accelerators,* New York, 1993, McGraw-Hill.
CNS, Central nervous system.
*Beam use at two multimodality departments.

sets of jaws may be desirable. A sharp, nondivergent field edge is obtained by closing one of the jaws to the beam's central axis (Fig. 13-20, *A*) thereby shielding half the radiation field. This eliminates the need for heavy cerrobend custom blocks. Use of the independent jaw motion necessitates accurate and precise treatment positioning to avoid treatment-field overlap. This technique may be useful in the treatment of the central nervous system, breast, sarcoma, and other sites requiring abutting fields. The dosimetry, treatment planning, and specifications of these asymmetrical fields are much more complex.[18,23,24]

Multileaf collimation is designed to reduce the use of lead or cerrobend custom-made blocks (Fig. 13-21). A simulation is performed conventionally, and the simulation radiograph is sent to the radiation oncologist for blocking identification. The dosimetrist or physicist then digitizes (processes the information through a computer in numerical form) the outlined blocking into the treatment-planning computer with a software package designed to convert the digitization into pulse or motion coding for the MLC shaper. During treatment the MLC information is transferred and duplicated in the treatment room without the therapist entering the room to change blocks between treatments. The MLC replaces the need for custom blocking in many but not all situations.

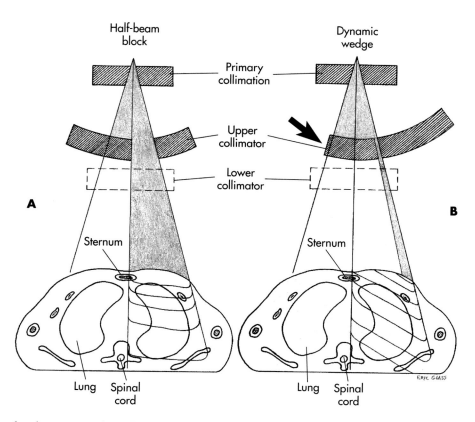

Fig. 13-20 **A,** Independent jaws create a beam in which half the field is blocked. **B,** The upper collimator moves during treatment to create a dynamic wedge effect. (Courtesy Varian Associates, Palo Alto, California.)

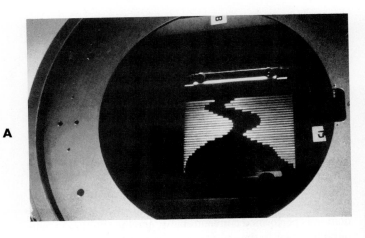
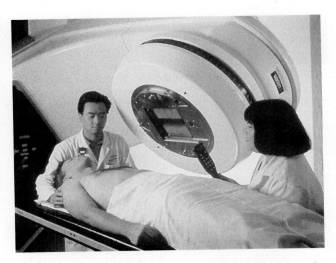

Fig. 13-21 **A,** MLC mounted on the treatment head. (Courtesy Siemans Medical Systems, Concord, California.) **B,** Initial setup of the patient with MLC. (Courtesy Varian Associates, Palo Alto, California.)

Several MLC systems exist that shield blocked area by using approximately 52 to 80 leaves. These heavy, metal collimator rods slide into place to form the desired field shape by projecting 1- to 2-cm beam widths per rod.[17] Mostly used for lung, humerus, head and neck, pelvic, and brain setups, the MLC is also available for stationary or rotational therapy. Fig. 13-22 compares several treatment fields that use multileaf collimation and custom cerrobend blocks. Fig. 13-23 compares the dose distribution for a prostate treatment field with multileaf collimation and custom cerrobend blocks. Equivalent dose distributions are achieved with both methods.

Dynamic wedges are designed in such a way that wedge-dose distributions using varying fields sizes yield excellent wedged-isodose distributions compared with physical wedges.[17] This design relies quite strongly on computer software to vary the dose rate and mechanical motion of the collimator during treatment. When the beam is turned on, the dose rate and collimator setting are automatically set according to a pregenerated treatment plan. The field size changes to generate the desired wedge angle (Fig. 13-20, *B*).

Electronic portal imaging is another of the latest methods of improving treatment-field accuracy and verification. With conventional portal systems, cassettes are positioned in the slot under the treatment couch for anteroposterior (AP) films or placed in a cassette holder for posteroanterior (PA), lateral, and oblique field positions. With this new technology, correct positioning of internal anatomical structures can be observed during the entire treatment process or checked by pretreatment imaging with the aid of computer software. Most electronic portal-imaging systems are lightweight and come with a retracted arm along the gantry's axis (Fig. 13-24). The arm is equipped with an image intensifier to improve the quality of the image. Despite the poor image quality common with regular port films (as a result of

Compton and pair-production interactions), comparable quality images are possible (Fig. 13-25).

Stereotactic radiation therapy

Linear-based **stereotactic radiation therapy** (radiosurgery) involves the aiming and delivery of a well-defined narrow beam to extremely hard-to-reach places.[1-10,12,13,19,28] Because of the relatively high doses per fraction, stereotactic radiosurgery must at the same time spare surrounding healthy tissue. Brain tumors and arteriovenous malformations (AVMs) are conditions that benefit from this technology because of their anatomical location and the tendency for complications to arise with conventional treatment. Most of the time necessary to complete a stereotactic treatment is spent in preparation, whereas the actual treatment time is comparatively small. The procedure is usually noninvasive, other than the impingement of the halo into the skull (small burr holes are drilled into the skull in several locations to secure the halo device). The halo device is used in immobilization and aids in treatment positioning. A finely collimated field is precisely aimed at the tumor volume. Here, a high dose of radiation is quickly delivered in a wide arc, thus ensuring an even dose distribution to the tumor volume (Fig. 13-26).

Computer-driven technology may provide more precise and accurate treatment in the future as more hospitals and clinics use these new technologies. As the technology becomes more available and costs are reduced, more patients will benefit from their use.

The sophisticated computer-driven linear accelerator can provide the patient with the benefits of these new technologies. Some of the equipment is expensive. Dual asymmetrical jaws act as beam splitters, thus eliminating the use of heavy custom-shaped blocking in some situations. The asymmetrical jaws and dynamic-wedge software costs approximately $200,000. MLCs that allow increased num-

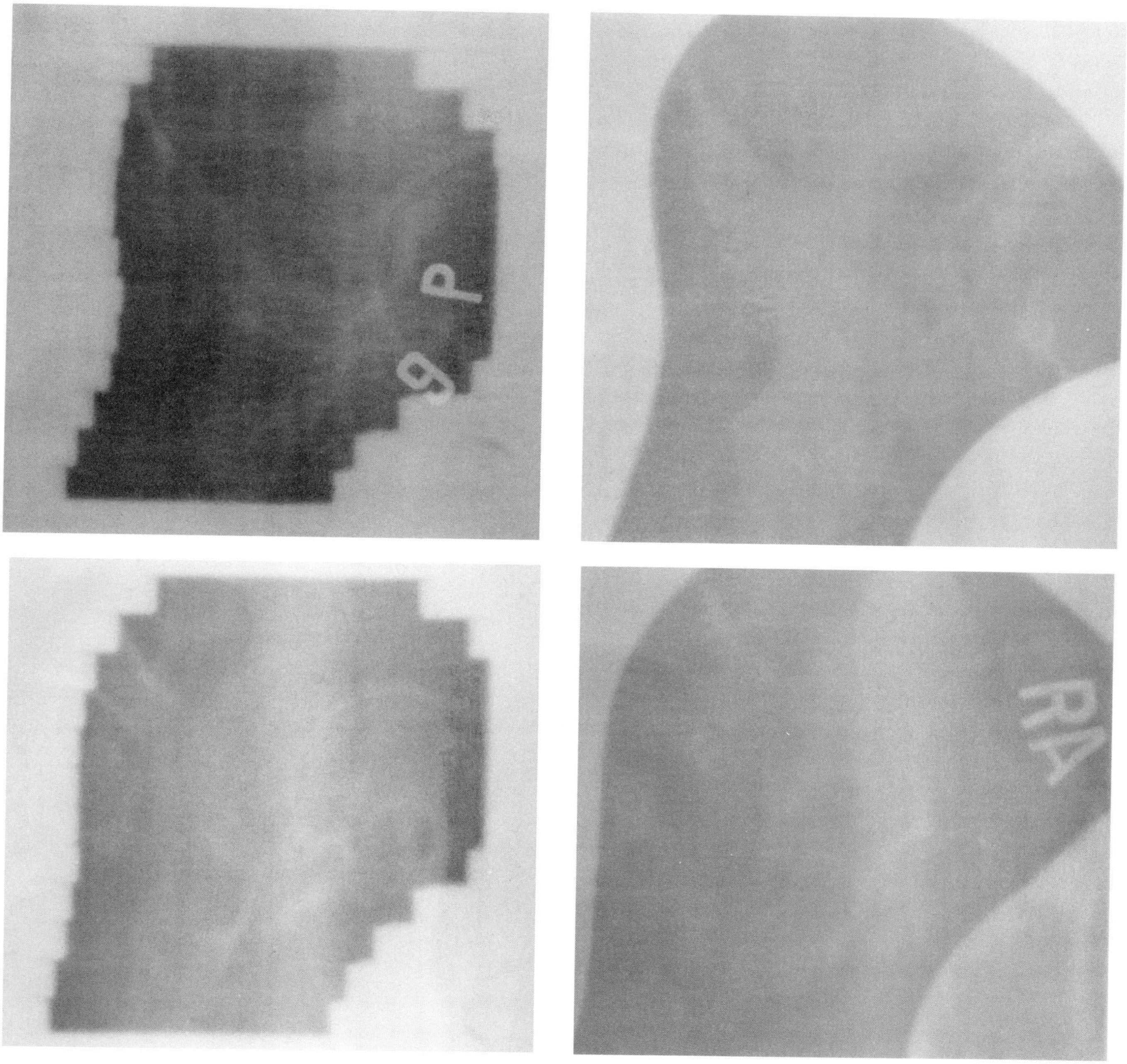

Fig. 13-22 Comparison of several treatment fields using MLC and custom cerrobend blocks (CCB). Note the smooth borders with the custom blocking versus the scalloped edges with MLC. **A,** Right posterior oblique using MLC; **B,** Right posterior oblique using CCB; **C,** Right anterior oblique using MLC; **D,** Right anterior oblique using CCB.

Continued on page 208.

bers of treatment fields and at the same time reduce custom blocking, may cost about $350,000 and can be retrofitted on some accelerator models. Clinical evidence demonstrates that increased cure rates result from increased tumor doses above 7000 cGy in prostate cancer.[27] With the help of MLC and electronic portal imaging, multiple fields and increased doses are achievable. In addition, sophisticated computer software allows the precise and accurate administration of stereotactic radiosurgery.

With the addition of computer-generated technology comes the added responsibility for quality assurance and safety. Equipment failure in linear-accelerator treatment units can result in serious radiation accidents, including overexposure.

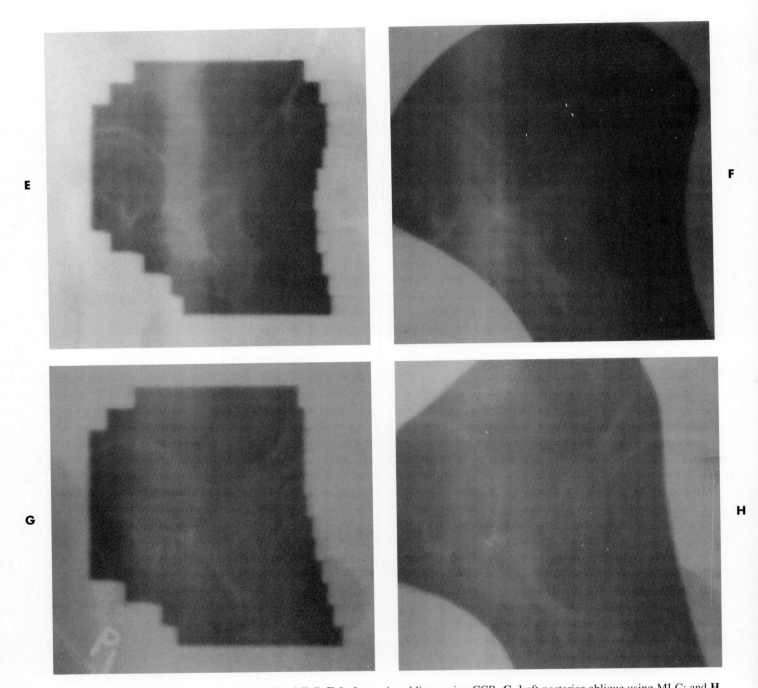

Fig. 13-22, cont'd.   **E,** Left anterior oblique using MLC; **F,** Left anterior oblique using CCB; **G,** Left posterior oblique using MLC; and **H,** Left posterior oblique using CCB. (Courtesy Varian Associates, Palo Alto, California.)

MEDICAL ACCELERATOR SAFETY CONSIDERATIONS

With the increased use of multimodality treatment units, potential hazards exist that usually are not present in single-modality treatment units.[14,25] Monitoring and controlling safe operating conditions for a computer-driven linear accelerator is more difficult than for the more conventional, electromechanical type.

Emergency procedures

Emergency procedures, if implemented properly, can prevent a serious accident and possibly save a patient's life. Written emergency procedures should be located at or near the treatment-control console. (Some state regulatory agencies require this.) Radiation therapists should be familiar with written procedures in the event of a patient emergency. Knowing the location of emergency stop buttons (inside and outside the

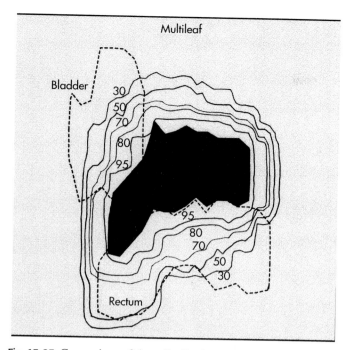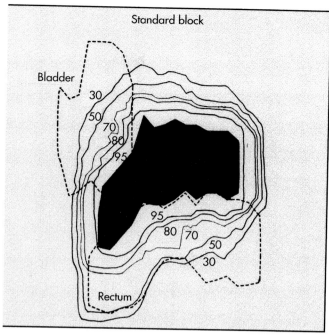

Fig. 13-23 Comparison of dose distributions for lateral prostate treatment fields using MLC and dose distribution for lateral prostate fields using CCB. The isodose distributions are extremely similar. (Courtesy Varian Associates, Palo Alto, California.)

treatment room) is critical in the event of a machine malfunction. Other emergencies involving the patient's medical condition may also require the therapist's attention.

Safety considerations

Electrical, mechanical, and radiation-safety considerations must be more elaborate with multimodality treatment units because of the accelerator's increased flexibility. An example may better portray the need for more elaborate safety considerations.

The failure of some software can allow the delivery of large doses. For example, if a large electron-beam current intended for x-ray production is used for an electron treatment, an extremely large dose rate can result. If the scattering foil is in place or the beam scanning operational, an estimated dose comparable to a typical 2-Gy dose fraction can be delivered to a patient in about 0.03 second at 4000 Gy/min. This dose rate can create hazards for the patient. To address this type of problem, digital logic and microprocessors have been incorporated into the linear accelerator control and monitor functions.[25]

Potentially dangerous problems can result from misadministration of a prescribed radiation dose. A **misadministration** (incorrect application or delivery of a prescribed dose of radiation therapy) can be minor or major and may cause death or serious injury to the patient depending on the extent of the dose. The Food and Drug Administration defines an accident that can cause death or serious injury as a class I hazard. If the risk of serious injury is low, due to human error or a linear accelerator malfunction, the accident is classified as a class II hazard.[25]

The American Association of Physicists in Medicine (AAPM) Radiation Therapy Committee Task Group Number 35 has developed a list containing most of the causes of potentially life-threatening problems associated with electrical, mechanical, human, and software errors involving medical linear accelerators[25] (Table 13-5).

Computer-operated linear accelerators provide more options for the radiation oncologist in treating benign and malignant disease. For example, electron arc therapy, x-ray arc therapy, and high-dose-rate total-skin electron therapy are available on some units.[25] However, with the increased flexibility comes an added responsibility to ensure safe and proper operation of this equipment.

Linear accelerators continue to gain in popularity throughout the United States. Some authors estimate that in the industrialized world, over 75% of the treatment machines are linear accelerators.[16]

A comprehensive understanding of and familiarization with the design, characteristics, performance parameters, and control of the linear accelerator is essential for many of the members of the cancer-management team. In addition, the mechanical, electrical, software, and radiation-safety considerations are critical to applying the theory and operation of a linear accelerator to patients needing treatment.

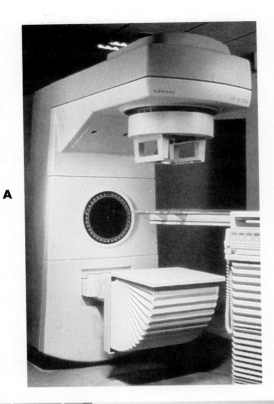

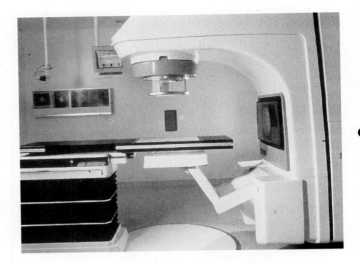

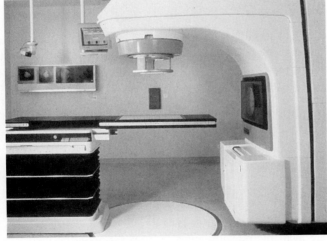

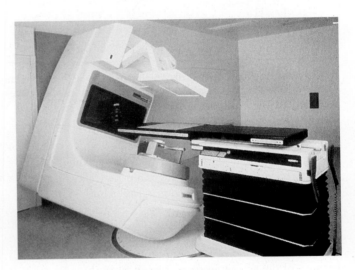

Fig. 13-24 **A,** A fully retractable and collapsible gantry-mounted detector used in an electronic portal-imaging system. **B** to **D,** A retractable arm at various positions provides unrestricted room for patient positioning with an electronic portal-imaging system. (**A,** courtesy Siemens Medical Systems, Concord, California; **B** to **D** courtesy Varian Associates, Palo Alto, California.)

Table 13-5 Medical accelerator hazards

Type	Cause	Consequences
Incorrect dose delivered	Electrical, software, and therapist	Serious injury, increased complications, genetic effects, second primary, and compromised tumor control
Dose delivered to the wrong area	Mechanical, software, patient motion, and therapist	Serious injury, increased complications, genetic effects, second primary, and compromised tumor control
Machine collision	Mechanical, software, patient motion, and therapist	Significant injury and death
Incorrect beam	Electrical, software, and therapist	Serious injury, increased complications, genetic effects, secondary primary, and compromised tumor control
General hazards	Electrical and mechanical	Significant injury and death

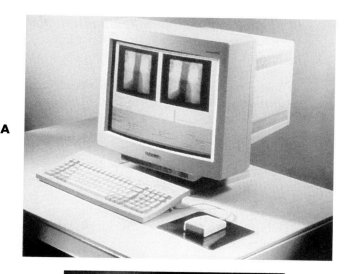

A

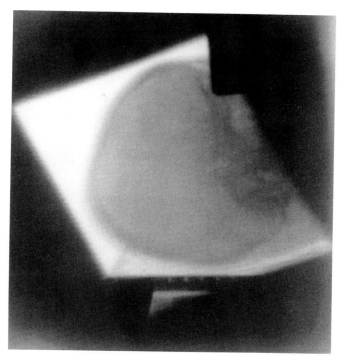

B

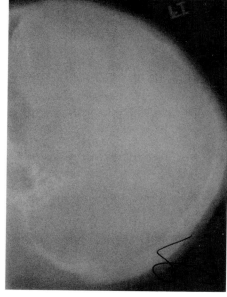

C

Fig. 13-25 **A,** A monitor from Siemans Beamview Plus portal-imaging system demonstrates two processed images. **B,** A processed whole brain portal image from Siemans Beamview Plus portal-imaging system. **C,** A posttreatment whole brain port film taken with three to five monitor units on a 6-MV linear accelerator. (**A** and **B,** courtesy Siemans Medical System, Concord, California.)

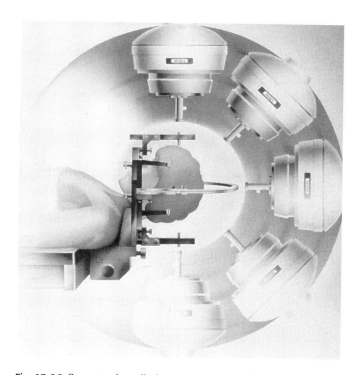

Fig. 13-26 Stereotactic radiation treatment to an intracranial tumor from several angles. (Courtesy Varian Associates, Palo Alto, California.)

Review Questions

Multiple Choice

1 When were linear accelerators first commercially available for clinical use?
a. 1895
b. 1930s
c. 1950s
d. 1970s

2. A scattering foil is placed in the path of the beam when which of the following are used for treatment purposes?
a. Protons
b. Electrons
c. X-rays
d. All of the above

3. A target is placed in the path of the beam when which of the following are used for treatment purposes?
a. Protons
b. Electrons
c. X-rays
d. All of the above

4. How do linear accelerators generate high-energy treatment beams?
a. By accelerating charged particles in a circular path
b. By accelerating charged particles in a linear path
c. By producing electromagnetic pulses used to influence protons and neutrons
d. By inhibiting photons from gaining too much energy

5. What does a klystron or magnetron produce?
a. Microwave power
b. Alternating current
c. Accelerated electrons and photons
d. Magnetic fields used to bend the beam

6. Trace the path of an electron in a linear accelerator by selecting the best route from the following:
I.   Electron gun
II. Collimator
III. Accelerator guide
IV. Bending magnet
a. I, II, III, IV
b I, III, IV, II
c. II, I, IV, II
d. III, I, II, IV

Questions To Ponder

1. Briefly describe the history of the linear accelerator, including the klystron.
2. Discuss the integration of computerization and linear accelerator operation. What are the benefits and drawbacks?
3. Analyze the need, design, and operation of a linear accelerator cooling system.
4. What is ergonomy? Can you give some examples of other ergonomically designed tools in your department? What is the benefit of ergonomic designs?
5. Is there any difference between a magnetron and klystron? When is a magnetron rather than a klystron used in a linear accelerator?

6. Discuss the major components of the linear accelerator, including the klystron, waveguide, circulator, electron gun, accelerator guide, and bending magnet.
7. Describe the difference between a beam-flattening filter and a scattering foil.
8. List and describe four hazards associated with the use of a medical linear accelerator.
9. What are the advantages and disadvantages of dual asymmetrical jaws, MLCs, and electronic portal imaging?
10. What is the purpose of a circulator?

REFERENCES

1. Betti O: Personal communication, 1988.
2. Betti O: Treatment of arteriovenous malformations with the linear accelerator, *Appl Neurophysiol* 50:262, 1987.
3. Betti O, Derechinsky V: Hyperselective encephalic irradiation with linear accelerator, *Radiother Oncol* 33:385-390, 1984.
4. Bomford CK, Walton L: The physics of stereotactic radiosurgery. *Fifth Varian European Clinac Users Meeting* 1(1):183-187, 1987.
5. Cierego G, Marchetti M, Avanzo RC: Dosimetric considerations on multiple arc stereotaxic radiotherapy, *Radiother Oncol* 12(2):141-152, June 1988.
6. Colombo F, Benedetti A, Pozza F: Radiosurgery using a 4 MV linear accelerator, *Acta Radiol Suppl* 369:603-607, 1986.
7. Colombo F et al: External stereotactic irradiation by linear accelerator, *Neurosurgery* 16(2):154-160, 1985.
8. Colombo F et al: Linear accelerator radiosurgery of arteriovenous malformations, *Appl Neurophysiol* 50(1-6):257-261, 1987.
9. Colombo F et al: Linear accelerator radiosurgery: clinical experience over five years, *Riv Neuroradiologia* 1(1):17-35, 1988.
10. Colombo F et al: Stereotactic radiosurgery utilizing a linear accelerator, *Appl Neurophysiol* 48(1-6):133-145, 1985.
11. Gington E: An informal history of the microwave electron accelerator for radiotherapy. *Proceedings Tenth Varian Users Meetings* 1(1):11-19, 1984.
12. Heifetz MD, Wexler M, Thompson R: Single-beam radiotherapy knife: a practical theoretical model, *J Neurosurg* 60(4):814-818, 1984.
13. Houdek PV et al: Stereotaxic radiotherapy technique for small intracranial lesions, *Med Phys* 12(4):469-472, 1985.
14. Karzmark CJ: Procedural and operator error aspects of radiation accidents in radiotherapy, *Int J Radiat Oncol Biol Phys* 13:1594-1602, 1987.
15. Karzmark CJ, Morton RJ: *A primer on theory and operation of linear accelerators in radiation therapy*, Madison, Wis, Medical Physics Publishing Corporation (originally published in 1981 by the Bureau of Radiologic Health).
16. Karzmark CJ, Nunan CS, Tanabe E: *Medical electron accelerators*, New York, 1993, McGraw-Hill.
17. Klein E: Higher doses, greater precision, *RT Image* 7(39):4-5, 1994.
18. Klemp PFB et al: Commissioning of a linear accelerator with independent jaws: computerized data collection and transfer to a planning computer, *Phys Med Biol* 33:865-871, 1988.
19. Lutz W, Winston KR, Maleki N: A system for stereotactic radiosurgery with a linear accelerator, *Int J Radiat Oncol Biol Phys* 14(2):373-381, 1988.
20. Miller RA: Personal communication, January, 1995.
21. Owen JB: Personal communication, March, 1995.
22. Owen JB, Coia LR, Hanks GE: Recent patterns of growth in radiation therapy facilities in the United States: a patterns of care study report, *Int J Radiat Oncl Biol Phys* 24:983-986, 1993.
23. Palta JR et al: Characteristics of photon beams from Philips SL 25 linear accelerators, *Med Phys* 17:106-116, 1990.
24. Palta JR et al: Electron beam characteristics of a Philips SL 25, *Med Phys* 17:27-34, 1990.
25. Purdy JA et al: Medical accelerator safety considerations: report of AAPM Radiation Therapy Committee Task Group no. 35, *Med Phys* 20:1261-1275, 1993.
26. Rajan G: *Advanced medical radiation dosimetry*, New Delhi, India, 1992, Pentice-Hall of India Private Limited.
27. Sandler HM, McShan DL, Lichter AS: Potential improvement in the results of irradiation for prostate carcinoma using improved dose distribution, *Int J Radi Oncol Biol Phy* 22(2):361-367, 1992.
28. Smith V, Schell MC, Larson DA: *The role of tertiary collimation for linac-based radiosurgery.* American Association of Physicists in Medicine Annual Meeting, Memphis, Tenn, 1989.

Cobalt Unit

Linda S. Wingfield
Dennis T. Leaver

Outline

Key terms

PERSPECTIVE
Background

Currently, 315 cobalt 60 (^{60}Co) units are used for the treatment of cancer in the United States. This is a decrease of approximately 48% from the 1980s, when ^{60}Co units were the mainstay of most radiation oncology departments.[9] The decrease began in 1960s with the introduction of the linear accelerator. Linear accelerators provided better isodose distribution (greater dose to the tumor and less dose to normal tissue), faster dose rate, and more manageable radiation protection concerns. Despite the decline in popularity of ^{60}Co units in the United States, they are the backbone of many radiation therapy departments in developing countries. This is probably due to the units' cost, simper design, and reliability.[13]

In the early 1950s, ^{60}Co units became popular because they could deliver a significant dose of radiation below the skin surface. Compared with earlier teletherapy (treatment at some distance) units such as radium and cesium treatment machines, ^{60}Co units were faster at delivering the dose and more cost effective at producing and using the isotope. At the time, mining the ore necessary to produce a small amount of radium was extremely expensive. The ^{60}Co units were the first practical radiation therapy treatment units to provide a significant dose below the skin surface and simultaneously spare the skin the harsh effects of earlier methods. This allowed the radiation oncologist and radiation therapist to deliver larger doses of radiation to greater depths in tissue. When a greater percentage of dose occurs below the skin surface, the term **dose maximum (D_{max})** is used to describe the process. D_{max} is the depth of maximum buildup, in which 100% of the dose is deposited. For ^{60}Co, D_{max} occurs at 0.5 cm below the skin surface. This was a tremendous advantage over the other types of equipment (especially orthovoltage) used to treat cancer at the time.

This chapter includes a discussion of the historic development of the ^{60}Co treatment unit, an examination of the design of the machine, and a comparison of some of the characteristics of the isotope. More specifically, some of the properties of the source (including its capsular design, half-life, **penumbra,** and beam quality) are discussed. An introduction to radiation-safety procedures involved with the safe application of ^{60}Co provides the radiation therapist with an overview of its importance in accurately delivering a prescribed course of radiation therapy.

Description of early equipment

Unlike other types of equipment available in the early days of radiation therapy, ^{60}Co units were mechanically simple, compact, and reliable, usually requiring little maintenance.[13] Early radiation therapy equipment, such as the betatron or Van de Graaff generator, required a lot of space. In addition, most equipment (including some cobalt units) were stationary or wall mounted (Fig. 14-1). For this reason, much of the early equipment was limited to a vertical beam direction. This meant the patient had to be positioned relative to the stationary equipment. Treatment with lateral beams (as in the case of head and neck cancer) was compromised somewhat because patients had to be placed on their sides and moved between the treatment fields.

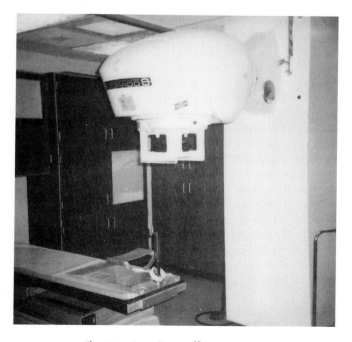

Fig. 14-1 A stationary ^{60}Co machine.

To compensate for this shortcoming, some manufacturers designed stationary *and* rotational treatment models. With rotational units the source moved around the patient, thus improving positioning reproducibility and isodose distribution. These units rotated around an axis at a constant distance from the source, called the *isocenter.* Today, this type of unit is installed with wall and ceiling lasers that are designed to aid in accurately positioning a patient. The laser lights produce thin beams of light that intersect at the axis of rotation or isocenter and correspond to external patient marks. Linear accelerators operate on the same principle by using a rotational gantry in order to deliver multiple treatment fields from various angles (all aimed at the same target volume.)

To protect personnel, the ^{60}Co source must be shielded when the source is in the off position. Compared with linear accelerators and other electrically operated therapy equipment, these machines constantly emit radiation. A great deal of high-density material, such as lead or depleted uranium, surrounds the source in the head of the machine (Fig. 14-2). To help the machine rotate smoothly and provide additional shielding, it must have a counterweight. In part, this is to balance the lead shielding in the head of the machine housing the radioactive ^{60}Co source. This counterweight, extending from the opposite end of the gantry in which the source is housed, is called a *beam stopper.* With the addition of a beam stopper, walls and ceilings in the treatment room do not require as much shielding. The beam stopper absorbs a significant amount of the radiation transmitted through the patient. Although it provides additional shielding and acts as a counterweight, the beam stopper has a number of drawbacks, including the difficulty associated with working around this cumbersome extension. The large beam stopper limits movement around the head of the gantry and can be a challenge at positioning a stretcher next to the treatment couch with the machine in the lateral position.

Application

Before the widespread distribution of linear accelerators, ^{60}Co units delivered radiation therapy treatments to all types of tumors. Because of its unique beam characteristics, the ^{60}Co unit is commonly used today to treat cancers of the head and neck area, breast, spine, and extremities. In addition, areas just below the skin surface (where a deep penetration of the beam is not necessary) can be effectively treated with ^{60}Co.

Anatomically, the head and neck area is not extremely thick. Therefore a ^{60}Co beam can provide an adequate distribution of dose by using parallel opposed fields (two fields treated 180 degrees from one another). The ^{60}Co beam is ideal in treating lymph nodes, which are superficially located in the cervical and subdigastric area. In addition, lymph nodes located in the axillary and supraclavicular areas, which may be involved with breast cancer, lie just below the skin

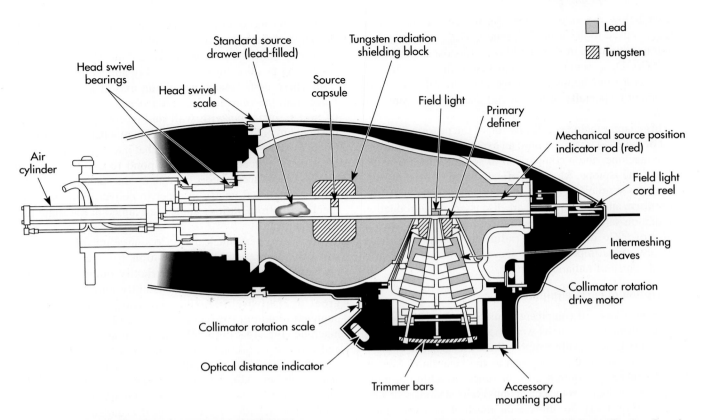

Fig. 14-2 A cross section of typical ^{60}Co components. (Courtesy Atomic Energy of Canada Limited, Medical Products, Kanata, Ontario, Canada.)

surface and may require treatment only with a single portal field. Bone metastases from other primary sites commonly occur in the spine and extremities, thus making ^{60}Co a good choice for treatment in which a single portal field may be used. Some radiation therapy departments with several treatment units find the ^{60}Co unit provides a good balance to the treatment of a wide variety of diseases.

PRODUCTION
Change of atomic number

^{60}Co is an artificially produced isotope. Like many other isotopes used in the diagnosis and treatment of disease, ^{60}Co becomes radioactive when its atomic number is altered. This may happen in a particle accelerator called a *cyclotron* or *nuclear reactor*. The production of ^{60}Co begins with the stable form of cobalt, which has an atomic-mass number of 59. The atomic-mass number is the sum of protons and neutrons in the nucleus. After ^{59}Co is bombarded or irradiated in a nuclear reactor with slow neutrons, the nucleus of ^{59}Co absorbs one neutron and becomes radioactive ^{60}Co. This can be expressed in the following formula:

$$^{59}\text{Co} + ^{1}\text{n} \cong {}^{60}\text{Co}$$

As in any radioactive substance, ^{60}Co emits radiation in an effort to return to its more stable state.

Volume and size

^{60}Co activity may be expressed in **curies (Ci)**, the historical unit of radioactivity, which equals 3.7×10^{10} Bq.[10] **Becquerel (Bq)**, the Standard International (SI) unit of radioactivity equals 1 disintegration per second.[2] Most sources have an activity of 750 to 9000 Ci and may be referred to as *kilocurie sources*.[11] In addition, the activity may be defined in Rhm units (1 rhm unit represents 1 roentgen per hour at 1 m). The quality of the radiation produced by the source does not depend on the number of curies or rhms. With a 3000-Ci source the equipment can be operated at an 80-cm distance and have a 10-cm depth dose of 56%.[3,5,7] Sources used in radiation therapy typically range from 3000 to 9000 Ci and have a specific activity of 75 to 200 Ci/g.

Specific activity is the number of transformations per second for each gram of radionuclide decaying at a fixed rate. *Specific activity* is the number of Ci per gram. The specific activity for a ^{60}Co source can be as high as 400 Ci/g, but for radiation therapy treatment, it is usually 200 Ci/g. A smaller source at the standard 80 source-skin distance (SSD) produces a beam of lower intensity requiring longer treatment time.

Capsule

The radioactive ^{60}Co source and its shielding (in the form of a protective casing) is referred to as the *cobalt capsule*. The

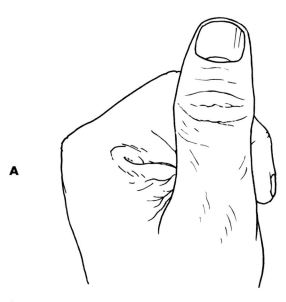

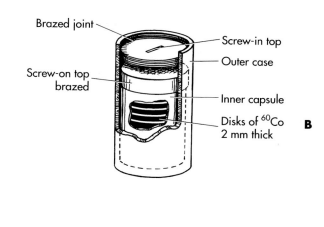

Fig. 14-3 A, The radioactive ^{60}Co source or capsule can be compared in size to the end of a person's thumb. **B,** A double encapsulated teletherapy ^{60}Co source. (From Meredith WJ, Massey JB: *Fundamental physics of radiology,* Chicago, 1977, Year Book Medical Publishing.)

diameter of the capsule can range from 1 to 3 cm (Fig. 14-3). For radiation therapy purposes, 1.0 to 2.0 cm is preferred. The radioactive cobalt source contains disks, slugs, or pellets grouped in a cluster or solid cylinder, encased in a stainless steel capsule, and sealed by welding. The capsule is placed inside a second steel capsule that is also welded. The multiple layers of metal prevent leakage of the radioactive material and absorb the beta particles produced during the decay process.[7]

CHARACTERISTICS
Gamma ray

The radioactive ^{60}Co nucleus emits ionizing radiation in the form of high-energy gamma rays. ^{60}Co decays by first emitting a beta particle with an energy of 0.31 MeV that is absorbed in the source's steel capsule. After emitting the beta particle, the nucleus enters an excited state of nickel 60. The nickel 60 decays to a ground state by emitting two gamma rays per disintegration. Of the two gamma rays emitted, one has an energy of 1.17 MeV and the other 1.33 MeV.[11] The beam can be considered polyenergetic or heterogeneous because more than one energy is decaying from the isotope. For practical purposes the two energies are averaged to give an effective energy of 1.25 MeV.

Half-life

Because ^{60}Co is a radioactive isotope, it has a **half-life ($T_{1/2}$)**, the time necessary for a radioactive material to decay to half or 50% of its original activity. ^{60}Co decays to 50% of its activity after a half-life of 5.26 years.[7] To compensate for the reduction in beam output each month, a correction factor of approximately 1% per month must be applied to the output.

The correction factor increases the treatment time necessary to deliver the appropriate dose. To maintain adequate output for patient treatment and thus eliminate longer treatment times, the ^{60}Co source should be replaced at least every 5.3 years. Replacing the ^{60}Co source can be an extremely expensive procedure, costing approximately $25,000. This financial disadvantage may be offset by the low operating maintenance of the machine.

Dose maximum

D_{max} occurs when the energy of electrons in motion equals the energy of the electron coming to rest. This process occurs mainly with high-energy radiation beams because much of the scatter radiation produced during beam interaction with tissue is in the forward direction. In low-energy beams such as superficial and orthovoltage, the scatter is backward or to the side.

Electron equilibrium is another term used to describe D_{max}. As energy increases, so does the depth of electron equilibrium. For ^{60}Co, this point occurs at 0.5 cm below the skin surface. Table 14-1 describes the depth of D_{max} for a variety of beams.

Penumbra

Penumbra is the area at the edge of the radiation beam at which the dose rate changes rapidly as a function of distance from the beam axis.[4,7] Penumbra describes the edge of the field having full radiation intensity for the beam, compared with the area at which the intensity falls to 0.[14] Compared with the sharper field edge produced with linear accelerators, penumbra is a definite disadvantage in using ^{60}Co beams for radiation therapy treatments. Fig. 14-4 demonstrates the dif-

Table 14-1	Depth of maximum dose for various photon energies	
Beam Energy	**D_{max} (cm below skin surface)**	
Superficial	0.0	
Orthovoltage	0.0	
Cesium 137	0.1	
Radium 226	0.1	
Cobalt 60	0.5	
4 MV	1.0	
6 MV	1.5	
10 MV	2.5	
15 MV	3.0	
20 MV	3.5	
25 MV	5.0	

From Stanton R, Stinson D, Shahabi S, editors: *An introduction to radiation oncology physics,* 1992, Madison, Wis, Medical Physics Publishing.

ference between a ^{60}Co beam and a 6-MV linear accelerator beam. The sharp edge of the linear accelerator beam compared with the fuzzy edge of the cobalt beam should be noted.

The radioactive-source size contributes greatly to the degree of penumbra. The larger the source size, the larger the penumbra. The following formula is used to determine the penumbra (P equals the penumbra size, S equals the source size, SSD equals the source-to-skin distance, and SDD equals the source-to-diaphragm [collimator] distance):

$$P = S \times \frac{(SSD - SDD)}{SDD}$$

Penumbra can be applied in two ways. The first is geometric penumbra. This is the place where a lack of sharpness or fuzzy area occurs at the edge of the beam. The geometric blurring of the field edge occurs at the skin surface and

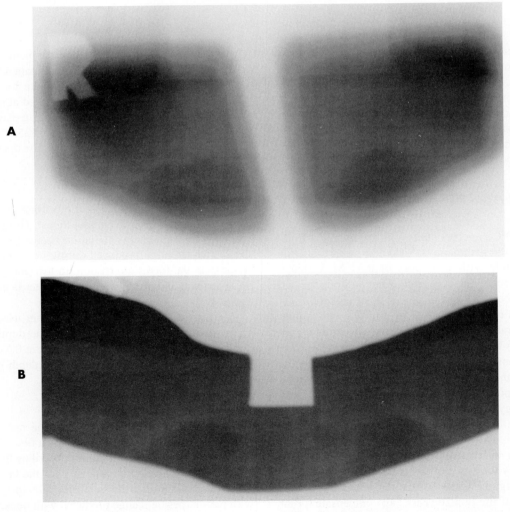

Fig. 14-4 A, Port film taken with a ^{60}Co beam demonstrates the fuzzy field edges or penumbra. **B,** Port film taken with a 6-MV beam demonstrates the sharpness at the field edges or lack of penumbra.

greater depths in tissue. The geometric penumbra should be considered during the planning of the patient's treatment, especially where treatment fields will abut or match. An example can be made with the simulator. During the planning process on the simulator, the field-defining wires of the simulator outlines the treatment volume. The wires outline the treatment area anatomically on a radiograph and visibly on the patient's skin. Different field sizes (slightly larger with the cobalt unit) are necessary to cover the same amount of tissue adequately on the cobalt machine as compared with a linear accelerator (Fig. 14-4).

The second type of penumbra, transmission penumbra, occurs as the radiation passes through the edge of the primary collimators. Transmission penumbra also occurs at the edge of the patient's shielding blocks mounted or placed below the collimator. The transmission penumbra correlates with the size of the collimator opening. Greater transmission penumbra occurs with larger collimator openings. As a result, larger field sizes have more transmission penumbra. If the inner surface of the collimator or shielding blocks are parallel to the edge of the beam, the transmission penumbra can be reduced (Fig. 14-5).[13]

To reduce this penumbra, a second set of smaller collimators (called *satellite collimators, penumbra trimmers,* or *trimmer bars*) can be added (Fig. 14-2). Trimmers are metal bars that attenuate the edge of the beam, thus providing a sharper field edge. Trimmer bars should be located no closer than 15 cm from the patient's skin to reduce electron contamination by the metal devices.[10] The 15 cm of air between the trimmer bars and patient's skin provides enough distance for the secondary electrons produced by the trimmer bars to lose sufficient energy. If electron contamination occurs, it may add significantly to the patient's skin dose.

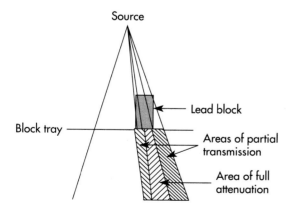

Fig. 14-5 Three areas of beam transmission. Blocks were placed in a manner in which the reflected light was blocked out, but because of beam divergence, areas shielded from radiation receive a considerable amount of dose. (From Stanton R, Stinson D. In Shahabi S, editor: *An introduction to radiation oncology physics,* Madison, Wis, 1992, Medical Physics Publishing.)

Half-value layer

The **half-value layer (HVL)** is the thickness of a specific material (i.e., lead) that reduces the intensity of the beam by 50%. The half-value layer thickness for ^{60}Co is 1.2 cm of lead.[2] By increasing the number of half-value layers in the beam's path, the amount of radiation reaching the patient is decreased by a constant percentage. For example, 1 HVL decreases beam intensity to 50%, 2 HVLs decrease by 25%, and 3 HVLs decrease by 12.5%. The recommended minimum thickness of lead for blocking a ^{60}Co beam is between 4 to 5 HVLs, which allows ≤ 5% transmission of the beam, thus shielding > 95% of the beam. For a beam to be considered fully blocked, this amount is required.

For radiation therapy beams, including ^{60}Co, shielding blocks are most commonly made of Lipowitz metal. Cerrobend is a form of Lipowitz metal used for designing custom shielding blocks and consists of 50.0% bismuth, 26.7% lead, 13.3% tin, and 10.0% cadmium.[6,12] Cerrobend melts (70° C) at a much lower point than lead (327° C). Therefore Cerrobend is easier and safer to use. However, cadmium (a toxic metal) can get into the bloodstream of individuals working with Lipowitz metal. At a considerable greater expense, some manufactures have introduced a type of Lipowitz alloy without cadmium.

The Cerrobend used in custom block fabrication hardens quickly depending on the amount and degree of cooling applied to the alloy. Using the density ratio of Cerrobend to lead, a factor of 1.21 can be applied to the thickness of lead needed to attenuate ≤ 5% of the primary beam. For the most common megavoltage beams, a thickness of 7.5 cm of Cerrobend is used. This is equivalent to about 6 cm of lead.[7]

Divergent, or custom-made, Cerrobend blocks offer little advantage for beams with large, geometrical penumbra. For ^{60}Co the sharpness at the beam cutoff at the block edge is not significantly improved by using divergent blocks.[7] This is the reason many departments have nondivergent blocks of various sizes and shapes for clinical use. Many radiation therapy departments had or still have a ^{60}Co treatment unit. The nondivergent blocks may have been purchased or fabricated for the ^{60}Co unit. Still, these types of blocks are convenient to use on any type of treatment unit with simple field designs, in emergency situations, or until custom blocks can be made. Many of the various square and rectangular nondivergent blocks have a short, threaded bolt protruding from the center of the block. This bolt is used with a wing nut to fasten the block securely to a plastic tray.

MACHINE DESIGN AND COMPONENTS
Source positioning

Of the five methods to position the radioactive ^{60}Co source shown in Table 14–2, the two most commonly used are the rotating-wheel (Fig. 14-6) and air-pressure (piston) methods (Fig. 14-7). The rotating-wheel method moves the ^{60}Co source into the on position by rotating a metal disk 180 degrees while a motor holds the source in position over the

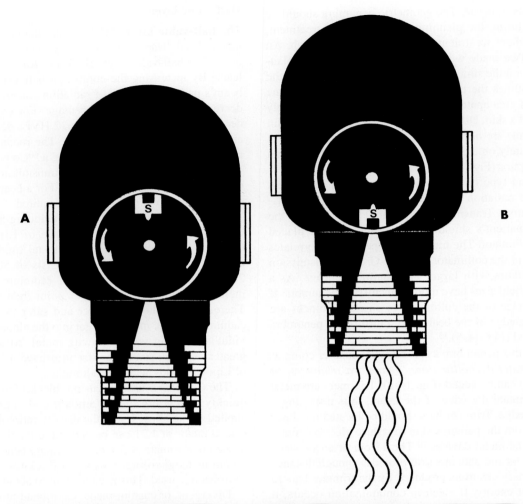

Fig. 14-6 A, A rotating wheel for ^{60}Co in the off position. **B,** A rotating wheel for ^{60}Co in the on position.

Table 14-2	Five methods to expose the ^{60}Co source

Type	Method
Air pressure (piston)	The compressor generates air pressure by pushing the source horizontally into position over the collimator opening (often referred to as the *sliding drawer*).
Rotating wheel	The motor rotates a wheel 180 degrees by placing the source over the collimator opening.
Mercury reservoir	Mercury is withdrawn or returned to a reservoir located below the source at the collimator opening.
Chain driven	A sphere that is chain driven rotates a stationary source 90 degrees to place it at the collimator opening.
Moving jaws	Lead jaws located below the source open and close for exposure or shielding.

collimator opening. If power is interrupted, the spring-attached wheel returns the source to the off position. The air-pressure method pushes a piston and thus the ^{60}Co source into the on position. A sliding draw allows the source to be positioned over the collimator opening. In the off position the source retracts back into the treatment head. In case of power failure the air-driven piston automatically returns the source to the off position.[3]

Travel time

The time necessary to deliver the source from the off, on, or treatment position is defined as the **travel time.** To compensate for the travel time, a correction (shutter error) must be added to the calculation to deliver the prescribed dose. The shutter error allows for the total advancement and retraction of the source from the off position to the on position and back to the off position again. Depending on the manufacturer and method of source delivery, this may take place in less than 1 second. If the travel time is neglected in the cal-

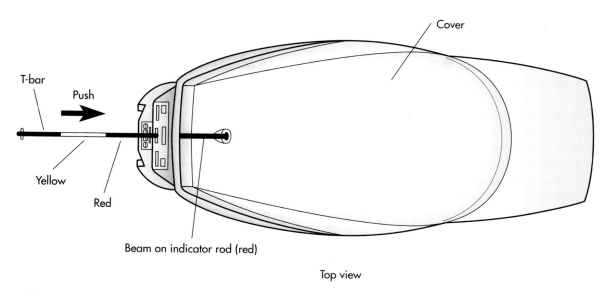

Fig. 14-7 A ^{60}Co air-pressure (piston) drawer in the on position. (Courtesy Atomic Energy of Canada Limited, Medical Products, Kanata, Ontario, Canada.)

culation used to deliver the prescribed dose, a small underdose may occur. Of course, the greater the number of fractions used to deliver the total dose, the greater the error in dose delivered.

Noises

If the source is exposed through the air-pressure or rotating-wheel method, loud or unusual noises associated with the delivery of the source can occur. The radiation therapist should inform the patient of noises that may occur during the course of treatment. The sudden noise caused by the compressor in the air-pressure method may not occur during each treatment. Because it is intermittent, the loud noise may occur when the patient is in the room receiving treatment. Therefore a patient should be educated before the start of treatment about all aspects of the course of treatment.

Shielding

Because it constantly emits radiation, the ^{60}Co source must be shielded in a protective housing. The housing used for shielding and containing the device for positioning the source is referred to as the **source head** (Fig. 14-8). The source head is a steel shell filled with lead or an alloy of lead, tungsten, and depleted uranium.[6] For adequate shielding the housing may be up to 2 feet in diameter.[11] Radiation leakage around the source head should conform to Nuclear Regulatory Commission (NCR) guidelines.

Machine components

A multivaned or interleaf collimator (Fig. 14-9) is constructed as part of the source head to shape the size of the radiation beam (Fig. 14-2). The collimator assists in reducing the penumbra associated with the source size. Trimmers or satellite collimators may be added to further sharpen the radiation-beam edge. Field size is defined by a light beam reflected from a light bulb to a small mirror. A tray holder is added below the collimators for field shaping by hand-placed lead or customized Cerrobend shielding blocks. Wedges made of lead, brass, or copper are placed in the path of the beam and shift or tilt the dose distribution from its normal shape. When needed, they are positioned in a separate slot in the block tray assembly.

RADIATION-SAFETY PROCEDURES
Regulatory agencies

In 1928 the International Commission on Radiological Protection (ICRP) was formed to develop standards for radiation protection. The ICRP is a group of international experts who publish recommendations for protection from ionizing radiation. The United States has a group of radiation experts who make recommendations and develop standards for radiation called the National Council on Radiation Protection and Measurements (NCRP). Neither of these agencies has the power to make regulations, only recommendations. Therefore they are considered *advisory*. The United States NRC and individual states establish radiation regulations in the United States. These regulations are incorporated into federal and state laws. Individual states may enter into an agreement with the NRC to assume the responsibility of enforcing regulations for ionizing radiation. These states are considered **agreement states.** States that are not agreement states with the NRC have the responsibility of enforcing ionizing radiation regulations.[13]

Licenses must be maintained on the ^{60}Co unit through the NRC or agreement states. Licenses are extremely costly and may include the following estimates[16]:

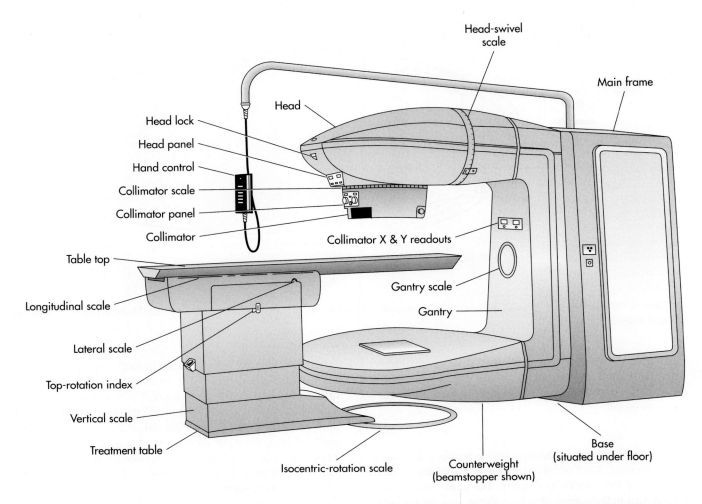

Fig. 14-8 An atomic Energy of Canada Limited Theratron 780C cobalt 60 unit. (Courtesy Atomic Energy of Canada Limited, Medical Products, Kanata, Ontario, Canada.)

1. Application for a new license ($3700)
2. Renewal ($1200)
3. Amendment ($500)
4. Inspections ($8700)

The NRC and agreement states specifically define which individuals are qualified to work on and perform testing on ^{60}Co units. For installation, maintenance, exchange, and removal of the ^{60}Co source, all persons or organizations performing services must be licensed by the NRC or the state licensing agency. The ^{60}Co unit must have a 5-year service and maintenance inspection performed by persons or organizations specifically licensed to do so by the NRC or state licensing agency. A qualified expert must perform the annual full calibration. A qualified expert is defined in the license that details the necessary training and experience.[1]

Calibration and leakage

A qualified radiation physicist must perform full calibration testing for radioactive ^{60}Co units annually. Full calibration may be done more frequency if (1) the source is replaced, (2) a 5% deviation is noticed during a spot check, and (3) a major repair requiring the removal or restoration of major components is done. A monthly output calibration should be done for a set of standard daily operating conditions. Measurements taken during a full calibration include the following[1]:

1. Radiation and light field coincidence
2. Timer accuracy
3. Exposure rate or dose rate to an accuracy of ± 3% for various field sizes
4. Accuracy of distance-measuring devices used for treatment

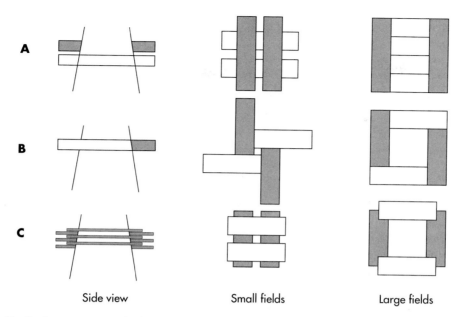

Side view   Small fields   Large fields

Fig. 14-9 Adjustable diaphragm systems: **A,** double plane; **B,** single plane; **C,** interleaved. (From Walter J, Miller H, Bomford CK: *A short textbook of radiotherapy,* New York, 1979, Churchill Livingstone.)

5. Uniformity of the radiation field and its dependence of the orientation of the useful beam

With the source always emitting radiation or continually active, the levels of radiation in the treatment room are always higher than background radiation.[15] Radiation therapists should therefore limit their time in the treatment room, especially the amount of time close to the source. The average leakage rate in the off position around the head of the unit cannot exceed 2 mrem/hr at 1 m, with a maximum of 10 mrem/hr at 1 m at any measurable location. The maximum permissible leakage in the on position cannot exceed 0.1% of the useful beam at 1 m from the source. The 0.1% of the useful beam is the percent of the actual output of the ^{60}Co source in cGy/min. For example, if the useful beam has an output of 197.3 cGy/min for the month of January, the maximum permissible leakage in the on position at 1 m from the source is 0.197 cGy/min.

A **wipe test** (or leak test) must be done twice a year on the sealed ^{60}Co source. If a source's seal is broken and leaking, it may have radiation contamination on the interleaf collimators. A wipe test is done, using long forceps, wiping the collimator edges with a filter paper, cloth pad, or cotton swab moistened with alcohol. A background radiation reading is done by using a survey meter calibrated with the same type material as the one being tested. A reading is then taken of the wipe to determine its activity, with the acceptable level of activity less than 0.005 μCi. If the activity is higher, radiation contamination or leakage may have occurred and the

unit must be removed from service until decontamination and repair can be completed.

Radiation monitoring and light system

Because it is a radioactive source that emits ionizing radiation, ^{60}Co requires not only a light system to show when the machine is on and off, but also a monitoring system to detect radiation. The machine on-and-off indicator lights must be on the console, at the head of the machine, and at the entrance to the treatment room. If the machine is on, a red light must be lit. When the machine is off, this light should show green. A radiation detector must be located in the treatment room. The detector is wired to a light outside the room near the console and door (Fig. 14-10). The light must be blinking red if radiation is present and must be in view of the radiation therapist. Before entering the room, the therapist must be sure the off light is green and the blinking red light has stopped. Because a moment is necessary for the ^{60}Co source to retract into its off position, the green light comes on first, before the blinking red light stops. If the red light continues to blink for longer than a few seconds, the therapist must be ready to carry out an established emergency procedure. The source may not have retracted fully or properly.

Emergency procedures

Emergency procedures must be established during the machine commissioning and before the unit is used for treatment. The emergency procedures must be posted at the

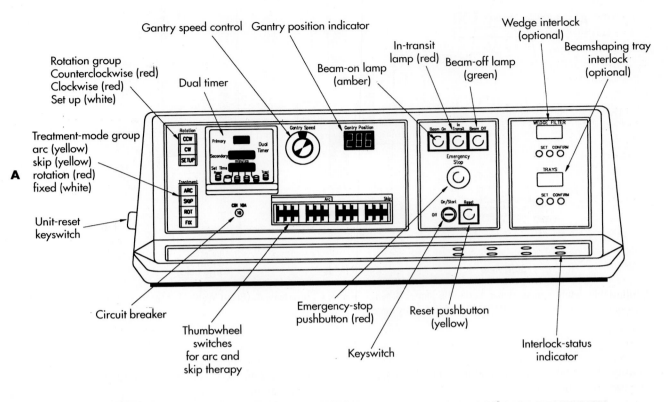

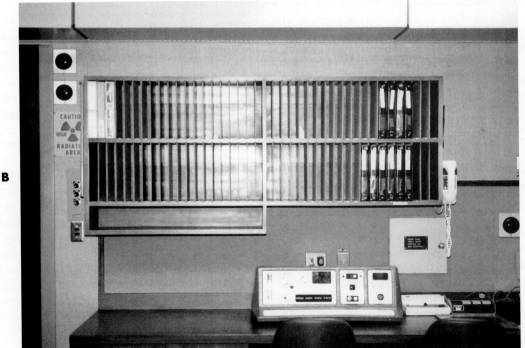

Fig. 14-10 A, A master control panel with a light system for a ^{60}Co unit. **B,** A console area with a radiation-detector monitoring system for the ^{60}Co unit. (**A,** Courtesy Atomic Energy of Canada Limited, Medical Products, Kanata, Ontario, Canada.)

machine console. These procedures must be developed by the radiation safety officer or radiation physicist and communicated to the radiation therapist and personnel responsible during a radiation emergency. No universal emergency procedure exists for a source that fails to return to the off position. Each department should develop and post emergency procedures. A sample procedure posted at the machine console is shown in the box.

Another procedure may include retracting the ^{60}Co source into the head source area with a T-bar. A T-bar is a steel rod 18 to 24 inches in length shaped like a T. The first 7 inches opposite the end of the T is painted red with the next 7 inches painted yellow (Fig. 14-7). In case of an emergency in which the source does not retract, the T-bar is placed in the source drawer at the top of the machine or source head. With the T end of the bar held in hand, forward pressure is applied to push the drawer backward into the off position. The ^{60}Co source can be considered relatively safe if no red paint is showing on the T-bar outside the machine or source-head cover. Before the ^{60}Co source is in the fully safe position, the yellow portion of the bar must be entirely inside the machine or source-head cover. Because of the complexity of this procedure, any radiation therapy personnel performing it may be exposed to a higher dose of radiation than under normal working conditions.

Room shielding

Because ^{60}Co is a radioactive source, primary, secondary, and leakage radiation must be considered in determining appropriate thickness for shielding. Depending on the strength of the source and distance of the walls and ceiling to the ^{60}Co beam, some concrete walls, floors, and ceilings may be up to 3 feet thick.

Warmup procedures

Warmup procedures for a ^{60}Co unit are relatively simple compared with those of a linear accelerator. The cobalt unit must be turned on and off to check whether the source is retracting properly. In addition, this provides an evaluation of the light (red and green) and radiation-monitoring system.

Several other components of the machine must be checked. The ^{60}Co uses a timer system to determine the time the source is in the on position. The timer can be in minutes and hundredths of minutes or minutes and actual seconds and can be checked by using a stopwatch. The door interlock should also be checked daily. If the door is opened while the machine is running, the machine automatically shuts off and the source retracts. Other treatment-machine parameters such as field size, optical-distance indicator, laser system, gantry, and collimator rotations must be evaluated.

Radiation Therapist Procedure for Cobalt 60 Emergency

A. If the console timer fails to terminate exposure, do the following:
  1. PUSH EMERGENCY OFF BUTTON.
  2. TURN CIRCUIT BREAKER OFF.
B. If the source drawer fails to close by shutting off electrical circuits, do the following:
  1. OPEN TREATMENT ROOM DOOR.
    a. Use the hand crank if electrical power is off and if using a pneumatic door.
  2. REMOVE PATIENT FROM ROOM.
    a. Verbally request that the patient get off the table and come to the treatment door.
    b. If the patient is unable to respond to a verbal command, enter the treatment room and quickly remove the patient. Do not stand in the path of the primary beam.
  3. CLOSE TREATMENT ROOM DOOR.
    a. Use the hand crank if electrical power is off and if using a pneumatic door.
C. Notify the attending physician and radiation safety officer.
D. Secure the room against unauthorized entry by placing a DO NOT ENTER sign on the door, and secure or lock the door.
NOTE: This machine shall not be used unless the operating and emergency procedure manual is available in the control area. Operating personnel should familiarize themselves with this manual before operating this machine.

SUMMARY

Although ^{60}Co units are mechanically simple, easy to operate, and relatively inexpensive, most radiation oncology departments in the United States are replacing these units with the more versatile linear accelerator. In developing countries, ^{60}Co treatment units enjoy more popularity than linear accelerators.[5] Cobalt units historically played a major role in radiation oncology by allowing the radiation oncologist and radiation therapist to deliver the dose below the skin surface. In the last 10 to 20 years, technology has advanced in the area of high-energy x-rays and electrons, thus providing doses at greater depths in tissue, a wider range of beam energies, and more sophisticated methods of delivering the dose. Despite the high cost of licensing, potential emergency situations, and limited beam characteristics, ^{60}Co still has a place in the field of radiation oncology.

Review Questions

Multiple Choice

1. What is the half-life of ^{60}Co, a radioactive isotope?
   a. 1.25 years
   b. 5.25 years
   c. 10.5 years
   d. 30 years
2. What is the average energy with which ^{60}Co emits gamma rays used for radiation therapy treatments?
   a. 1.17
   b. 1.25
   c. 1.33
   d. 2.50
3. Because of the decay of the ^{60}Co source, a patient calculation correction of what percent must be made monthly?
   a. 0.1%
   b. 1.0%
   c. 5.0%
   d. 10.0%
4. The maximum permissible leakage for the ^{60}Co source at 1 m in the on position is what percent of the useful beam?
   a. 0.1%
   b. 1.0%
   c. 5.0%
   d. 10.0%
5. What is the average leakage of the ^{60}Co source at 1 m in the off position?
   a. 1 mrem/hr
   b. 2 mrem/hr
   c. 5 mrem/hr
   d. 10 mrem/hr
6. Which of the following is a disadvantage in using a ^{60}Co beam for radiation therapy treatments?
   a. Penumbra
   b. Sharp field edge
   c. No skin sparing
   d. None of the above

Questions to Ponder

1. Analyze the need for a radiation-detector lighting system for ^{60}Co units?
2. Why must a monthly calculation correction be made for the ^{60}Co unit?
3. Discuss an emergency procedure for a source that fails to retract.
4. Compare and contrast the daily warmup procedure for a ^{60}Co unit and linear accelerator.
5. Discuss the rationale for performing biannual leak or wipe tests on a ^{60}Co unit.

REFERENCES

1. Arkansas State Board of Health: *Rules and regulations for control of sources of ionizing radiation*, Little Rock, Ark, 1994, The Board.
2. Coia L, Moylan D: *Introduction to clinical radiation oncology*, Madison, Wis, 1991, Medical Physics Publishing.
3. Hendee W: *Radiation therapy physics*, Chicago, 1981, Year Book Medical Publishing.
4. Internal Commission on Radiation Units and Measurement: *Determination of absorbed dosed in a patient irradiated by beams of x and gamma rays in radiotherapy procedures*, ICRU report 24, Washington, DC, 1976, The Commission.
5. Jackson S: *Radiation oncology: a handbook for residents and the allied health professions*, St Louis, 1985, Warren H Green.
6. Johns H, Cunningham J, Friedman M, editors: *Physics of radiology*, ed 2, Springfield, Ill, 1974, Charles C Thomas.
7. Khan F: *Physics of radiation therapy*, Baltimore, 1994, Williams & Wilkins.
8. Nais A: *An introduction to radiobiology*, New York, 1990, John Wiley & Sons.
9. Owen JB: Personal communication, July 1995.
10. Rafla S, Rotman M: *Introduction to radiation therapy*, St Louis, 1974, Mosby.
11. Selman J: *Basis physics of radiation therapy*, ed 2, Springfield, Ill, 1976, Charles C Thomas.
12. Shahabi S: *Blackburn's introduction to clinical radiation therapy physics*, Madison, Wis, 1989, Medical Physics Publishing.
13. Stanton R, Stinson D, Shahabi S, editors: *An introduction to radiation oncology physics*, Madison, Wis, 1992, Medical Physics Publishing.
14. Stryker J: *Radiation oncology*, New Hyde Park, NY, 1985, Medical Examination Publishing.
15. Travis E: *Primer of medical radiobiology*, ed 2, St Louis, 1989, Mosby.
16. United States Nuclear Regulation Commission: *Rules and regulations, part 170*, Washington, DC, 1994, The Commission.

CHAPTER

15

Other Therapeutic Equipment

Linda Alfred
Dennis T. Leaver

Outline

Historical overview
Equipment development
Characteristics of kilovoltage
   x-ray equipment
   X-ray tube
   Specification of beam quality
   Half-value layer measure
      ments
   Filtration
Clinical applications of kilovolt-
   age equipment
   Grenz-ray therapy
   Contact therapy
   Superficial treatments
   Orthovoltage therapy

Megavoltage equipment
   Betatron
   Van de Graaff generator
   Proton accelerator
Remote afterloading
   Historical perspective
   Pioneers and the arrival of
      remote afterloading
   High dose rate and low dose
      rate
   Radiobiology of high dose
      rate
Summary

Key terms

Betatrons
Bragg peak
Contact therapy
Cyclotron
Grenz rays
Half-value layer
High-dose-rate (HDR)
  brachytherapy
Isodose curve
Kilovoltage units
kVp

Linear accelerator
Low-dose-rate (LDR)
  brachytherapy
mA
Megavoltage equipment
Orthovoltage therapy
Positron emission tomography
  (PET)
Superficial therapy
Van de Graaff

HISTORICAL OVERVIEW

The discovery of x-rays by Wilhelm Roentgen in 1895 and the subsequent therapeutic use of radiation has generated a variety of equipment. The features of each system mirrored the technology of the day while addressing the radiobiological needs of the patient as closely as deemed necessary with the knowledge then available. In the relatively short period since the discovery of these mysterious rays, a great deal of specialized equipment has emerged. The application of this equipment has had most of its success in the treatment of malignant diseases.

This chapter discusses several aspects of related radiation therapy equipment, including many characteristics of this specialized equipment. Low-energy machines such as grenz rays, contact therapy, superficial equipment, and orthovoltage machines are discussed. In addition, an overview of high-energy machines, including the Van de Graaff generator, betatron, and cyclotron, are introduced. (Separate chapters have been developed for the linear accelerator and cobalt 60 treatment units.) This chapter concludes with a discussion of positrion emission tomography (PET) studies, remote afterloading, and future outlooks concerning radiation therapy equipment.

EQUIPMENT DEVELOPMENT

Conventional low-energy equipment, which typically uses x-rays generated at voltages up to 300 kVp, have been used in radiation therapy since the turn of the century. These **kilovoltage units** (low x-ray voltage radiation therapy treatment machines) include grenz, contact, superficial, and orthovoltage machines. The use of this equipment dramatically decreased after 1950. This was due in part to the increased popularity of cobalt 60 units and subsequent development of the **linear accelerator** (a radiation therapy treatment machine that uses high-frequency electromagnetic waves to accelerate charged particles such as electrons to high energies via a linear tube). However, kilovoltage equipment is still part of many departments today, partly because of the low cost and simplicity of design compared with megavoltage units. The primary application of kilovoltage equipment is in the treatment of superficial lesions.

The introduction of megavoltage therapy equipment, which generated x-ray beams of 1 MV or greater, was a natural progression from low-energy units. Although kilovoltage units were and are beneficial, they still have two principle limitations that are clinically essential: They could not reach deep-seated tumors with an adequate dosage of radiation, and they did not spare skin and normal tissue. As a result, manufacturers began concentrating their efforts on addressing these and other shortcomings of low-energy equipment.

The early to middle part of the twentieth century marked a period of tremendous development of equipment used to treat tumors (Fig. 15-1). The physics community began experimenting with the acceleration of electrons, protons, neutrons, and heavy ions. The attempt was being made in medicine to find a better way to deliver a lethal dose of radiation therapy. In North America the Van de Graaff (1937), betatron (1941), cobalt 60 (1951), and linear accelerator (1956) were introduced.[12]

The clinical application of the cyclotron, which could accelerate several types of particles, began around 1938. Patients received treatments from a variety of particles. Neutrons *and* protons were used with limited success, a stationary beam of protons was used to treat patients as early as 1946, and neutron treatments began in the United States around 1938. However, the first hospital-based (as opposed to physics-based) rotational cyclotron was not operational until about 1982.[12]

Until the early to mid 1950s, most cancer patients undergoing radiation therapy were treated with low-energy equipment. Physicians did their best with the equipment available to them. Surgery was still the treatment of choice for most cancers.

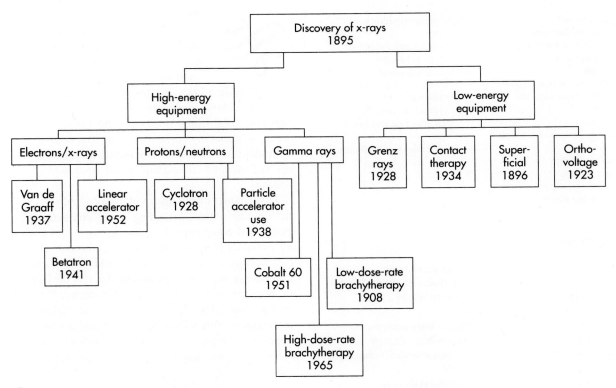

Fig. 15-1 A timetable chart illustrates the development of high- and low-energy treatment equipment since the discovery of x-rays in 1895. Every effort has been made in researching the accuracy of the information in this table. However, several sources and experts in the field sometimes disagree about the exact dates that equipment was introduced clinically. (For more information, refer to the following: Bentel C: *Radiation therapy planning,* New York, 1993, McGraw-Hill; and Grigg EM: *The trail of the invisible light,* Springfield, Ill, 1965, Charles C Thomas.)

CHARACTERISTICS OF KILOVOLTAGE X-RAY EQUIPMENT
X-ray tube

The design criteria and operation of conventional kilovoltage x-ray units are based on standard stationary and rotating anode tubes and circuitry to produce therapeutic rays (Fig. 15-2). Low-energy x-rays were produced and applied to extremely superficial tumors. Skin lesions benefited most as a result of the low-energy x-rays' lack of penetrating ability. (See Chapter 12 for further details on the construction of the x-ray tube and production of x-rays.)

Specification of beam quality

For a discussion of the penetrating characteristics of an x-ray beam, a method of specifying beam quality (strength) is useful. This allows a comparison of one beam with another. Beam quality is important in deciding which type of kilovoltage equipment to use in specific clinical situations. Weak beams are generally used for extremely superficial tumors, and strong beams are reserved for deep-seated tumors.

The quality of x-rays can include the accelerating potential (kVp) and half-value layer (HVL) measurements. Each method describes the penetrating ability of the beam. The **half-value layer** of an x-ray beam is the thickness of absorbing material necessary to reduce the x-ray intensity to half its original value. The more the beam penetrates matter, the higher the energy and HVL. HVL is the best method for specifying x-ray quality, mainly because variations in penetrating ability with changes in **kVp** (x-ray voltages measured in kilovoltage peak [l kV equals 1000 V of electric potential]) and filtration are not simple relationships. Obtaining the HVL involves measuring an absorption curve of the radiation in the specified material and interpolating the thickness corresponding to 50% absorption.[19]

Central-axis-depth dose *and* physical penumbra are related to beam quality. In treatment planning, the central-axis-depth dose distribution for a specific beam depends on the energy (Fig. 15-3). The depth of an isodose curve increases with beam quality. For example, a 50% **isodose curve** (a line representing various points of similar value in a beam along the central axis and elsewhere) for a 200-kVp beam reaches a deeper tumor than a 50% isodose curve of a 100-kVp orthovoltage beam. The shape of the isodose curve also bulges sideways, as illustrated in the isodose distribution for the 200-kVp x-ray beam in Fig. 15-3. Orthovoltage beams show increased scatter dose to the tissue outside the treatment region, thus exhibiting a marked disadvantage compared with megavoltage beams.[19] In other words, the absorbed dose in the medium outside the primary beam is greater for low-energy beams than for those of a higher energy[18] (Fig. 15-3). In orthovoltage radiation, isodose curves become distended and tend to bulge sideways. Conversely, limited scatter outside the field for megavoltage beams occurs because of predominantly forward scattering of the beam. This is illustrated in the isodose distribution for the 25-MV beam in Fig. 15-3.

Half-value layer measurements

Experimentally determining HVL involves the measurement of exposure at a selected point in a beam as increasing thickness of material is placed in the beam.[16] Two facts should be noted before the experiment is performed: (1) The ionization

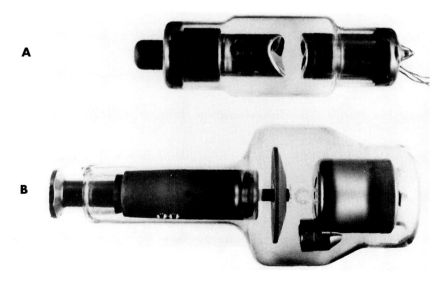

Fig. 15-2 X-ray tubes used in low-energy kilovoltage machines can be classified by the type of anode they contain: **A,** stationary or **B,** rotating. (From Bushong S: *Radiologic science for technologists,* ed 5, St Louis, 1993, Mosby.)

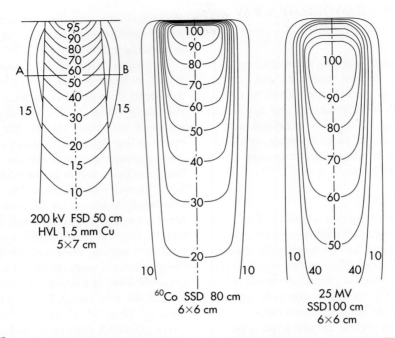

Fig. 15-3 Isodose distributions for several beams: *left,* 200 kVp, HVL 1.5 mm Cu, SSD 50 cm, field size 5 × 7 cm; *middle,* cobalt 60, SSD 80 cm, field size 6 × 6 cm; *right* 25 MV, SSD 100 cm, 6 × 6 cm. (Redrawn from Johns HE, Cunningham JR: *The physics of radiology,* ed 4, Springfield, Ill, 1983, C Thomas.)

chamber wall is air equivalent over the range of measured photon energies (i.e., the same chamber cannot be used for 10 kVp *and* 10 MV), and (2) the penetrating ability of the beams greatly varies (therefore the choice of absorbing material is extremely important). One of several ways to determine HVL is by using the following basic components: the x-ray tube, a radiation detector, and a graded thickness of filter, usually aluminum (Fig. 15-4). The beam-collimation size should be small enough to cover the ionization chamber, referred to as the *detector.* The source-filter distance should approximate the filter-detector distance and be greater than the range of electrons emitted from the filter material. A guide to performing the procedure is provided in the following steps:

1. Find the x-ray intensity with no absorbing material.
2. Determine the x-ray intensity equal to half the original intensity, and locate this value on the y, or vertical, axis of the graph (Fig. 15-5, *A*).
3. Draw a horizontal line parallel with the x-axis from the point identified in step 2 until it intersects the curve.
4. From this point of intersection, drop a vertical line to the x-axis.
5. On the x-axis, read the thickness of absorber required to reduce the x-ray intensity to half its original value. This is the HVL.[5]

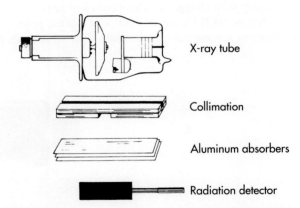

Fig. 15-4 A common experimental arrangement for determining HVL. (From Bushong S: *Radiologic science for technologists,* ed 5, St Louis, 1993, Mosby.)

If the exposure is not accurate with one monitor chamber, a second chamber can be used on the tube side of the small beam collimator. This second monitor detects the variation in the exposure incident on the filters added to the experiment.[5] Again, the beam collimation must fit the size of the chamber. This is crucial to minimize the radiation scattered by the added filter because of an unnecessarily large beam of radiation.[19] Fig. 15-6 illustrates the relationship between kVp and HVL from 50 to 150 kVp.

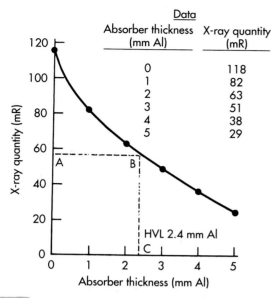

Data

Absorber thickness (mm Al)	X-ray quantity (mR)
0	118
1	82
2	63
3	51
4	38
5	29

HVL 2.4 mm Al

Fig. 15-5 A graph showing a typical plot of data relating to HVL measurements. The data demonstrates an HVL of 2.4 mm. (From Bushong S: *Radiologic science for technologists,* ed 5, St Louis, 1993, Mosby.)

kVp	HVL (mm Al)
50	1.9
75	2.8
100	3.7
125	4.6
150	5.4

Fig. 15-6 An example of the relationship between HVL and kVp for a fixed radiographic unit that uses 2.5-mm Al total filtration. (From Bushong S: *Radiologic science for technologists,* ed 5, St Louis, 1993, Mosby.)

Filtration

Two types of filtration are used with diagnostic x-ray beams: inherent filtration and added filtration. When specifying filtration, a clear distinction exists between the two. *Inherent filtration* is a product of the glass envelope and insulating oil of the x-ray tube. *Added filtration* is described in clinical practice. Thin sheets of an absorber, usually aluminum or copper, align between the protective tube housing and collimator. Inherent filtration increases as the tube ages because the tungsten metals of the target and filament vaporizes and becomes deposited on the inside of the glass envelope. Added filtration hardens the beam because most low-energy x-rays are attenuated. This results in a beam with a higher effective energy, thus greater penetrating ability and higher quality. Adding filters also results in an increased HVL.[19]

Clinically, extreme care should be exercised in correctly placing the proper filter. Grave errors can be made in the placement of the wrong filter. The patient's prognosis may be compromised if an incorrect filter is used. This may result from underdosing or overdosing the treatment area.

CLINICAL APPLICATIONS OF KILOVOLTAGE EQUIPMENT
Grenz-ray therapy

In 1923 Gustav Bucky constructed an x-ray tube with a lithium borate window (Lindemann glass). The window permitted the transmission of long wavelength x-rays, the physical properties of which Bucky later studied. Consequently, the rays became Bucky rays, or **grenz rays** (low-energy x-rays having an energy of 10 to 15 kVp). This term comes from *grenz,* a German word meaning "border." This was an accurate description because grenz rays were thought at the time to lie within a grey zone between x-rays and ultraviolet radiation.

The construction of a grenz-ray tube and superficial tube is similar. In a grenz-ray tube, the envelope is glass and the window is beryllium. Inherent filtration is approximately 0.1 mm aluminum (Al). Like the superficial and orthovoltage units, the quality of grenz-ray measurements in terms of HVL is expressed in millimeters of aluminum. Sometimes in dermatology, copper is the metal used to designate the HVL. The intensity of the radiation decreases when the kVp and mA decrease. This intensity also decreases when the distance is increased as a result of the inverse square law. Grenz rays are almost entirely absorbed in the first 2 mm of skin and have a useful depth-dose range of about 0.5 mm. The intensity falls off rapidly after this. Less than 2% is capable of reaching the sebaceous glands of the skin.

The application of grenz rays characteristically is safe and painless for the patient and often yields visible results in 48 to 72 hours. The recommended fractionation involving approximately 200 roentgens (R) per session at weekly intervals totals 800 to 1000 R, followed by a 6-month period before additional treatment may occur. Grenz rays are especially effective for the treatment of inflammatory disorders, namely those involving Langerhans' cells. Grenz rays have also yielded positive results for Bowen's disease, patchy-stage mycosis fungoides, and herpes simplex.[8]

Contact therapy

Clinical data on contact therapy is scarce. Fig. 15-7 illustrates a handheld **contact therapy** unit. Historically, contact therapy was primarily used to treat superficial skin lesions. The treatment machine derived its name because the treatment unit actually came in contact with the patient. Another use of contact therapy relates to endocavitary treatments for curative intent. This involves a limited group of patients with cancers of the low to middle third of the rectum.

The rectal cancers treated are confined to the bowel wall in most situations. Papillon has established several criteria

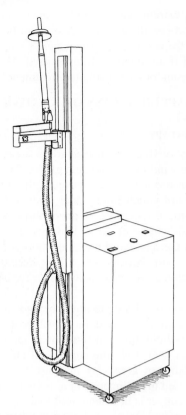

Fig. 15-7 A handheld contact-therapy machine used to treat superficial skin lesions. The operators, one to monitor the patient and the other to hold the applicator, must wear protective shielding during the treatment application.

for treating rectal lesions by using low-energy x-rays.[21] These criteria are as follows: a maximum tumor size of 3 × 5 cm, a mobile lesion with no significant extension into the anal canal, and a well differentiated to moderately well differentiated exophytic tumor that is accessible by the treatment proctoscope ($\leq$ 10 cm from anal verge). This treatment is especially desirable for the patient because it preserves the anal sphincter. (This may not be true with other methods.) On an outpatient basis, patients received four treatments of 3000 cGy each, separated by a 2-week interval. Papillon used a 50-kVp Philip's contact unit. The source-skin distance (SSD) used was 4 cm with 0.50 to 1.0 mm aluminum filtration at a dose rate of 1000 cGy per minute. A 3-cm applicator cone can deliver treatments directly to the rectal mucosa via the rectum. Overlapping fields existed if the size of the lesion exceeded the diameter of the applicator.[21] Chapter 10 of volume III provides additional details about the use of contact therapy in the treatment of rectal lesions.

Historically, Chaoul contact therapy was the treatment of choice for hemangiomas, especially in the dermatology department of the University Hospital in Munich, Germany. Fractionated doses of 300 to 500 R and total doses ranging from 1200 to 1500 R were delivered to patients in intervals of several days. Most patients showed visible improvement as evidenced by diminished lesion size and less elevation within 8 weeks of treatment. The Chaoul radiation technique was less hazardous than previously used orthovoltage techniques.[9] The popularity of this technique has decreased dramatically since 1975 because large studies have proved conclusively that spontaneous involution of strawberry angiomas (hemangioma simplex) occurs in 95% of cases after several years.[9]

Superficial treatments

Superficial therapy relates to treatments with x-rays produced at potentials ranging from 50 to 150 kV. Usually, 1- to 6-mm thick aluminum filters insert in a slot in the treatment head to harden the beam to the desired degree. The degree of hardening, as with other units, is measured in HVLs. Typical HVLs used in superficial treatments range from 1 to 8 mm of Al.[18] Superficial-treatment administration uses a cone or applicator. Cone sizes are generally 2 to 5 cm in diameter. Lead cutouts are tailored to fit the treatment area if needed. The cone lies directly on the skin or lead cutout and generally provides an SSD of 15 to 20 cm. Skin cancer and tumors no deeper than 0.5 cm are treated as a result of the rapid falloff of the radiation.

Three parameters are set at the console area for treatment delivery: kVp, **mA** (x-ray current measured in milliamperes), and treatment time. Superficial treatment and orthovoltage units are extremely reliable and free of eletromechanical problems. This contributes to a lack of downtime, which is a problem more often with linear accelerators. The main difficulty encountered with the use of superficial units arises from having to lock down the unit after the cone is in position. Usually, the unit has a variety of handles or knobs (depending on the model) that require tightening while keeping the cone in place. This can be a challenge. Because no standard treatment table comes with the system, the patient can lie on a stretcher or sit in a chair for treatment, thus amplifying the difficulty of locking down all the knobs[13] (Fig. 15-8).

Orthovoltage therapy

Orthovoltage therapy describes treatment with x-rays produced at potentials ranging from 150 to 500 kV. Most orthovoltage equipment operates at 200 to 300 kV and 10 to 20 mA. Much like the superficial units, orthovoltage units use filters designed to achieve HVLs from 1 to 4 mm Cu.[18] Orthovoltage units can use external or del Regato cones to collimate the beam. In addition, a movable diaphragm consisting of lead plates can be used to adjust the field size. Conventionally, the SSD is 50 cm.

The types of tumors treated with orthovoltage units include skin, mouth, and cervical carcinoma (with the use of cones inserted into the patient). As with superficial treat-

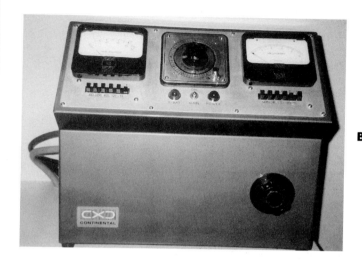

Fig. 15-8 **A,** A continental superficial machine with a treatment couch at Great Plains Regional Cancer Center, Elk City, Oklahoma. **B,** A control panel used to regulate the kVp and mA. (Courtesy Great Plains Regional Cancer Center, Elk City, Oklahoma.)

ments, the average treatment time can be seconds to several minutes depending on the filtered kV, prescribed dose, collimator, or cone size. The penetrating depth depends on the kV and filter. Usually, orthovoltage units experience limitation in the treatment of lesions deeper than 2 to 3 cm.[4]

Orthovoltage units are still popular in many clinics and hospitals. They are reliable alternatives to the use of electrons in the treatment of many superficial skin lesions. Most skin lesions treated with orthovoltage units are squamous cell and basal cell cancers. Some clinicians prefer the orthovoltage unit for treating skin tumors because of beam characteristics, especially treatments requiring small fields.

In many departments in which kilovoltage equipment still exists, several treatment units may operate out of the same treatment room. Much of the equipment is older, compared with the design and appearance of modern megavoltage equipment. Historically, when orthovoltage was the highest energy available, treatments were limited by the skin's radiation tolerance. This limitation made the skin-sparing properties of cobalt teletherapy especially desirable and became the major reason for the modern trend to megavoltage beams.

MEGAVOLTAGE EQUIPMENT

X-ray beams of 1 MV or greater can be classified as **megavoltage equipment.** Examples of clinical megavoltage machines are accelerators such as the Van de Graaff generator, linear accelerator, betatron, and cyclotron. Teletherapy units such as cobalt 60 are also classified as megavoltage treatment units. For a variety of reasons, linear accelerators are growing in popularity in the United States. The development of dual-energy machines allows for treatment with two x-ray energies and a variety of electron energies on the same machine. Computerization has ushered in an era of more complex treatments using ancillary devices such as record and verify systems, electronic portal imagers, and multileaf collimators. As the goal of true conformal therapy becomes the standard rather than the exception, the complexity and popularity of linear accelerators is sure to continue (Fig. 15-9).

Because earlier chapters provide detailed descriptions of the cobalt 60 unit and linear accelerator, the remainder of this section focuses on a brief overview of the betatron, Van de Graaff generator, and cyclotron.

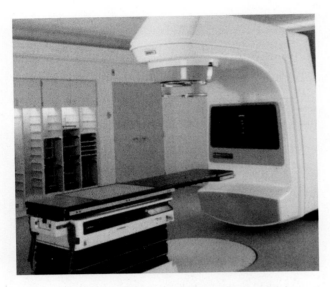

Fig. 15-9 A linear accelerator, the 2300 CD. (Courtesy Varian Associates, Palo Alto, Calif.)

Betatron

The first betatron, developed by Kerst in 1941, produced x-rays of 2 MV.[21] **Betatrons** (megavoltage treatment units that can provide x-ray and electron therapy beams from less than 6 to more than 40 MeV) were initially used for radiation therapy in the early 1950s.[18,19] Besides medical uses, betatrons were applied to industrial radiography. Betatrons were used especially during World War II, when they provided the energy to x-ray thick castings and other metal sections of equipment used in wartime.

The operation of the betatron is based on the principle that an electron in a changing magnetic field experiences acceleration in a circular orbit (Fig. 15-10).

> The accelerating tube is shaped like a hollow doughnut and is placed between the poles of an alternating current magnet. A pulse of electrons is introduced into this evacuated doughnut by an injector at the instant that the alternating current cycle begins. As the magnetic field rises, the electrons experience acceleration continuously and spin with increasing velocity around the tube. By the end of the first quarter cycle of the alternate magnetic field, the electrons have made several thousand revolutions and achieved maximum energy. At this instant or earlier, depending upon the energy desired, the electrons are made to spiral out of the orbit by an additional force. The high energy electrons then strike a target to produce x-rays or a scattering foil to produce a broad beam of electrons.[1]

One advantage of the betatron is the production of electrons for use with superficial tumors. In addition, x-rays can be used for hard-to-reach tumors at great depths. Betatrons capture and transport a smaller-than-average beam current compared with linear accelerators and are most often used for electron therapy.[17] However, medical betatrons can produce x-ray beams with energies over 40 MV.[22]

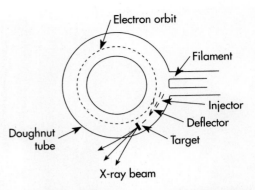

Fig. 15-10 A schematic illustrating the operation of the betatron. (From Khan F: *The physics of radiation therapy*, ed 2, Baltimore, 1994, Williams & Wilkins.)

The betatron generally used Lucite cones of various sizes, ranging from 15 × 15 to 8 × 8 at 100 SSD. Common tumors treated with the betatron included mostly gynecological, bladder, and prostate carcinomas. The treatment times depended on the prescribed dose and diameter of the patient. They usually averaged 3 to 5 minutes and used a dose rate of 200 cGy/minute. To compensate for the characteristically noisy machine, therapists applied cotton balls and ear mufflers for patients wanting some noise reduced during treatments (Fig. 15-11).

Betatrons are suitable for electron production but cannot compare with the x-ray dose rates of a linear accelerator. Linear accelerators are also capable of much larger field sizes and electron therapy energies up to 20 MeV. The bulky and noisy betatrons will most likely continue to diminish in popularity as medicine demands more sophisticated and flexible equipment.

Van de Graaff generator

In 1937 R.J. Van de Graaff, while working at the Massachusetts Institute of Technology, developed the first electrostatic linear accelerator. Accelerators may be circular or linear, and the linear type is electrostatic (such as the **Van de Graaff**) or electronic.[11]

> The Van de Graaff is a constant potential electrostatic generator developed around the physical principle illustrated by the classical Faraday "ice bucket" experiment. The hemispherical high-voltage dome is analogous to the ice bucket (Fig. 15-12). In the ice bucket experiment, electrons deposited inside the electrically conducted metal bucket (presumably used for carrying ice in earlier days) quickly move to the outside. The process can continue until a specified potential is attained or until there is a coronal breakdown of the air outside the bucket.[18]

These 2-MV units have a steel dome of about 3 feet in diameter and 5.5 feet in height and are constucted non-isocentrically. Van de Graaff units use an external blocking tray to hold hand-placed blocks. Because no standard table is

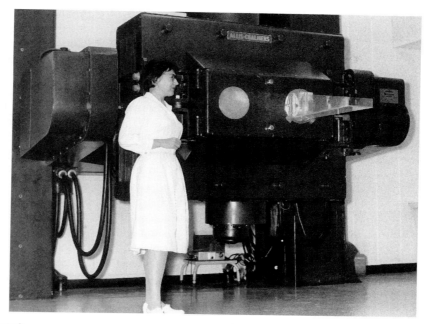

Fig. 15-11 Fig. 15-11 The Allis-Chalmers betatron. (Courtesy M.D. Anderson Cancer Center, Houston, Texas.)

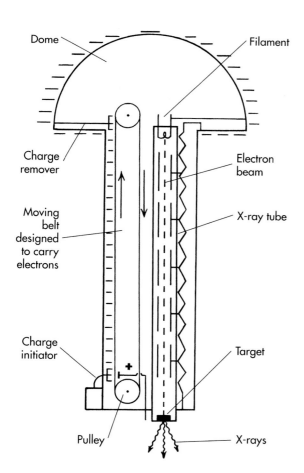

Fig. 15-12 A schematic diagram of the Van de Graaff generator.

affixed to this unit, the patient lies on a stretcher underneath the machine or can even be placed in a chair if necessary. Blocking can be dangerous because blocks frequently require stacking to approximate the treatment area. Van de Graaff units can operate at 200 cGy/minute and provide a standard SSD of 100 cm, but they can also approximate much greater treatment distances. This was extremely useful in the treatment of extended fields needed to treat a variety of malignancies. The Van de Graaff unit (Fig. 15-13) was routinely used to treat seminoma (a lengthy field in the abdomen and pelvis used to treat a type of testicular cancer), whole brain, and mantle field (used to treat lymph nodes in the neck and thorax for Hodgkin's disease).

Arcing was frequent for radiation therapists warming up these units, which could sometimes require as long as 1 hour. When setting up a patient for treatment, the therapist used a front-pointer device to measure the distance to the patient. No optical distance indicator was available.[15] However, the Van de Graaff unit could treat any tumor that other megavoltage equipment could treat. Its bulk made it cumbersome to use, and it was destined to be replaced by the isocentric linear accelerator and cobalt 60 treatment units, which are more popular today.

Proton accelerator

In 1928, E.O. Lawrence developed the cyclotron.[11] A **cyclotron** is a charged particle accelerator used often for nuclear research. Early on, the use of the cyclotron for medical purposes was explored. Its use primarily relates to accel-

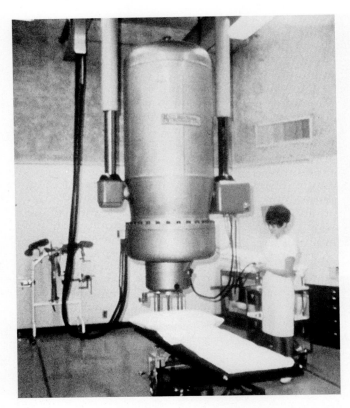

Fig. 15-13 The Van de Graaff unit at the University Hospital in Oklahoma City, Oklahoma, was routinely used to treat seminoma, whole brain, and mantle fields. (Courtesy University Hospital, Oklahoma City, Oklahoma.)

erating protons, neutron beams, light ions, and heavy charged particles used in radiation therapy.[25] In this section, three specific medical uses of the cyclotron are discussed briefly. This includes the production of radionuclides applied primarily in nuclear medicine and the use of neutrons and protons in radiation therapy.

Radionuclides. The cyclotron has been used recently as a particle accelerator for the production of radionuclides used in **positron emission tomography (PET).** This is a scanning technique that involves the systemic administration of a radiopharmaceutical agent labeled with a positron-emitting radionuclide. PET scanners are used in nuclear medicine studies to measure important physiological and biomedical processes such as blood flow, oxygen, glucose and metabolism of free fatty acids, amino acid transport, pH, and neuroreceptor densities. A cyclotron is required to produce radionuclides such as carbon 11, nitrogen 13, and oxygen 15, which all have short half-lives. Today, nuclear medicine PET scanning occurs at over 90 research centers around the world.[3]

Clinical application and characteristics of PET procedure. Unlike conventional radiographic or computed tomography scanners that use x-rays passing through a person, PET scanners use radiation emitted from within the patient to produce images. While the patient is alert and conscious, distinct areas of the brain, for example, can be evaluated in microscopic detail. Patients receive a small amount of a radioactive pharmaceutical agent that closely resembles a substance naturally found in the body (such as sugar). The amount of radiation a patient receives varies with the radiopharmaceutical agent used. The most widely used radionuclides are listed in Fig. 15-14. Oxygen, carbon, and nitrogen are essential atoms to a majority of the body's physiological processes.

PET imaging involves positrons emitted during the breakdown of the nuclei of certain radioisotopes. Pure energy, released as gamma rays, is a result of the collision and subsequent annihilation of matter and antimatter. Radiation from the positron-emitting isotope is detected by the PET scanner and displays in microscopic detail the chemical processes occurring. Two gamma rays of equal energy are produced when a positron meets an electron going in the opposite direction. The information is then delivered into a computer that performs complex algorithms, thus resulting in a detailed picture.[2] PET will probably expand to include the evaluation of patients with malignancy and those with psychiatric illnesses.[7,10]

Although the data strongly support the clinical applications of PET in certain brain and heart disorders, the future of PET will directly relate to reimbursement for these procedures. Other factors relate to the expense of a cyclotron, which can easily approach $1 million and is expensive to install and operate.[3]

The outlook for cyclotrons, PET studies, and clinical applications. The potential of PET imaging in the diagnosis of medical disorders is still being discovered. Cyclotrons are necessary components of a PET facility, mainly because many of the isotopes generated in the cyclotron have such short half-lives. This prohibits the transportation of the isotopes to any nonlocal distance. Most dedicated cyclotrons used in PET imaging are in place solely to produce PET radiopharmaceutical agents. Further advancements in superconducting technology may lead to smaller and more reasonably priced accelerators capable of heavy-particle radiation therapy using protons, neutrons, and heavy ions.

In addition to isotopes used for PET studies, cyclotrons produce the radiopharmaceutical agents used every day in hundreds of nuclear medicine departments for liver, bone, and other valuable diagnostic scans. These pharmaceutical agents include iodine 123, thallium 201, gallium 67, indium 111, and others.[28]

Components of the cyclotron. The cyclotron consists of a short metallic cylinder divided into two sections, which are usually referred to as *Dees,* partly because of their shapes. These Dees are highly evacuated and placed between the poles of a direct-current magnet producing a constant magnetic field. An alternating potential is applied between the two Dees.[18]

Radionuclide	Half-life
Carbon-11	20 min
Nitrogen-13	10 min
Fluorine-18	110 min
Oxygen-15	2 min
Gallium-68	68 min
Rubidium-82	1.3 min

Fig. 15-14 Chart of radionuclides used in PET studies. (From *J Nuclear Med* 32[1]:26N, 1991.)

An RF oscillator applies a high RF voltage to the dees. The voltage gradient in the gap between the dees reverses each time the dee polarities change. Inside each dee there is no electric field, but a particle is still subject to the magnet's field and therefore travels in a circular path. When the particle reaches the gap, it accelerates through the electric potential between the dees, and then coasts in a circular path through the other dee. By the time the particle has traveled 180 degrees, the oscillator has reversed the dee's polarity, so again, the particle accelerates through the gap. At each acceleration the radius of the orbit increases, so the particle spirals outward. The particles' final energy is the sum of the energy gained at each gap crossing.[20]

The machine does not have unlimited energy potential because of the theory of relativity. According to this theory, further acceleration causes the particle to gain mass. This increase in weight causes the particle to slow down, thus ultimately causing the particle to be out of sync with the frequency of the alternate potential applied to the dee. This phenomenon is the reason electrons cannot accelerate in a cyclotron.[20]

Neutrons. As mentioned earlier, the cyclotron has been used not only for nuclear physics research, but also to produce particles for clinical usage. To produce neutron beams, deuterons (2/1 H+) are accelerated to high energies and then forced to strike a suitable target (usually beryllium), thus producing neutrons (subatomic particles equal in mass to protons but without electrical charge) via nuclear reactions. Because neutrons possess no electric charge, they are extremely effective in penetrating nuclei and producing reactions by a process termed *stripping*.[11] Fast neutrons were first used by Stone in 1938. Unacceptable late complications, mostly in fatty tissue in the patients treated, caused the study to be abandoned. These complications were due to the high concentration of hydrogen in the fatty tissue.[22]

Partly because of their inferior depth doses, neutrons are not used as much as protons in radiation therapy. One program that has used neutrons in clinical practice is the M.D. Anderson Cancer Center located in Houston, Texas. This center's cyclotron (a negative ion machine built by the Cyclotron Corporation) generated a neutron beam by using a 42-MV beam impinging on a 6-mm-thick beryllium target. The primary neutron beam was flattened with Teflon filters and hardened with a 3.3-cm thickness of polyethylene.[14]

The unit provided a treatment distance of 125-cm SSD and used a set of collimators of fixed field sizes ranging from 4 × 4 to 20 × 20 cm. Extremely awkward and heavy external cones were the norms, as were Teflon wedges, which shaped the radiation field and created wedged isodose curves. Modification of the field sizes occurred with tungsten blocks that were 3 HVL thick (7.5 cm) in the direction of beam axis. This cyclotron was capable of sending a beam into two separate treatment rooms.[20]

Clinical application of fast neutrons. In the 1930s, when Stone undertook fast-neutron radiation therapy, a vast majority of long-term survivors experienced severe radiation side effects in the normal tissue surrounding the tumor sites. Many patients suffered from extremely high doses of radiation because of lack of information concerning relative biological effectiveness (RBE) values. Clinical trials resumed in the 1960s at Hammersmith Hospital in London. Hundreds of patients with advanced disease achieved good responses to therapy. Because of the success of these trials, clinical trials with fast neutrons increased in popularity throughout the world. A few of the centers that conducted patient treatments in the United States were the M.D. Anderson Cancer Center; the University of Washington; the Manta facility at George Washington University in Washington, DC; the Glanta facility in Cleveland, Ohio; and the Fermi laboratory in Bactavia, Illinois.

The trials conducted on patients from the late 1970s to mid 1980s suffered from physical limitations of physics laboratory-based machines of the era. These limitations included (1) poor depth-dose characteristics; (2) poor skin sparing; (3) fixed horizontal treatment beams; (4) inadequate collimation, beam-film capabilities, and treatment simulation; (5) difficult logistics; and (6) frequent accelerator breakdown.

Beginning in the mid 1980s, high-energy, isocentric neutron therapy systems in hospitals performed patient treatment. They could deliver dose distributions comparable to conventional megavoltage equipment. Disease sites treated with neutrons have included brain tumors (glioblastoma multiforme), squamous cell carcinoma of the head and neck, salivary gland tumors, lung cancer, prostate tumors, and soft-tissue sarcomas. Since 1992, approximately 10,000 patients worldwide have undergone neutron therapy.[22]

Protons. A proton is a positively charged particle in the nucleus of all atoms that relates to the atomic number of the atoms. One of the earliest proton-producing, hospital-based cyclotrons was installed in 1949 at the Harvard Cyclotron Laboratory in collaboration with Massachusetts General

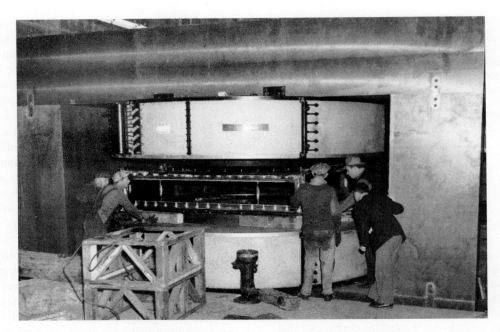

Fig. 15-15 Construction of the 160-MeV synchrocyclotron at the Cyclotron Laboratory at Harvard University in 1947. Several workers are inspecting the coils, yoke, and dee. Although it was originally designed for physics research, the unit has treated thousands of patients with proton beams since 1961. (Courtesy Cyclotron Laboratory, Harvard University, Cambridge, Massachusetts.)

Hospital and the Massachusetts Eye and Ear Infirmary (Fig. 15-15). A brief description of the production of protons at the Harvard cyclotron is presented to provide a basic understanding of the complex process of a proton accelerator (in this case a sychrocyclotron):

In order to produce a usable beam of protons, we start with hydrogen gas. The basic unit, or atom, of hydrogen is composed of one proton and one electron. We strip off the electrons by subjecting the hydrogen gas to an electric current, which leaves us with an abundant supply of protons. These protons are then subjected to both an oscillating electric field which accelerates them up to about 1/2 the speed of light (approximately 300,000,000 miles/hour) and to a strong magnetic field which keeps them contained in an ever-widening spiral configuration. At the end of each cycle (which takes 3/1000 of a second) the protons are channeled off into a beam pipe which then leads into the treatment area. By using several magnets placed at various points along this beam pipe, the final proton beam attains a diameter about the size of a pencil and an intensity of some 109 protons/cm2/sec (that's 1,000,000,000 protons hitting an area about 1/2 inch square in one second's time).[6]

Proton radiation has proved effective in the treatment of benign and malignant lesions.[27] In 1961, under the direction of Dr. Raymond Kjellberg, the proton beam irradiated benign tumors of the pituitary gland. The program grew to include the treatment of arteriovenous malformations. Almost 3000 patients have received a single high dose of radiation to a small, precise area with satisfactory results since the program ended in 1993.[26] Today, over 6000 patients have received treatment to a variety of sites, including ocular melanoma; soft-tissue and bone sarcomas; and prostate, head and neck, and other miscellaneous and metastatic tumors. Plans are underway to complete a new proton accelerator with a rotational gantry in the Boston area by 1998. Several other new facilities for proton and ion therapy have been proposed worldwide. Table 15-1 describes current and proposed clinical programs using a variety of charged particles for the treatment of benign and malignant disease.

Protons are a valuable tool for clinical use for the following reasons: (1) They are precision-controlled; (2) scattering is minimal compared with that from x-rays, neutrons, and cobalt radiation; (3) they have a characteristic distribution of dose with depth; and (4) most of their energy is deposited near the end of their range, where the dose peaks to a high value and then drops rapidly to zero. This sudden change in dose distribution with depth is called the **Bragg peak**. Fig. 15-16 illustrates the Bragg peak and compares two proton beams with a 10-MV x-ray beam. These reasons helped establish proton therapy as the treatment of choice for lesions close to sensitive areas of the body.[26]

| Table 15-1 | Current and proposed clinical programs using protons for the treatment of benign and malignant disease* |

Facility	Location	Type	Energy	Date of first treatment
Harvard	Massachusetts	Synchrocyclotron	160 MeV	1961
Moscow	Russia	Synchrotron	200 MeV	1969
St. Petersberg	Russia	Synchrocyclotron	1000 MeV	1975
Chiba	Japan	Cyclotron	70 MeV	1979
PMRC, Tsukuba	Japan	Synchrotron	500 MeV	1983
PSI (SIN)	Switzerland	Cyclotron	72 MeV	1984
Dubna	Russia	Synchrocyclotron	660 MeV	1987
Uppsala	Sweden	Synchrocyclotron	180 MeV	1989
Clatterbridge	England	Cyclotron	62 MeV	1989
Loma Linda	California	Synchrotron	250 MeV	1990
Louvain-la-Neuve	Belgium	Cyclotron	90 MeV	1991
Nice	France	Cyclotron	65 MeV	1991
Orsay	France	Synchrocyclotron	200 MeV	1991
N.A.C.	South Africa	Cyclotron	200 MeV	1993
Indiana Cyclotron	Indiana	Cyclotron	200 MeV	1993
UC Davis	California	Cyclotron	70 MeV	1994
P.S.I.	Switzerland	—	200 MeV	1994†
TRIUMF	Canada	Cyclotron	520 MeV	1994†
Berlin	Germany	Cyclotron	72 MeV	1995†
Munich	Germany	—	64 MeV	1995?†
ITEP, Moscow	Russia	—	—	1996†
Julich (KFA)	Germany	—	—	1997†
KVI Groningen	Netherlands	—	200 MeV	1997?†
NPTC, Harvard	Massachusetts	New facility	—	1998†
NC Star	North Carolina	Synchrotron	70-300 MeV	1999?†
Novosibirsk	Russia	—	180-200 MeV	?†
PDNA	Illinois	Private facility	250 MeV	?†
Clatterbridge	England	Upgrade	—	?†
Tsukuba	Japan	—	230 MeV	?†
Krakow	Poland	—	60 MeV	?†

Courtesy Janet Sisterson, Harvard Cyclotron Laboratory, Cambridge, Mass.
*This information is taken in part from *Particles* (vol 15, 1995), a biannual newsletter published for those interested in proton, light-ion, and heavy-charged-particle radiation therapy, vol 15, 1995.
†Proposed programs.

Before treatment begins, a great deal of preparation is necessary. Patient positioning and immobilization are essential. Necessary pieces of equipment include various immobilization devices, an aperture (a 5-cm-thick brass cutout with a custom-shaped opening determined by the tumor volume [Fig. 15-17]), a modulator, and often a Lucite bolus compensator. The aperture has a purpose similar to custom-shielding blocks used with x-rays and gamma rays. With a compensator (a milled block of plastic carved out to various depths [Fig. 15-18]) and modulator, the aperture controls the distance protons penetrate (Fig. 15-19). A spinning, circular Lucite modulator is positioned in the treatment beam to spread out the Bragg peak over a greater distance. This allows a larger volume of tissue to be irradiatied because the treatment depth can be precisely controlled (Fig. 15-16).

The treatments take approximately 2 minutes, but the setup time may vary from 30 minutes to 1 hour. Large fractions are usually given to extremely precise tumor volumes for which accuracy in millimeters is crucial. For example, a modulated proton beam can be directed to a tumor surrounding the brain stem and stopped within millimeters. As many as three localization films (taken from separate angles by using three x-ray tubes) are compared and evaluated with the simulation radiographs before each treatment is delivered. Positioning the patient is a challenge because the proton beam is stationary. The patient needs to be positioned relative to the beam. Therefore many patients are treated in the sitting position. Large-field and small-field ocular melanoma treatments have been treated with good results at the Harvard Cyclotron Laboratory since 1974 and 1975, respectively.

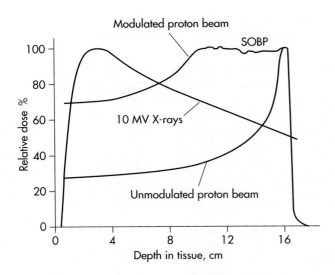

Fig. 15-16 Depth-dose curves showing a Bragg peak (unmodulated) for a monoenergetic 160-MeV proton beam and an example of a modulated or spread-out Bragg peak (SOBP). Included for comparison is a depth dose curve for a 10-MeV x-ray beam. (Courtesy LJ Verhey and J Munzenrider, Boston.)

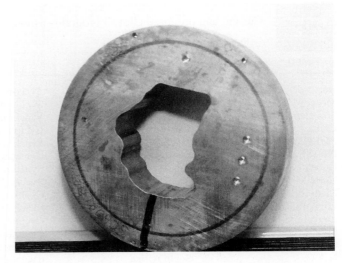

Fig. 15-17 A brass aperture similar to custom-shielding blocks used with a linear accelerator is constructed individually for each patient treated with protons. This aperature measures about 8 cm in diameter and 5 cm in thickness and shapes the beam to conform to the tumor volume.

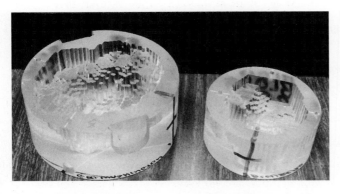

Fig. 15-18 The Lucite bolus compensator, which is a milled circular piece of plastic, is used to even the dose distribution of the proton beam because of variations in tissue thickness and density.

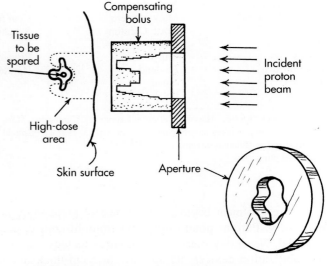

Fig. 15-19 A cross section of a beam-defining aperture and compensating bolus, used with a high-energy proton beam, shape the proton beam. (Courtesy Janet Sisterson, Harvard Cyclotron Laboratory, Cambridge, Mass.)

REMOTE AFTERLOADING
Historical perspective

Radiation exposure to staff members is still a concern in the application of brachytherapy isotopes used in radiation therapy. However, with low- or high-dose remote afterloading, radiation exposure is dramatically reduced. In the early days of brachytherapy an active radioisotope was preloaded in an applicator before being placed in a patient. Radium (the most common isotope used then) was sealed in a platinum tube, which sometimes bent or broke. Because radium has an extremely long half-life of 1620 years, a compromise of the tube presented a major radiation-safety problem. In the 1950s, afterloading applicators were developed. This allowed dummy sources to be evaluated radiographically for their proper position before the actual sources were loaded, thus reducing exposure to personnel. Cesium 137 began to substitute for radium during this time, mainly because of its shorter physical half-life of 30 years. Developments of new applicators (including the Fletcher-Suite, Henschke, and Ter-Pogossian instruments) also occurred.[24] Many radionuclides commonly used in radiation therapy are listed in Fig. 15-20.

Radionuclide	Half-life	Proton energy (MeV)	Half-value layer (mm lead)	Exposure rate constant Rcm²/mCLh
^{225}Ra *Radium*	1600 years (0.83 avg)	0.047-2.45	8.0	8.25*†
^{222}Rn	3.83 days (0.83 avg)	0.047-2.45	8.0	Rcm²/Ci-h 10.15*†
^{60}Co *Cobalt 60*	5.26 years	1.17, 1.33	11.0	13.07‡
^{137}Cs *Cessium*	30.0 years	0.662	5.5	3.26‡
^{192}Ir *Iridium 192*	74.2 days (0.38 avg)	0.136-1.06	2.5	4.69‡
^{198}Au *Gold*	2.7 days	0.412	2.5	2.38‡
^{125}I *Iodine 125*	60.2 days	0.028 avg	0.025	1.46‡

*In equilibrium with daughter products.
†Filtered by 0.5 mm Pt.
‡Unfiltered.

Fig. 15-20 A chart of radionuclides used in brachytherapy. (From Khan F: *The physics of radiation therapy,* ed 2, Baltimore, 1994, Williams & Wilkins.)

Pioneers and the arrival of remote afterloading

Rolf Sievert, in an attempt to further decrease radiation exposure by performing manual source handling through mechanical means, is credited with developing the idea of remote afterloading. Ulrich Henschke of Memorial Sloan Kettering Cancer Center in New York and Basil Hilaris developed a high-dose-rate remote-afterloading system in 1964. The Catheton, using cobalt 60 pellets, was developed in 1963 and became popular in the European market. Other varieties include the cesium 137 Curietron and iridium 192 Buchler. A newer model, the Selectron, demonstrated a higher level of dose optimization not realized with radium, cesium, or cobalt pellets. One disadvantage of using iridium is that the source needs replacing every 3 months because of the short 74-day half-life of iridium 192.[24]

High dose rate and low dose rate

Parameters for **low-dose-rate (LDR) brachytherapy** versus **high-dose-rate (HDR) brachytherapy** are established in several ways. International Commission on Radiation Units and Measurement (ICRU) report 38 sets the range for LDR at 40 to 200 cGy per hour, a middle range at 200 to 1200 cGy per hour, and HDR at greater than 1200 cGy per hour or more than 20 cGy per minute. Brachytherapy sources such as iridium, cesium, cobalt, and radium are usually administered at dose rates of 50 to 500 cGy per minute. This rate commonly parallels that of a linear accelerator.[24]

Clinical considerations. Several important clinical considerations affect the decision to convert an established low-dose-rate brachytherapy program to one using HDR. Advantages for the high-dose-rate system are as follows: (1) Treatment can be given on an outpatient basis; (2) treatment time is extremely short compared with that of an LDR system; (3) with this short treatment time the implant repro-

ducibility is more precise than with manual systems; (4) complete radiation protection exists for staff members; (5) no general anesthesia or bed rest, which decreases complications, is needed; (6) the system has the ability to treat a large clinical patient volume; (7) individualized treatment can be done with source optimization; and (8) an increased level of comfort exists for the patient.[23]

LDR and HDR systems can improve dose distribution through multiple dwell positions. Optimum tumor dose distribution can be achieved while the normal tissue exposure is minimized. The danger of afterload applicators shifting in the pelvis, for example, during the several days usually involved in low-dose-rate treatment can negatively affect dose distribution. In HDR therapy the instruments are secured into place after the desirable position is attained. Packing or retracting protects the vaginal wall, bladder, and rectum over the several minutes of actual treatment time. A disadvantage of HDR therapy is that treatment plan changes are difficult to make before the treatment is completed because the time of treatment is several minutes instead of several days as with LDR. HDR is extremely labor intensive because it requires a complement of physicists, dosimetrists, therapists, nurses, and physicians for each insertion.[24]

Radiobiology of high dose rate

Careful consideration of biological effects must be included in the decision to move from LDR to HDR brachytherapy. HDR rates can be high enough that the exposure can be less than the repair half-time of sublethal damage (sometimes shorter than 2 hours). Ideally, the duration of an exposure does not exceed a small portion of the repair time for sublethal radiation injury (i.e., a few minutes).[24]

A successful compromise between radiobiological considerations, patient convenience, and staffing realities is defined by persons at the University of Wisconsin, who routinely combine HDR brachytherapy with teletherapy. Four fractions of external-beam therapy are given at a rate of 1.7 Gy per fraction per week. This is coupled with one HDR insertion per week for a total of five HDR fractions.[24] Patient comfort is a definite advantage of HDR over LDR. Before the procedure, the patient cannot eat or drink for 8 to 12 hours before the treatment time.

In the treatment of a head and neck tumor, for example, several preparatory procedures are necessary. Intravenous access is obtained after the patient's arrival to give the physician easy access for medications that may be required during the procedure. An endoscopic nurse helps the patient gargle and spray the nostrils with a special solution to numb that region in anticipation of scope insertion. The scope guides the catheter to the tumor site at which the radiation is directed. During the procedure the patient's heart and pulse are monitored, and oxygen is administered through the nostrils. An x-ray machine is positioned over the patient's head for localization purposes. After the scope is in place, a smaller tube (called a *catheter*) passes through the scope before scope removal. The scope is secured with tape, and then a radiograph is taken to verify position. The patient is moved from the examination room to the treatment room. The catheter, connected by tubing to the HDR unit, transports the appropriate radiation sources (Fig. 15-21). After the treatment is finished and the source secured, the patient is taken to the recovery room for usually less than 1 hour.[17] This is a typical HDR application for a tumor in the head and neck region.

HDR brachytherapy has been used successfully to treat tumors of the brain, esophagus, and rectum; tumors obstructing the biliary system; and gynecological cancers (most notably, cervical carcinoma). Further work is needed to identify radiobiological differences of this therapy compared with conventional LDR interstitial and intracavitary techniques.

SUMMARY

Ionizing radiation (in one form or another) has been used in the treatment of cancer almost from the time x-rays and radium were discovered. The equipment and competencies of the staff members involved in the quality delivery of patient treatments have undergone and will undergo continuous changes to keep pace with increasingly sophisticated treatment regimes. Historically, equipment evolved from low-energy, low-skin-sparing, unsophisticated systems (such as orthovoltage units) to today's computerized, megavoltage linear accelerators and cobalt 60 units that can treat a variety of deep-seated tumors. New protocols are being formulated to reflect the enormous capabilities of radiation oncology equipment. The goal is to spare more normal tissue and deliver higher doses to the actual tumor volume. This will hopefully result in decreased morbidity and increased cure rates.

Many changes are yet to come concerning protons, PET studies, and remote afterloading that mirror the changing health care environment as much as the patient's needs. These changes will directly affect whether cyclotrons become realistic to operate and whether high-dose remote afterloading can rightly replace LDR facilities or become a practical boost alternative on a grander scale.

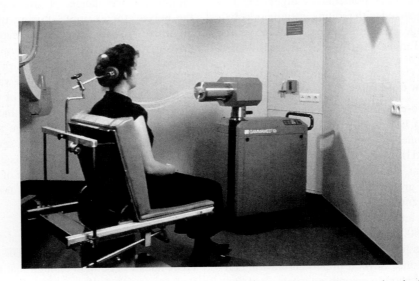

Fig. 15-21 A remote afterloading system used to store and deliver high-dose-rate brachytherapy sources. Sources are delivered via a catheter located in the center of this portable device. Treatment time is generally in the range of minutes. (Courtesy Gammamed and Frank Barker Associates, Pequannock, NJ.)

Review Questions

Fill in the Blank

1. Two major clinical limitations of kilovoltage units are _____ and _____.
2. Neutrons are not used as much as protons in radiation therapy, primarily because of their _____ _____ _____ depth dose.
3. A 1- to 6-mm-thick _____ is inserted in a slot in the treatment head of superficial units to harden the beam to the desired degree.
4. The _____ is used to accelerate neutrons and protrons in the treatment of cancer patients.
5. The operation of the betratron is based on the principle that an electron in a changing _____ _____ experiences acceleration in a circular orbit.

Multiple Choice

6. Which of the following does not relate to beam quality?
   a. Penumbra
   b. kVp
   c. Central-axis depth dose
   d. mA
7. Which of the following is considered an electrostatic linear accelerator?
   a. Betatron
   b. Van de Graaff
   c. Cyclotron
   d. All of the above

8. Protons are a valuable tool for clinical use for all except which of the following reasons?
   a. They have a characteristic distribution of dose with depth
   b. Scattering is minimal compared with x-rays, neutrons, or cobalt radiation
   c. Their energy range is similar to that of x-rays
   d. None of the above
9. Which of the following units lacked an optical distance indicator?
   a. Van de Graaff
   b. Linear accelerator
   c. Cobalt
   d. None of the above

Matching

10. Neutrons _____
11. Dees _____
12. Proton _____
13. Bragg peak _____
14. mA _____
    a. A positively charged particle that is a basic component in the nucleus of atoms
    b. A measurement of electric current
    c. A sharp maximum in the dose-distribution curve of a charged particle occurring at a particular depth
    d. A short, metallic cylinder divided into two sections in a cyclotron
    e. A subatomic particle equal in mass to a proton but without an electric charge

Questions to Ponder

1. List and discuss three specific medical uses of the cyclotron.
2. Describe and compare the production of a radiographic image that uses a PET and CT scanner.
3. Discuss the application and use of the contact, superficial, and orthovoltage treatment units in radiation therapy.
4. Briefly explain the reason a clinical radiation facility may consider switching from an LDR to HDR brachytherapy program.
5. Discuss the relationship of HVL and selection of an appropriate treatment beam.

REFERENCES

1. Ames JC: Personal communication, January 18, 1994.
2. Applied Research, Triumf: *Pet scanner.* Internal Publication, Canada, July 1992.
3. Bernier DR, Christian PE, Langan JK: *Nuclear medicine technology and techniques,* ed 3, St Louis, 1994, Mosby.
4. Bogardus C Jr: Personal communication, June 5, 1994.
5. Bushong SC: *Radiologic science for technologists: physics, biology, and protection,* ed 4, St Louis, 1988, Mosby.
6. Coggeshall A, Johnson K, Sisterson J: *HCL: the Harvard Cyclotron Laboratory,* Cambridge, Mass, 1987, Harvard Cyclotron Laboratory.
7. Coleman E et al: The future of positron emission tomography in clinical medicine and the impact of drug regulation, *Semin Nucl Med* 22(3):193-200, July 1992.
8. Edwards IK Jr, Edwards EK, Edwards SR: Grenz ray therapy, commentary, *Int J Dermatol* 29:17-18, January-February 1990.
9. Falco-Braun O, Schultze U: Contact radiotherapy of cutaneous hermangiomas *Arch Dermatol Res* 253-254:237-246, 1975.
10. Freeman L, Blaufaro DM: Letters from the editors, *Semin Nucl Med* 22(3):1-2, July 1992.
11. Grigg FRN: *The trail of the invisible light: from x-olyahlen to radio (bio)logy,* Springfield, Ill, 1965, Charles C Thomas.
12. Hansen WF: The changing role of the accelerator in radiation therapy, *IEEE Trans Nucl Sci* 30(2):1781-1783, April 1983.
13. Herbel L: Personal communication, June 14, 1994.
14. Horton JL, Otte VA, Schultheiss TE: Physical characteristics of the M.D. Anderson Hospital clinical neutron beam, *Radiother Oncol* 13:17-22, 1988.
15. Ingram J: Personal communication, May 11, 1994.
16. Johns HE, Cunningham JR: *The physics of radiology,* ed 4, Springfield, Ill, 1983, Charles C Thomas.
17. Jordan LN, Buck SS: A teaching booklet for patients receiving high dose rate brachytherapy, *Oncol Nurs Forum* 18(7):1235-1238, 1991.
18. Khan FM: *The physics of radiation therapy,* Baltimore, 1994, Williams and Wilkins.
19. Klevehagen SC, Thaites DI: *Radiotherapy physics in practice,* Oxford, England, 1993, Oxford University Press.
20. Mallory MI: Personal communication, January 18, 1994.
21. Papillon J: *Rectal and anal cancers: conservative treatment by irradiation: an alternative to surgery,* Berlin, 1982, Springer-Verlag.
22. Perez CA, Brady LW: *Principles and practice of radiation oncology,* ed 2, Philadelphia, 1992, JB Lippincott.
23. Speiser B: Advantages of high dose rate remote afterloading systems: physics or biology, *Int J Radiat Oncol Biol Phys* 20:1133-1135, 1991.
24. Stitt JA: High-dose-rate intracavitary brachytherapy for gynecologic malignancies, *Oncology,* 49:59-70, January 1992.
25. Suit H, Vrie M: Review, proton beams in radiation therapy, *J Natl Cancer Inst* 84(3):159, February 1992.
26. Travers M: Personal communicaton, May 5, 1994.
27. Verhey LJ, Munzenrider JE: Proton beam therapy, *Ann Rev Biophys Bioengin* 11:331-357, 1982.
28. Winn J: Personal communication, May 10, 1994.

16

Treatment Procedures

Annette Coleman

Outline

Key terms

Beam modifiers
Bolus
Carfusion
Collimation
Compensators
Critical structures
Daily treatment record
Elapsed days
Electron shields
Electronic portal imaging devices
Feathering
Fractionation
Gaps
Hinge angle
Immobilization devices
Interlocks
Isocenter

Isodose lines
Localization
Penumbra
Portal verification
Positioning devices
Protraction
Quality-assurance (QA) program
Random errors
Shielding blocks
Systematic errors
Target volume
Transmission filters
Treatment console
Treatment field
Treatment number
Treatment technique
Universal precautions
Wedges

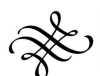

Grounded in the planning, simulation, and administration of a prescribed course of radiation therapy, the professional practice of radiation therapy is a primary component of quality oncologic care.[1] Conscientious attention to precision in simulation and treatment administration and to the physiological and psychological needs of patients highlights the radiation therapist's contributions to the cancer-management team.

Maintenance of quality patient care requires knowledge in a variety of basic science and patient care principles and an understanding of and respect for the legal considerations of practice. Successful coordination of individual patient treatments in the context of a varied patient load requires the application of well-developed organizational and communication skills.

As members of the treatment team, radiation therapists contribute to the achievement of goals of the **quality-assurance (QA) program**. The QA program (see Volume II, Unit I, Chapter 5) consists of activities and documentation performed with the goal of optimizing patient care. Primarily dependent on the written records of each member of the treatment team, computerized patient-monitoring systems are rapidly becoming integrated into the fabric of radiation oncology QA. These systems monitor and document experiences of the patient with the department, including past treatments, current treatment-plan delivery, scheduling, and billing. The radiation therapist's primary role in the QA program is to ensure accuracy in the delivery of the radiation-treatment plan as prescribed by a radiation oncologist. This requires reviewing patient records, monitoring the functioning of radiation-producing equipment, maintaining accuracy in the reproduction of treatment parameters, monitoring changes in patient status, and maintaining complete and accurate treatment records. The radiation therapist communicates with the radiation oncology team through activities such as weekly chart reviews and through maintaining open verbal lines of communication. Because their participation in QA activities is integral to the accomplishment of program goals, radiation therapists are represented on the departmental QA committee.[7,12]

Conventional external-beam radiation therapy is accomplished through the use of technically advanced linear accelerators producing high-energy x-ray beams or isotopic units that house radioactive cobalt 60 (^{60}Co) sources. These machines are engineered to facilitate the precise application of radiation beams to well-defined treatment volumes. The goal of radiation therapy treatment planning is to deliver an evenly distributed radiation dose to the **target volume** (area of known and presumed tumors) while minimizing the dose to surrounding normal tissue. To achieve this, the majority of treatment plans require treatment with more than one field. Areas in which treatment beams overlap receive an increased radiation dose relative to areas that receive radiation from only one field. (For a detailed discussion of radiation dose distribution, see Volume II, Unit III, Chapter 12.) Modern treatment units are installed with the ability to rotate around a fixed point. This point, or **isocenter,** is the point of intersection of the three axes of rotation (gantry, collimator, and base of couch) of the treatment unit (see Volume I, Unit II, Chapters 13 and 14 for descriptions of isocentric-treatment units). Precision in the reproduction of the treatment plan is facilitated by the ability to direct multiple treatment fields to a constant point in the tumor without repositioning the patient.

Advances in imaging and treatment-planning computers encourage continued development in the precise planning of external-beam radiation treatments. With increasing confidence the physician, dosimetrist, and radiation therapist can focus beams to the target volume while minimizing the radiation delivered to surrounding normal tissues. Record and verification systems communicate with the treatment unit to check and document the reproduction of treatment-unit parameters for individual patients. The clinical significance of these technical advances, however, will always be limited by the ability to translate them to the patient. Unfortunately, accuracy in the reproduction of treatment-volume **localization** (identification of internal anatomy relative to surface landmarks) has not increased at the same rate.[11] Precision in the reproduction and immobilization of the treatment position, stability of surface landmarks, and exactitude in alignment of light fields with these landmarks contribute greatly to variation in daily treatment delivery and thus represent the greatest obstacle to the application of advances in treatment planning. Management of these factors is also the radiation therapist's primary technical challenge.

Accurate treatment delivery depends on the needs of the patient and the specialized knowledge and skills of the radiation therapist in the operation of equipment. The ability to reproduce daily treatment setups depends on abilities and limitations imposed by the equipment and geometry of the treatment beam and by the patient.

Daily patient treatment constitutes the foundation of the practice of radiation therapy. Proficiency in technical and patient care skills and a knowledge base in oncology, treatment planning, physics, and radiation biology are prerequisite to the formation of good clinical judgment. These are primary characteristics of the professional practice of the radiation therapist. The development of an action plan in the approach to treatment delivery assists the radiation therapist in ensuring thoroughness. A task analysis (outline of tasks) provides a simple method for organizing a plan of action (see the box).

TREATMENT CHART

Separate from the individual's medical chart, the treatment chart remains in the radiation oncology department as a record of the patient's radiation therapy history. It is the legal document of the patient's radiation treatment. Therefore its completeness, organization, and legibility are critical. Each page must clearly identify the patient by name and hospital identification number. The radiation therapist recognizes the ethical and legal responsibility to maintain the patient's privacy and right to confidentiality of medical records.

Quality-management programs require that the treatment chart include information regarding the patient's history, including a diagnostic evaluation, rationale for treatment, detailed description of the treatment plan, and documentation of informed consent and the treatment delivered.[5,7,12] Individual departments may identify specific documentation

Task Analysis of Treatment Procedures

1. Review the chart.
2. Prepare the room.
3. Identify and prepare the patient.
4. Assist the patient onto a treatment table and locate surface landmarks.
5. Raise the couch, thus bringing the patient to correct source-skin distance (SSD).
6. Refine the patient position relative to the isocenter by using lasers.
7. Align the field light to surface landmarks.
8. Position beam-shaping accessories (blocks) and verify by using the light field.
9. Position beam modifiers (wedge, compensator, and bolus).
10. Inform the patient you are leaving and treatment will begin.
11. Monitor the patient.
12. Set appropriate machine controls and review the record and verification system.
13. Initiate the beam-on setting and monitor patient and equipment function.

When multiple fields are to be treated, do the following:

14. Enter the room and check the patient and field position.
15. Rotate to the next field and repeat steps 6 through 13 for all fields at the completion of treatment.
16. Assist the patient from the couch and room.
17. Complete a daily treatment record.
18. Prepare the room for the next patient.

procedures demonstrating these requirements and quality-control procedures to verify their internal compliance. Normally, the radiation therapist does not begin treatment if any of this information is unavailable.

Rationale for and documentation of treatment

The rationale for radiation treatment includes a written patient history documenting the results of diagnostic and staging procedures. Before receiving treatment, patients must receive an explanation of their status, treatment alternatives, and consequences associated with and without treatment. This information must be presented in a manner that is understandable to the patient.[5] As the patient advocate, the radiation therapist verifies that departmental procedures are followed in regard to the receipt of documentation ensuring informed consent.

The physician also documents patient progress during and after the course of treatment. Notes from weekly on-treatment visits, records of the patient's weight, blood counts, and other indicators of treatment response are maintained. Other members of the treatment team such as nurses, nutritionists, and social workers may also contribute in this area.

Treatment record

The information necessary for the reproduction of the course of treatment by a qualified professional must include the patient's identification, a signed prescription, treatment-planning data, and the daily treatment record.[5,12] The daily treatment record documents the delivery of treatments, administration of daily and cumulative doses, use of portal films, and implementation of prescribed changes.

Before initiating daily treatment, the radiation therapist performs a review of the treatment section of the chart. A photograph of the patient should be included, thus providing a visual identification for caregivers. The treatment prescription, detailed patient- and equipment-positioning information, dosimetric plans, and calculations must be reviewed for completeness and accuracy. Any changes in the treatment plan must also be identified.

The chart review includes a check to verify the accuracy of previous entries. The most common charting errors are those of addition, and any corrections must leave the original entry legible. One line is drawn through the entry, followed by the correction, initials of the correcting individual, and the date. Because the chart is the primary document referenced in litigation processes, changes must be legible and accompanied by reasonable explanations. The use of correction fluid and other correction methods that hide original entries are viewed with suspicion and must therefore be avoided.

The treatment chart is the primary record of radiation delivery to the patient, but with the use of record and verification systems, this is changing. Radiation therapists will soon see the emergence of the paperless radiation oncology department. Until then, the accurate recording of an individual's radiation treatment depends on the conscientiousness and integrity of the radiation therapist.

Prescription

Radiation may be delivered only under the direct order of the radiation oncologist. Similar to drug and other therapies, orders are written as prescriptions that must be signed by the radiation oncologist before the initiation of radiation treatment. No exceptions are allowed. The prescription must provide specific information to allow its interpretation by other qualified professionals, including the radiation therapist. The anatomical site and total radiation dose to be delivered with its **fractionation*** and **protraction†** schedule must be clearly stated. The prescription also identifies the **treatment technique‡** to be applied.[5] Information specifying beam energy, portal sizes and entry angles, and beam modifiers may be included in the prescription and with patient-positioning information. The physician's signature and date must accompany any changes in the prescription or treatment plan.

*Individual treatment doses.
†The time over which the total dose is to be delivered.
‡The number and orientation of treatment fields.

The radiation therapist must immediately review the prescription before the delivery of each treatment fraction. Changes in the treatment plan may be made anytime during the course of treatment, and the radiation therapist is responsible for ensuring that changes are implemented as ordered. Common changes include fractionation and total dose, or the addition or deletion of a bolus or blocks.

Isodose distributions and monitor-unit calculations prepared by the dosimetrist are included in the review of the treatment plan. All calculations should be reviewed and signed by at least two members of the treatment-planning team. Before treatment, the radiation therapist ensures the accuracy of the calculation. Field sizes, beam modifiers, and treatment depths must match those identified on the daily treatment setup instructions.

As the dispenser of the radiation prescription, the radiation therapist accepts a great responsibility. Radiation therapists must be knowledgeable of the effects of radiation on their patients, tumor-lethal doses, and limits of radiation tolerance for normal tissue. Prescriptions appearing to exceed these limits or deviate from standard practice should be reviewed with the physician before their implementation. Care must be taken to eliminate any errors and the delivery of unsafe treatment.

Treatment description and simulator instructions

The radiation therapist reviews the treatment description to ensure the availability of sufficient information for treatment-plan reproduction before the initiation of the treatment. If a record and verification system is in place, written information must be checked against parameters on the computer. Instructions include descriptive information with diagrams and/or photographs illustrating patient positioning and immobilization. Surface landmarks used to localize* the target volume must also be clearly identified. If adjustments have been made to the original information, they must be clearly identified, signed, and dated by the radiation therapist and reported to proper authorities.

Each **treatment field,** or portal, is assigned a number and described relative to the anatomical site and direction that it enters the body (Fig. 16-1). Field numbers are assigned only once to each patient, and new treatment fields are numbered sequentially as they are added to the patient record. The field description must include the field size,† angle of entry, and **beam modifiers‡** to be used. Subletters may be used to denote changes in the field size or shape from the original field. Changes involving beam direction or the placement of the isocenter generally are identified as *new treatment fields.*

*To identify a hidden structure relative to observable or palpable surface landmarks.
† Portal dimensions are identified in centimeters, width by length.
‡Devices that change the shape of the treatment field or distribution of the radiation at depth.

Daily treatment record

The treatment plan and prescription direct the treatment, and the **daily treatment record** documents the course of its implementation. An inspection of the daily treatment record directs each subsequent treatment. Records for individual treatments identify the date of treatment, **treatment number** (number of treatments delivered), and **elapsed days** (total time over which treatment is protracted). The daily and total dose delivered must also be included. The radiation therapist records the radiation dose and parameters under which it was delivered at the completion of each day's treatment. Notations are made regarding procedures completed on a particular treatment day, such as **portal verification** films and the addition or deletion of a block. All treatment-record entries must be accompanied by the treating therapist's signature or initials and the date.

During this review the radiation therapist asks the following questions:

- "When was the last treatment delivered?"
- "How far along is the patient in the course of treatment?"
- "Are verification films necessary?"
- "Have any changes in the treatment plan or prescription been ordered by the physician?"

By verifying the total dose delivered to the patient thus far, the radiation therapist appropriately monitors the administration of the radiation treatment. Radiation therapists maintain awareness of the dose being delivered to the target volume and critical structures* near or in the treatment volume and respond to or initiate necessary changes in the treatment plan through consultation with the radiation oncologist. The radiation therapist must document and sign treatment-plan changes in the daily treatment record.

Attention to the dose delivered also provides the therapist with expectations of the patient's physical reactions to the treatment. As the member of the treatment team who sees each patient daily, the therapist has a significant responsibility in monitoring these reactions. The radiation therapist possesses a firm understanding of radiation reactions and intervention methods for their management. The entire treatment team (including the oncologist and nursing staff members) monitor radiation reactions through review of blood counts, observation, and questioning of patients regarding their nutritional intake, skin reactions, and other associated symptoms. This understanding provides the foundation for the decision to withhold treatment pending consultation with the radiation oncologist.

Portal films

The radiation therapist fulfills the need for field verification through portal imaging. Portal images perform a critical role in quality assurance by providing the means to evalu-

*Normal tissue with radiation dose tolerances that limit the deliverable dose.

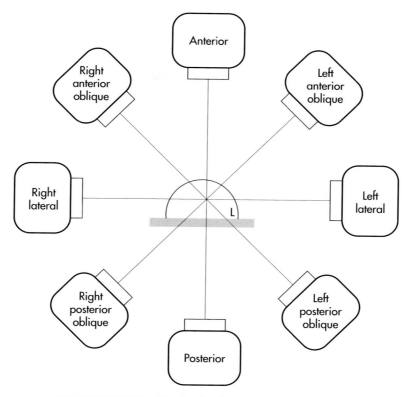

Fig. 16-1 Field identification by direction of beam entrance.

ate and document accuracy in the reproduction of treatment localization. Whereas portal images are taken at the start of treatment and at regular intervals during its course, frequency is based on departmental policy and professional judgment and varies among institutions. Partially based on historical studies showing a reduction in treatment errors associated with increased portal imaging, weekly portal imaging for radical cases has become an accepted, though not universally implemented, standard.[6,8] Some clinical situations, such as unstable localization landmarks or the proximity of the treatment volume to **critical structures,** may make increasing the frequency of portal imaging necessary. The professional judgment of the therapist is central in determining an appropriate imaging schedule with the radiation oncologist.

Care must be taken in the evaluation of portal films to differentiate between systematic and random setup errors. **Systematic errors** are those resulting from variations in the translation of the treatment setup from the simulator to the treatment unit and remain constant through the course of treatment if not corrected. Portal images taken before the first treatment generally assess systematic errors. These include the localization of the isocenter relative to surface landmarks and the position and shape of blocks. Corrections may be made for these errors by adjusting setup parameters or blocks. **Random errors** are inherent variations in daily setup. The range of random errors varies

with the anatomical site and must be accommodated in target-volume planning. A random error is minimized by careful patient positioning and treatment-plan reproduction. Increasing the rate of portal filming demonstrates the consistency of errors.

Traditional film methods of portal imaging are accomplished by using single- or double-exposure techniques. Cassettes provide stability for the film, may be hard or soft, and are usually lined with lead to reduce film fog caused by backscatter. Films must be positioned perpendicular to the central ray of the treatment beam. The double-exposure technique yields a visualization of the treatment field and surrounding anatomy, thus increasing the number of landmarks available for interpretation. This technique is accomplished by producing a short exposure of the treatment area. Then a second exposure is taken after the removal of field-shaping blocks and opening of the collimators. Single-exposure films may be used in situations in which sufficient landmarks for verification are visualized in the treatment area.

Time factors, poor image quality, and subjectivity in evaluation introduce limitations to precision with the use of traditional film portal imaging techniques. Films often are evaluated after treatment, even on subsequent days, and offer no opportunity to correct for treatments already delivered. Even when portal films are taken immediately before treatment delivery, patient movement is possible while patients wait for the film evaluation. The time-consuming nature of the filming process also has an affect on patient flow. Images created by megavoltage beams have poor contrast, thus making landmarks difficult to delineate. Portal film interpretation is mostly a subjective process with room for variation in assessment between individuals.[3] Finally, weekly portal filming cannot document variations in daily positioning of treatment fields. A review of daily portal images taken with **electronic portal imaging devices** (EPID) has shown variations of greater than 1 cm in fields demonstrating excellent reproduction based on assessment of weekly films.[11] Awareness of these limitations spurs the desire for increased frequency and precision in portal imaging.

Portal imaging systems that create static or real-time images of treatment volumes provide a means to improve daily treatment accuracy. A detector mounted opposite the head of the gantry converts the x-ray information into digital information that can be displayed as an image on a computer screen or through a laser printer to produce a hard-copy image. Portal imaging offers many advantages to the practice of radiation therapy by allowing the therapist to verify portal field alignment and make adjustments much more quickly and accurately. Images are produced in seconds and displayed on a terminal at the **treatment console,** thus minimizing movement factors and the affect of frequent filming on the patient schedule. Computer manipulation of gray scales can enhance contrast. Some systems can superimpose simulation and on-treatment images to display measured variations from the simulation to the therapist. With this tool, therapists can implement precise adjustments before treatment delivery.

Portal images must be reviewed with the radiation oncologist for approval. The radiation therapist implements and documents any modifications indicated on the images. The radiation oncology department maintains portal images as part of the permanent treatment record.

TREATMENT PREPARATION
Treatment room

The treatment room of the standard linear accelerator or ^{60}Co room is engineered around the isocenter. Lasers projecting horizontally from the walls and vertically from the ceiling (or opposite the gantry) intersect at the isocenter, thus providing visual guides to identify its location.

A well-planned treatment room facilitates accessibility to treatment accessories and movement by the therapists around its focal point, or isocenter. Shelves and storage cabinets form the perimeter of the room. Tables and counters do not obstruct access to and from the treatment unit. Treatment accessories are stored in consistent places and at heights that do not require therapists to use step stools or ladders. An organized system for custom block storage facilitates quick retrieval. The radiation therapist accepts responsibility for the maintenance of the treatment room as part of the department's QA program.

Treatment rooms are lit with standard and dim lights. Standard lighting provides safety for patients entering and exiting the room and assists radiation therapists in locating accessory equipment. Reducing the light in the treatment room improves the visualization of lasers and field light, thus promoting patient positioning and treatment setup. While treatment is in progress, full lights are on for visualization of the patient on the monitors.

Treatment unit

The isocentric mounting of modern treatment units facilitates the reproducibility of complex treatment plans. The accurate positioning of the treatment-unit isocenter relative to that of the treatment plan allows the rotation of the treatment unit (redirecting the treatment beam) to treat the target from multiple directions without moving the patient. These versatile units can treat extremely complex field arrangements.

Many preparations are necessary before the arrival of the patient. The field area, gantry, collimator, and table positions are confirmed. This is done by referring to manual scales or digital readouts located in the treatment room or at the control panel. Clean linens cover the treatment table, except over the treatment window. Treatment accessories, **positioning devices,** and **immobilization devices** matching those used at the simulation are prepared and placed in accessible places. These may include blocks, **wedges,** a **bolus, compensators,** sponges, casts, masks, and bite blocks.

Standard **collimation** systems using adjustable, divergent, and opposing jaws allow the customizing of fields into a square or rectangle. Field size (sometimes referred to as *jaw size*) indicates the size and dimensions of the radiation field at the isocenter. Individualization of treatment volumes is accomplished through the use of **shielding blocks.** Whereas a supply of standard lead blocks may be maintained to accommodate emergency situations, modern radiation therapy requires the fabrication of custom shielding blocks. To create custom blocks, molds are cut and filled with low-melting lead alloys. Cutting systems mimic the geometrical arrangement of the treatment beam, thus ensuring proper divergence and magnification at the treatment site. Drawbacks of these systems include space requirements for fabrication and storage and hazards associated with lifting heavy equipment and exposure to hazardous chemicals.

Multileaf collimation (MLC) systems allow the customization of field shape without the use of shielding blocks. These systems contain an additional set of jaws that have been sliced into a series of opposing leaves. Each of these leaves measures 1 cm at the isocenter and can be positioned independently, thus producing a variety of treatment field shapes. By reducing the need for the positioning of heavy blocks, MLC promises to improve customization of treatment volumes with reduced treatment time and increased safety for patients and radiation therapists.

THE PATIENT
Identification

At least two methods of identification should be used to confirm patient identity because many factors contribute to the possibility of misidentification. Patients may have the same or similar names, and illness or anxiety may hinder their ability to respond to their own name. As a result, the radiation therapist must be extremely cautious when identifying new patients. The consequences of misidentification can range from discontent in the waiting room to misadministration of treatment if the error is not discovered before treatment delivery.

The treatment chart includes an identification photo for visual confirmation. Patients may be asked to state their own name. The most important piece of identification on inpatients is their wrist bracelet, which is checked before the patient is moved into the treatment room.

PATIENT PREPARATION AND COMMUNICATION

As a professional caregiver, the radiation therapist seeks to establish with the patient a relationship that encourages confidence and cooperation. Patients must entrust the radiation therapist with their care. The nature of the illness and anxiety surrounding the dangers of radiation make this no easy task. An individual may be treated over a period ranging from 2 to 8 weeks. Over this time the therapist has the responsibility to develop a constructive patient-professional relationship, which may provide the radiation therapist insight into the individual's experience and coping mechanisms. Observations of changes in patient behavior may also indicate changes in the disease state. In the event of such changes the physician must be notified. As a radiation oncology team member having daily contact with the patient, the radiation therapist becomes a liaison by directing the patient to resources designed to meet physical and psychosocial needs.

The radiation therapist demonstrates respect for the patient through the clear communication of directions at a level understandable to the patient. Age, mental status, and native language must be considered in the determination of the way messages can be presented most effectively. An understanding of what is expected during treatment empowers patients, thus fostering increased cooperation through feelings of mutual respect. Every effort must be extended to maximize patients' feelings of security. At the outset the patient is shown the audio and visual monitoring systems. Patients must be informed about safeguards to their privacy and reassured that although radiation therapists leave the room, contact will be maintained at all times.

If departmental practice requires the patient to undress before entering the treatment room, an explanation is given before the first treatment. The patient is informed of the necessity of removal of restrictive clothing that may alter the position of skin marks and inhibit reproduction of the patient's position. The location of gowns or robes and a secure place for their belongings is identified.

Radiation therapists greet patients and direct them into the treatment room. Here the radiation therapist initiates the rapport that characterizes the therapist-patient relationship. Throughout the course of treatment, the radiation therapist is a resource for the patient. The radiation therapist has a great deal of control over the extent of this relationship and hence the quality of care perceived by the patient. With this control comes the responsibility to create an environment sensitive to the patient's questions and concerns. At the same time, anticipation of these questions and concerns assists the radiation therapist to ease the anxiety associated with radiation treatments.

Patients must be counseled from the start of treatment in the proper maintenance of skin marks, general skin care, and nutritional guidelines. Radiation therapists provide these services while being mindful of the limitations of their scope of practice and make professional referrals when appropriate. Questioning skills may be used to discover the onset or severity of acute radiation reactions. Questions are chosen to encourage dialogue, and brief answers by the patient may be followed with gently probing questions to develop a fuller picture of the patient's reactions to treatment. The radiation therapist is responsible for assessing the patient's verbal and observable responses (e.g., skin reactions, weight change, changes in demeanor) and evaluating whether treatment should continue or be withheld until the patient may be seen by the physician.

PATIENT TRANSFERS

Patients require varying assistance onto the treatment table, or patient-support assembly (PSA). Many ambulatory patients may require only a stool to reach the top of the table. Some treatment units are equipped with an extended-range treatment table, which may be lowered closer to the floor than a traditional PSA, thus eliminating the need for step stools. Some patients may need a supportive arm to assist walking, whereas others may arrive in wheelchairs or on stretchers.

In evaluating the situation before transferring the patient onto the treatment table, the radiation therapist is mindful of the variety of auxiliary medical equipment the patient may be using. Although this equipment is most likely to be extensively used with inpatients, outpatients are not infrequently treated with oxygen or nutritional support and chemotherapy. Tubes and catheters must be recognized and carefully handled so as not to disrupt their placement or introduce infection.

Universal precautions are practiced with all patients. The radiation therapist is conscious that undiagnosed infections may be present in any individual, and the therapist handles all blood and body fluids as if they are infectious. Therapists also remember the immunodeficient state of their patients and take responsibility for the prevention of disease transmission. The most important practice toward this goal is thorough hand washing after patient contact. Linens must be replaced, and the treatment table and positioning accessories must be cleaned with disinfectant cleaners after each use.

For safe transfer of the patient to the treatment table, proper body mechanics of the patient and radiation therapist must be considered. In the initial planning of a patient transfer, the radiation therapist must assess the need for assistance. This is critical to the safety of the caregiver and patient. General rules for lifting require the maintenance of a wide base of support with the feet apart and one foot placed slightly in front of the other. The weight to be moved is kept close to the lifter, who bends at the knees and hips rather than at the waist while maintaining the normal curve at the lower back. Lifters should never twist nor bend sideways while supporting the weight.[9]

In the planning of any transfer the patient should be included when possible. Patients may be able to move themselves or have pain they wish the therapist to consider. They may also have other suggestions to facilitate their safe transfer.

Wheelchair transfers

For patients unable to stand unassisted, the therapist prepares for the transfer by positioning the chair parallel to the table and locking the wheels. Foot rests are raised and the radiation therapist stands facing the patient. With the patient's feet together and therapist's feet on either side, the radiation therapist leans forward, bends at the knees and hips, and maintains the natural curve of the lower spine. The patient reaches around the radiation therapist's shoulders while the radiation therapist reaches under the patient's arms. The radiation therapist's arms are then locked around the patient's back. Patients are raised to their feet and pivoted 90 degrees so that their back faces the table. Next, the patient is eased into a sitting position. With an arm behind the patient's shoulders and the other behind the knees, the therapist turns and eases the patient into the supine position in one smooth motion.

If for any reason (e.g., paralysis, pain) the patient requires more assistance onto the table, the patient should be transported to the department with a stretcher. This is a safety consideration for the patient and caregivers.

Stretcher transfers

Stretcher transfers should be completed with a minimum of two caregivers. The stretcher is placed alongside the treatment table with the side rails lowered and wheels locked. The table is positioned at the same level as the stretcher. If the patient can slide over, one therapist may secure the stretcher while the other therapist stands opposite the treatment table, thus providing assistance and ensuring that the patient does not fall.

Immobile patients may be lifted from a stretcher to a table through the use of a draw sheet. The width of the treatment table next to the stretcher forces the lifters to breach some of the rules of good body mechanics. Specifically, at some point the weight is held away from the lifter's own center of gravity, and some have to push rather then pull the weight. The reach may also make maintaining proper pos-

ture difficult. Therefore the therapist uses the assistance of as many trained individuals as needed to transfer the patient in a safe manner. The appropriate number of lifters depends on factors such as the size of the patient or special considerations such as pain.

The use of a slide board for transferring stretcher patients reduces the risk of injury to the people performing the transfer. This option is preferred when insufficient staff members are available for a safe transfer. Slide boards are large enough to support the patient but are generally used to bridge the space between the stretcher and treatment table so that the patient may be pulled rather than lifted from one to the other. Patients are positioned with their hands on their chest. The slide board is positioned by rolling the patient from the treatment table and placing the board under the draw sheet. After the patient is eased back onto the slide board, the board is pulled to the treatment table or the patient is slid across the bridge created over the gap between the stretcher and treatment table. The slide board must be removed if it is in the path of a treatment beam. Slide boards should not be used if rolling places the patient at risk for injury. In this situation, lifters must position themselves to maintain support of the patient's head, shoulders, hips, and feet during the entire lift. Sheets are rolled and gripped firmly, and the team leader counts (usually to three) so that everyone moves at the same time. The patient is lifted just high enough to clear the treatment table and stretcher surfaces, moved over, and eased down. The radiation therapist ensures that the patient and any accessory equipment is secure before moving the stretcher away. Intravenous lines, catheters, oxygen, and other tubing is secured away from moving treatment machine parts.

PATIENT POSITION, ISOCENTER, AND FIELD PLACEMENT

The isocenter of the treatment unit is defined in a static position. The radiation therapist is responsible for reproducing daily the position of the patient relative to this point. Because neither the isocenter nor its planned position in the patient can be directly visualized during treatment setup, external tools must be used to guide the process. These tools are the localization landmarks and lasers. Localization landmarks are references that can be readily identified on the patient's surface. Lasers are aligned with the isocenter on the vertical and horizontal axis of the gantry's rotation. Lasers shine on the patient's surface, thereby forming references to be aligned with the localization landmarks.

Identification of localization landmarks

While patient dignity is maintained with drapes, surface landmarks are located by using the treatment description as the reference. Landmarks may be maintained in a variety of permanent and nonpermanent forms. Permanent references include visible and palpable anatomical landmarks (bones or other identifiable points that can be seen or felt and point to the location of hidden anatomy) or tiny tattoos placed on the patient. Semipermanent inks such as felt tip markers and **carfusion** may be used during treatment to outline the field or mark the field center and corners. Carfusion, a dyelike liquid, varies in its formulation but generally contains silver nitrate and phenol in a fuchsin base, thus producing a magenta liquid that can be painted onto patients by using thin sticks or swabs. Marks created by this inklike fluid are less easily removed than those of other markers. Concerns about toxicity have limited the use of carfusion in many centers.

Patient positioning

Patients are positioned with the treatment area over the appropriate table window. Treatment couches are generally designed with two window options to allow various treatment fields to reach the patient without intercepting the couch. The primary window is supported by bars on either side of the table, thus providing stability while leaving an opening that allows treatment of posterior fields. The second window is supported down the center of the table, thus allowing treatment of oblique or rotational fields that intersect the side bars of the primary treatment window. A mylar sheet covers windows to support the patient, and this support may be enhanced by a tennis racket beneath the mylar.

The positioning of patients with the isocenter of their treatment plan as close as possible to the center of the table provides the maximum clearance for techniques that require 360-degree gantry rotation around the patient.[7] Many oblique or tangential fields may be accommodated without rotation of the treatment table by making lateral shifts of the patient (consequently isocenter) relative to the table surface. For example, small angles off the vertical axis such as those used for lung boost fields may be accommodated by biasing the patient toward the side that the anterior field enters, or larger angles off the vertical axis (such as those used in breast tangents) may be accommodated by moving the patient closer to the treatment side.

Localization landmarks and tattoos are then identified. The treatment description in the chart is used to reproduce a position consistent with that prescribed at the simulation (see Volume II, Unit II, Chapter 9). Configurations of positioning aids and immobilization devices (Volume II, Unit II, Chapter 7) must match those used at the simulation. Tools assisting reproduction include descriptive statements such as supine versus prone, arm placement, names and location of sponges or other positioning devices are given. Measurements indicating the relative position of anatomy (e.g., chin to suprasternal notch or slope of the sternum) may be used. Photographs taken at the simulation are often used to illustrate written descriptions. The precise reproduction of the treatment position is critical to the maintenance of the orientation of surface landmarks to internal targets.

Comfort is central in the patient's ability to maintain the treatment position. Care is taken at the simulation to define a treatment position that the patient can tolerate for daily treatment. Considerations at the simulation include the general condition of the patient (e.g., age, disability, pain), location of normal structures, skin folds in the treatment fields, ability to treat all fields in one position, and reproducibility. For treatment the responsibility is to reproduce the planned position to ensure the coincidence of surface landmarks relative to the internal target. Even with the best planning, however, discomfort is not avoided for every patient. In these situations the radiation therapist accommodates the patient's needs while maintaining the integrity of the planned position.

Many techniques are used to reproduce the treatment position and placement of the isocenter. The complexity of this task varies depending on the mobility of the anatomical site. Immobilization devices that reproduce the treatment position while restricting movement are necessary for head and neck and extremity treatments for which reproduction is obviously the most difficult. Yet, as treatment planning and portal image evaluation methods improve, these tools are finding increased application in all treatment sites.

The common three-point positioning technique defines the plane of treatment on the patient and provides references with which the radiation therapist aligns the treatment plane with the axis of the gantry's rotation. With the patient in the approximate treatment position and the localization landmarks identified, the treatment table (PSA) is positioned to bring the patient close to the location for treatment. The room lights are dimmed, and patient position is refined by using lasers and the treatment-field light. Through the alignment of three localization landmarks on the patient relative to three external references, the treatment position is reproduced.

A breast bridge (a two-legged device with a spirit level [Fig. 16-2]) may be used to reproduce the position of two points relative to one another. For example, the rotation of

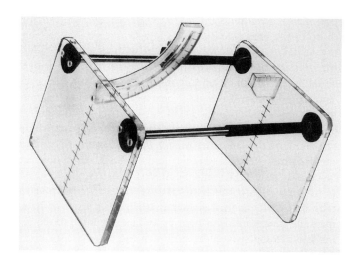

Fig. 16-2 A breast bridge. (Courtesy Arthur Swayhoover, Nuclear Associates, Carle Place, New York.)

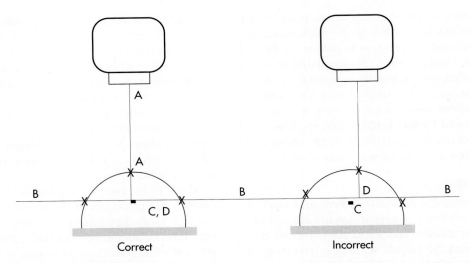

Fig. 16-3 Three-point positioning: tattoos (x) *A*, crosshairs; *B*, lasers; *C*, planned location of the isocenter; *D*, actual location of isocenter.

the pelvis can be measured by placing each leg of the bridge on the anterior superior iliac spines of the pelvis. The incline of the thorax can be measured by placing one leg on the suprasternal notch and the other leg at the base of the sternum.

Reproduction of isocenter localization

With the patient in the precise treatment position, the isocenter is positioned relative to the localization landmarks. In some situations the intersection of the planes identified by the three positioning points coincides with the localization points for the isocenter (Fig. 16-3). For many clinical situations, however, this is not practical. Anatomical references are seldomly so conveniently located, and many sites do not lend themselves to the reproducible placement of localization marks. Examples include mobile skin surfaces such as those of the breast, axilla, and older or obese persons; sloping surfaces such as those treated with tangential fields; irregular surfaces; and areas covered by dressings. For these situations a landmark and coordinate system may be used. The reproduction of isocenter placement is accomplished by identifying a stable surface landmark and specific treatment-couch motions from that point. The SSD distance positions the depth of the isocenter relative to the landmark. Several methods may be used to determine the SSD. An optical-distance indicator (ODI), or rangefinder, consists of a light that is projected onto the patient's skin and intersecting the crosshairs. Mechanical-distance indicators consist of incrementally marked rods or measuring tape mounted to the collimator assembly extended to touch the patient's surface at the center of the treatment field. Horizontal (in-and-out, right-to-left) movements direct the positioning of the isocenter, as shown in Fig. 16-4.

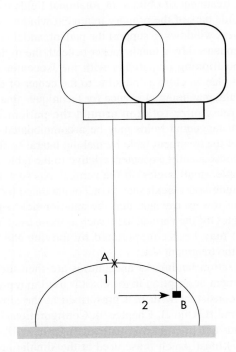

Fig. 16-4 Landmark and coordinate method: *A*, surface landmark (tattoo); *B*, planned location of isocenter; *1*, shift to depth; *2*, lateral shift.

Beam direction

The gantry, collimator, and couch are positioned to reproduce field requirements defined in the treatment plan. Before accepting the beam placement, the radiation therapist evaluates its accuracy. Using their knowledge of anatomy and information provided by the portal imaging, therapists

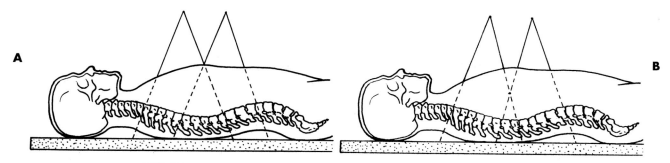

Fig. 16-5 Matching adjacent treatment fields: **A,** abutting a hot match; **B,** a calculated gap.

assess the reproduction of the treatment setup daily. Considerations such as the sparing of a strip of tissue to preserve lymphatic drainage or sufficient flash for tangential fields must be verified in this assessment. Portal films must be taken if any question exists about the accuracy of the treatment-field placement.

Adjacent fields

The divergence of the radiation beam poses geometrical problems during the alignment of adjacent treatment fields. Matching methods vary with changing clinical objectives. Methods include abutting fields at the surface and the use of **gaps** between fields with or without coplanar alignment of treatment-beam edges. **Feathering** (migration of the gap through the treatment course) may be used to blur dose inhomogeneities in the gapped area. The choice of gap technique and positioning of the gap depends on the location of tumor and critical structures.

Abutting field edges produces a hot match in which the diverging beams overlap immediately below the surface (Fig. 16-5, *A*). This may be necessary in situations in which the tumor lies close to the skin surface near the position of the match. The primary example of this application is the treatment of head and neck cancer. The area of overlap must be carefully evaluated for the presence of critical structures and the dose delivered to them with this technique. Care must be taken to avoid the overdose of critical structures.

When an area of low dose is acceptable at and near the surface, adjacent fields may be separated by a gap (Fig. 16-5, *B*). Treatment fields overlap at a prescribed depth in the patient. The exact length of the gap must be calculated by knowing the length of each treatment field and depth at which the intersection of the fields is to be positioned (Volume II, Unit III, Chapter 11).

Some clinical situations demand a precise alignment of the radiation beam. Areas of overdose and underdose arising from variations in the amount of overlap or space between fields may be unacceptable in these situations. Common examples include tangential breast techniques with and without matching supraclavicular fields and craniospinal irradia-

tion (CSI). In each of these treatment techniques, positioning the planes of field edges coincident (coplanar) to one another is useful. This may be accomplished through the use of blocks, independent jaws or a gantry, a collimator, and couch rotations.

A nondivergent beam edge is achieved through the placement of an independent jaw at the isocenter or through the use of a block to the same point (Fig. 16-6, *A*). These blocks may be called *half-beam blocks, central-axis blocks,* or *beam splitters*. Two fields with nondivergent beam edges may be abutted or separated by a standard* gap. Limitations to the application of this method include techniques covering large target volumes because jaw openings must be double the length of the treatment area and concerns regarding beam transmission through blocks.

For large field sizes such as those used in CSI, the flexibility of motion designed in the treatment unit is used. The rotation of the gantry, collimator, and table can be used in the effort to align treatment-field edges. With CSI as an example the inferior field edges of the opposing cranial fields can be made coplanar through the rotation of the couch while a rotation of the collimator aligns the same edge with the divergence of the posterior spine field (Fig. 16-6, *B* and *C*). Although the abutting of these geometrically matched fields theoretically provides a perfect match without the inhomogeneity of other techniques, the risks of variations in daily setup must be recognized. Abutting may be desirable in clinical situations in which risks are low, but the presence of critical structures at the match may require the addition of a gap.

The use of a gap between geometrically aligned fields creates a low-dose area, or cold spot. This is reduced through the application of the feathering technique. The feathered gap moves through the course of treatment, thus varying the low-dose area and increasing the total dose the area of the gap receives. Many methods are used with varied sequences, number of migrations, and gap sizes.[4]

*Noncalculated because beam geometry no longer creates an overlap at depth.

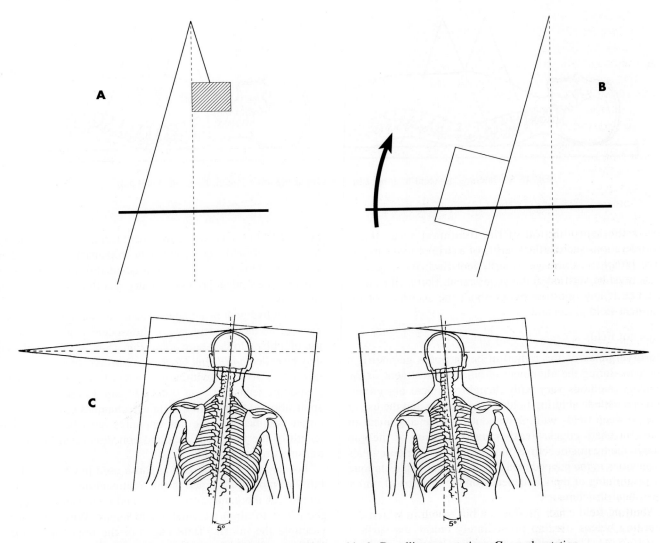

Fig. 16-6 Geometrical field matching: **A,** half-beam block; **B,** collimator rotation; **C,** couch rotation.

BEAM-SHAPING AND MODIFYING DEVICES

Treatment units are designed to produce square and rectangular treatment fields delivering consistent doses of radiation across a field perpendicular to the central ray of the beam. Individuals and tumors, however, do not appear as squares and rectangles with flat surfaces. Customization of the radiation dose delivery requires the use of devices that modify the shape and distribution of the radiation dose to meet individual patient needs.

Modification devices for photon beams must be secured a minimum of 15 cm from the surface of the patient. The interaction of the photon beam with materials of beam modifiers produces scatter electrons that contaminate the photon beam and produce increased skin doses for patients. These low-energy electrons are absorbed in 15 cm of air.

Treatment accessories are often heavy and awkward. Mounted on trays with sharp edges and square corners, they pose a hazard to patients and radiation therapists if dropped or mishandled. Care must be taken to avoid the positioning of accessories over patients.

Blocks

Shielding blocks, used to shape photon fields, take several forms. Materials range from spent uranium to lead and lead alloys used in the production of customized shielding blocks. Blocks rest on or are screwed to plastic trays inserted into the accessory tray of the treatment-unit head. The shape and position of blocks are verified before the initiation of treatment by using portal imaging. The required thickness of actual blocks varies based on the energy of the treatment beam. However, full shielding blocks are constructed to transmit less than 5% of the original beam.

A supply of standardized lead blocks are among the necessary accessories in the treatment room. These occupy little space and accommodate emergency treatments until custom blocks are created. Limitations include minimal variability in shape and size. Perpendicular block sides produce an increased **penumbra*** along the blocked field edges (see Fig. 14-3). Standardized lead blocks are often placed on trays without a means of being secured to the tray, and the radiation therapist is always careful to remove them before changing the gantry position.

Customized shielding blocks use lead alloys with low melting points. These materials allow molds to be cut from styrofoam to match the size and shape defined by the physician at the simulation. Block edges are parallel to the divergence of the treatment beam, thus reducing the penumbra caused by beam absorption through changing block thickness (Fig. 16-7). These molds are filled with the molten alloy and allowed to cool. After completion of the individual's treatment, blocks are melted and the alloy is reused.

Shielding blocks may be mounted on trays or left loose for use in an individual's treatment. Mounting blocks produce several advantages. After portal-film verification, the treatment setup time decreases and daily block placement is consistent. By securing blocks to the tray, the risk of injury to patients and staff members caused by a block falling or being dropped is greatly reduced.

Unmounted blocks must be positioned on the holding tray before the treatment of each field. Reproduction of block placement is accomplished through the use of templates identifying the shape and position of each block relative to the central axis. Small variations in alignment with tray markings are magnified at the treatment distance, thus reducing the precision of daily treatment. This limitation may be reduced by creating templates at the treatment distance; however, this is often not practical.

The practice of mounting all blocks requires stocking more materials and considerable storage space in the treatment room. These considerations must be taken into account when determining departmental practice. Improvements in accuracy, safety, and treatment time argue strongly in favor of mounting treatment blocks.

Bolus

In radiation therapy, *bolus* refers to materials whose interactions with the radiation beam mimic those of tissue. Bolus comes in many forms and has many applications. Acceptable materials include paraffin wax, Vaseline gauze, wet gauze or towels, and water bags. Commercially available products developed specifically for use in radiation therapy are available in sheets of variable thicknesses and

*Dose gradient caused by geometrical or physical factors.

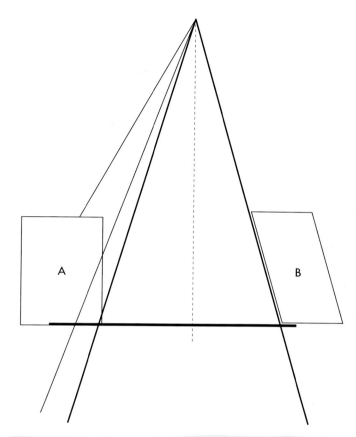

Fig. 16-7   Blocks: *A,* nondivergent (clinical); *B,* divergent (custom).

powder forms that can be mixed with water and formed to meet specific needs. Flexibility in shaping is an advantage because bolus must conform to the treatment surface without air gaps (Fig. 16-8).

Bolus of a thickness equal to the depth of maximum dose eliminates the skin-sparing effect of megavoltage photon beams. Bolus may be applied with this goal over entire treatment areas or simply over scars, superficial nodes, or other areas of concern. When bolus is applied in this fashion, the buildup of dose occurs within it, thus bringing the area of maximum dose deposition to the patient's surface.

Bolus may also be used to compensate for variations in surface contour or eliminate air gaps in cavities. For example, surgical procedures leaving anatomical defects such as those used for the removal of sinus malignancies produce significant irregularities. Filling the cavity with bolus material such as Vaseline gauze or a water-filled balloon significantly improves the dose distribution in the target volume. This application is only useful in situations in which the loss of skin sparing is acceptable or desired. When skin sparing is to be maintained, the creation of individualized compensators should be evaluated.

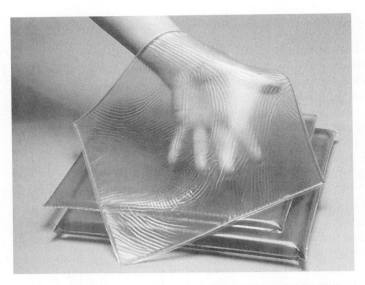

Fig. 16-8 Bolus example: Superflab. (Courtesy MED-TEC, Inc, Orange City, Iowa.)

Compensators

The design of megavoltage treatment units produces a radiation beam delivering a relatively even dose across the plane perpendicular to the radiation beam. Patients, however, rarely provide a flat surface parallel with this ideal. Skewing of dose distribution caused by irregular surfaces can be compensated by using bolus material to produce a level treatment area; however, a loss of skin sparing accompanies this technique. To retain this important effect, compensating filters may be positioned in the head of the treatment unit, thus modifying the radiation beam to accommodate the contour of the patient. Compensating filters can be made from a variety of materials as long as the materials' equivalence to tissue absorption is known. Common materials include copper, brass, lead, and lucite.

Tissue deficits in need of compensation are usually most significant over one dimension (width or length), and a set of standardized two-dimensional compensators meets the needs of many treatment situations. Custom compensators can easily be built for special situations. Strips of attenuating materials of known thicknesses are layered and mounted onto a tray. Compensating material is carefully oriented on the tray to the air gap at the treatment distance.

Three-dimensional compensators are created by using square blocks or special cutting units to complement the contour of the surface across the width and length dimensions. Care must be taken to position compensating materials on the tray so that their projection at the treatment distance corresponds to the area of tissue deficit. The complexity of their creation limits their use in most facilities. Alternative methods of creating three-dimensional compensators use equipment that can transfer the surface contour to a router system forming a styrofoam mold designed to be filled with a specific compensating material such as bolus or Lipowitz metal (cerrobend).

Wedges

The primary goal of treatment planning is to treat a target volume* to an even (homogenous) dose while minimizing the dose delivered to normal tissue. The orientation of multiple fields to one another during treatment may produce inhomogeneous dose distributions over the target volume. The **isodose lines**[†] of a single treatment field on a flat surface are relatively parallel to the surface. When a second beam is positioned directly opposite this beam, the combined dose distribution is relatively even throughout the volume. However, as the **hinge angle**[‡] (Fig. 16-9) decreases, doses delivered to overlapping areas vary significantly, thus creating areas of high- and low-dose regions in the desired target volume.

Wedges appear similar to compensator filters; however, their application differs significantly. The wedge is designed to change the angle of the isodose curve relative to the beam axis at a specified depth. Wedges reduce the dose in areas of overlap between fields that have hinge angles less than 180 degrees. The thick end of the wedge, referred to as the *heel*, attenuates the greatest amount of radiation, thus drawing the isodose lines closer to the surface. Attenuation decreases along the wedge to the thin end, or toe where the dose delivered to the patient will be relatively greater than the dose at

*An area of known and presumed tumor.
[†]Lines connecting points of equivalent relative radiation dose.
[‡]The measure of the angle between central rays of two intersecting treatment beams.

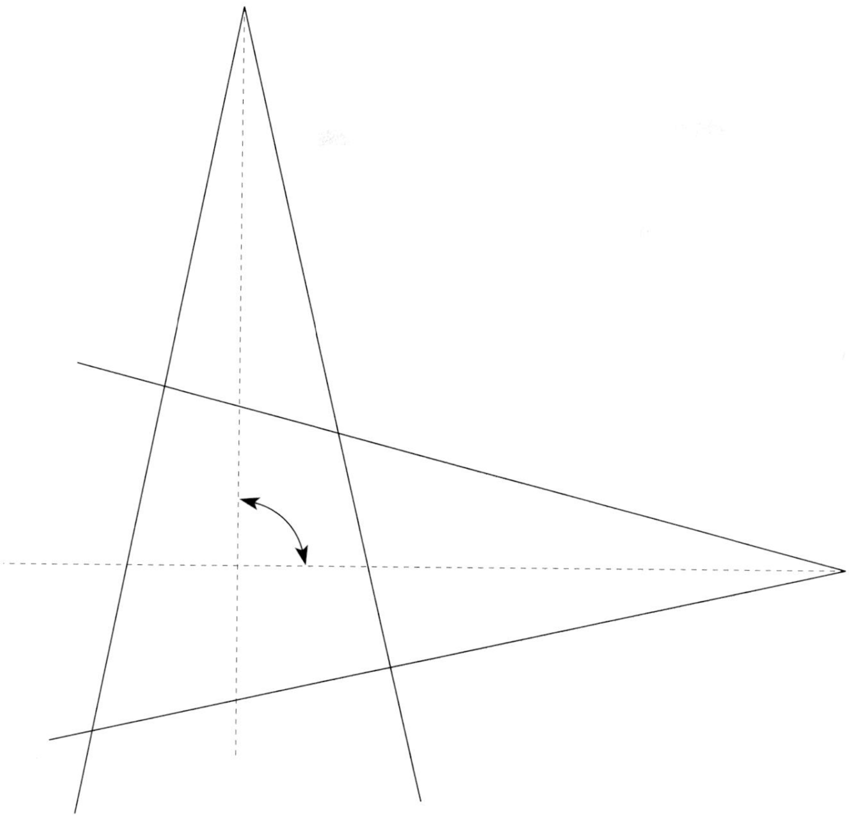

Fig. 16-9 A 90-degree hinge angle.

the opposite side of the treatment field. When wedges are used, heels should always be positioned together.

Standard wedge systems use externally mounted wedges that the radiation therapist must position when required by the treatment plan. The manufacturer usually provides these wedges, which are customized for specific treatment units. Standard wedge sizes are 15, 30, 45, and 60 degrees.

Some treatment units use internal wedging methods, which allow customizing of the wedge angle for each treatment plan. One system uses a 60-degree universal wedge placed in the beam path for a specified number of monitor units. The beam is interrupted to remove the wedge, and the remaining monitor units are delivered. Other systems use a dynamic jaw system in which a moving jaw starts at one side of the field and opens to a full field over the course of dose delivery (see Fig. 13-20). This effectively delivers a range of dose over the field. The side of the field at which the jaw starts its movement correlates with the wedge toe.

Field sizes are limited with the use of compensators and wedges. Care must be taken to ensure that treatment fields do not extend beyond the heel or sides of either beam-modification device. (Flash or extension beyond the toe is acceptable.)

Transmission filters

Transmission filters are designed to allow the transmission of a predetermined percentage of the treatment beam to a portion of a treatment field and may be used throughout the course of the treatment. This allows the physician to treat structures that have varying radiosensitivity in proximity to one another at different dose rates. For example, whole-abdomen radiation therapy induces significant gastrointestinal effects. By reducing the daily dose to the upper portion of the abdomen through the use of the transmission filter, patient tolerance is improved. The pelvis receives the dose at a higher rate, thus effectively completing the boost dose concurrently with the whole-abdomen treatment. When using a transmission filter, daily fraction and total doses for each area must be written in the prescription and documented separately in the daily treatment record.

ELECTRON BEAM
Collimation

The mass and charge of the electron give rise to increased interactions in air compared with those of the photon beam. This scattering of the electron beam makes the extension of collimation close to the treatment surface necessary. Secondary collimation systems for electron therapy usually take the form of cones or trimmer bars attached to the treatment-accessory tray of the gantry. This equipment is usually secured before the patient is positioned (Fig. 16-10).

Electron cutouts

Field-shaping requirements for electron-beam therapy differ significantly from photon requirements. Unlike photon shielding blocks, **electron shields,** or cutouts, collimate and shape treatment fields. Electron beams are attenuated much more efficiently than photon beams. Full shielding requires lead thicknesses of several millimeters. Shields may be cut and molded to the patient surface except in instances in which the field area makes weight uncomfortable (general rule: $^1/_2$ energy in mm lead).

As discussed earlier, collimation of electron beams is accomplished through the use of electron cones or trimmer bars. Electron cones or trimmer bars bring the collimation of these beams closer to the patient's surface, thus improving radiation-dose distribution by sharpening the dose gradient at the beam edges. Cones are limited to a few selected field sizes, generally squares. Trimmer bars attached to the collimator provide greater flexibility in field size, but the increased distance from the patient increases penumbra. To customize field areas, field-shaping cutouts can be designed to fit directly inside the electron cone or molded to fit the patient's contour, thus providing tertiary collimation at the treatment site. Planning of these field-shaping cutouts may be accomplished by using the simulator or a clinical procedure. For clinical customization the required field shape is drawn on a template positioned on the patient's surface with localization landmarks for later treat-

ment reproduction. The template is then used to form a mold for creation of a cerrobend cutout (Fig. 16-11), which fits inside the base of the cone.

Internal shielding

Treatment sites such as the nares, auricle, eyelids, and lips are often treated with electron therapy. These structures are thin, and underlying normal tissue such as the medial nasal membranes, skin behind the ear, optic lens, and gingiva must be protected from unnecessary radiation exposure. Shields may be produced to achieve this goal. The interaction of the electrons with the metal of these shields, however, produces low-energy scatter radiation that increases the dose and reaction at the incident tissue surface. To absorb this low-energy scatter radiation, the shield must be covered with a low Z number material such as aluminum, tin, or paraffin wax.

Bolus

Although the materials used for bolus in electron therapy are the same as those used with photons, the applications differ. Three applications for bolus exist in electron therapy. First, because the dose deposition for electrons differs from that of photons,* bolusing to eliminate skin sparing is only applied for low-energy electron beams. Second, the depth at which dose fall-off occurs can be customized by the choice of electron energy and by the use of bolus to decrease the depth of penetration. Third, irregular surfaces and air cavities play havoc with the dose distribution of electron beams, and bolus may be used to fill in these irregularities.

*The depth of maximum dose decreases with increasing energy followed by an area of homogenous dose and ending with an area of rapid fall-off.

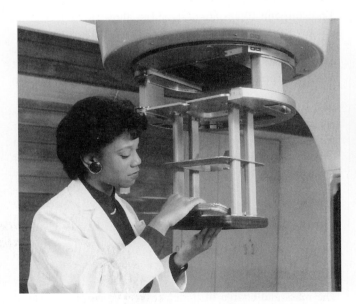

Fig. 16-10 Electron cones. (Courtesy Varian Associates, Palo Alto, California.)

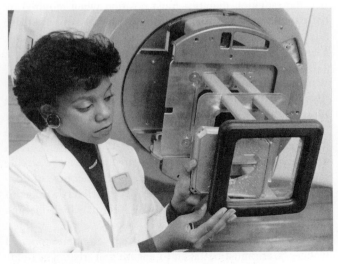

Fig. 16-11 Electron cutouts. (Courtesy Varian Associates, Palo Alto, California.)

ASSESSMENT AND ACCEPTANCE OF TREATMENT PARAMETERS

The radiation therapist performs a final review of the treatment setup, verifying the patient positioning, beam direction, and use of beam modifiers. If arc therapy is being applied, the therapist ensures free clearance for gantry motion throughout the treatment rotation. After being satisfied that the set parameters meet those prescribed by the treatment plan, radiation therapists notify the patient that they will exit the treatment room to administer the radiation. The therapist reminds and reassures patients that they are being monitored at all times. An indication of the approximate time that the beam will be on is also reassuring. On confirmation that the patient is the only person in the treatment room, the radiation therapists exits and securely closes the door.

Console

Radiation delivery is controlled at the treatment console located outside the treatment room. The configuration of the console varies widely among treatment units, from simple cobalt units with two timers and beam on-off lights to complex computer-controlled screens displaying multiple treatment unit parameters.

Calculated treatment times for cobalt units or monitor-unit settings for linear accelerators are set on the console in preparation for treatment delivery. Backup timers may be manually or automatically set depending on the sophistication of the treatment unit. These backup timers function as safety **interlocks** by terminating the beam if the primary timer malfunctions.

The console provides information to the radiation therapist regarding the operation of the treatment unit. The use of beam modifiers such as wedges may require verification of placement to release a safety interlock for treatment. Interlocks assist in meeting many safety parameters for treatment delivery, including (but not limited to) the closing of doors, placement of proper beam modifiers (wedges, compensators, electron cones), and machine-operation requirements (water, Freon). A lack of agreement with the requirements of any of these interlocks triggers a fault indicator on the console. Fault-light panels provide diagnostic information regarding proper functioning and the source of problems in the treatment unit. The radiation therapist sets the parameters for treatment delivery, including the calculated primary and backup monitor unit (or timer) settings. Primary, secondary, and backup timers function to interrupt the treatment beam after the prescribed dose has been delivered. Gauges and light panels provide further information regarding machine operation, including the dose rate during beam operation. Although the maintenance of equipment is ultimately the responsibility of the radiation physicist, the monitoring of equipment functioning and reporting of problems to the physics or engineering department is a critical responsibility of the radiation therapist.[7] Any equipment malfunctions or setup errors affecting treatment delivery must be reported to the radiation oncologist, and corrective actions must be documented in writing.

Record and verification systems

Record and verification (R & V) systems are increasingly being used in radiation oncology. These systems compare machine setup parameters with those most recently prescribed for a particular field, thus preventing the initiation of the treatment beam if settings vary outside a certain tolerance range. Parameters typically monitored include monitor units, gantry position, collimator aperture and rotation settings, table position, arc versus fixed treatment, and use of beam modifiers.[10] Care must be taken that parameters set on the first day of treatment are accurate because errors will continue on subsequent treatments. To reduce the risk of replicating an error of this type, patient setups should be completed by using the simulator, rather than R & V information provided in the treatment chart. The use of R & V systems in this manner has been recommended by the American Association of Physicists in Medicine (AAPM).[7] After the radiation therapist performs a final review of treatment parameters, the treatment beam is turned on and the prescribed radiation dose delivered.

TREATMENT DELIVERY
Beam on and beam off

The initiation of the treatment beam requires turning a key, pressing a switch key, or both. The console displays the dose rate and time or number of monitor units administered. Lights in and outside the treatment room flash red, which indicates the presence of radiation in the treatment room.

In the event of movement by the patient, improper machine motion, or failure of the unit to cease treatment at the prescribed dose, interruption of the treatment beam is necessary. Options for beam interruption include pressing the beam-off key, turning the operation key to the off position, and opening the door to the treatment unit. If these actions fail to stop the beam, an emergency off switch must be used, thereby completely turning off the treatment unit. The use of the emergency off switch usually requires a warmup period before reuse of the machine.

Geiger counters are required equipment in ^{60}Co treatment units. Visual (flashing light) and audible (clicks) indicators inform the radiation therapist of the radiation level in the treatment room. Source-position indicators located on the front of the treatment-unit head may include a dial for rotating sources or rod for sliding-drawer sources. A note must be made upon entry into the treatment room after each exposure of the return to normal exposure rate in the ^{60}Co room. If the radiation source does not retract, radiation therapists must react quickly to ensure the safety of the patient and themselves. While staying out of the primary beam, the therapist moves the patient out of the beam's path and closes the collimator opening. An attempt may be made to manually retract the source by turning the dial on the head of the treatment unit or using a T-bar that fits over the rod and pushing the source into the retracted position. Any extra exposure time the patient receives must be noted in the chart.

Patient-monitoring systems

To protect the radiation therapist from radiation exposure, the patient must be left alone in the treatment room for the radiation delivery. However, to maintain patient safety and accuracy of treatment, audio and visual contact must be maintained at all times. A stop at the console area before the patient's first treatment allows the radiation therapist to demonstrate monitoring systems, thus ensuring patients that they are being monitored during treatment delivery and their privacy is being protected.

In some situations (orthovoltage or other low-energy treatments), the therapist may monitor treatment directly through leaded glass windows. This becomes impractical with megavoltage units, however, and indirect monitoring systems must be used. For standard radiation therapy treatment, at least two cameras are used to maintain visual contact with the patient. One camera provides a long view of the whole patient, thus allowing observation of general distress or movement. Another camera zooms in, thereby providing a closer view on the treatment field to observe subtle patient movement.

A two-way communication system between the treatment room and console must remain audible to the operator. A switch allows the communication into the treatment room when necessary.

Multiple fields

The majority of treatment plans require radiation delivery through more than one port to achieve sufficient dose homogeneity through the target volume. Accuracy in multiple-field irradiation is greatly enhanced with the use of isocentric treatment techniques. With the isocenter of the treatment unit precisely positioned in the target volume, radiation beams can be aimed at the target volume from many directions without the patient being moved and accuracy compromised. The areas of overlap from these fields receive an increased dose relative to tissues receiving radiation from only one portal.

After radiation delivery to the first treatment port, the radiation therapist must assess the position of the patient and treatment unit for each subsequent field. Field size, table, gantry, and collimator angles are set, and treatment accessories are positioned. Although often accomplished by reentry into the treatment room, the setup of subsequent fields from the console may be allowed by some computer-controlled linear accelerators. The patient is informed that the radiation therapists are leaving the room for treatment delivery. With everyone except the patient out of the treatment room, the beam is turned on. This process is repeated until all fields have been treated.

The choice of field arrangement depends on the location of the tumor and nearby critical structures. As a member of the treatment-planning team, the radiation therapist works with the radiation oncologist and dosimetrist to plan field arrangements that cover target volumes while avoiding critical structures.

The most basic multiple-field technique is the parallel opposed portal, or POP. *POP fields* are defined as those with a hinge angle of 180 degrees. These fields may enter the patient from any two directions relative to the patient and are often identified by those directions. Examples include right-and-left laterals (laterals), anteroposterior and posteroanterior (APPA), and anterior oblique and posterior oblique (obliques). These are used for a great variety of treatment sites and usually require few treatment accessories other than blocks and compensators. In the treatment of head and neck cancer with lateral ports, patients who have metal fillings may benefit from the addition of internal shielding to reduce the dose on the buccal mucosa and tongue produced by increased electron scatter near the metal surface. A mouth guard made of wax and inlaid with a thin layer of tin can be prepared before the simulation and used throughout the treatment course to attenuate this scatter without significantly altering the dose distribution.

The four-field technique, sometimes referred to as a *four-field box* or *brick*, is commonly used in the treatment of deep-seated tumors of the pelvis or abdomen. These fields are arranged 90 degrees from one another and generally require no more than blocks for optimal dose distribution in the target volume.

The wedge-pair technique changes the volume receiving radiation by decreasing the hinge angle between two treatment fields. The relative dose in the area formed between the narrowing hinge angle increases. Overlapping isodose lines are not parallel to one another, and combining them produces extremely high dose deposition in the shallow portion of the target volume relative to the dose deposited more deeply. By reducing the amount of radiation delivered to this region, wedges distribute the dose more homogeneously throughout the target volume. Three-field techniques also often require the use of wedges to achieve the same dose-homogeneity goal.

Total body irradiation (TBI) is accomplished through a variety of techniques. Patients must be positioned at an extended distance to produce a sufficiently large field size. On treatment units not specifically designed for this purpose, this usually means lying on the floor or standing or sitting against a treatment-room wall with the gantry rotated 90 degrees. To achieve dose homogeneity, patients must be treated with POP fields requiring repositioning halfway through the treatment. Several dedicated TBI treatment machines have been developed in centers with a high demand for this treatment. These machines simplify treatment by using fixed, extended distance, double-headed treatment units to deliver radiation through both surfaces with the patient in a comfortable, constant position.

Arc therapy demonstrates the ultimate multiple-field technique. In standard arc therapy, radiation is delivered as the gantry moves through its arc of rotation, thus effectively delivering radiation through a continuous sequence of individual overlapping treatment portals. Verification of clearance of the patient; accessory medical equipment; the treatment table; and all stretchers, chairs, and stools must be completed before initiating the treatment beam. Visual monitors must be positioned so that the patient and motion of the gantry can be observed. The changing gantry angle must not obstruct monitoring of the treatment at any time.

Stereotactic radiosurgery or radiation therapy uses sophisticated localization methods to reproduce the placement of the isocenter in the cranium with an accuracy of less than 1 mm. Multiple noncoplanar arcs are directed at the tumor by changing the treatment-table rotation between treatment arcs. By distributing the dose delivered to normal tissue over an even greater area, the area of high relative dose is increasingly focused on the target volume. In radiosurgery a single large fraction of radiation dose can be delivered to the target without overdosing nearby normal brain tissue. With stereotactic radiosurgery the radiobiological benefits of fractionation is combined with advances in localization and definition of dose distribution.

Treatment-room maintenance

Maintenance of the treatment room and its contents is the domain of the radiation therapist. In addition to monitoring the performance of the treatment unit, the radiation therapist must inspect treatment accessories for signs of wear or damage. Supplies of nonreusable or disposal items such as tape, laundry, and some bolus materials must be monitored.

Cleanliness and orderliness are essential to providing a safe treatment and work environment. Treatment accessories and positioning or immobilization devices coming in contact with patients must be cleaned and disinfected after each use. Sufficient shelf and cabinet space must be available to securely store equipment off the floor, and proper lighting

levels must be maintained. Any unsafe conditions must be reported and corrected promptly.

SUMMARY

Through participation in the treatment-planning process and daily delivery of treatment the radiation therapist has a primary responsibility to the quality of care delivered to the patient. To meet the goals of treatment, whether palliative or curative, the radiation therapist remains vigilant in the accurate reproduction and administration of the treatment as prescribed by the physician. As the expert in treatment delivery, the radiation therapist is highly skilled in the use of megavoltage treatment units and accessories used to customize treatments for each patient. Through the documentation of treatment, monitoring of treatment-unit function, and inclusion on the departmental QA committee, radiation therapists actively participate in the ongoing goal of the radiation oncology team to continuously improve patient treatment and care.

As the treatment team member interacting with the patient on a daily basis, the radiation therapist applies knowledge of the physical and emotional reactions to radiation treatment by addressing the needs and concerns of patients within the guidelines of the scope of practice. Patients are directed to the physician or other professionals as specific needs are demonstrated.

Technical advances in diagnostic imaging, treatment-planning computers, and megavoltage treatment units have created great flexibility in the complexity of treatment plans that can be developed. Tumor volumes are identified and localized with greater confidence, and treatment beams are focused more narrowly. Normal tissue is increasingly spared from radiation exposure and damage. However, translation of the computer-generated plan to a living, breathing individual is still the primary challenge to reaping the benefits of these advances. Reduction in daily setup errors through the development and application of improvements in positioning, immobilization, and localization landmarks is attained through the diligence and precision of the radiation therapist.

Review Questions

Multiple Choice

1. Which of the following includes the area of a known and presumed tumor?
   a. Tumor volume
   b. Irradiated volume
   c. Critical volume
   d. Target volume

2. Beam modifiers that simulate tissue include which of the following?
   I. Compensator
   II. Wedge
   III. Bolus
      a. I and II
      b. I and III
      c. II and III
      d. I, II, and III

3. What is the identification of the isocenter and field borders in relation to surface or bony landmarks?
   a. Definition
   b. Localization
   c. Dosimetry
   d. Simulation

4. Which of the following is included in the daily treatment record?
   I. Treatment number
   II. Cumulative dose
   III. Patient position
      a. I and II
      b. I and III
      c. II and III
      d. I, II, and III

5. The period over which radiation is delivered is referred to as which of the following?
   a. Fractionation
   b. Exposure time
   c. Protraction
   d. Treatment time

6. Overlap of adjacent fields can be eliminated by using which of the following techniques?
   a. Half-beam blocks
   b. Gaps
   c. Feathering
   d. Abutting fields

7. The feathering technique is used to do which of the following?
   a. Eliminate overlap
   b. Increase dose to gapped region
   c. Decrease dose to gapped region
   d. Decrease dose in abutted fields

8. Patients are monitored during treatment delivery with megavoltage treatment units by using which of the following?
   I. Closed-circuit television
   II. Direct visual
   III. Two-way audio
      a. I and II
      b. I and III
      c. II and III
      d. I, II, and III

9. What is the angle between the central axes of two treatment beams?
   a. Central angle
   b. Gantry angle
   c. Wedge angle
   d. Hinge angle

10. What are used to shape electron fields?
    a. Cutouts
    b. Blocks
    c. Compensators
    d. Transmission filters

Questions to Ponder

1. Describe the way an immobilization device differs from a positioning aid.
2. Analyze information to be included in the radiation therapy treatment chart.
3. Discuss factors contributing to decisions regarding portal imaging frequency.

REFERENCES

1. American Society of Radiologic Technologists: *The scope of practice for radiation therapists,* Albuquerque, 1993, The Society.
2. Bentel G: Collimator and couch design in radiation therapy equipment, *Radiat Ther* 1(1): 250-258, 1992
3. Denham JW et al: Objective decision-making following a portal film: the results of a pilot study, *Int J Radiat Oncol Biol Phys* 26:869-876, 1993.
4. Digel C et al: Dosimetric comparison of five craniospinal techniques, *Radiat Ther* 3(2):95-102, 1994.
5. Glatstein E: Radiation oncology in integrated care management, *Report of the Intersociety Council for Radiation Oncology*, December 1991.
6. Herman MG et al: Clinical use of on-line portal imaging for daily patient treatment verification, *Int J Radiat Oncol Biol Phys* 28(4):1017-1023, 1994.
7. Kutcher GJ et al: Report of AAPM radiation therapy committee task group 40, *Medical Phys* 21(4):581-618, 1994.
8. Marks JE et al: The value of frequent treatment verification films in reducing localization error in the irradiation of complex fields, *Cancer* 37:2755, 1976.
9. Miller G, Hebert L: *Taking care of your back,* Bangor, Maine, 1984, IMPACC.
10. Podmaniczky KC et al: Clinical experience with a computerized record and verify system, *Intl J Radiat Oncol Biol Phys* 11(8):1529-1537, 1985.
11. Reinstein LE, Pai S, Meek AG: Assessment of geometric treatment accuracy using time-lapse display of electronic portal images, *Int J Radiat Oncol Biol Phys* 22(5):1139-1146, 1992.
12. Wizenberg MJ: *Quality assurance in radiation therapy: a manual for technologists*, Chicago, 1982, American College of Radiology.

Patient Care

17

Education

Pamela J. Ross

Outline

Key terms

Accreditation
Advocates
Communication
Critical thinking
Karnofsky score

Life experiences
Protocol
Radiation therapy domain
Randomization

Education is a vital part of radiation oncology because it seeks to dispel myths and overcome years of misunderstandings. Only recently have efforts become pronounced to remove stigmas attached to cancer. However, fears associated with radiation therapy are still prevalent. Therefore the importance of education cannot be overemphasized.

Education has two main components: the formal setting, which is composed of standard classroom learning at varying levels, and informal education, which consists of a large range of **life experiences**. *Life experiences* can be described as information gathered through a normal day's activities that are useful to enhance an existing knowledge base. Using the basic concepts of formal education as a foundation, life experiences play varying roles. In the 1990s, interactive education has evolved to enhance the learning experience through the acceptance, assimilation, and sharing of ideas and responsibility for learning between the educator and student. Life experiences are equally important as or possibly more so than formal education because they often pertain directly to day-to-day living and have a strong connection with continuing education.

The educational evolution of radiation sciences can be traced as far back as 1646 with the invention of the first particle vacuum.[10] The study of radiation science was further advanced in the late nineteenth century when Antoine-Henri

Becquerel discovered radioactivity. These discoveries opened the door for Marie and Pierre Curie, who in 1898 performed scientific research on radioactive materials. Also during this time, in 1895, Wilhelm Roentgen discovered x-rays. The first therapeutic use of x-rays was in 1896, when Dr. Emil Herman Grubbe used them to treat a breast cancer patient.[6] Despite the early history, education in radiation therapy lagged for many decades, mainly because of a lack of specialty identification. Professionals working in the field of radiation oncology continued the endeavor for recognition, and this field has now advanced scientifically to a point at which it functions as an important part of the study and treatment of cancer. As radiation therapy emerged as an independent area of practice, the need for educated personnel became apparent and the evolution of the radiation therapist commenced.

Approximately a quarter million people were treated with radiation therapy in 1995 in the United States. The radiation therapist is a key member in the medical care of the oncology patient; thus a need exists for the therapist to have a strong and varied education. Radiation therapists are highly respected professionals and an integral part of the scientific community because they serve as a resource for the education of others. The subsequent discussion describes the educational background of the radiation therapist, credentialing agencies in radiation therapy, and necessary issues in radiation oncology that the radiation therapist must be capable of addressing.

EVOLUTION OF THE RADIATION THERAPIST

In the United States, radiation therapy education has been "recognized as a separate discipline within radiologic technology since 1964, when the first certifying examination was administered by the American Registry of Radiologic Technologists (ARRT)."[5] The first set of essentials for a formal school of radiation therapy technology were adopted by the American College of Radiology (ACR), American Society of Radiologic Technologists (ASRT), and American Medical Association (AMA) in 1968. The essentials applied only to 1-year programs because almost all technologists entering the field of radiation therapy at that time were recruited from radiography and nursing. In 1972 the ACR, ASRT, and AMA provided guidelines for the first 2-year programs by adopting essentials for programs with a minimum entrance requirement of a high school diploma.[5] The 1968 didactic essentials for the first 1-year programs are compared with the 1994 didactic essentials in the box at the top of the page.

The first radiation therapy education programs in the United States were strongly influenced by the earlier growth of radiation therapy courses in England. The Royal Marsden School of Therapeutic Radiography offers a 3-year program for radiation therapy that began in 1963 with the faculty of science of Kingston University (department of radiography

---

Essentials

School of Radiation Therapy curriculum (1968)	Radiation Therapy curriculum (1994)*
• Introduction to course • Physics • Mathematics • Elementary pathology • Radiobiology • Anatomy • Treatment planning • Nursing procedures • Radiation therapy • Protection and shielding • Ethics	• Orientation to radiation therapy technology • Medical ethics and law • Methods of patient care • Medical terminology • Human structure and function • Oncology pathology • Radiobiology • Mathematics • Radiation physics • Radiation protection • Radiation oncology technique • Radiographic imaging • Clinical dosimetry • Quality assurance • Introduction to hyperthermia • Introduction to computers

*The curriculum for radiation therapy programs has been revised over the years to reflect an increase in the necessary skills of the therapist. The radiation therapist is regarded as an important part of the radiation therapy team; therefore the educational background of the therapist must reflect the scientific expanse of radiation therapy.

---

education). The program includes didactic and clinical education. The clinical education requirement for the program was and still is approximately 2000 hours. The didactic courses parallel those in the 1994 essentials that are found in the box with the additions of sociology of health, psychology of the sick, and research. Originally, the program graduates were awarded diplomas from the college of radiographers. Presently, the graduates are awarded a bachelor of science degree in therapeutic radiography from Kingston University.

Governing agencies

Three main agencies are directly involved in establishing educational standards, professional credentialing, and the exchange of professional information for the discipline of radiation therapy. These agencies are the Joint Review Committee on Education in Radiologic Technology (JRCERT), ARRT, and ASRT.

The JRCERT has been responsible for the development and review of educational standards in radiologic sciences since 1944. Not until 1964, 20 years after its inception, did the JRCERT recognize radiation therapy as a science distinguishable from other radiologic sciences. In 1975 the JRCERT established a set of essentials, which still governs today, that incorporated 1- and 2-year programs in radiation therapy technology.

The JRCERT has the authority to accredit all radiologic technology education programs. **Accreditation** is the process of credentialing a learning institution and giving formal approval to the merits of an existing program. The accreditation process includes a microscopic review of a program by an official agency and a comparison of the critiqued data with standards set by that agency. The primary objective is to assure the public that all accredited programs have attained a satisfactory level of performance with the ability to produce over time a therapist with the highest level of competence.

The accreditation process includes a self-study that is completed by the program staff members requesting accreditation. The report is then submitted to the JRCERT before the second step, which is a site visit.

The self-study is an all-inclusive document with the following six main divisions: (1) *sponsorship* (describes the institution or institutions supporting the program), (2) *resources* (includes specifics regarding the program director, clinical coordinator, clinical supervisor, medical director of the school, didactic staff members, clinical instructors, financial resources, physical resources, equipment, supplies, and library), (3) *curriculum* (includes the didactic courses offered and specifics of the competency-based clinical program, including quality assurance, simulation procedures, dosimetry, treatment procedures, patient care and management, and periodic evaluation of students), (4) *students* (describes the admissions criteria, program, health standards, and guidance available for students), (5) *operational policies* (describes fair policies and student records), and (6) *continuing program evaluation* (includes an ongoing internal review process).

The site visit is the on-site review by the accreditation staff of a newly proposed program or a program requesting renewal of accreditation. This visit serves two purposes: to examine the didactic program and competency-based clinical program and to compare the reality of the setting with the previously submitted self-study.

The JRCERT sets clinical standards that specify a set number of students per program. This number depends on the available education resources, including the number of registered therapists, treatment machines, and simulators. Usually two students are allowed per megavoltage unit, and one student is allowed per simulator. The program should have one registered radiation therapist for each two students.[5] The number of JRCERT-accredited programs has continued a steady growth since the 1960s, and as of December 1995, 120 radiation therapy programs were accredited by the JRCERT.

A student intent on becoming a radiation therapist can select one of four educational options: (1) a baccalaureate degree program in radiation therapy, (2) a college-based associate degree in radiation therapy, (3) a 2-year, hospital-based certificate program, and (4) a 1-year certificate program in radiation therapy offered to graduates of an accredited 2-year radiology technology program. All theses options afford the graduate an opportunity to become nationally registered and/or state licensed. An increasing emphasis is on the need for persons working in the field of radiation therapy to hold one or both of these official documents. A standardized and strict credentialing system will help secure the professionalism of the radiation therapist. Radiation therapists who pass the national registry examination are automatically awarded a state license in most areas in which such a license is available. The awarding of a state license is an individual matter that varies according to each state and should be investigated on a state-to-state basis. Presently, 30 states and Puerto Rico offer state licenses. In the next 2 years, three more states will also offer licenses in the field of radiation therapy.

The ARRT is responsible for the credentialing examination that allows the radiation therapist to become nationally registered. The ARRT has the objective of "encouraging the study and elevating the standards of radiologic technology, as well as the examining and certifying of eligible candidates and periodic publication of a listing of registrants."[2] The ARRT was formed in 1922 after the Radiologic Society of North America (RSNA) agreed that x-ray technicians needed an organization to monitor education standards. The RSNA and the American Roentgen Ray Society (ARRS) worked together to form the ARRT.[6] Currently, the governing board of the ARRT consists of nine members, five of which are technologists appointed by the ASRT and four of which are physicians appointed by the ACR.[4] The ACR took over the responsibilities relating to the ARRT from the RSNA in 1944. In 1962 the ARRT recognized radiation therapy as a separate discipline from radiology and initiated the first examination. The first year that graduates from a radiation therapy program satisfied the essentials for the examination was 1964, when 108 candidates took the examination with a passing rate of 81%. The passing rate over the past 15 years has increased to 86%, which is a credit to the present education standards. Fig. 17-1 shows the obvious growth of radiation therapy through a comparison of the number of candidates accepted to take the registry examination at 10-year intervals over 30 years. Currently, approximately 10,000 radiation therapists are registered as a result of the continuous growth of education in the field of radiation oncology. The eligibility requirements for a student to take the registry examination include a satisfactory completion of a formal radiation therapy course in a JRCERT-accredited school. Candidates without an education from a JRCERT-accredited program may take the examination if they meet special eligibility requirements set forth by the ARRT. These requirements are equal to or beyond those requirements necessary for a graduate of an approved program. Special eligibility will no longer be offered as an option after the year 2000.

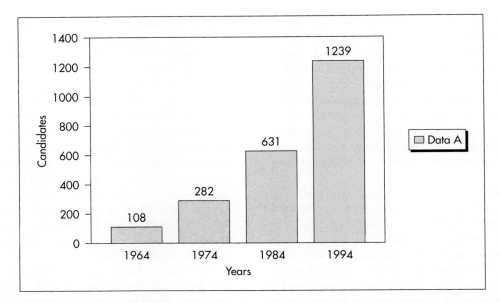

Fig. 17-1 ARRT examinations (1964-1994). The national registry in radiation therapy has experienced a 91.3% growth in the number of applicants accepted to take the registry examination over a 30-year period. The inaugural examination was given in 1964, with sequential examinations showing a steady and continuing increase up to the most recent examination in 1994. The most rapid growth seems to have taken place during the last decade.

The registry examination is administered 3 times per year, on the third Thursday of March, July, and October at 4:00 PM. The examination is made widely available in over 100 locations in various parts of the country. A policy enacted in 1994 limits the number of times a candidate can fail the examination to three before the candidate must show proof of remediation. The specific areas of the core content of the examination are continually updated and made available to program directors. These changes are instituted to reflect the evolving needs of the radiation therapist and advancement in radiation therapy.

The ARRT established a code of ethics for registered technologists and applicants for the registry examination. The radiation therapist should have a full understanding of the code and its implications to apply it on a daily basis. A more detailed explanation of the code of ethics is addressed in Chapter 4.

The ASRT is a national organization that encompasses technologists in radiology, radiation therapy, nuclear medicine, and sonography. The Society originated in Chicago in October 1920 as the American Association of Radiologic Technicians (AART) and underwent a name change in 1930 to the American Society of Radiographers because of the possibility of confusion over the acronyms AART and ARRT. The society changed its name yet again in 1934 to the American Society of X-Ray Technicians (ASXT), and in July 1963 the Society changed once more to the present name, the ASRT. The final name change was meant to signify the pro-

fessional status of the technologist and eliminate the connotation of on-the-job training.[3]

The first journal published for members of the Society was in 1929 under the title *The X-Ray Technician*. Later the publication title was changed to reflect the new name of the Society; thus the title became *Radiologic Technology*.[6] The advent of radiation therapy evoked a new journal, *The Radiation Therapist*, which is primarily concerned with the science of radiation oncology and technical aspects of radiation therapy.

An important organizational step occurred in 1966 when the president of the ASRT, Leslie Wilson, stated that the Society would attempt to restrict professional status to technologists graduating from a formal 2-year program. A major development in increasing the standing of the professional status occurred in 1981 when President Reagan signed the Consumer-Patient Radiation Health and Safety Act, which "established standards for accreditation of educational programs and for certification of those who administer ionizing radiation procedures."[3] In 1984 the Society added an educational foundation, which uses contributions for projects focused on strengthening educational programs. The ASRT gained more momentum in 1992 when it was able to gain a majority of representation of technologists on the boards of the ARRT and JRCERT. This majority ensures that only technologists will have a major voice in setting standards of practice. The ASRT, which started with 13 technicians from the United States and Canada, has grown to a current membership of over 40,000. This figure includes national and international members. The chapter system, which was created in 1993, allows the creation of specific focus groups such as radiation therapy, management, and education. Keeping up with the times and the needs of its members, the ASRT now offers assistance with mandatory continuing-education credits.

Educational background of the radiation therapist

The role of the radiation therapist was created as a result of a specific need in the medical community. The education of the radiation therapist evolved from on-the-job training to condensed 12-month courses to a comprehensive 24-month program. A student in an accredited radiation therapy program will be educated in two separate areas that merge and complement each other. The schooling consists of a didactic section as outlined in the 1994 essentials and a competency-based clinical section.

The clinical program is based on technical competencies that are divided, according to the complexity of a setup, between first- and second-year students. Students are evaluated with regard to specific tasks and graded according to their ability to complete a particular task. The clinical evaluation process differs from program to program, but the goal is the same. The basic concept of any program involves an evaluation system based on the adeptness and efficiency with which the student performs a task. Aside from the technical aspect, the evaluation should also include the social and communicative skills between the student and patient and the student and therapist. The ARRT created a task-inventory list that outlines responsibilities of the radiation therapist. Individually, each item seems banal, but collectively the items create a masterful therapist. The clinical aspect of radiation therapy should always be strengthened by didactic portions of the program. The combination of cognitive powers and technical abilities helps to reinforce accuracy and reproducibility incumbent daily on the radiation therapist.

The didactic and clinical areas of the program are each evaluated on their own merit and must be passed with a minimum grade for the candidate to graduate and be eligible to take the registry examination.

Education in radiation therapy must empower the practitioner and afford experiences that foster analytical and critical-thinking skills. Rote memorization and recounting of facts and figures provide a basis for task-oriented scopes of practice. However, in today's health care environment, the radiation therapist must be able to solve problems and function effectively as a health care team member. Outcome-based education is a desirable form of instruction giving a radiation therapist an awareness that resolution involves organized analytical decisions and judgments.

The prescriptive methods of early educational philosophies are currently being replaced by outcome-based methodologies. This approach offers educators and educational institutions flexibility in developing educational curricula that suit their individual resources and philosophies in achieving the final product, a well-rounded therapist who is able to think critically.[11] Long learning curves after the completion of the educational process are not acceptable with the rapidity in health care delivery changes. Instead, a radiation therapist must have an ability to relate diverse experiences encountered in practical clinical education settings to a broad knowledge base obtained during didactic and clinical courses. A variety of experiences provide the therapist with opportunities to develop practical problem-solving skills, which are essential in practice today.

Radiation therapists who are able to think critically are open-minded and therefore capable of analyzing and evaluating situations. **Critical thinking** can be defined as the freedom to use the cognitive process to allow mastery of theory and practical experiences. Critical thinking incorporates the use of cognitive, affective, and psychomotor domains. The art of critical thinking helps the therapist question and critique each step of a patient's treatment, thereby ensuring an understanding and accurate administration of the treatment. The therapist must be able to understand the function of the treatment plan and relate it to the function of the available equipment to ensure feasibility. As a part of the radiation therapy team, the radiation therapist must have the ability to make technical judgments, offer alternative treatment arrangements, and relate all of this to other members of the team.

The hierarchical ladder of the cognitive domain (Fig. 17-2) describes the steps demonstrated in the domain. The lower parts of the ladder correspond to lower levels of learning consistent with the cognitive foundation. Students on this level are asked to memorize and give the information back. The higher parts require mastery of the foundation levels to perform more evaluative tasks. Educators should spend more time on the higher levels. This is the only way to infuse the educational curriculum and student with critical thinking skills.

Critical-thinking skills, such as reasoning and intuitiveness, give the therapist a knowledge base that allows a proactive approach to patient care. Higher thinking skills and diverse experiences allow the practitioner to anticipate problems. The evolution of education and educational standards that promote higher learning has greatly enhanced the effectiveness of today's practitioner.[12]

Educational advancement

Students who have successfully graduated from a JRCERT-accredited radiation therapy program and received a certificate from the ARRT by passing the national registry examination with a grade of 75% or better have only just begun their learning experiences. After a student has achieved the professional status of radiation therapist, the student may continue formal education and training to become a

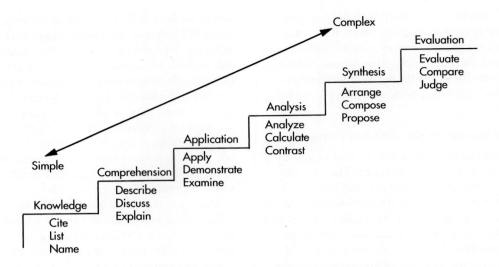

Fig. 17-2 A representation of the cognitive domain of learning. (Modified from Ford C: *Clinical education for the allied health professions,* St Louis, 1978, Mosby.)

dosimetrist or physicist. Another option is to continue education in management and administration for career opportunities in these fields. Therapists may elect to teach their own specialty. Teaching may include didactic or clinical radiation therapy or both and could eventually lead to a qualified individual becoming a program director. Some radiation therapists have chosen to pursue a medical degree and specialize in radiation oncology. Although career choices are myriad, many therapists prefer to continue in the technology-based patient care area as radiation therapists. The career choice is an individual one and need not be immediate because options are continually available. A therapist may take the opportunity to gain as much knowledge as possible during the clinical practice of radiation therapy over a period of several years before deciding to pursue a different career. A new graduate has a great deal of growth to achieve before becoming an accomplished radiation therapist and should benefit from all resources available. The therapist acts much the way an orbiting electron does, by interacting with various people including patients, colleagues, and physicians. As the electron does, so the therapist goes through an endless process of absorbing useful information and participating in an infinite number of critical chain reactions.

The year 1994 was significant for the radiation therapist because it marked yet another advancement toward increasing professional status. The therapist now has an opportunity to do this through mandatory continuing education. A therapist must show evidence of obtaining 24 continuing-education credits over a 2-year period to renew the registry certification. A therapist can obtain evidence of continuing education (ECE) in several ways. The therapist may obtain and record credits through services that the ASRT makes available to its members.

Attendance at conferences is an excellent way to acquire necessary credits. The ASRT assists the therapist by examining conference material and assigning appropriate credits to each conference that contributes suitably to the therapist's education. The therapist may attend conferences outside of the department setting or use existing programs in the department or hospital setting. Therapists who have the support of their institution or department may be allowed to attend national conferences such as the American Society of Therapeutic Radiologists and Oncologists (ASTRO) and RSNA meetings. These large conferences consist of many meetings that are approved for continuing education. Also, throughout the year, local societies organize numerous smaller conferences that offer meetings accredited for continuing education.

A therapist who works in an institution that has other educational programs may benefit by attending conferences arranged through the institution. An example of this is to use a program that is operational under residency programs in oncology disciplines, especially radiation oncology. Many of these meetings are already accredited by the AMA. A request can be made to the ASRT for approval of a meeting that can be attended by a number of therapists. If the request is accepted, the ASRT assigns reference numbers to each course. The establishment of such a program assures the department that the therapists are following an organized plan for continuing education and thus minimizes the chances that a therapist will lose certification from the ARRT.

In addition, the ASRT offers directed readings in the journals that equal approximately 12 credits per year when the corresponding paperwork is properly completed and submitted. This alone is enough to cover the necessary credits requested by the ARRT. The introduction of the *Radiation Therapist Journal* will increase the number of directed readings and include a greater number of articles focused on the science of radiation oncology. The ASRT also offers continuing-education credits for articles and directed readings that are submitted to the ASRT and accepted for publication in the journals *Radiologic Technology* or *Radiation Therapist.*

The ASRT provides a tracking service of credits for its members by requiring the therapist to submit proof of attendance of any accredited conferences to the ASRT along with the therapist's name and social security number. The ASRT sends a letter to members the month preceding their birth month; the letter enumerates the credits by title, date, and number of credits. This summary alleviates the process of reporting the continuing-education credits to the ARRT.

Using directed readings and attending in-house programs to obtain ECEs shows good faith to hospital and department administrators. This is important because continuing education is the responsibility of the therapist. Therapists should show self-motivation and intense interest in their professionalism through initiating participation in educational activities. After this has been accomplished and self-motivation established, the technologist has a firm basis to request funding to attend outside society meetings.

Continuing education is an important concept that helps broaden the perspective of the radiation therapist. The purpose of continuing education is to stay on the crest of the wave of the constantly changing technology. Therefore the therapist should pursue learning of new technical developments such as stereotactic radiosurgery, dynamic wedging, and conformal radiation therapy. The therapist must join the computer revolution because most of radiation therapy revolves around computerization through treatment planning, record and verification systems linked to treatment machines, or technical operation of much of today's equipment. Other areas in which the therapist must be well versed are the critical aspects of patient care. To apply the best care possible, the therapist should thoroughly understand the rights of the patient. Therapists, by virtue of their position in the community, are expected to be leaders in the education and health awareness of the residents. The therapist should be able to address today's social concerns of medical cost reduction. A therapist who is a member of a health team in an institution that is active in graduate medical education must understand and be ready to participate in relevant research aspects.

Radiation therapists should focus their attention on the object of concern (the patient) and delivery of premium patient care. The therapist can meet many of these objectives through a clear understanding of the Patient's Bill of Rights. The components of the Bill of Rights are meant to protect the patient and raise awareness in the medical community of the patient's medical needs. A dissection of the Bill of Rights illuminates the areas of interest that apply to the oncology patient and radiation therapist.

PATIENTS' RIGHTS

Anyone who has the misfortune to suffer from an ailment that requires medical attention undergoes a transformation from a well person to a patient, a status that may be accompanied by a sense of loss of control over life and possibly of dignity. As a result, to protect the rights of the individual, the Patient's Bill of Rights evolved. For example, the components as made available in New York in accordance with New York State public health law are listed in the box on p. 274. The Patient's Bill of Rights is distributed to each hospitalized patient or a representative at the time of admission. An outpatient has access to the Bill of Rights, which is posted in various areas of the hospital, including the emergency room and all ancillary outpatient departments. The Patient's Bill of Rights must be available in multiple languages appropriate for the patient population of the hospital. The language selections are made by using a mathematical analysis that is based on the acquisition of information from the U.S. Bureau of the Census regarding the demographics of the hospital's service area. Any non-English-speaking group that constitutes more than 1% of the patient population should have translator services and the Bill of Rights available in that group's language. An expert in communicating with the visually and hearing impaired should be available to relay the Patient's Bill of Rights to that population of patients. The Patient's Bill of Rights reinforces the fact that patients are people and should not be treated differently from individuals not confined to a hospital setting. Today's hospitals have an array of patient **advocates** who are responsible for ensuring that patient's needs are fulfilled and their rights enforced. The advocate is a supporter who can act as a protector and a friend.

Patient advocates

The patient representative is on the forefront of ensuring the patient's rights during a hospital visit. The purpose of the patient representative as related by The New York Methodist Hospital's Department of Patient Representation[9] is "to assure that patients are provided with quality care given in a considerate, courteous and individualized manner without discrimination as to race, color, religion, sex, national origin, sexual orientation, or source of payment." The patient representative should assist the patient, family, and friends in understanding hospital policies. The patient representative is responsible for providing the patient, family members, and friends with a means for referring matters that occur between the hospital personnel and patient, including any allegations of mismanaged health care and medical negligence. The patient representative may intervene in discussions regarding the signing of legal documents and activation of such documents as *do-not-resuscitate* (DNR) orders *health care proxy* documents, and *living wills.*

A second group of hospital personnel, called *social workers,* has goals specifically focused on fulfilling the needs of patients. These needs change as the health status changes. Social workers have the responsibility to care for the con-

Patients Bill of Rights*

1. The patient has the right to understand and use these rights. If for any reason the patient does not understand or needs help, the hospital must provide assistance, including an interpreter.
2. The patient has the right to receive treatment without discrimination as to race, color, religion, sex, national origin, disability, sexual orientation, or source of payment.
3. The patient has the right to receive considerate and respectful care in a clean and safe environment free of unnecessary restraints.
4. The patient has the right to receive emergency care if necessary.
5. The patient has the right to be informed of the name and position of the doctor in charge of the hospital care.
6. The patient has the right to know the names, positions, and functions of any hospital staff members involved in the care and to refuse their treatment, examination, or observation.
7. The patient has the right to a no-smoking room.
8. The patient has the right to receive complete information about the diagnosis, treatment, and prognosis.
9. The patient has the right to receive all the information necessary to give informed consent for any proposed procedure or treatment. This information shall include the possible risks and benefits of the procedure or treatment.
10. The patient has the right to receive all the information necessary to give informed consent for an order not to resuscitate. The patient also has the right to designate an individual to give this consent if the patient is too ill to do so. For additional information the patient may ask for a copy of the

pamphlet *Do-Not-Resuscitate Order—A Guide for Patients and Families.*
11. Patients have the right to refuse treatment and be told what effect this may have on their health.
12. The patient has the right to refuse to take part in research. In deciding whether or not to participate, the patient has the right to a full explanation.
13. The patient has the right to privacy while in the hospital and confidentiality of all information and records regarding the care.
14. The patient has the right to participate in all decisions about the treatment and discharge from the hospital. The hospital must provide the patient with a written discharge plan and written description of the way patients can appeal their discharge.
15. The patient has the right to review the medical record without charge and obtain a copy of the medical record, for which the hospital can charge a reasonable fee. Patients cannot be denied a copy solely because they cannot afford to pay.
16. The patient has the right to receive an itemized bill and explanation of all charges.
17. The patient has the right to complain without fear of reprisal about the care and services received and to have the hospital respond with a written response if requested. If patients are not satisfied with the hospital's response, they can complain to the New York State Health Department. The hospital must provide the patient with the Health Department telephone number.

Modified from the Health Care Association of New York State: *Your rights as a hospital patient,* New York, 1994, The Association.
*The Patient's Bill of Rights is made available in accordance with the New York State Public Health Law and is distributed and posted in all public areas of the hospital in observance of this law.

crete portion of the patient's needs. The social worker intervenes when the needs of a patient lean toward psychosocial assessment, counseling, crisis intervention, financial problems, housing or home placement, home care, and support groups.[9] The social worker usually assists the patient who is recuperating from an illness and for whom the prospect exists of leaving the hospital. Serving both inpatients and outpatients, the social worker assists the patient in applying for financial help with Medicaid or discovers other available financial resources. Patients who need continued outpatient services can be steered toward grants that can help pay for services such as home care assistance and transportation between the home and hospital. The social worker can assist the patient if family support and the patient's medical condition warrant admission to an adult care facility. In addition, the social worker can assist the family with necessary counseling about fears of unknown treatment and problems caused by the interruption of daily life caused by an illness. The social worker is particularly important to oncology

patients because this group of patients tends to have a great number and variety of needs. The National Association of Oncology Social Workers was formed to better fulfill the large scope of these needs.

The radiation therapist plays an important advocacy role for the oncology patient. The chances of a patient successfully completing a course of radiation therapy can be enhanced by the establishment of a strong patient-therapist relationship. The therapist can help create a comfortable environment for the patient by creating an atmosphere of respect and understanding. The first step toward this is for therapists and patients to understand the way each item in the Patient's Bill of Rights influence them. The first right with specific consequence to the therapist-patient relationship is as follows[7]:

The patient has the right to understand and use these rights. the hospital must provide assistance to the patient to enhance understanding by way of patient representation and an interpreter when necessary.

Communication

The therapist must possess good **communication** skills and should be aware of outside resources that are available to enhance communication between the patient and therapist. Communication is the art of transferring concrete and abstract information from one person to another. Humans communicate in two main ways: through verbal and nonverbal communication. Verbal communication uses verbalization of the thought process in such a way that a concept passes from one person to another with the same basic meaning. Nonverbal communication is a way to exchange mental images through body language by using facial expressions, physical animation, or written dialogue.

The health care worker deals with such an array of people of different nationalities that verbal communication often yields to nonverbal communication as a matter of need. The health care worker can communicate in a variety of ways with a patient who does not speak English. The hospital may have a language roster enumerating different staff members who can translate different languages. These staff members can be contacted and, if available, will assist in communication. Each department in the hospital may have direct access to translators through its own personnel, some of whom may be able to translate a variety of languages. The AT&T language phone can assist in communication by accessing translators for multiple languages and dialects over a phone line.

Patients who are hearing impaired may need the support of staff members who are trained in the use of sign language and can also communicate through a relay teletype phone service. A radiation therapist can also use nonverbal communication to express ideas to the hearing impaired.

Patients who are unable to speak because of the removal of the larynx can use written communication. A means of written communication should be easily accessible to the patient.

Communication offers a way for patients to become involved in their own health care. Solid and honest communication can initiate and solidify a trusting relationship between the radiation therapist and patient, thereby allowing treatment steps to proceed smoothly and effectively. Communication is paramount, as is evident by the following tenet of The Patient's Bill of Rights[7]:

> The patient has the right to know the names, positions, and functions of any hospital staff members involved in the care and to refuse their treatment, examination, or observation.

The radiation therapist is only one in a line of personnel that the patient meets during the course of radiation therapy treatments. Good communication skills must prevail, and all appropriate introductions between staff members and patients should be made at the earliest possible time. The patient interacts with various people in the radiation department at different times. The nurse obtains basic information from the patient and explains the consultation process to the patient. The physician, attending or resident, obtains a history from the patient and examines reports and a variety of x-ray or computed tomography (CT) scans, and magnetic resonance images (MRIs). The physician goes through a decision-making process and then discusses findings with the patient. The decision to treat with radiation alone or in combination with other modalities such as surgery, chemotherapy, hormones, or immunotherapy is given to the patient and family. If the patient agrees to accept radiation as a treatment modality, the physician arranges a schedule for the patient to start the treatment portion of the regimen. The patient is scheduled for a simulation and returns to the nursing staff. The nurse, physician, or therapist may give the appointment to the patient. After a treatment plan has been outlined, the nurse or therapist can give the patient more specific information regarding reactions that can be expected and instructions to follow for site-specific areas to be treated. The nurse or therapist can give the patient written information about the specific areas of treatment and make arrangements for regular visits with a dietitian and social worker. The nurse may assist the patient with transportation arrangements to and from treatments. The nurse can assess the needs of patients from their **Karnofsky score**, from the area to be treated, and from the expected number of treatments. The therapist, physicians and nurse should have continuous interaction regarding the patient's care. A smaller department may be void of a nurse, dietitian, or social worker. The absence of any or all these critical personnel places additional responsibilities on the radiation therapist. The therapist must understand the individual practices of each profession and be ready to assume these duties.

The need for consistently good communication skills appears in yet another right of the patient[7]:

> The patient has the right to receive complete information about the diagnosis, treatment, and prognosis.

This prerogative gives patients the right to a clear understanding of the radiation treatment that they are undergoing and the effects of the treatment. This right is particularly important because oncology patients undergoing radiation treatments need specific instructions regarding diet and skin care and a full explanation of the treatment regimen. The radiation therapist's role is only one component of the health care team, which is led by the radiation oncologist. The radiation oncologist carries the ultimate responsibility for the patient's care. Members of the radiation therapy team include the radiation oncologist, radiation therapist, nurse oncologist, dietitian, and others, depending on the particular disease and needs of the patient

The patient usually starts the course of radiation treatments with a simulation. The therapist working in the simulator should know the patient's type of cancer, area to be treated, and general condition. This prepares the therapist for the amount and type of care the patient needs. The therapist should start the simulation by explaining to the patient the steps involved in the procedure. The intervention of the family or friend may be required if the patient is unable to understand. Instructions should be simple and clear so that the patient does not need to use a complex thought process, which may cause confusion and distress. The patient should be told only pertinent information about the simulation procedure. The following information should be detailed to the patient:

1. The names of personnel involved in the simulation
2. The use of x-ray films taken
3. The positions and movements of the machine
4. The positioning and cooperation required of the patient
5. Necessary radiopaque contrast materials, such as barium and Gastrografin
6. Markers that may be inserted, such as rectal and vaginal markers
7. Marks on the patient, including tattoos
8. Contouring procedures
9. The time necessary to complete the task

The therapist should allow the patient to ask questions, and assess the patient's comprehension level. The therapist working in the simulator is the patient's first contact. This initial therapist can help the patient begin to accept the reality of radiation therapy treatments. Therefore the patient must be treated with care. At the completion of the simulation, the therapist should stress the following to the patient:

1. The fact that patient has been simulated in preparation for treatment
2. The reason for maintaining the skin marks
3. The purpose of the tattoos
4. The necessary skin care
5. Dietary and nutritional considerations depending on the area being treated and availability of the dietitian
6. Expected reactions from the treatment depending on the area being treated

The therapist should set the next scheduled appointment for an additional simulation or the first radiation therapy treatment, discuss necessary transportation arrangements, and refer the patient to the appropriate person for those arrangements. In addition, the therapist should allow the patient to ask questions and should assess the patient's comprehension level. Usually, the patient next meets the therapist assigned to the treatment machine. The patient interacts with this therapist daily. Depending on the scheduling of therapists and size and organization of the department, the treating therapist may vary and may be the same therapist who worked in the simulator. The treating therapist should explain to the patient that all therapists are equally adept at the procedures. An attempt should be made to introduce as many of the involved therapists as possible before treatments are started. The treating therapist should speak openly to the patient about the treatments and should make the patient feel as comfortable as possible. A relaxed person tends to absorb more information and be more cooperative than an unnerved person. The therapist should discuss the following with the patient:

1. An introduction of the involved personnel
2. An explanation of the way the machine will move and whether it will at any time touch the patient
3. Noises that the patient can expect to hear and the frequency
4. Visual monitoring that the therapist performs
5. The available verbal communication system
6. Reactions to expect during the course of the treatment specific to the area of treatment
7. Skin care necessary during treatment and the purpose
8. Diet and nutrition recommended during the treatment and the availability of a dietitian
9. The way patients should react if they need something during the treatment
10. Radiation oncologist visits and availability during the course of the treatment
11. Convenient scheduling for the patient over the course of the treatment
12. Transportation needs

The therapist should allow the patient to ask questions and repeat necessary information after the first treatment, especially if the patient's comprehension is noted to be limited. Redundancy is apparent and purposeful. The patient absorbs only small portions of information, especially during periods of stress. The purpose of the repetition is to ensure the patient's full understanding regarding all aspects of the radiation therapy treatments. This repetition is generally enhanced by the issuance of similar instructions by physicians and nurses. The therapist should behave in a friendly and familylike manner while maintaining the professionalism necessary to gain the patient's respect and cooperation with instructions.

The daily interaction should foster a bond between the patient and therapist that helps gain the confidence and openness of the patient. This interaction allows the therapist to monitor firsthand the physical reactions and mental stability of the patient. The therapist has the duty of informing the relevant department personnel of any physical, psychological, or mental changes noticed in the patient. The therapist should be aware of the various services available to the patient in the hospital or the community and offer advice when the occasion arises. In addition, the therapist can assist the patient by describing various forms of available help, such as literature, videos, self-help support groups, social services, community education groups, financial support, and national groups that lend assistance through patient education such as the American Cancer Society and the National Cancer Institute. Therapists can ensure that written information is displayed in a convenient manner and available in a variety of languages suiting the demographic needs of the hospital. A connection should be established between the radiation therapy department and a community cancer service group. In addition a connection should be established for transportation of the patient to and from treatments. The more involved the therapist is in the overall care of patients, the more patients trust the therapist with their well-being.

SOCIAL PERSPECTIVES RELATED TO THE RADIATION THERAPIST

The radiation therapy department is usually secluded from other departments and other hospital personnel because of the use of high-energy x-rays and the danger of unnecessary exposure to other personnel, patients, and visitors. By its nature, this seclusion affects the behavior of staff members and patients. For long periods of time the radiation therapy department becomes the home of the patient and staff members. The term **radiation therapy domain** describes the confines and socialization process of a radiation therapy department. The radiation therapy domain is a limited physical environment in which a wide sample of people gather daily and create a miniature society. Social perspectives become an issue for the therapist because persons of a variety of ages, races, and nationalities all suffering from cancer coexist daily and must maintain harmonious interdependence. Many social interactions occur among clusters of patients and between patients and staff members illuminating the rights of the patient, which state the following[7]:

> The patient has the right to receive treatment without discrimination as to race, color, religion, sex, national origin, disability, sexual orientation, or source of payment. The patient has the right to receive considerate and respectful care in a clean and safe environment free of unnecessary restraints.

The professional commitment made by radiation therapists obligates them to fulfill this right, which is difficult as a result of the complexion of the patients.

Oncology patients commonly enter the department traumatized by a diagnosis of cancer. The most intelligent person is often unable to assimilate explanations and instructions while digesting a diagnosis of cancer. Difficulties arise because the oncology population has decreased in age because of an emphasis on cancer education and detection. This young patient category has a set of special problems: family responsibilities, financial burdens, job obligations, and all other activities associated with being the head of a household. These patients' needs (scheduling, child care, counseling, and others) must be accommodated to ensure patient compliance with treatment requirements and allow an adequate quality of life. Patients have an advantage because they posses *the right to know,* which allows them to question all aspects of the impending treatment. Patients may find quietude by knowing the educational background of radiation therapists and their credentials. Patients may question the abilities of a therapist; the question must be handled calmly and without detriment to other colleagues. The protracted length of the treatment schedule makes it imperative that the radiation therapist gain the confidence of the patient technically and professionally.

The radiation oncology patient is scheduled for a series of treatments over a period of 2 to 8 weeks. Appointment times for each patient usually remain the same during the entire course of treatment. This arrangement gives patients a way to develop relationships (some lasting, some short term) with people who share similar circumstances. The patient may take this opportunity to extract information from others to acquire a knowledge base for the purpose of comparing personal treatments and reactions to the disease. The daily waiting time is often unpredictable and variable, but during this time the personality of patients emerges and they may assume different roles. Family members and more capable patients become caregivers by helping less able patients. The freedom given to patients to fit into the radiation therapy domain as members of the extended family leaves them relaxed and amiable. This feeling allows for acceptance of the circumstances and often helps encourage patient compliance with treatment schedules and with adherence to necessary recommendations regarding care during various procedures. After patients experience this feeling of familiarity, they are able to set aside fears about daily treatments.

Radiation oncology departments are responsible for the patient's basic needs during treatment and should ensure some activities for the patient during the day. A television-viewing area with a VCR may be set up for education or entertainment purposes, and reading material should be available. The patient should have access to a variety of refreshments. The department should provide available resources to accommodate patients by providing comfortable areas for relaxation. This becomes particularly important for a patient receiving multiple daily fractions of radiation. The fraction schedules vary, but in all situations the time the patient is in the department is substantially increased. These patients spend many hours interacting with radiation staff members and should be given special consideration for their circumstances.

The compliance of the patient to instructions and to treatment schedules is affected by the demeanor of the patient. The deportment of the patient is based on the way the patient visualizes the treatments and will affect the patient's mental and emotional attitudes. Patients' views of their treatment will vary according to the patient population. Patients can initially be categorized according to one or more of the following three criteria: (1) age, (2) Karnofsky score, and (3) type of treatment (curative or palliative). This criteria is helpful to formulate an impression of the patient, but because of the unpredictability of patients it cannot be relied on without incorporating the individual peculiarities of each patient. It is difficult to guess the way each patient will respond to the course of treatments and the way each will view the ordeal. Obviously, a positive response and view of treatments would be that of a young patient who has a high Karnofsky score* and is undergoing a curative course of treatment.

---

*The Karnofsky score is based on a standardized numerical rating scale that describes the performance status of a patient. A patient is assigned a numerical value from 0 to 100 depending on daily functionality.

Unfortunately, patients are not that predictable. A competent therapist will individualize each situation by using the previously mentioned criteria as a base to begin a compassionate understanding of the patient. Patients make their wishes for recovery known by complying with the treatment schedule. The attitude of patients and the social support they receive from family members and friends can affect the outcome of treatments. A patient who has a good physical and psychological support system is better able to withstand the dehumanizing effects of the illness.

Patients begin a new learning experience when they are diagnosed with cancer. This diagnosis invariably alters the patient's behavior. Behavioral scientists have formulated many theories to explain human behavior. Abraham Maslow's theory, called the *hierarchy of needs,* bases all human behavior on needs.[8] The needs are divided into five categories: (1) physiological, (2) safety, (3) socialization, (4) esteem, and (5) self-actualization. Theoretically, persons move consecutively from one category to the other and may at times revert back to a previous category, depending on their needs. Patients undergoing cancer therapy basically start from scratch on the hierarchy-of-needs chart. They must first fulfill *physiological* and *safety* needs by ensuring that the family receives care, financial problems are addressed, and housing needs are solidified. Then the patient can move to the category of *socialization.* During this stage, a patient may look for support and camaraderie from family and friends. Patients may seek people in similar situations to whom they can relate and on whom they can depend for social interaction. The next level on the hierarchy of needs is *esteem.* The patient looks for approval of the effect of the treatment from the physician and therapist to gain a feeling of empowerment over the disease. The last step in the needs theory is called *self-actualization,* the highest level of behavior. It is the most individualized of all the categories because its outcome depends on the personal aspirations and standards of the individual. Maslow indicated the belief that many people never reach this level because each time they approach it, they psychologically change their ideals. Therefore this level is unattainable for many. It may be unrealistic because it does not exist in a concrete form.

Legal prerogatives of patients

The factors in the Patient's Bill of Rights, which are important for the therapist to understand, clarify the patient's freedom to affect the outcome of treatment. This freedom applies to all aspects of patient care, including radiation therapy. The radiation therapist must learn to deal with the patient on various levels. The therapist can be properly prepared by becoming familiar with aspects of the health care system not directly related to radiation therapy but affecting the patient.

Patients have the legal right to affect the outcome of their treatment through the use of DNR orders, living wills, and health care proxies. Although the radiation therapist may not be directly involved in the administration of these docu-ments, awareness of them enhances the therapist's ability to respect the patient's wishes and offer some insight into the patient's circumstances.

The patient has the right to receive a copy of the pamphlet, *Do-Not-Resuscitate Order.*[7]

A *DNR order* is a complex document, which, depending on the mental and physical capacities of the patient, can be signed by the patient, health care agent, or physician. A DNR order is a part of the Public Health Law and allows a legal avenue to withhold cardiopulmonary resuscitation in circumstances that warrant it if proper consent has been obtained. DNR policies may vary from hospital to hospital, and all personnel should familiarize themselves with the administrative directives regarding DNR as they relate to specific hospitals. The therapist should be aware of patients who have DNR orders signed to clearly understand the way to respond if the patient needs immediate and extreme medical care to sustain life.

The patient has the right to refuse treatment and be told what health effects this may have.[7]

As long as they are of sound mind, patients have the complete and full authority on rights regarding decisions that affect their future. Family members' wishes, although they are important and should be respected, cannot override a patient's legitimate decisions. Patients may elect various means to express their wishes. A *living will* is one of the means by which people may take control over their future. A legal document may be completed at any time during the course of a lifetime. This document clearly states the wishes of the person initiating the will. A hospital must follow these wishes as long as the document is valid. The living will usually begins, " Being of sound mind, if I become incapacitated and there is no hope for my future recovery, I do not wish to be kept alive by extraordinary means."[9] This can be stated generally or more specifically by listing a variety of artificial means: cardiac resuscitation, respirator, tube feedings, and antibiotics. The living will may also include the refusal of life-sustaining treatment such as radiation therapy and chemotherapy. Many states have a standardized living will form that can be easily used; if this is not available, a legal document between the initiator and a lawyer may be created.

Persons may take affirmative action to ensure that their medical wishes are carried out by using a document called a *health care proxy.* A health care proxy is a legal document that appoints a person referred to as the *health care agent,* who may be a family member or friend. The health care agent is a legal appointee who has the authority to make critical decisions in the event that the initiator of the health care proxy becomes unable to make such decisions. The health care agent can make all medical decisions as they relate to treatment. The agent follows written instructions such as a living will and is obliged to follow the instructions in this document. In the absence of a living will the health care agent is bound to follow the moral and religious beliefs of the initiator of the proxy. This document may be written by a lawyer, or a standardized form can be used. Consideration should be given for early preparation of this document before its use may become necessary. A health care proxy is activated in the event that the initiator lacks the ability (mentally or physically) to make decisions regarding medical care. A health care agent is authorized to sign a consent form for radiation therapy on behalf of the patient.

These three documents allow patients to retain dignity during an illness by giving them responsibility for health care decisions.

Informed consent

All documents, including those previously discussed, must be channeled through the proper personnel for signatures. The document called the *consent form* gives the patient the right to understand fully all tests or procedures that are part of the health care regimen and to accept or refuse them individually. The consent form protects the rights of the patient *and* integrity of the physician.

> The patient has the right to receive all the information necessary to give informed consent for any proposed procedure or treatment. This information shall include the possible risks and benefits of the procedure or treatment.[7]

The radiation oncologist has the full responsibility to explain to the patient all aspects of the radiation treatments, which include possible problematic conditions that can occur during the course of the treatment and late effects that can cause long-term complications. The explanation should include possible treatment options in combination with or separate from radiation therapy. The consent form can be written to be site-specific to ensure pertinent information is given to the patient, or it may be presented in a more general form. The consent form may also request permission to take photographs during the course of the treatment. The consent form must be signed by the patient or appointed health care agent before the initiation of radiation therapy. The signature should be requested after the physician gives the patient or health care agent a complete disclosure of facts surrounding the radiation therapy treatments. The therapist at times may be asked to sign the consent form as a witness. In this situation the therapist should be a party to the discussion that takes place between the physician and patient or health care agent. If not witnessing the consent, the radiation therapist is responsible for ensuring that an appropriate consent form is completed before starting the course of radiation.

Clinical research

Clinical research is an important activity, especially in academic departments that have residency-training programs. Clinical research usually entails treating patients according to a predetermined plan. Clinical studies offer the opportunity for eligible patients to be assigned to a particular study regimen according to random selection. Clinical trials may be conducted through national study groups or intramurally. The most prominent national study group for cancer-related trials is the Radiation Therapy Oncology Group (RTOG).

A clinical trial may compare existing treatments in different combinations or may compare new treatments or techniques with existing treatments. The goal of a clinical trial is to improve the patient's possibility of survival and quality of life through the discovery of more effective cancer treatments. Patients who meet the established requirements and agree to participate in clinical research are introduced to a component of the study called a **protocol.** A protocol is a specific regimen that dictates the type of treatment and manner in which it is administered to a patient. A protocol is divided into arms, which are specific formats of treatment. Patients are assigned randomly to participate in specific arms. This process is called **randomization.** There are no set number of arms per protocol; rather, the number depends on the objectives of the study. The process of randomized selection ensures that the patient's treatment-arm selection is chosen in a fair and equitable way. Patients may be informed about clinical trials from the primary physician, medical oncologist, or radiation oncologist. Information regarding trials can be acquired from physicians, community organizations, or professional organizations such as the National Cancer Institute. The patient has a right to a full disclosure of anticipated side effects and pros and cons of the treatment being offered through the protocol.

The Patient's Bill of Rights addresses the issue of clinical research and the prerogative the patient has in governing the selection of experimental treatments.

> The patient has the right to refuse to take part in research. In deciding whether or not to participate, the patient has the right to a full explanation.[7]

Patients who agree to participate in clinical research must sign an additional consent form specific to the protocol; however, this does not negate the patient's right to withdraw from the project anytime during the course of the treatment. The physician may also stop the treatment anytime during the course if the patient is not responding well to treatments.

The recruitment of many patients for clinical trials is important to ensure the participation of a substantial population of acceptable patients, make the trials meaningful, and increase the efficacy of future treatments. The therapist plays an important role in clinical research through the proper administration of radiation therapy. The treatment protocol is extremely specific regarding the patient's treatments, including describing the simulation, specifying exact areas that should and should not be treated, setting the daily and total treatment dose and number of fractions per day, and detailing any adjuvant therapy. The simulation and port films are sent for review to the coordinators of the trial and must comply with stipulations of the protocol. The therapist must ensure that all technical components of the protocol are followed precisely because any deviation can cause the department to be penalized and can jeopardize the validity of the study.

COMMUNITY EDUCATION

Addressing the education of the professional without also discussing the larger expanse of community education is impossible. Therapists can play an integral part in community education with their strong background in a variety of radiation technologies. The bill of rights written for the patient can be further expanded to be the bill of rights for the public. The public's right to be informed regarding cancer-risk reduction, the availability of cancer screenings, and various modalities of cancer therapy should be the objective of community education. Approximately 1,300,000 new cancer cases are expected to be diagnosed in 1996, and almost half this number of victims will die with some malignancy every year.[1]

Cancer is a disease that can often be linked to an active agent. Epidemiological data have led to the belief that the number of many forms of cancers can be reduced through behavioral and environmental modification. The belief that the best offense is a good defense holds true in the world of medicine. The defense against malignancies through strong scientific data reduces the incidence of cancer and thus suffering and eventually benefits the society financially. Cancers that develop regardless of behavior and environmental modification have a greater probability of eradication and better potential for control of the disease when the illness is diagnosed at an early stage. Human beings have the intellectual capability to make choices and therefore have the potential to reduce the risk of cancer or allow an early diagnosis. Humans can also exercise the privilege of an informed choice of therapy. The goal is to allow an aggressive and definitive course of treatment as early as possible after the diagnosis of a malignancy. The participation of the therapist in community education can be achieved through hospital-based programs, from programs in various free-standing institutions, and through professional organizations such as the American Cancer Society and National Cancer Institute.

Risk reduction

The term *cancer prevention* is misleading because it insinuates that measures capable of preventing cancer are available. *Risk reduction* is a more realistic term because it implies a greater chance of cancer prevention if people are willing to follow scientifically based advice. Risk reduction is one element of community education, the goal of which is to enlighten a large population. The phrase *cancer prevention* may defeat this purpose.

Educating people in risk reduction is a twofold process: (1) to raise public awareness of a specific cause and effect and (2) to increase the awareness of primary care physicians and the public of recommendations for screening examinations made by nationally recognized cancer authorities such

as the National Cancer Institute and American Cancer Society (Table 17-1). To be effective, the concept of risk reduction must reach a wide and varied population. This can be done by promoting cancer-risk reduction in existing groups, such as church meetings, rotary clubs, Kiwanis clubs, parent-teacher organizations, groups helping homeless persons, and schools, or by setting up meetings to target a specified group of people.

Risk reduction can be targeted at different age groups, starting with early childhood. Children may be trained to develop healthy eating habits, and teenagers may be taught specifically about the links between lifestyle (such as smoking and early sexual activity) and certain cancers (such as lung cancer and cancer of the uterine cervix). If children are educated during their most impressionable years to lead low-risk lifestyles, behavior modification may not be necessary when these children become adults. Pertinent areas of adult education include these risks and relevant aspects of early cancer detection and awareness. Community education includes the presentation of recommendations made by established professional organizations such as the American Cancer Society and National Cancer Institute. These organizations give fact-based information regarding screenings, follow-up examinations, and early warning signs of cancer and the way they affect an early diagnosis of cancer.

Communication can be achieved through various forms: the routine verbal and written methods and newer methods such as video tapes and computer programs through the internet, set up as patient information systems. These mediums can be combined to best meet the needs of a particular audience.

Community screenings

Community screenings are another subdivision of the community education program. Cancer screenings are offered in the community through various hospital-based programs or community organizations. Organizations offer screenings based on the population they are serving, the means available to do the screenings, and the value of the examinations available. Screening programs are set up to offer the patient the appropriate physical examinations. They also offer an excellent forum for educating participants. The American Cancer Society approves of screening programs that are believed to have direct links to specific cancers and have an effective clinical or pathological examination. The American Cancer Society's recommended screenings listed in Table 17-1 can be timed to draw maximal attention by having screenings tied in with national awareness months. The primary awareness months are April (cancer), September (prostate cancer), and October (breast cancer). Community or hospital screening programs can take advantage of this national exposure as free advertisement to emphasize the critical nature of timely medical care and the importance of an informed population.

Screenings benefit individuals in the community and those persons involved in the examinations. Screenings are

Table 17-1	American Cancer Society early-detection recommendations

Test or procedure*	Gender	Age	Frequency
Sigmoidoscopy	Male and female	50 and over	Every 3 to 5 years
Stool blood test (guaiac)	Male and female	50 and over	Annually
Digital rectal examination	Male and female	40 and over	Annually
Mammography	Female	By age 40	Baseline
		40 to 49	Every 1 to 2 years
		50 and over	Annually
Breast physical examination	Female	20-40	Every 3 years
		40 and over	Annually
Breast self-examination	Female	20 and over	Every month
Prostatic antigen blood test	Male	50 and over	Annually
Papanicolaou test	Female	18 and over	Annually
		At inception of sexual activity if younger than 18	Annually
Pelvic examination	Female	18 and over	Annually
		At inception of sexual activity if younger than 18	Annually
Endometrial tissue sampling	Female	Women at high risk	At menopause
Skin self-examination	Male and female	Adult	Every month
Cancer checkup and counseling	Male and female	20 and over	Every 3 years
		40 and over	Annually

Modified from American Cancer Society: *Cancer facts and figures*, Atlanta, 1995, The Society.
*Screening examinations that are recommended by the American Cancer Society have been proved to have a direct relation to specific cancers. The aim of screening examinations during regular checkups is to increase the early detection of cancer.

offered free of charge and are usually run by volunteers. These volunteers include physicians, nurses, technologists, radiation therapists, and lay persons. The hospital or community organization that runs screenings and educational programs can raise money through grants established by professional organizations or from the government, or it can receive from the public through various types of fund raisers. Fund raising is sometimes an unpleasant and difficult task; however, it is necessary if medical awareness is to continue in an organized and constructive fashion in the community.

The radiation therapist can become involved in screening programs as part of the educational segment or can serve various other functions such as registering patients or assisting other professionals in preparation for the examination of the patient. The involvement of the radiation therapist in community screenings is yet another learning experience and gives the therapist a different perspective regarding care of the patient with cancer.

THE FUTURE OF THE RADIATION THERAPIST

The advancement of education and technology in radiation oncology is the responsibility of each successive generation of radiation therapists. Conceptually, the idea is to avoid complacency and pursue refinement and scientific advancement in radiation therapy. This pursuit can be an individual or collaborative effort. The objective is to have a radiation therapist with a strong scientific interest and thorough knowledge of job requirements. The therapist should be familiar with multiple facets of radiation therapy that directly or indirectly affect the role of the radiation therapist. The ability of the therapist to excel in numerous areas and have an effect on some component of radiation therapy raises self-confidence. Radiation therapists who have a high opinion of their professional status are able to play a direct, important role in the future direction and enrichment of the science of radiation therapy.

Review Questions

Fill in the Blank

1. Education can be accomplished by means of _____ or _____ .

2. Radiation therapy education was recognized as a separate discipline from radiography in _____ _____ .

3. The three main agencies responsible for governing the discipline of radiation therapy are _____, _____, and _____ .

4. The radiation therapist is educated through _____ and _____ mediums, two separate yet equally important components.

5. The three legal documents that afford persons control over the outcome of their medical care are the _____ , _____, and _____ .

6. Communication can be achieved through the use of _____ or _____ method of expression.

7. The radiation therapist should play the role of an _____ for the patient.

8. Community screenings and risk reduction are important components of _____ .

9. The American Cancer Society gives credence to particular screening programs based on _____ and _____ .

10. The majority representation of the technologist on the board of the ARRT and the JRCERT took place in _____ .

Questions To Ponder

1. How did the formal division of radiation therapy from radiology affect the evolution of the field of radiation therapy as a science and the radiation therapist as a professional?

2. Continuing education is mandatory for the ARRT to recertify the radiation therapist. How will continuing education affect the field of radiation therapy? How will continuing education affect the radiation therapist as a professional? How do you envision a viable continuing education program? What areas do you consider important for the radiation therapist to pursue when completing the necessary studies for continuing education?

3. Does the radiation therapist have a role in medical research? If so, how do you visualize this role? Why should the radiation therapist have an interest in the pursuit of data collection that could lead to presentations and/or scientific publications?

4. Does the Patient's Bill of Rights have a direct affect on the relationship between the radiation therapist and patient? How does The Patient's Bill of Rights affect the patient? How does The Patient's Bill of Rights affect other medical staff? How has The Patient's Bill of Rights changed overall patient care? In your opinion, was The Patient's Bill of Rights a positive or negative step in the history of medicine, and why?

5. How can community education, including community screenings and instruction in risk reduction, affect reduction of medical costs? Does the extreme emphasis on medical cost reduction accentuate the need for community education? Does society have an obligation to attempt to reduce the incidence of cancer by following recommendations based on scientific data made by the American Cancer Society or National Cancer Institute? At what point should the government intervene and institute laws that would accomplish the same thing?

6. Practical exercise: Perhaps the best route to giving excellent patient care is to picture oneself caring for a relative. This mental trick can help to ensure that the radiation therapist always gives quality care to a patient. The consciousness of therapists can be further heightened by using the same theory but picturing themselves as the patient. Put yourself in the place of the patient. Try to associate with similar circumstances that the patient may be experiencing. Extract personal information from the patient to draw a correlation between yourself and the patient. Select five patients in different age categories.

   After 1 month, determine whether placing yourself in the shoes of the patient makes you feel different about your approach to work. How does it make you feel? Does the age of the patient make a difference in the way you feel? Would you feel this way without placing yourself in the circumstances of the patient? Does knowing more details about the patient (other than name, age, and disease status) affect the way you deal with the patient? Is it better or worse? What do you feel is the best way to ensure quality patient care?

REFERENCES

1. American Cancer Society: *Cancer facts and figures: 1995,* Atlanta, 1995, The Society.
2. The American Registry of Radiologic Technologists: *ARRT educator's handbook,* Mendota Heights, Minnesota, 1990, The Registry.
3. The American Society of Radiologic Technologists: *The American Society of Radiologic Technologists historical background sketch,* Albuquerque, 1995, The Society.
4. ARRT majority representation, *Wavelength* 3:1,9, 1992.
5. Fay M et al: *JRCERT handbook for educational programs,* Chicago, 1991, The Joint Review Commission on Education in Radiologic Technology.
6. Grigg ERN: *The trail of the invisible light,* Springfield, Ill, 1965, Charles C Thomas.
7. Health Care Association of New York State: *Your rights as a hospital patient,* New York, 1994, The Association.
8. Hersey P, Blanchard KH : *Management of organizational behavior,* ed 5, Englewood Cliffs, NJ, 1988, Prentice-Hall.
9. The New York Methodist Hospital: *Policies and procedures,* New York, 1992, 1994, The Hospital.
10. Rafla S, Rotman M: *Introduction to radiotherapy,* St Louis, 1974, Mosby.
11. Washington CM: *Multiskilling, critical thinking and the radiation therapist: changing paradigms in education.* Prepared for Varian's Fifteenth Users Meeting, Session IV, Palo Alto, Calif, May 1995, Varian Associates.
12. Washington CM: Profession undergoing change. In *Radiography: the second century,* Albuquerque, 1995, American Society of Radiologic Technologists.

18

Infection Control In Radiation Oncology Facilities

Lana Havron Bass

Outline

Key terms

The concept of trying to control infectious disease in medical settings has a relatively long history and is associated with famous names such as Florence Nightingale and Joseph Lister. The focus remains the same today; that is, health care workers promote the surveillance, control, and prevention of infectious disease. This chapter emphasizes measures taken to protect the health care worker, patient, and public. Also, regulatory agencies and legal aspects of infection control are briefly discussed.

DEFINITIONS

In the hospital setting the epidemiology department is responsible for infection control. The term **epidemiology** is historically related to the study of epidemics, such as the bubonic plague of the Middle Ages.[71] Today, *epidemiology* may be defined as the study of the distribution and determinants of diseases and injuries in human populations. To familiarize oneself with terminology pertinent to epidemiology, the following definitions need to be reviewed.

Infection involves the reproduction of microorganisms in the human body. The related clinical signs and symptoms associated with the infectious agent or unknown etiology are collectively known as *disease.* If a person develops an infection but has no clinically observable signs or symptoms, the infection is referred to as *subclinical.* A subclinical infection initiates an immune response in the body. On the other hand, infection is also possible without an immune response, which is a condition that is known as **colonization.** A person who is colonized but not ill is known as a **carrier.** People who are ill, those with subclinical disease, and carriers are all capable of spreading disease. The presence of microorganisms on the body or on inanimate objects is known as *contamination.*

Workers in the health care environment are especially interested in **nosocomial** infections. The term *nosocomial* refers to an infection that develops in the hospital or to an infection that is acquired at a hospital but does not develop until after discharge. Nosocomial infections may be acquired not only by patients, but also by health care workers and visitors. Infections caught before a hospital admission, but in which symptoms do not become apparent until after admission, are not nosocomial; they are community related rather than hospital related. The primary goal of the epidemiology department is to decrease all preventable nosocomial infections. The hospital epidemiology team continuously monitors the number of infections that occur and investigates any abnormal occurrence or frequency to determine if some action could have been taken to prevent the infection.

The Centers for Disease Control and Prevention (CDC) has estimated that the nationwide nosocomial infection rate is 5.7%.[45] Investigators of the Study of the Efficacy of Nosocomial Infection Control (SENIC) project estimated that nearly 2.1 million nosocomial infections occur annually. These infections cost more than $1 billion and lead to 25,000 deaths each year.[43] The results of the SENIC project also suggested that an effective hospital infection-control plan reduces nosocomial infections by 20%.[45]

INFECTION CYCLE

Infectious disease cannot occur without the presence of an infectious agent, or pathogen, which is any of a wide range of small, primitive life forms. Pathogens may exist as bacteria, viruses, fungi, protozoans, or algae or lesser known agents such as chlamydiae, rickettsiae, and prions[36] (Fig. 18-1). Of these, bacteria and viruses are most often the sources of nosocomial infections, with fungi next and rarely protozoa or the other forms.[10] Several terms are associated with a disease and the infectious agent. **Pathogenicity** describes the ability of an infectious agent to cause clinical disease. In other words, some agents readily cause clinical disease, and others may be present but not cause clinical disease. The

term **virulence** describes the severity of a clinical disease and is typically expressed in terms of morbidity and mortality. *Dose* refers to the number of microorganisms; thus an *infective* dose is one in which enough microorganisms are present to elicit an infection. Microorganisms are also selective as to their host, or the location at which they cause disease. The infectious agent may cause disease in animals but not humans, vice versa, or in both. This selectivity is known as *host specificity.*

To remain viable, all microorganisms require a source and a reservoir; these may be the same or different. The *reservoir* is where the microorganism lives and reproduces. For example, the polio viral reservoir is human, never animal, whereas the rabies viral reservoir can be human or animal. The place from which the microorganism comes is known as the *source.* From the source it moves to the host; this transfer from the source to the host may be direct or indirect. In the case of the common cold transmitted through a sneeze, the reservoir and source are the same. An example in which the reservoir and source are not the same is histoplasmosis, which is a fungal infection. In this situation a chicken can serve as the reservoir. The chicken's fecal droppings are deposited on soil and serve as the source. Then the wind carries the remains of the droppings, and they are inhaled by a human. Another example might be a case of hepatitis A, in which the reservoir is a cafeteria cook who handles food. The food serves as the source of the infection.

A *host* is the person to whom the infectious agent is passed. Whether the host develops clinical disease depends on the body location at which the infectious agent is deposited and on the host's immune status and related defense mechanisms. If disease develops in the susceptible host, the host goes through three disease phases: **incubation,** clinical disease, and **convalescence.** Depending on the specific disease, a person may be infectious to others during any or a combination of the three disease phases. In some diseases, such as hepatitis B, in which a chronic carrier state exists, a person who is apparently well can actually be disseminating disease. For disease to be passed to others, a *portal of exit* is necessary. Examples include the respiratory tract, gastrointestinal tract, blood, and skin.

After an exit portal is reached, transmission can take place. *Transmission* is defined as the movement of the infectious agent from the source to the host.

Transmission modes or routes vary from one disease to another. Four transmission routes are identified: contact, common vehicle, airborne, and vectorborne. The box that is located on p. 286 displays an outline of transmission routes. A specific disease may use one or more transmission modes.

Contact spread can be direct, indirect, or by droplet. The susceptible host makes contact with the source of infection. Person-to-person spread is an example of direct contact. Mononucleosis transmitted through kissing or acquired immunodeficiency syndrome (AIDS) spread through sexual intercourse represents transmission via direct contact.

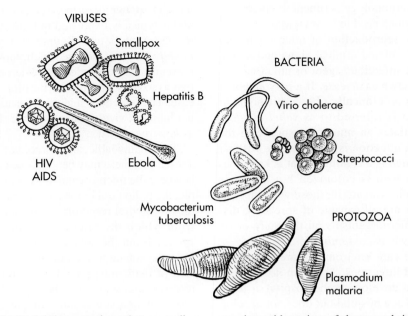

Fig. 18-1 Microorganisms that cause disease come in a wide variety of shapes and sizes.

Indirect contact involves an intervening object that is contaminated from contact with an infectious agent, which then comes into contact with another individual and results in a single infective episode. An example is a needle stick to a health care worker after it has been used in a patient infected with human immunodeficiency virus (HIV). Transmission by droplet involves the rapid transfer of the infectious agent through the air over short distances, such as in talking, coughing, or sneezing close to someone's face. The droplets consist of large particles and thus are spread over short distances, typically 3 feet or less. Measles, colds, and influenza are commonly transmitted in this fashion. Another route of transmission is common vehicle spread. This type of transmission involves a contaminated inanimate vehicle that acts as the common **fomite** for transmission of the infectious agent to multiple persons. The number of people infected distinguishes this type of transmission from indirect contact, which involves the spread of infection to only one person. In common vehicle spread, all the people are infected from a common vehicle. An example is blood contaminated with HIV or hepatitis B that goes to several people.

Airborne spread is transmission that involves an infectious agent using the air as its means of dissemination and typically involves a long distance of more than several feet. These airborne pathogens are the remains of droplets that have evaporated. The infectious agent is contained in the **droplet nuclei,** dust particles, or **skin squames** (the superficial skin cells). Agents may also remain in the air for hours or even days. Tuberculosis has spread in hospitals in this fashion because of air recirculation and low air-flow rate.[42] *Histoplasma capsulatum,* the infectious fungal agent of the

Transmission Routes	

1. Contact
  • Direct
  • Indirect
  • Large droplet
2. Common vehicle
  (fomite)
	3. Airborne
	  • Droplet nuclei
	  • Dust particles
	  • Skin squames
	4. Vectorborne

disease histoplasmosis, grows as a mold in soil containing bird droppings, such as in a chicken coop or pigeon roost. On a windy day the dust containing the spores of this infectious fungal agent can be carried for miles to the susceptible host.[8] Legionnaires' disease made the headlines again in 1994 when 1200 passengers were evacuated from a Royal Caribbean cruise ship. This acute bacterial disease is associated with air-conditioning cooling towers and evaporative condensers.[59] Skin squames have been blamed in several outbreaks of streptococcal wound infections that were eventually traced to hospital staff personnel.[10]

Vectorborne transmission involves a **vector** that transports an infectious agent to a host. An example is a fly that transports an infectious agent on its body or legs, or an *Anopheles* mosquito, which carries the malaria sporozite, a protozoan parasite.[11] The malaria sporozite enters the bloodstream of the human victim bitten by the mosquito. Other examples include Lyme disease and Rocky Mountain spotted fever, which are carried by ticks containing the infectious agent.

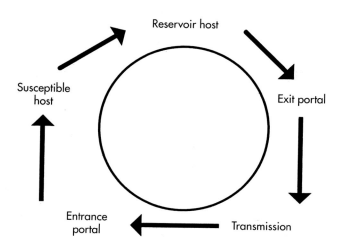

Fig. 18-2 Diagram of the infection cycle. To stop disease, the cycle can be broken at any point.

To cause disease, the infectious agent must gain entrance to the body. The entrance portal can be through normal skin such as in the contraction of hepatitis B, or through broken skin such as with a needle stick in the transmission of HIV. Agents also gain access through the respiratory system, gastrointestinal tract, urinary tract, or transplantation. Transmission of an infectious agent through these entry portals is also often associated with medications or equipment such as scopes or catheters. The complete cycle of infection is shown in Fig. 18-2.

DEFENSE MECHANISMS
Nonspecific defense mechanisms

To establish an infection, the pathogen must successfully get by the host's defense mechanisms. The human body comes equipped with a wide variety of nonspecific defense mechanisms. For example, skin serves as a mechanical barrier and contains secretions that have antibacterial qualities. The upper respiratory system is full of cilia that facilitate the removal of pathogens. If the cilia are not successful, mucus aids in catching and removing pathogens. The respiratory system also protects against invasion through its secretions and defensive white cells that engulf and destroy pathogens. The gastrointestinal and urinary tracts are acidic and thus serve as a hostile environment to possible invaders. Even tears exhibit antibacterial activity and aid in the removal of pathogens.

Other nonspecific defense mechanisms include local inflammatory action and genetic, hormonal, and nutritional factors. Personal hygiene and behavioral habits also influence the likelihood of developing disease. The age of a person also plays a role, with the extremely young and extremely old being most at risk. Alterations of any nonspecific defense mechanism through a skin break, surgery,

chronic disease such as diabetes or immune deficiency disorders, or even medication to treat some diseases influence the host's susceptibility by lowering resistance to infectious disease processes.

Specific defense mechanisms

Immunity plays a critical role in reducing host susceptibility. Immunity exists in two forms: natural and artificial. The box above displays an outline of the different types of immunity. Natural immunity develops as a result of having acquired a certain disease. For example, children who have had rubella will never have it again. This is a fairly general rule for most acute viral infections, and such immunity usually persists for the life of the host. Natural immunity can also develop after subclinical disease, in which no readily apparent disease is observed. Unfortunately, all pathogens do not initiate lifelong immunity. Herpes simplex virus (cold sore) is a good example. After a herpes attack, the virus lies dormant until some event triggers another painful attack.

Artificial immunity can be further subdivided into active and passive immunity. Active immunization via vaccines against diphtheria, tetanus, and pertussis has been a mainstay of U.S. public health for many decades. Later, vaccines against poliomyelitis, measles, mumps, and rubella came along. More recently, a vaccine against hepatitis B was developed and must be offered to at-risk health care providers. Currently, immunologists have worked for over a decade trying to develop an effective vaccine against HIV to curtail the worldwide AIDS epidemic. To date, several experimental vaccines have been developed, although their effectiveness has yet to be determined.

Vaccines come in several forms: killed, toxoid, and attenuated live vaccines. Active immunization consists of the altered pathogen or its products. In any event the vaccine serves as the **antigen** (foreign substance) and thereby triggers the human body's immune system to create **antibodies.** Antibodies are specific; they work only against a specific antigen. The physiological basis of this specificity resides in the unique sequences of amino acids, which makes an antibody distinct from other antibodies. T and B lymphocytes are the key white cells in the body's immune system. The immune response is far too complex for this chapter; how-

Forms of Immunity

1. Natural immunity: active disease
2. Artificial immunity
   - Active immunity: vaccine
   - Passive immunity
     Maternal antibodies
     Antibody transferral to susceptible host

ever, it is well established that the B lymphocyte transforms itself into a plasma cell. Simply put, this cell is a highly active factory that synthesizes its own genetically unique type of antibody and sets it free into the body's fluids. The antibody then seeks the specific invading antigen. With some vaccines a booster is necessary after a period of time because the number of antibodies (**titers**) drops to a level insufficient to provide adequate protection.

Passive immunity, another form of artificial immunity, is defined as the transferral of protective antibodies from one host to a susceptible host. Examples include the administration of **immune serum globulin** (ISG; e.g., a serum-containing antibody) for the prophylaxis of measles, tetanus, and hepatitis A (infectious hepatitis). The transfer of maternal antibodies to the fetus through the placenta is another form of passive immunity. Other substances available for passive immunization include antiserum against rabies administered after animal bites and antibiotics in known contacts of cases of tuberculosis (TB), gonorrhea, and syphilis. Although it protects the individual from the disease in most cases, passive immunization does not protect against infection, nor does it prevent spread to others. Passive immunization typically has a short duration, usually several months at most,[10] and thus active immunization is preferable whenever possible, such as in tetanus active vaccination.

Environmental factors contributing to nosocomial disease

Environmental factors such as air flow, temperature, and humidity also influence links in the cycle of infection because they directly affect the pathogen and host. For example, measures directed at minimizing the risk of tuberculosis transmission within a hospital include the appropriate adjustment of air flow in designated rooms so that in any high-risk area, negative pressure air flow occurs within the room. With the recent increase of classic TB, AIDS-related TB, and antibiotic resistant strains of TB, the CDC has modified its guidelines. Hospitals are taking far greater protective measures to reduce the transmission of TB in the hospital environment.[15] Host susceptibility is also affected by environmental factors. For example, in winter, health care workers tend to stay indoors more often, with doors and windows tightly closed. The central heat tends to dry protective mucous membranes. This combination of reduced air circulation and dry membranes increases the risk of airborne diseases.

Many other environmental factors can contribute to nosocomial disease. A person may enjoy the comfort and beauty of carpets in a radiation oncology department, but carpeting greatly increases the microbial level when compared with linoleumlike surfaces. Fresh flowers in water may enhance the beauty of surroundings but harbor a multitude of microorganisms such as spores and bacteria. For this reason, flowers and fruit are often banned from areas such as bone marrow transplant wards and intensive care units. Ideally, flowers and fruit should be banned from any area in which immunosuppression is a concern.

Laundry is a nosocomial concern only if used. Health care workers should use caution in handling used laundry by making sure it is not vigorously shaken and never handling it without gloves if it is contaminated with blood or other body fluids. Fresh linen or paper should always be used for each patient.

Other items routinely used in radiation therapy should also be considered as possible hazards. Bite blocks should be disinfected between each use on a single patient and then dried and stored in a clean, closed container. Like treatment tables, slide boards for transferring patients should also be cleaned between uses. Tattooing or placing permanent ink dots is a routine procedure. The ink bottle must be treated as a sterile container. Each patient must be tattooed with a fresh syringe and needle. After being used, the needle should never be reintroduced to the ink container. Likewise, drawing ink into a syringe and then changing needles between the tattooing of patients is an unacceptable technique. Ideally, bolus sheets should not be used on multiple patients. If bolus is to be reused, it should be wrapped in flexible plastic film or latex to prevent the bolus material from being contaminated during use and then thoroughly disinfected before rewrapping for use on a subsequent patient. Another item often used on more than one patient is a pen or marker for drawing in a treatment port. If an item is contaminated by use on one patient, any harmful microorganisms can easily be spread to subsequent patients who need their treatment port markings reinforced. Some departments have solved this problem by issuing each patient a marker and placing it in a plastic, sealable bag that is kept with the patient's radiation treatment chart. The repeated use of marking pens and bolus would provide interesting data for epidemiological studies.

To summarize, the best defense is a good offense. Health care workers should take good care of their bodies to keep nonspecific defense mechanisms healthy, practice good personal hygiene and behavioral patterns, take advantage of active immunizations, and pay close attention to the work environment. Any strategy workers can take to break a link in the cycle of infection helps protect not only themselves, but also those for whom they care.

DRUG USE AND DRUG-RESISTANT MICROORGANISMS

Antibiotics have been in use for over 50 years and have served as the main weapon in the medical world's arsenal against disease. Many of the once terrifying killer diseases have become mere health inconveniences that, if diagnosed early enough, can be cured with pills or injections. Not too long ago, some people envisioned a future free of infectious disease. Then things began to change. Mutated germs and diseases such as AIDS, once unheard of, began making the media headlines. This led to many questions about the origins of these new and resurgent diseases, and the reasons for antibiotics not working as they once did. The answers to these questions require a review of the evolution of the use of antibiotics and other medications and a new understanding of the way microorganisms function.

By changing their genetic makeup, microorganisms have found ways to resist the effects of medications. Many microorganisms have mutated and developed the ability to manufacture cell products that destroy the drugs that used to

kill them[50,59] (Fig. 18-3). Mutations arise much faster in microorganisms than in man because the time for a new generation to be created may be a matter of minutes compared with decades in man. If in their relatively short evolutionary process mutations develop that are beneficial in the struggle to survive against medications, the mutants are better suited to live and reproduce. Others have picked up protective genes from other microorganisms[52,59] (Fig. 18-3). People have also unwittingly helped in the development of drug-resistant microorganisms by not finishing prescribed medica-

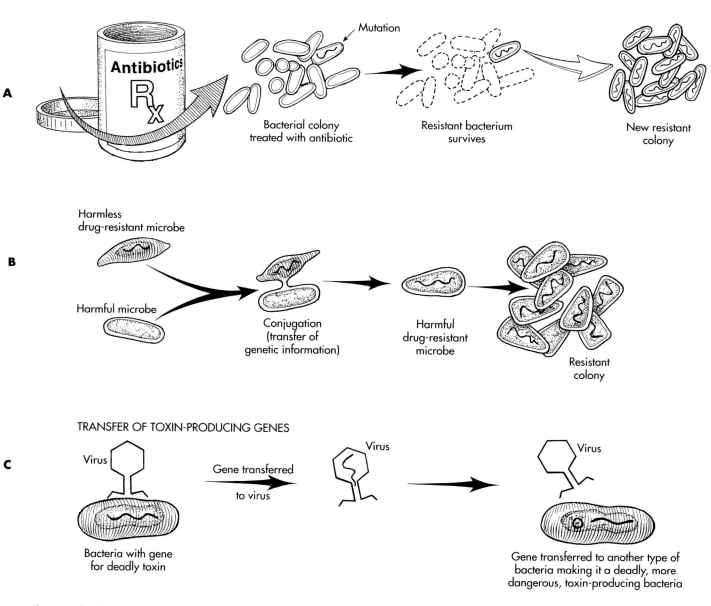

Fig. 18-3 **A,** When antibiotics are used to treat a bacterial infection, most will die. However, a mutated bacteria may survive, and it goes on to produce more drug-resistant clones. **B,** The transfer of a drug-resistant gene from a harmless microbe to a harmful microbe through the conjugation process. **C,** A virus can carry a harmful trait to other types of bacteria, making them dangerous.

tions and by demanding and receiving inappropriate antibiotics for illnesses. The tougher, remaining pathogens endure as the most fit to survive. Vaccines, like antibiotics, are challenged by mutating pathogens. This has been part of the problem in developing a successful vaccine for the continuously evolving HIV.

Because massive quantities of antibiotics and other drugs are used in medical settings, logic dictates that a large proportion of these new mutating pathogens are responsible for nosocomial infections. This causes great concern because the patients who are the sickest are also the poorest equipped to fight these "super infections." This is also alarming for health care workers and should serve as notice regarding the importance of the epidemiology department in helping to protect workers and their patients. The CDC's Hospital Infection Control Practices Advisory Committee has also been discussing approaches to control resistant microorganisms in hospitals.[13,14] Through stringent adherence to infection-control protocols, nosocomial infections can be reduced, thus lowering the overall cost of health care.

HEALTH CARE FACILITY EPIDEMIOLOGY

The CDC is based in Atlanta, Georgia, and funded by the federal government. Over time the Hospital Infections Branch of the CDC was established to help hospitals deal with nosocomial infections. Today's hospitals are required to establish an epidemiology division if they wish to be accredited by and meet the standards of the Joint Commission on Accreditation of Healthcare Organizations (JCAHO).[54] Even in non-JCAHO-accredited facilities, state health departments or public health codes must be met for licensure, and requirements typically include some form of epidemiological oversight.

State laws also govern the reporting of specific infectious diseases and the disposal of medical waste. In the past decade the Occupational Safety and Health Administration (OSHA) has focused its attention on health care facilities and the health care worker more than ever before. In fact, OSHA mandated that employers of health care workers must offer the workers the hepatitis B vaccine.[29] Although current mandates do not specifically address students, common sense suggests that students are also at risk and should be vaccinated. Today's health care worker can expect to undergo an employment physical, an epidemiological-related health and safety orientation, ongoing inservices on a regular basis, and routinely offered health services such as TB testing and checking of disease-related titers.

Even hospital reimbursement by third-party payers such as Medicare or Blue Cross/Blue Shield is affected by a health care facility's attention to the quality of care and quality assessment (QA). This reimbursement association is influenced by external reviewers such as the Health Care Financing Administration. A staff radiation therapist, chief radiation therapist, or manager in a radiation oncology department can expect to participate at some level in the development or implementation of a QA or quality continuing improvement (QCI) program, with infection control being just one portion of the overall program.

PERSONNEL AND STUDENT HEALTH SERVICES AND PERTINENT INFECTIOUS DISEASES

The employee health clinic and the epidemiology division of a health care facility have a vested interest in their health care workers because the workers are at risk of exposure to infectious disease in the work place and the community. If workers develop an infection, they pose a risk to patients, coworkers, friends, and family members. Because of the nature of their chosen profession, health care workers have frequent and prolonged direct contact with patients who harbor a multitude of infectious agents; thus health care workers are at great risk of exposure.

A health placement evaluation should be completed for hiring or for a new student before contact is made with patients. Such an examination should determine that the potential health care worker is able to perform the essential physical and mental functions of the position to ensure the safe and efficient performance of duties. The examination should also determine the worker's immunization status and medical history. A listing of recommended vaccines for health care workers is shown in the box on the next page. The following text highlights specific diseases that are of utmost importance in protecting workers and their patients.

Hepatitis B virus (HBV) infection is the major infectious occupational hazard of health care workers. Its transmission occurs through contact with blood and body fluids. HBV is a highly transmissible virus, and evidence has shown that this potentially deadly virus can live on surfaces at room temperature for 7 days.[9] In response to health care workers' concerns, the Department of Labor, OSHA, and the Department of Health and Human Services[28] issued a Joint Advisory Notice in 1987 and began the rule-making process to regulate HBV exposure. In 1987 the CDC recommended that health care workers be vaccinated. The final rule proposed by OSHA was printed in the *Federal Register* on December 6, 1991, and mandated that the HBV vaccine be made available to all at-risk health care workers.[29] Workers should understand that the HBV vaccine protects only against hepatitis B, not hepatitis C, D, E, and so on, for which no vaccine is available at this time.[62] As with any rule, an implementation deadline is set; thus mandatory implementation did not occur until July 6, 1992.

In the recent past, the CDC estimated that the total number of people infected annually in the U.S. with HBV was 280,000, with 8700 of these being health care workers. The annual CDC mortality rate for health care workers has been approximately 200.[29] Morbidity associated with HBV includes chronic hepatitis, which is highly associated with hepatocellular (liver) cancer and other types of progressive liver damage or associated complications such as liver failure and liver cirrhosis, both of which can lead to death.[12] In

Recommended* Vaccines for Health Care Workers

- Hepatitis B
- Influenza
- Measles
- Mumps
- Rubella

- Tetanus
- Pertussis
- Diptheria
- Chickenpox

*Should not be viewed as all inclusive.

1992, 5020 health care workers were infected. Of this number, 6 persons died with acute cases and 300 developed chronic hepatitis.[62]

A safe HBV vaccine derived from human plasma became available in the U.S. in 1982 and is effective in producing an HBV antibody in the majority of healthy, susceptible people. In 1987 a **recombinant deoxyribonucleic acid** (DNA) vaccine became available.[29] Both vaccines are remarkably free of side effects, the most common being soreness at the injection site.[68] The HBV vaccine is of no use in HBV carriers or individuals who are immune to HBV.[70] Postvaccine testing should be performed 1 to 6 months after the three-part vaccination series to ascertain that immunity was conferred. Approximately 90% of healthy vaccinees develop protective antibodies after the series of three injections.[67] With the HBV vaccine available by law to all at-risk health care workers, the morbidity and mortality rates in these workers will undoubtedly drop quite significantly.

Of increasing concern is the hepatitis C virus (HCV), which was identified in 1989.[1] As previously mentioned, no vaccine exists for HCV. Although the risks of transmission remain undefined, HCV appears to be transmitted not only through contact with blood and body fluids, but also through household contact. Obviously, nosocomial and occupational exposure are of concern. Of particular importance is that HCV is associated with an extraordinarily high frequency of chronic infection leading to cirrhosis and primary hepatocellular carcinoma. The Food and Drug Administration (FDA) has recommended plasma screening for HCV since 1992.[1] Ongoing research should soon lead to the development of a vaccine.

Other diseases for which immunizations are recommended for health care workers are influenza, measles, mumps, rubella, pertussis, tetanus, and diphtheria. In diseases for which no vaccine is available or for which the health care worker has not received a vaccine or does not respond to a vaccine, prompt prophylaxis is advised. Diseases included in this group are hepatitis A, hepatitis B, hepatitis C, meningococcal disease, and rabies.

At the turn of the century, TB was one of the top causes of death. As a result of improved housing and nutrition, TB decreased in frequency until 1985, at which time the decline

leveled off. Since 1985, TB has made a dramatic reappearance.[41] To a large degree, its emergence is related to the AIDS epidemic. In a study conducted at Parkland Memorial Hospital in Dallas, Texas, and published in 1989, one patient admitted to the hospital's emergency department in April 1983 contributed to the development of active TB in six employees and one other patient as well as positive conversion in at least 47 other employees.[42] Recirculation of air was deemed a major contributing factor in this specific transmission case. Based on the Parkland experience and CDC recommendations, many hospitals have redesigned air flow systems, and the employee health clinics of such hospitals have begun making TB surveillance among health care workers a high-level priority.

Because of patient noncompliance with prescribed medications and lost follow-ups, multiple drug resistance (MDR) strains of TB have developed. Even more frightening is the fact that the CDC has documented numerous cases of MDR TB in health care workers. Some of these cases have resulted in death.[41] No effective vaccine exists for TB. The bacille Calmette-Guérin (BCG) vaccine, widely used outside the U.S. for several decades, confers varied and questionable degrees of protection, ranging from some degree to no protection at all.[8] The CDC has issued several publications in recent years in response to the increase of TB. Titles include *Guideline for Infection Control in Hospital Personnel*[72]; *Guidelines for Preventing the Transmission of Tuberculosis in Healthcare Settings, With Special Focus on HIV-Related Issues*[16]; and the most recent, *Guidelines for Preventing the Transmission of Mycobacterium Tuberculosis in Health-Care Facilities.*[15] OSHA has also focused its attention on job-related transmission of TB. Jokes in the past about Darth Vader masks already have the ring of reality in the health care setting. For now, all new health care workers, including those with a history of BCG vaccination, should receive an intradermal **Mantoux tuberculin skin test** (purified protein derivative [PPD] of tuberculin) unless a previously positive reaction or completion of adequate therapy can be documented. The four-prong tine test is not recommended and has been deemed almost useless.[41] Health care workers who document a positive history should be exempt from further screening unless they develop symptoms suggestive of TB. Periodic retesting of PPD-negative health care workers should be conducted to identify those who convert to positive. Current guidelines recommend at minimum an annual test for all health care workers and more frequent tests (as often as every 3 months) for those workers who are at high risk.[15] A positive screening Mantoux test is identified by a significant reaction, usually defined as 10 mm or more induration at the injection site, read 48 hours after injection.[12] Positive conversion is typically treated prophylactically with isoniazid (INH) for 6 months to 1 year with a monthly follow-up, whereas active TB is treated with at least two drugs such as INH, pyrazinamide (PZA), ethambutol (EMB), streptomycin (SM), or rifampin (RIF).[4]

All persons with a history of TB or positive TB test should be alerted that they are at risk of developing the disease in the future and thus should promptly report any pulmonary symptoms. Health care workers with active TB pose a risk to others and should be removed from work until adequate treatment is administered, cough has resolved, and sputum is free of bacilli in three consecutive smears.[68] In the majority of infected workers or patients, respiratory secretions are no longer infective 10 days after effective treatment.[66]

With other diseases, infected health care workers should be removed from direct patient contact for variable time frames. These diseases include conjunctivitis, epidemic diarrhea, streptococcosis, hepatitis A, herpes simplex of exposed skin areas such as the hands, measles, mumps, pertussis, rubella, rabies, *Staphylococcus aureus* skin lesions, and varicella zoster.

Of these diseases, varicella zoster virus (VZV) deserves special attention in a radiation oncology department. VZV is the pathogen that causes varicella zoster (chickenpox) and herpes zoster (shingles). VZV has an extremely high degree of communicability and is transmitted by the inhalation of small droplet nuclei or by direct contact with respiratory droplets or vesicle fluid.[44]

For children, chickenpox usually consists of a mild illness characterized by fever and a vesicular rash mainly on the body trunk. The rash may range from one or two vesicles to hundreds; thus extremely light or subclinical infections may go undiagnosed. The skin lesions appear in groups at different times, so late and early lesions can be seen at the same time. In adults, chickenpox is typically more severe and the risk of complications is higher. Infection early in pregnancy is associated with neonatal complications and congenital malformations. In cancer patients, chickenpox can be life threatening in children and adults as a result of an impaired immune system. If a cancer patient is exposed, varicella zoster immune globulin (VZIG) can be given to modify the disease.[21]

Shingles is a local manifestation of a recurrent, reactivated infection by the same virus. After a person has chickenpox, the VZV is thought to remain dormant in the cells of nerve root ganglia. Shingles usually is seen in middle age; however, children and even infants occasionally develop shingles. Lesions appear on the skin area supplied by the affected nerve. Clinically, especially in adults, pain and severe itching occurs and often lasts for long periods after the lesions have crusted over and healed. A significant number of transplant or cancer patients, especially those with leukemia, lymphoma, or AIDS-related cancers, develop shingles as a result of immunosuppression.[12]

Because VZV can be life threatening to cancer patients, health care workers, especially those in oncology or transplant departments, should have had documented varicella or should be able to show serologic evidence of immunity. Certainly only those workers who have a positive history should care for patients with VZV. If susceptible health care workers are exposed to persons with chickenpox or shingles, these workers should be considered potentially infective during the incubation period. They should be excluded from work beginning on the tenth day after exposure and remain away from patient contact for the maximum incubation period of varicella, which is 21 days. Also, infected workers should not return to work until all lesions have dried and crusted, which is usually 6 days from the onset of the rash. VZIG can be used after exposure in susceptible health care workers to lessen the severity of the disease if they develop it. If a worker receives VZIG after exposure, the incubation period is prolonged; thus the worker must be reassigned or furloughed for a longer time, typically 28 days after exposure.[21] A VZV vaccine has been available for many years outside the U.S. In March of 1995, the FDA approved a vaccine by the trade name of Varivac for use in the U.S.[7]

Viral respiratory infections are another major source of nosocomial infections. Although most people do not associate influenza specifically with the work environment, the issue should be addressed. Respiratory diseases, such as influenza, are associated with significant morbidity and mortality in older patients, patients with chronic underlying disease, and immunocompromised patients. In other words, patients of all ages seen in a radiation therapy department are at high risk for influenza and other respiratory viral infections.

Respiratory viruses are spread through three major transmission modes: (1) direct contact via large droplets over a short distance; (2) airborne transmission, consisting of small droplet nuclei that can travel long distances; and (3) self-inoculation after contact with contaminated materials (this usually involves the hands transferring the virus to the mucous membranes of the eye or nose).

The common cold, croup, and viral pneumonia are all examples of infections caused by the influenza virus. Influenza is spread mainly by the airborne route via small particle aerosol, thus explaining explosive seasonal outbreaks of the flu. Two major types of influenza are recognized: type A and type B.[8] These two types of influenza are among the most communicable diseases of humans. Shedding of the influenza virus from an infected individual usually lasts 5 to 7 days after the onset of symptoms.[33] Because of the constantly changing nature of these viruses, new subtypes appear at irregular intervals. This translates to the need to develop different influenza vaccinations that will be effective against new mutated subtypes. Prevention of winter influenza outbreaks consists of immunization programs initiated each year before the influenza season strikes. Vaccination programs are typically aimed toward older persons, those with chronic disease states, those with respiratory diseases, and health care workers. Vaccine effectiveness ranges from 60% to 90%.[22] In persons not fully protected the vaccine appears to reduce the severity of symptoms. Adequate serologic response typically takes place a couple of weeks after vaccination.

Unfortunately, health care workers often do not take advantage of free or low-cost vaccinations offered by employers. The workers are apparently reluctant to participate because of misinformation regarding the influenza vaccine's effectiveness and side effects. Famous quotes such as, "The flu shot gave me the flu," and "Flu shots don't work," simply cannot be substantiated. On the other hand, substantial evidence supports the vaccine's effectiveness in preventing and decreasing morbidity.[22] The most commonly reported side effect is soreness at the injection site, which lasts less than 24 hours. Surely this temporary discomfort, which does not occur in all people, is better than a week's sick leave, possible loss of income, and the health risk imposed on patients who are far more likely to develop serious complications, including death. Perhaps with better educational programs, health care workers and the public would participate in greater numbers. In the event that an individual is not inoculated with the influenza vaccine, drugs such as amantadine hydrochloride and rimantadine hydrochloride are 70% to 90% effective in preventing influenza A to the same level of a vaccine or, if administered after the fact, decrease the length of illness.[17] Amantadine and rimantadine are not effective against influenza B.[17,63]

UNIVERSAL PRECAUTIONS AND ISOLATION SYSTEMS

Nosocomial infections have been a serious problem ever since sick patients were placed together in a hospital and a long time before the term *nosocomial* came about. Even in biblical times the need to isolate or quarantine persons with leprosy was recognized. In the early part of this century, health care workers wore special gowns, washed their hands with disinfectant agents, disinfected contaminated equipment, and practiced a wide variety of isolation or quarantine measures to contain contagious diseases such as TB. In 1970 the CDC published its first guidelines for nosocomial infections and isolation techniques.[18] These guidelines recommended the use of isolation categories based on the routes of disease transmission. Because all diseases in a given category did not require the same degree of precautions, this approach, although simple to understand and apply, resulted in overisolation for many patients. Over the next decade, it became evident that although this approach helped prevent the spread of classical contagious diseases, it neither addressed new drug-resistant pathogens or new syndromes nor focused on nosocomial infections in special care departments. Thus in 1983 the CDC again published new guidelines.[38] In this edition, many infections were moved or placed under new isolation categories. Three new categories were added: contact isolation, acid-fast bacilli (AFB, another name for TB), and blood and body fluids. The protective isolation category was deleted. These significant changes encouraged the hospital's infection-control committee to choose between category-specific and patient-specific isolation categories.

Then came AIDS. The onset of the HIV pandemic has drastically altered the way health care workers practice overall infection-control procedures. For the first time, emphasis was focused on applying blood and body fluid precautions (now known as *universal precautions*) to all persons. According to this new infection-control approach, all human blood and certain body fluids are to be treated as if known to be infectious for HIV, HBV, and other bloodborne pathogens. Universal precautions were intended to supplement rather than replace long-standing recommendations for the control of nonbloodborne pathogens. Although the old blood and body fluids isolation category was negated, the earlier CDC category-specific or disease-specific isolation precautions remained intact. The 1987 CDC universal precautions recommendations also addressed the prevention of needle sticks and the use of traditional gloves and gowns and placed new emphasis on masks and eye protection and other protective equipment and procedures.[20]

Another system, known as *body substance isolation (BSI)*, was proposed in 1987 by two hospitals, one in Seattle and the other in San Diego.[61] BSI differs from universal precautions in that the focus of universal precautions is placed primarily on blood and body fluids implicated in the spread of bloodborne pathogens, whereas BSI focuses on the isolation of all moist body substances in all patients. In other words, the term *universal* refers to all patients, not to all body fluids or all pathogens. Universal precautions do not apply to tears, sweat, saliva, feces, vomit, nasal secretions, or sputum unless visible blood is present.[19,20,24] On the other hand, BSI deals with all body fluids.

On December 6, 1991, OSHA published in the *Federal Register*, "29 CFR Part 1910.1030—Occupational Exposure to Bloodborne Pathogens, Final Rule."[29] Although previous CDC recommendations on universal precautions or BSI recommendations were just that—recommendations—the rules and regulations of the Department of Labor and OSHA are enforceable in terms of occupational exposure. OSHA chose to adopt the universal precautions concept rather than the BSI concept. Major details of these OSHA requirements implemented on July 6, 1992, are addressed in the following text.[29]

Universal precautions—OSHA style

At minimum, universal precautions must be followed precisely by all health care workers who are at risk of occupational exposure. Enforcement protects the workers and those for whom they care. In addition, the medical facility can be faced with substantial fines and penalties for failure to comply with OSHA rules and regulations. OSHA requires that employers provide new health care workers with occupational-exposure training at no cost and during working hours before the initial assignment to tasks in which occupational exposure can take place. Employers must also make the hepatitis B vaccine available at no cost to the health care worker within 10 working days of the initial assignment. If workers decline the hepatitis B vaccine, they are required to sign a waiver. If the workers change their mind later, the employer must make the vaccine available at that time. Annual in-service training of health care workers is required within 1 year of previous training.[29]

The components of universal precautions and their required application under a medical facility's exposure control plan include engineering controls, work-practice controls, personal protective equipment, and housekeeping. Major highlights of OSHA's rules and regulations regarding bloodborne pathogens are shown in the box on the next page.

Body substance isolation

As mentioned earlier, BSI is an alternative isolation concept. As its names implies, BSI concentrates on the isolation of all body fluids for all patients through protective equipment such as gloves. BSI also addresses the transmission of non–body-fluid associated pathogens such as those transmitted exclusively or in part by airborne transmission. In the BSI system, if a patient has an airborne infectious agent, a "stop" sign is placed on the door of the patient's room with further instructions to check with the nurse's station. The decision regarding the type of protective action to be taken is based on the specific patient, with the informed decision being made by the professional practitioners in charge of that patient. Decisions are guided by CDC isolation category-specific or disease-specific recommendations. Overall, many aspects of BSI are identical or extremely similar to the universal precautions concept and to OSHA's version of universal precautions. However, one major difference is the guideline for wearing gloves and washing hands. In the BSI system, hand washing is not required after removing gloves unless the glove's integrity has been broken and the hands are visibly soiled. This difference has been interpreted by some as a disadvantage of using the BSI concept.

COMPLIMENTARY ISOLATION CATEGORIES

Additional isolation categories are recommended by the CDC and are needed to supplement BSI, universal precautions, and OSHA rules and regulations. These category-specific isolation categories include the following: strict isolation, contact isolation, respiratory isolation, AFB (TB) isolation, enteric precautions, and drainage and secretion precautions.[38] As previously mentioned, the earlier CDC blood and body fluids category was superseded by the adoption of universal precautions. The term *isolation* should be noted at the end of each category. Isolation usually indicates the need for a private room, whereas the term *precautions* is used when a private room is not needed or is optional. A brief description of each isolation category follows and includes protective gear and related specific pathogens as examples. Table 18-1 on p. 297 highlights basic requirements of category-specific infection-control measures.

Strict isolation

Strict isolation is specified to prevent the transmission of highly infectious or extremely severe infections that can be transmitted through contact or air. A private room with a closed door is necessary. The only exception is that two people with the same pathogen can share a room. In addition to keeping the door closed, special ventilation (negative air flow) of the air within the room is desirable. Anyone entering the room should wear a mask, gown, and gloves. Hand washing must follow glove removal after the person exits the room. Contaminated articles must be discarded or bagged and labeled as necessary if being sent for decontamination and reprocessing. Disease examples in this category include the following: pharyngeal diphtheria, pneumonic plague, varicella zoster (chickenpox), and disseminated herpes zoster (shingles).

Contact isolation

Contact isolation is specified to prevent the transmission of highly transmissible infections that do not justify strict isolation. Diseases in this category are spread by close or direct contact. Thus a private room is necessary. However, two people with the same pathogen may share a room unless contraindicated. Protective equipment includes masks if close contact takes place, gowns if contamination is likely, and gloves if there is touching of any infectious material. Materials that are contaminated must be discarded or bagged and labeled before being sent for decontamination and reprocessing. Diseases included in this category are rabies, newborn gonococcal conjunctivitis, herpes simplex, staphylococcal skin infections, and scabies.

Respiratory isolation

Respiratory isolation is specified to prevent the transmission by large droplets of infectious pathogens over short distances. A private room is necessary (except in the case of two people with the same pathogen) unless otherwise indicated. Masks are needed if close contact occurs. Gowns and gloves are not needed, but hands should be washed immediately after the patient or potentially contaminated materials are touched. Contaminated materials should be discarded or bagged and labeled before being sent for decontamination and reprocessing.

AFB (TB) isolation

Acid-fast bacilli (AFB) is used rather than the word *tuberculosis* to protect the patient's privacy. The transmission mode of AFB is airborne. Any patient suspected of having active TB should be placed in respiratory isolation in a private room until shown to be negative for TB. If the AFB test results are positive, the patient should be placed in a private room with negative pressure air flow, which should be vented to the outside of the building and away from any person or intake vents. Ideally, this type of room should be used

Major Highlights of the OSHA Rules and Regulations on Occupational Exposure to Bloodborne Pathogens

1. Gloves that meet the FDA standard for medical gloves should be worn in any patient-contact situation in which blood or other specified body fluid contact is possible. Other body fluids defined by OSHA are semen, cerebrospinal fluid, pericardial fluid, peritoneal fluid, pleural fluid, synovial fluid, amniotic fluid, saliva in dental procedures, vaginal secretions, any body fluid visibly contaminated with blood, and all body fluids in situations where it is difficult or impossible to differentiate between body fluids. Other potentially hazardous materials include any unfixed tissue or organ from a human, cell or tissue cultures, and tissues from experimental animals infected with HIV or HBV. When touching any mucous membrane or broken skin surface, the person should wear gloves. The person should also wear gloves when handling any equipment or surface contaminated with blood or body fluid previously listed when performing any vascular or invasive procedure. Gloves should be changed after each patient and/or procedure. After the gloves are removed, the hands should be washed immediately.

2. Some people are allergic to regular gloves. If this is the case, the employer must provide hypoallergenic gloves, glove liners, powderless gloves, or other suitable alternatives.

3. Employers are required to provide readily accessible hand-washing facilities. If this is not feasible, the employer is required to provide an appropriate antiseptic hand cleanser. If such a hand cleanser is used, employees should wash their hands with soap and running water as soon as possible.

4. Hands and any other skin surface should be washed thoroughly and immediately if accidentally contaminated with blood or any of the listed body fluids.

5. Extreme care should be taken when handling needles or any sharp instrument capable of causing injury. Contaminated needles or sharps should not be recapped, bent by hand, or removed from a syringe. Needles, sharps, and associated disposables should be placed in closable, leak-proof, puncture-resistant, specially labeled, or color-coded containers. If reusable needles must be used, recapping or needle removal must be done with a mechanical device that protects the hand or by using a one-handed technique. In general, it is always best to avoid using reusable sharps if possible. Reusable needles and sharps should likewise be placed in closable, leak-proof, puncture-resistant containers for transport to the sterilization department.

6. Masks and protective total-eye shields or whole-face shields must be worn to protect the mucous membranes of the eyes, nose, and mouth in any procedure in which spraying, spattering, or splashing with blood or other potentially infective materials could occur.

7. Personal protective equipment also includes gowns or, preferably, waterproof aprons that should be worn in any procedure in which spraying or splashing with blood or specified body fluid could occur. General work clothes are not considered protective. Surgical caps or hoods and shoe covers or boots must be worn in situations in which gross contamination can be reasonably foreseen.

8. Mouthpieces, resuscitation bags, or other ventilation devices should be available and used in any area in which the need for resuscitation is predictable. Health care workers should not perform mouth-to-mouth resuscitation; instead, they should take a moment to get the appropriate equipment. (NOTE: There is no documentation of transmission following mouth-to-mouth resuscitation.)

9. Eating, drinking, smoking, applying cosmetics or lip balm, and handling contact lenses is prohibited in work areas having potential exposure hazards.

10. Contaminated laundry should be handled as little as possible with no shaking or other forms of agitation and bagged at the location at which it was used. The bag must be labeled or color-coded sufficiently to permit identification of the bag's contents. The bag should be leak proof if the laundry is wet. Contaminated trash such as used bandages is to be handled with the same general precautions as laundry. The exceptions to labeling and color-coding requirements are when the medical facility takes the BSI approach or considers all laundry and trash to be contaminated.

11. Potential infectious hazards must be communicated to employees through warning signs and labels. OSHA requires that the biohazard label be affixed to containers of regulated waste under specific conditions. The biohazard sign is displayed in Fig. 18-4. The biohazard labels are fluorescent orange or orange-red, with the lettering or symbols in contrasting color. Red bags or red containers are acceptable as substitutes for labels. If the medical facility practices BSI and it is understood that all specimens, used linen, and reusable equipment are treated as if potentially infectious, additional biohazard labeling or colored bags are not necessary.

12. OSHA mandates also address procedures that must be followed if a health care worker is exposed.

Modified from the Department of Labor, Occupational Safety and Health Administration: Occupational exposure to bloodborne pathogens, final rule, 29 CFR Part 1910.1030, *Federal Register* 56(235):64004, Washington, DC, 1991, The Department.

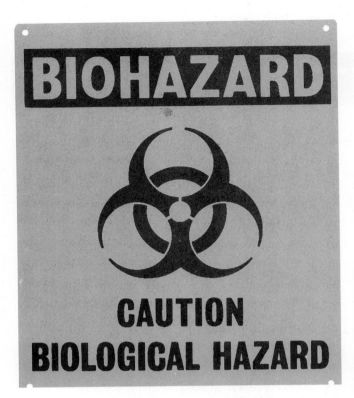

Fig. 18-4 The biohazard symbol is used in order to remind health care workers to be cautious in areas in which the possibility of contamination exists. These reminders can be found anywhere infection control warrants them. The biohazard symbol is orange or orange-red, except in special cases in which white, black, and red combinations are used. A sign using the symbol is shown here.

for any patients suspected of having TB. Doors to the room should remain closed. Surgical masks, although certainly better than no mask, have been deemed ineffective in recent studies.[15,40,42] Thus, the current recommendation is that health care workers wear a particulate respirator, which provides a tighter fit and better filtration. Particulate respirators are especially needed in cases of MDR TB. At this time, OSHA rules state that if health care workers use a respirator, they must be instructed in its use.[15] Newer OSHA guidelines and possible mandates are forthcoming in the near future; in fact, proposed rules have already been published.[64] The National Institute for Occupational Safety and Health (NIOSH) has also shown concern by funding a study directed at the prevention of transmission of TB to and among health care workers.[30] Gowns are not needed unless gross contamination is likely to occur. Gloves are not necessary, but hands should be washed immediately after contact with a patient or materials. Materials are rarely involved in the transmission of TB; nevertheless, they should still be discarded or disinfected.

Enteric precautions

Enteric precautions are necessary in infections transmitted by direct or indirect contact with fecal material. A private room is not needed unless the patient has poor hygiene. Masks are not necessary, and gowns are needed only if the health care worker is at risk of being contaminated. Gloves are needed for touching any potentially infectious material. Hands must be washed immediately after the removal of gloves. Contaminated materials should be discarded or bagged and labeled if being sent for decontamination and reprocessing. Disease examples in this category are infectious diarrhea, amebic gastroenteritis, conditions caused by *Escherichia coli*, salmonellosis, and hepatitis A.

Drainage and secretion precautions

Drainage and secretion precautions are necessary to prevent infections transmitted by direct or indirect contact with purulent (pus-forming) material or with secretions or drainage from an infected body site. Diseases in this category include any infection that produces a discharge that is not included in another category requiring more stringent precautions.

Disease-specific isolation categories

Disease-specific isolation categories are an alternative to the category-specific isolation concept. Instead of grouping disease into categories that require similar precautions, each disease and its specific isolation requirements are treated as a unique entity. The CDC's disease-specific isolation guidelines list precautions for approximately 150 common infectious diseases that are found in the U.S.[38] Ongoing updates have been and will be necessary to address emerging diseases such as that caused by the *Hantavirus,* a mysterious respiratory illness with a high mortality rate that was recently reported in the southwestern part of the U.S.[51]

As addressed previously, a health care facility is not under any mandate to adopt the category-specific or disease-specific isolation system. The only obligation is to meet OSHA's infection-control mandates. To be accredited by JCAHO, a facility must adopt one of the two isolation systems. After meeting OSHA requirements, some hospitals actually practice a combined disease-specific/category-specific isolation system. Other facilities, after meeting OSHA requirements, choose to adopt only a respiratory category that also addresses TB because they practice the BSI concept, which negates the need of some disease-specific or isolation categories recommended by the CDC. In this case, the health care facility and its professional practitioners are obligated to initiate precautions not addressed by policy, as indicated on a patient-to-patient need basis. Health care workers can expect changes in the future as further insights are gained into the transmission and prevention of infectious diseases and in response to the emergence of new drug-resistant pathogens and new pathogens. In fact, the CDC's Hospital

Table 18-1	Basic requirements of category-specific isolation categories

Category	Requirements
Strict isolation	Private room with a closed door
	Negative air flow
	Use of a mask, gown, and gloves (always)
	Hand washing after exiting
	Bagging of contaminated articles
Contact isolation	Private room with a closed door
	Use of a mask, gown, and gloves (if close contact)
	Hand washing after exiting
	Bagging of contaminated articles
Respiratory isolation	Private room with a closed door
	Use of masks (if close contact)
	Hand washing after exiting
	Bagging contaminated articles
AFB (TB) isolation	Private room with a closed door
	Negative air flow
	Use of a particulate respirator
	Use of a gown (if gross contamination)
	Hand washing after exiting
	Discarding, cleaning, and disinfecting of articles
Enteric precautions	Semiprivate room
	Private room (if poor hygiene)
	Use of gloves
	Use of gowns (if gross contamination)
	Hand washing after exiting
	Bagging of contaminated articles
Drainage and secretion precautions	Semiprivate room
	Private room (if poor hygiene)
	Use of gloves
	Use of gowns (if gross contamination)
	Hand washing after exiting
	Bagging of contaminated articles

Infection Control Practices Advisory Committee has already begun drafting proposals for revised isolation-practice guidelines.[13,14]

Other general infection-control measures

Hand washing is the most important way to prevent the spread of infections (Fig. 18-5). To be done properly, hand washing includes the use of antibacterial soap and running water. Health care workers should be cautious not to recontaminate their hands when turning off faucets by using several layers of dry paper towels to touch the faucet if foot-operated facilities are not available. The use of special antimicrobial products is not necessary, but these kinds of products do provide an extra degree of safety for those involved.

The use of masks is intended to prevent or decrease the risk of transmission of infectious agents through the air and applies to large-droplet and small-droplet nuclei. When a cloth or paper mask is worn, it gradually becomes damp with exhalation respiratory moisture. Because transmission risk increases with the degree of wetness, damp masks should be replaced with dry ones as needed.

Blood spills should be cleaned up immediately. Either a disinfectant approved by the Environmental Protection Agency or a 1:10 fresh solution of household bleach (sodium hypochlorite) should be used, with 1 part bleach and 10 parts water.[29] Disinfectants labeled as germicides should not be used because they are ineffective.

Students should receive instruction at the earliest stage of their professional education. Orientation to OSHA rules and regulations and medical facilities' overall infection-control programs and hazardous materials programs should take place before active participation in the clinical component of education. In some educational programs, students rotate through multiple health care facilities. These programs need to ensure that a student is thoroughly familiar with each facility's specific programs before any active participation occurs.

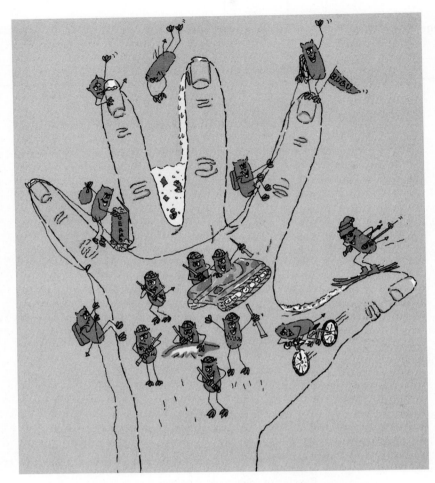

Fig. 18-5 Hand washing is the best way to prevent the transmission of disease. (Courtesy Brevis Co., Salt Lake City.)

HANDLING EXPOSURE INCIDENTS RELATED TO HIV

Names such as Rock Hudson, Ryan White, Kimberly Bergalis, Earvin "Magic" Johnson, and Greg Louganis are associated with the most significant epidemic of the twentieth century. The introduction in 1981 of the acronym AIDS (acquired immunodeficiency syndrome) and later the acronym HIV (human immunodeficiency virus) struck fear and anxiety in the community and in the health care setting. Since 1983, when the first case of occupational HIV-1 infection was documented, health care workers have been flooded with information and literature about the risk that accompanies caring for HIV-positive patients.[2] Because these patients do not always have obvious characteristics of the disease, the only logical approach that a health care worker can use for self-protection is to assume that all patients are HIV positive.

Because health care workers are human, accidents happen. When an exposure incident occurs, the first and most urgent question is, "What actions can be taken to decrease the risk of transmission?" Over the past decade, the CDC, OSHA and the scientific community have closely observed exposure incidents in health care workers. Although a multitude of questions and issues have not yet been resolved, these exposure incidents have aided in the development of guidelines for treatment. Before any guidelines and recommendations are addressed, the risk of acquiring HIV should be reviewed.

For perspective, the risk of acquiring HIV is commonly compared with the risk of acquiring HBV. As stated previously in this chapter, before the OSHA-mandated HBV vaccine, approximately 8700 HBV infections occurred annually in U.S. health care workers. These infections also resulted in approximately 200 deaths each year.[29] In contrast, as of December 1994, there were only 42 documented cases of occupationally acquired HIV infections since 1981.[23] The most glaring difference is that death is *possible* with an HBV infection and *expected* after an HIV infection because of the inevitability of acquiring of AIDS, for which no known cure exists at this time.

The risk of acquiring HBV has been statistically calculated to be 10 to 100 times greater than the risk of acquiring HIV. The risk of HBV after a needle stick involving blood from an HBV-positive patient has been estimated to be 5% to 43% compared with less than 0.3% (1 in 250) for HIV.[66] These statistics come from an ongoing prospective study of health care workers at the National Institutes of Health (NIH) and other prospective studies.[5,6,23,56] The risk from mucosal and nonintact cutaneous exposure is not zero; however, it is too low to be reasonably calculated at this time. No risk from contamination of normal skin or other types of casual contact exposure has been documented. Other risk factors that may affect transmission include the following: titer of virus in source fluid, volume of material involved, and viral viability.

The type of exposure appears to be highly associated with the risk of acquiring HIV. Percutaneous exposures account for 84% of occupationally acquired HIV cases, followed by mucocutaneous exposure (13%) and combined percutaneous and mucocutaneous exposure (3%).[23] To date, no additional routes of transmission have been proved in occupational HIV exposure,[6] and casual contact that occurs with infected patients apparently poses no risk to the health care worker.

After an exposure, the type and severity of the exposure must be recorded because this information may eventually provide better epidemiological data. For example, documenting the type of needle (e.g., hollow-core, surgical), gauge of the needle, depth of penetration, volume of blood or body fluid, and source of fluid (e.g., semen, amniotic fluid) helps provide better analysis.

Some hospitals have defined levels of HIV exposure to be used as guides in counseling the exposed health care worker and in initiating prophylactic treatment. Typical exposure levels are as follows[27]:

- Massive exposure—example: parenteral exposure to HIV laboratory animals with high viral titers
- Definite parenteral exposure—example: intramuscular "deep" injury with needle
- Possible parenteral exposure—example: subcutaneous "superficial" needle injury
- Doubtful parenteral exposure—example: prior wound or skin lesion contaminated with non–OSHA-specified body fluid
- Nonparenteral exposure—example: intact skin contaminated with blood or specified body fluid

A true occupational exposure requires documented seroconversion to take place. This means that the health care worker tested negative for HIV shortly after an exposure and subsequently developed clinical and/or serological evidence of HIV infection. This documentation is necessary to sort

health care workers who may have unknowingly been positive for HIV at the time of exposure as a result of nonoccupational factors.

Although no data are available demonstrating that first aid is effective in preventing the transmission of HIV, the use of first aid procedures is the only logical immediate management strategy. Health care workers should be instructed to initiate decontamination procedures immediately if possible. Percutaneous wounds should be irrigated with sterile saline, an antiseptic, or another suitable solution. Intact skin should at least be washed with soap and water. Oral and nasal mucosal surfaces should be forcefully rinsed with water. Eyes should be thoroughly rinsed with water, saline, or other suitable sterile solutions. The use of bleach, hydrogen peroxide, and other antiseptics for wound care are logical even if no scientific data support their use. A 1990 article reported a case in which a health care worker poured undiluted bleach over a cut that involved blood from an AIDS patient; in spite of this action the worker still converted to HIV positive.[48]

The management of exposed health care workers is extremely sensitive and complex. Workers should be treated on a priority basis in light of the extreme mental anguish associated with an HIV exposure. Psychological reactions include fear, anxiety, anger, depression, denial, sexual and sleep disturbances symptoms, suicide, and psychosis. Counseling must be available immediately and continuously for workers exposed to HIV. Some institutions have even set up 24-hour counseling hotlines for their exposed health care workers.[39]

The CDC recommends follow-up HIV antibody testing at 6 weeks, 3 months, and 6 months after exposure.[20] The Enzyme-Linked Immunosorbent Assay (ELISA) test is performed to detect HIV antibody. Because false-positive results occur, a positive ELISA test should be followed with a confirmatory test such as the Western Blot test.[25,29] Early tests for HIV antibody may be negative; however, infection can usually be documented at an early stage by less widely available tests such as measuring p24 antigen, by HIV cultures, or by gene-amplification studies.[39] *Delayed seroconversion,* defined as the appearance of the HIV antibody at greater than 6 months, has not yet been documented; however, some institutions test again at 12 months. The rationale for testing after 6 months is that treatment may delay seroconversion. In addition, later testing often reassures the health care worker.[39] Symptoms that are compatible with seroconversion include the following: an unexplained fever, lymphadenopathy, a rash, lymphopenia, and a sore throat.

Counseling of the health care worker should also address lifestyle changes that should be made until seroconversion occurs or until enough time has passed (typically 6 months) for the worker to be deemed free of HIV infection. Lifestyle changes include no exchanging of body fluids during sex; deferment of pregnancy; and cessation of breast feeding, intimate kissing, the sharing of razors and tooth brushes and the donation of blood, sperm, or organs. If the health care worker is involved in an accident that results in bleeding, surfaces that are contaminated should be promptly disinfected.

Chemoprophylaxis with zidovudine, more commonly known as *azidothymidine (AZT)*, is typically recommended after a significant occupational HIV exposure.[46] AZT is a drug approved by the FDA for use in the treatment of patients with AIDS. Although this drug does not cure AIDS, some evidence exists that AZT delays the progression of AIDS, prolongs survival, and decreases the incidence of opportunistic infections.[3] This evidence and data, derived from animal studies, are the rationale behind using AZT in occupationally exposed health care workers who provide informed consent. AZT is believed to possibly prevent the establishment of infection if the drug is administered soon after exposure.[58]

When an exposure incident occurs, the employer must make immediately available to the health care worker a confidential medical evaluation and follow-up. If the incident involves a source individual, who is defined as any person, living or dead, whose blood or other potentially infectious body materials may be a source of exposure, the identification of the source individual will be made except when doing so is infeasible or prohibited by law. In some states the source's blood can be tested to determine if the source is positive for HIV, but this is done only after consent is obtained.[39] Other states have passed legislation that allows HIV testing of the source after occupational exposure even if the source patient refuses to have the test performed.[47] Test results are to be made known to the health care worker, but the worker also must be advised on laws regarding the confidentiality of the source's identity, if known, and the infectious status.[29]

The blood of exposed health care workers should be tested if consent is obtained to establish an HIV baseline. OSHA rules further state that if the workers consent to blood collection but not to an HIV test, the sample must be preserved for at least 90 days in case the persons change their mind.[29]

The efficacy of AZT as a chemoprophylactic is unknown and difficult to determine because of the low risk of transmission. Prospective, randomized trials were attempted in 1988 by Burroughs Wellcome Co., but too few subjects were enrolled to justify continuing the trials.[39] The medical literature also documents cases in which health care workers were given AZT but later experienced positive conversion.[58,60] On the other hand, an encouraging 1991 study documented no seroconversions among 160 health care workers who chose to receive AZT after their occupational exposure.[46] Insufficient data exist to mandate providing AZT or other new drugs or to advise against their use after occupational exposure.

Although the use of AZT rarely induces serious toxicity, a wide variety of side effects is associated with its use. Side effects include headaches, nausea, fever, fatigue, gastrointestinal pain, bone marrow suppression, hepatomegaly, muscle weakness, and lactic acidosis. In addition, the optimum AZT time and dose relationship has yet to be determined. Health care workers who elect to receive AZT must be closely monitored. They must also be counseled in regard to issues such as pregnancy and breast feeding, and they must be medically evaluated to rule out conditions such as underlying renal insufficiency, which would contraindicate the use of AZT.[3]

In general, employees should be allowed to perform patient care duties except during times when their condition is infectious through nonbloodborne routes. For example, with infectious diarrhea, skin lesions, and pulmonary infections, work restrictions would be reasonable. In the case of a bloodborne infection status, such as HIV or HBV positive, employers are not allowed to discriminate against the employee. Employees are protected by section 504 of the Rehabilitation Act and the Americans with Disabilities Act, which prohibit discrimination against individuals with disabilities, including persons who are positive for HIV or HBV.[34] Employers must make every effort to maintain the employment of an individual as long as the individual is capable of performing the job and does not pose a reasonable threat of infection to others. At the same time, however, employees and students should take personal responsibility for their actions and not perform any procedure that could be dangerous to their coworkers or patients.

RIGHTS OF THE HEALTH CARE WORKER

Hopefully, today's health care worker will never have to wonder what to do if an employer does not provide proper protection equipment, but if this occurs, health care workers have legal rights. OSHA helps provide job safety and health protection for workers by promoting safe and healthful working conditions throughout the nation.[32] Health care workers can lawfully refuse to work in truly unsafe conditions and have the right to insist on wearing protective equipment. However, workers cannot leave their job if they want their rights protected. Health care workers must first inform their employer of the unsafe conditions. If an employer does not respond, the worker should contact OSHA to file a complaint and request that an inspection be conducted.[31] OSHA will withhold, on request, the name of the employee filing the complaint.[32] Before complaining, a health care worker should be sure that the unsafe condition is indeed serious (i.e., the situation could have caused death or serious harm).

The opposite situation can also coccur. On occasion, a health care worker may have unreasonable fears and be overly cautious. Examples include the worker who refuses to go anywhere near an AIDS patient or the worker who insists on wearing a full-body space suit. This type of reaction is usually caused by lack of proper education about the risk of transmission and proper protective actions workers should take. The employer should let the health care worker explain fears and perceptions and should then educate the worker with the necessary information in understandable language. The health care worker cannot be discharged or discriminated against in any way just because of a misperception or because of a complaint or a call to OSHA. Workers who believe they have been discriminated against should file a complaint with their nearest OSHA office within 30 days of the alleged discriminatory act.[32] However, if after counseling and if the situation is deemed to be reasonably safe and proper equipment was provided, and the worker still refuses to provide care as in the AIDS patient example, the employer may have the right to dismiss the worker.

Health care workers also have legal rights if they develop an occupationally acquired infection. Worker's compensation laws, determined by each state, are in place to protect the employee. To be compensated in cases in which workers are disabled or killed, the injuries must have occurred while the workers were practicing within their scope of practice. Bungee jumping off the seventeenth floor of the hospital during lunch hour, for example, would not be covered because it is outside the scope of practice of a radiation therapist. In most cases, workers do not have the right to file a negligence or criminal suit in addition to a worker's compensation claim unless they can prove that their employer intentionally disregarded an infection risk. The worker must be able to establish that the infection was actually acquired on the job, not in the community.

Another extremely important right health care worker's have is complete confidentiality. To protect the workers privacy, most health care facilities take special steps to avoid placing the health care worker's "patient" chart where other employees have access to it. In addition, such a diagnosis would not be placed on computerized charting systems.

ROLE OF THE CENTRAL SERVICES DEPARTMENT

In the past, medical supplies and equipment that needed to be sterilized were often sterilized in an autoclave unit housed in the radiation oncology department. With the concerns of bloodborne pathogens and emerging diseases, health care centers have learned that it is far better to leave the reprocessing of medical supplies and equipment in the hands of experts. This area of expertise typically is housed in a department known as *central services,* or *central supply.* The central service department (CSD) is accountable for preparing, processing, sorting, and distributing medical supplies and equipment required in patient care. This central location not only is economical, but also is subject to stringent levels of quality control according to JCAHO guidelines.[54]

A student tour through a major hospital's CSD can be an extremely enlightening and educational experience. Contaminated equipment is first precleaned and decontaminated by trained, specially clothed workers. This clothing includes items such as waterproof aprons and face shields. Reprocessing may include disassembly and sending equipment through devices that remind a person of a commercial car wash complete with a presoak cycle, wash cycle, and dry cycle. Instruments are then prepared for sterilization by the most appropriate method. Ideally, each package sterilized is labeled with a control number in case any item needs to be recalled. The labeling process may also identify the sterilizing unit used, its load, the time and date an item was sterilized, the item's expiration date, and sometimes even the individual who packaged the item (Fig. 18-6).

After a package has been disinfected or sterilized, it should be handled as little as possible and stored in a low-traffic, clean, dry, closed area. If an item comes into contact with something and becomes soiled, is exposed to moisture, or is physically penetrated, it is deemed contaminated and should not be used. Sterile items should be stored away from the floor, vents, pipes, doors, and windows. Closed shelves are preferred over drawers because the risk of damaging a sterilized package is greater in opening and closing a drawer than opening the door to a cabinet. If a closed cabinet is not an option, open shelves are a feasible solution. The chance of contamination can be decreased by placing a plastic dust cover over the sterilized packages. Each health care facility determines the amount of time a sterilized item can be stored. Important factors in determining shelf life include packaging material and an open or closed shelf design, both of which combined are more important than time alone. It is further assumed that after the opening of a sterilized package, sterile technique will be used and the date of expiration will be checked.

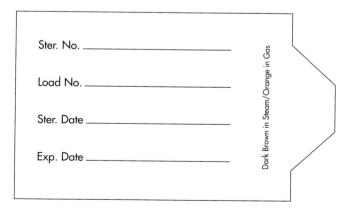

Ster. No. _____

Load No. _____

Ster. Date _____

Exp. Date _____

Dark Brown in Steam/Orange in Gas

Fig. 18-6 Sterilization labels are used as part of the quality-control program in a central services department. If an item needs to be recalled, it can be tracked by its control number.

STERILIZATION AND DISINFECTION TECHNIQUES

Because a radiation therapist needs to routinely practice infection-control techniques, an overview of sterilization and disinfection techniques is desirable and addressed in the following text. Every health care facility should have infection-control policies and experts available for consultation. Simple questions regarding whether radiation oncology supplies should be single-use disposables or reprocessed can be answered by these experts. In addition, experts can advise the most economical route and the best method or product for each situation. Expertise is readily available from an institution's CSD and/or epidemiology department. Any policy developed within a radiation oncology department should be reviewed by these experts before the policy's implementation.

In general, medical supplies and equipment can be divided into risk categories based on an item's use. *Critical items* are products or instruments inserted into normally sterile areas of the body or into the bloodstream and must be sterile for use. Items in this category include needles, surgical instruments, and implants. *Semicritical items* are those that contact mucosal surfaces but do not ordinarily penetrate body surfaces. These include items such as endoscopes and urinary catheters. It is preferrable to sterilize items in this category, but high-level disinfection may be used. *Noncritical items* do not ordinarily touch the patient or touch only the patient's intact skin; therefore they do not need to be sterile. This category includes items such as blood pressure cuffs.

The FDA requires that medical devices be sold with instructions stating whether the devices are single-use or reusable items, and the way they must be processed if reusable.[35] Sterilization is a process that destroys all microbial life forms, including resistant spores. Disinfection is a process that reduces microbial life forms and can range from high-level disinfection to low-level disinfection.[49] *Low-level disinfection* is synonymous with *sanitization*.

Antiseptics are different from disinfectants. The term *antiseptic* is reserved for antimicrobial substances applied to skin surfaces. Methods of sterilization and disinfection are addressed in the following text and differ with regard to the biocidal agent, biocidal action, contact between the biocidal agent and microorganism, and severity of treatment.[36]

Heat

The use of heat, moist or dry, is the most reliable, available, and economical method of destroying microorganisms. Boiling water (212° F, 100° C) is probably the oldest method used. Although boiling greatly decreases the number of microorganisms, it does not destroy all microorganisms such as spores; thus boiling fits into the category of disinfectants rather than sterilants. In fact, temperatures lower than boiling (50° to 70° C, 122° to 158° F) are sufficient to kill most

viruses, bacteria, and fungi.[49] HIV is destroyed by moist heat at 60° C (140° F) in 30 minutes, a temperature well below the requirement for boiling water.[26]

Steam under pressure, however, is capable of destroying all life forms, provided that a proper combination of temperature and time is achieved. Older textbooks typically quoted a specific time, temperature, and pressure combination, and the student accepted this combination as an absolute. In reality, steam sterilization works as an inverse relationship and many combinations are equally effective; thus steam sterilization is analogous to the various time-dose relationships used in treating cancer. Simply put, the time required for sterilization decreases as the temperature increases.

No life forms survive if exposed to steam under pressure at 15 pounds per square inch (psi) at 121° C (250° F).[49] The variable factor in this example is time. An exposure that lasts 15 to 20 minutes is adequate for killing most life forms; however, the Creutzfeldt-Jakob agent, a type of prion, requires 1 hour of exposure.[36] The term *prion*, which was introduced in 1982, is used to describe unique, infectious central nervous system agents composed of protein but lacking identifiable nucleic acid. Prions multiply and are extremely resistant to standard sterilization methods.[36] To summarize, sterilization combinations of pressure, temperature, and time are also influenced by the type of microorganism to be destroyed.

Steam sterilizers are commonly referred to as *steam autoclaves* and can be described as closed metal chambers. **Autoclaves** can be grouped into two general categories: gravity-displacement and mechanically evacuated devices. The gravity-displacement type requires a longer exposure time. Steam sterilization is the most commonly used method of sterilization used in health care facilities because of its low cost, its absence of toxic residue, and the fact that it can be used to sterilize an extremely wide assortment of materials. A drying cycle follows exposure to the steam and is often the slowest portion of the autoclave cycle. Another device known as a *flash sterilizer,* or *flash autoclave,* can be used in an emergency situation. This device is operated at a higher temperature, and exposure time is only a few minutes. Flash autoclaving should not routinely be substituted for standard autoclaving procedures.

Cotton fabric and special steam-permeable plastics or paper can be used as packaging materials. Other criteria essential to the selection of appropriate packaging materials for any sterilization method include the resistance to puncture and tears, penetration by microorganisms, and absence of toxic or biologically harmful particles. Care must be exercised in packing items for steam sterilization to ensure that the steam can reach all surfaces and cavities of a specific item. For example, lids must be taken off containers and many items may require disassembly. Items in a package must be arranged loosely because overpacking may lead to nonsterilization. Steam sterilization also has its limitations. Instruments with sharp points, such as needles, or cutting edges, such as scalpels, may be dulled. Oxidation and corrosion may also occur with certain metals. Powder and oil products should not be autoclaved because the steam has difficulty in penetrating such substances. Many products such as rubber and synthetic polymers are heat sensitive and could melt or deteriorate. Other products such as injectable solutions may lose their biological usefulness when subjected to high heat levels.

Because of packing precautions, packaging material differences, product sensitivity to heat, and JCAHO quality-control standards, comprehensive knowledge is required of anyone in charge of steam sterilization or any method of sterilization. For these reasons, sterilization should be done only by experts, the employees of the CSD.

Dry heat is also used for sterilization. Although its use has sharply declined since the introduction of single-use syringes and needles sterilized by other methods, dry heat is still quite useful for reusable needles, glass syringes, sharp-cutting instruments and drills, powders and oily products, and metals that oxidize or corrode with exposure to moisture. The advantage of dry heat is its ability to penetrate solids, nonaqueous powders or oils, and closed containers. Its primary disadvantage when compared with steam is that higher temperatures and longer exposure times are required to achieve sterilization. A commonly quoted temperature is 160° C (320° F) with a time of 1 to 3 hours.[49] As with steam sterilization, appropriate time and temperature combinations follow an inverse relationship. Similar to cooking in a home oven, aluminum foil or aluminum containers are commonly used for packaging. As with steam sterilization, items that are heat sensitive should be sterilized by other available techniques.

Incineration, another form of heat, is frequently applied to biohazardous waste materials generated in health care settings. Some incinerators are located on hospital grounds, but most are now located away from hospitals, residential areas, and high-occupancy buildings. Because incinerators are typically located some distance away, designated vehicles are required to transport biohazardous waste to the incinerator site.

Gas

Gas sterilizers are available for medical products that cannot withstand high temperatures. In recent times, the use of gas has become increasingly important in the health care setting and the commercial setting because of the use of a greater number of instruments and products that cannot tolerate high heat exposure. Ethylene oxide (ETOX) is the gas used in the vast majority of gas. In the past, ETOX was mixed with freon, but carbon dioxide (CO_2) is now used because of freon's harmful effect on the ozone layer. The operation of a gas sterilizer should be attempted only by qualified experts

because the gases present fire and explosion hazards. In addition, the gas has a toxic effect on humans, thus making it subject to OSHA regulations. Gas sterilizers are equipped with special detectors to alert personnel in the event of a gas leak. Packages sterilized by gas are typically exposed for 4 to 12 hours at temperatures of 25° to 60° C.[36,49] Other time and temperature combinations can be used because the process follows an inverse relationship.

Packages are then aerated in special closed cabinets for 12 to 24 hours by heated, high air flows to dissipate any residual ETOX because of its tissue toxicity.[49] Gas should not be used to sterilize products that can withstand heat because gas is slower and more expensive and has the possibility of toxic residue. Large medical institutions frequently cooperate and provide gas-sterilization access to medium and small medical institutions to assist with cost. Gas sterilization is not applied to liquids or products packaged in gas-impervious wrappers. Products can be wrapped in the same packaging materials used for steam sterilization.

Radiation

Although not used in the health care setting, ionizing radiation is widely applied at commercial industrial sites to heat-sensitive medical products and equipment. Gamma beams from cobalt 60 sources and electron beams are used. Electrons are more limited in use because of their poorer penetration, and beams over 10 MeV are not used because they can induce radioactivity in the sterilized product through artificial nuclide production.[36] Extremely high absorbed doses (kGy) are necessary because microorganisms are far more resistant to the effects of radiation than humans.[55] The time required for sterilization depends on the unit's output rate and the required absorbed dose. Packaging materials and the product contained within are sterilized. Caution must be employed in using radiation as a sterilant for medications because it may induce chemical changes by breaking chemical bonds and thus inactivate or modify some medications. An interesting student project is to check packages for a wide variety of single-use (disposable) products to see the number that were irradiated.

Radiation sterilization is routinely used in the autosterilization of a strontium (^{90}Sr) applicator. After the ^{90}Sr treatment for pterygium of the eye, the radioactive end of the applicator is wiped against a sterile alcohol pad to remove any biological debris and then rinsed with sterile water. The surface radiation output emitted by a typical 50-mCi ^{90}Sr source is approximately 50 cGy per second, a rate high enough that it sterilizes itself with a dose of over 4 million cGy in a 24-hour period.[53]

Nonionizing radiations such as ultraviolet and infrared light or microwave are capable of killing microorganisms, but the wavelengths are too low to allow any significant penetration; thus most are not used for sterilization purposes except in a few extremely limited applications.

Chemicals liquids

Using chemicals for sterilization or disinfection is a relatively easy process. Items need only to be placed in a basin deep enough to completely submerge the item, with care taken to ensure that the chemical can reach all inner and outer surfaces and crevices. Caution should also be exercised to ensure that the chemical does not damage the item to be processed or the basin containing the chemical itself. The most difficult part is selecting the best, most appropriate chemical. Therefore a radiation therapist should contact a qualified CSD expert for input in choosing products and protocols for their use. The assumption should not be made that oncology physicians or nurses have any more expertise in this subject than a radiation therapist. Chemicals have an extremely wide range of antimicrobial action. Few can sterilize; most cannot.

The CDC cannot endorse specific products, but it can provide guidance in choosing products.[37] Other professional groups such as the Association for Practitioners in Infection Control (APIC) also publish extremely useful guidelines.[69] Manufacturers are also responsible for furnishing recommendations on the reprocessing of items they produce. Thus the chemical to be used on a specific item is based on expert guidelines, scientific literature, and manufacturer product information. Reliance on labels alone is insufficient and at times even misleading. Therefore caution should be used with wording such as, "hospital strength disinfectant." "Hospital disinfectant" is preferred because this term indicates a higher level of disinfection. Many chemical products may have other terminology on their labels that provide useful information about effectiveness. For example, a bactericide or germicide is capable of killing nonsporing bacteria, fungicides kill fungi and their spores, sporicides are agents that can kill bacterial spores, virucides make viruses noninfective, and tuberculocides kill TB bacteria and other acid-fast bacteria. Commonly used chemicals are addressed in the following text.

Soap's usefulness as a disinfectant is limited because of its feeble antimicrobial action. The main merit of soap is that it aids in the removal of contamination buildup. Chlorine or chlorine compounds are widely used as disinfectants, and although they are extremely effective against most microorganisms (including HIV and HBV), they are ineffective against spores and have an irritating odor. Alcohol, ethyl and isopropyl, is also ineffective against spores and some viruses. Iodine or iodine compounds may have sporicidal activity. In addition, some people are allergic to it. Hexachlorophene is used for surgical hand disinfection but does not kill all microorganisms. Formaldehyde is effective against all microorganisms, but its vapors are extremely irritating. Alkaline glutaraldehyde (Cidex) can kill spores if they are exposed to it long enough, but it has a pungent odor and is temperature sensitive, which causes it to eventually lose effectiveness. Some chemicals, when old and/or too diluted, even encourage rather than retard the growth of microorganisms. Some chemical disinfectants are extremely short acting, and others continue to retard the growth of microorganisms for variable lengths of time. Few special-use chemicals are effective as true sterilants. Because of the wide variability in the effectiveness of chemicals and their potential hazardous risks to health care workers, CSD experts should be contacted for advice on each situation to achieve the appropriate degree of asepsis.

A special note of caution is that liquid disinfectants and sterilants should not be used to clean brachytherapy devices such as ovoids. These liquids are known to be capable of corroding the silver brazing that secures the ovoid to the ovoid handle.[57]

Sterility quality-control measures

A wide selection of chemical indicators is used externally and/or internally on packages subjected to a sterilization process. The purpose of the indicators is to alert a health care worker that something went wrong during the sterilization process. External indicators are commonly used in heat, gas, and radiation sterilization processes and typically consist of an adhesive tape that darkens or changes color if exposed to a sterilization process (Fig. 18-7). External indicators do not guarantee that sterility has been achieved; they indicate only that the package was exposed to the process. Internal indicators are strategically placed inside a package at a site that is least likely to be penetrated by steam or gas (Fig. 18-8). Like external indicators, internal indicators do not guarantee that all microorganisms have been destroyed. Different types of external and internal indicators are commercially available for the different specific sterilization processes.

Biological indicators are used to determine whether sterilization was achieved. A biological indicator is a specially prepared strip coated with hard-to-kill microorganisms such as spores and enclosed in a small container placed inside a test package. After the test package has gone through the sterilization process with other packages, a microbiologist or another qualified expert examines the biological indicator to determine whether all the microorganisms were killed. If not, all packages are recalled by their processing number. Routine use of biological indicators is required by external accrediting agencies such as JCAHO. These indicators are typically used daily in each sterilization unit cycle and after any repair on a particular unit. Biological indicators, external and internal indicators, and close attention to proper time and temperature combinations are all needed to ensure that products and equipment are safe for patient use.

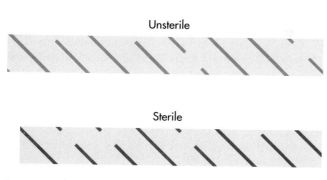

Unsterile

Sterile

Fig. 18-7 External indicators are placed on the outside of a package to be sterilized. After exposed to the sterilization process, the tape darkens or changes color. An external indicator does not guarantee sterility; it indicates only that the package was exposed to the process. Different types of tape are used in different sterilization processes (e.g., gas, steam).

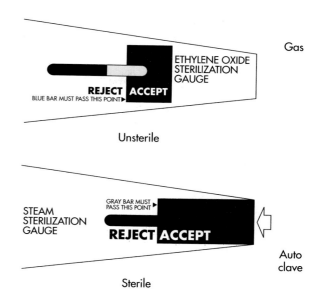

Fig. 18-8 Internal indicators are placed inside packages to be sterilized. They are placed in sites least likely to be reached by the sterilization process. Although they provide a higher degree of sterility assurance than do external indicators, internal indicators also do not guarantee sterility.

Review Questions

Fill in the Blank

1. _____ is the name of the medical science field that studies the incidence, distribution, and determinants of disease.
2. An individual who is colonized but shows no immune response is known as a _____.
3. _____ is the federal agency that oversees safety in the work place.
4. Two nosocomial infectious diseases for which no vaccine is currently available are _____ and _____.
5. AFB stands for _____.
6. The three phases that a susceptible host goes through are _____, _____, and _____.
7. _____ is the gas that is routinely used for gas sterilization.

Essay

8. What are the major differences between large droplet and droplet nuclei transmission?
9. If a health care worker develops hypersensitivity to latex gloves, what should be done?
10. What is sodium hypochlorite, and what is its use in the medical setting?
11. Define *delayed seroconversion*.

Questions to Ponder

1. Discuss the differences between universal precautions and body substance isolation.
2. Using documented research, identify 10 infectious diseases that, if caught, result in lifelong immunity.
3. Compare and contrast the differences between killed, toxoid, and attenuated live vaccines.
4. Develop an infection-control protocol for any clinical area task that needs to be addressed.
5. Compare labels on various liquid chemicals used for infection control in the medical setting and discuss what they can and cannot kill.

REFERENCES

1. Alter MJ: The detection, transmission and outcome of hepatitis C virus infection, *Infect Agents Dis* 2:155-156, 1993.
2. Anonymous: Needlestick transmission of HTLV-III from a patient infected in Africa, *Lancet* 2:1376-1377, 1984.
3. Barnhart ER, publisher: *Physician's desk reference,* ed 49, Montvale, NJ, 1995, Medical Economics Data Production.
4. Bartlett JG: *Pocketbook of infectious disease therapy,* Baltimore, 1991, Wilkins & Wilkins.
5. Beekman SE, Henderson DK: Health care workers and hepatitis: risk for infection and management of exposure, *Infect Dis Clin Pract* 1:424-428, 1992.
6. Beekman SE et al: Risky business: using necessarily imprecise casualty counts to estimate occupational risk of HIV-1 infection, *Infect Control Hosp Epidemiol* 11(7):371-379, 1990.
7. Beil L: FDA approves vaccine against chickenpox, 70 to 90% effectiveness expected, *Dallas Morning News,* p 1, March 18, 1995.
8. Benenson A, editor: *Control of communicable diseases in man,* 13 ed, Washington DC, 1981, American Public Health Association.
9. Bond WW et al: Inactivation of hepatitis B virus after drying and storage for one week (letter), *Lancet* 1:550-551, 1981.
10. Brachman PS: Epidemiology of nosocomial infections. In Bennett JV, Brachman PS, editors: *Hospital infections,* ed 3, Boston, 1992, Little Brown.
11. Campbell CC: Malaria. In Hoeprich PD, Jordan MC, editors: *Infectious diseases,* ed 4, Philadelphia, 1989, JB Lippincott.
12. Cawson RA et al: *Pathology: the mechanisms of disease,* ed 2, St Louis, 1989, Mosby.
13. Centers for Disease Control and Prevention, Hospital Infection Control Practices Advisory Committee: Agenda, *Federal Register* 58:103, 1993.
14. Centers for Disease Control and Prevention, Hospital Infection Control Practices Advisory Committee: Meetings, *Federal Register* 58:204, 1993.
15. Centers for Disease Control and Prevention: Guidelines for preventing the transmission of *Mycobacterium tuberculosis* in health-care facilities, *MMWR* 43(RR-13):69, 78-81, 1994.
16. Centers for Disease Control and Prevention: Guidelines for preventing the transmission of tuberculosis in healthcare settings, with special focus on HIV-related issues, *MMWR* 39(Re-17):1, 1990.
17. Centers for Disease Control and Prevention: Prevention and control of influenza: part II. Antiviral agents—recommendations of the Advisory Committee on Immunization Practices (ACIP), *MMWR* 43(No RR-15):1-10, 1994.
18. Centers for Disease Control and Prevention: *Proceedings of the First International Conference on Nosocomial Infections,* Atlanta, August 5-8, 1970, American Hospital Association.
19. Centers for Disease Control and Prevention: Recommendations for preventing transmission of infection in the human T-lymphotropic virus type III/lymphadenopathy-associated virus in the workplace, *MMWR* 34:681-695, 1985.
20. Centers for Disease Control and Prevention: Recommendations for prevention of HIV transmisssion in health care settings, *MMWR* 36(Suppl 2S):1-19, 1987.
21. Centers for Disease Control and Prevention: Recommendations of the Advisory Committee on Immunization Practices: varicella-zoster immune globulin for the prevention of chickenpox, *MMWR* 33:84-100, 1984.
22. Centers for Disease Control and Prevention: Recommendations of the Immunization Practices Advisory Committee: prevention and control of influenza, *MMWR* 39(No. RR-7):1-15, 1990.
23. Centers for Disease Control and Prevention: Surveillance for occupationally acquired HIV infection—United States, 1981-1992, *MMWR* 41:823-825, 1992. Personal Communication Update with CDC National AIDS Clearinghouse, 1995.
24. Centers for Disease Control and Prevention: Update: universal precautions for prevention of transmission of human immunodeficiency virus, hepatitis B virus, and other bloodborne pathogens in health care settings, *MMWR* 37:377-388, 1988.
25. Cooper JS: The role of radiation therapy in the management of patients who have AIDS. In Cox JD, editor: *Moss's radiation oncology: rationale, technique, results,* ed 7, St Louis, 1994, Mosby.
26. Cuthbertson B et al: Safety of albumin preparations manufactured from plasma not tested for HIV antibody (letter), *Lancet* 2(8549):41, 1987.
27. Department of Epidemiology, Baylor University Medical Center: *Human immunodeficiency virus (HIV) workplace guidelines,* Dallas, 1993, The Department.
28. Department of Labor, OSHA, and the Department of Health and Human Services: Joint Advisory Notice: Protection against occupational exposure to hepatitis B virus (HBV) and human immunodeficiency virus, *Federal Register* 54:41818, October 30, 1987.
29. Department of Labor, Occupational Safety and Health Administration: Occupational exposure to bloodborne pathogens, final rule, 29 CFR Part 1910.1030, *Federal Register* 56(235):64004, 1991.
30. Department of Labor, Occupational Safety and Health Administration: Proposed rules on TB transmission to and among HCWs, *Federal Register* 59(219):58884-58935, 1994.
31. Department of Labor, Occupational Safety and Health Administration: *Title 29, code of federal regulations, part 1977.12,* Washington DC, 1989, The Department.
32. Department of Labor, Occupational Safey and Health Administration: *Title 29, code of federal regulations, part 1903.2,* Washington DC, 1989, The Department.
33. Douglas RG Jr: Influenza in man. In Kilbourne ED, editor: *The influenza virus and influenza,* New York, 1975, Academic.
34. Equal Employment Opportunity Commission: *A technical assistance manual on the employment provisions (title 1) of the Americans with Disabilities Act,* Washington DC, 1992, The Commission.
35. Favero MS, Bond WW: Chemical disinfection of medical and surgical materials. In Block SS, editor: *Sterilization and preservation,* ed 4, Philadelphia, 1991, Lea & Febiger.
36. Gardner JF, Peel MM: *Introduction to sterilization, disinfection and infection control,* ed 2, New York, 1991, Churchill Livingstone.
37. Gardner JS, Favero MS: CDC guidelines for the prevention and control of nosocomial infections: Guideline for handwashing and hospital environmental control, 1985, *Am J Infect Control* 14:110-129, 1986.

38. Gardner JS, Simmons BP: CDC guidelines for isolation precautions in hospitals, *Infect Control* 4:245-325, 1983.

39. Gerberding JL, Henderson DK: Management of occupational exposure to bloodborne pathogens: hepatitis B virus, hepatitis C virus and human immunodeficiency virus, *Clin Infect Dis* 14:1179-1185, 1992.

40. Guvton HG, Decker HM: Respiratory protection by five new contagion masks, *Appl Microbiol*, 11:66-68, 1963.

41. Haley CE: *Drug resistant TB*. Lecture at Baylor University Medical Center, Dallas, February 25, 1994.

42. Haley CE et al: Tuberculosis epidemic among hospital personnel, *Infect Control Hosp Epidemiol* 10(5):204-210, 1989.

43. Haley RW: *Managing hospital infection control for cost*, Chicago, 1986, American Hospital Publishing.

44. Haley RW: The development of infection surveillance and control programs. In Bennett JV, Brachman PS, editors: *Hospital infections*, ed 3, Boston, 1992, Little Brown.

45. Haley RW et al: The efficacy of infection surveillance and control programs in preventing nosocomial infections in U.S. hospitals, *Am J Epidemiol* 121(2):182-205, 1985.

46. Henderson DK: Postexposure chemoprophylaxis for occupational exposure to human immunodeficiency virus type 1: current status and prospects for the future, *Am J Med* 91:(Suppl 3S):312-319, 1991.

47. Henderson DK: Zeroing in on the appropriate management of occupational exposure to HIV-1, *Infect Control Hosp Epidemiol* 11(4):175-177, 1990.

48. Henderson DK et al: The risk for occupatioanl transmission of human immunodeficiency virus type 1 (HIV-1) associated with clinical procedures: a prospective evaluation, *Ann Intern Med* 113:740-746, 1990.

49. Hoeprich PD, Jordan MC: *Infectious diseases: a modern treatise on infectious processes*, ed 4, 1989, JB Lippincott.

50. Holmberg SD et al: Health and economic impacts of antimicrobial resistance, *Rev Infect Dis* 9:1065, 1989.

51. Hughes JM: Hantavirus pulmonary syndrome: an emerging infectious disease, *Science* 262:850-851, 1993.

52. Jacoby GA, Archer GL: New mechanisms of bacterial resistance to antimicrobial agents, *N Engl J Med* 324:601, 1991.

53. James CJ: Personal communication, 1995.

54. Joint Commission on Accreditation of Healthcare Organizations: *Accreditation manual for hospitals*, Chicago, 1995, The Commission.

55. Kollmorgen GM, Bedford JS: Cellular radiation biology. In Dalrymple GV et al, editors: *Medical radiation biology*, Philadelphia, 1973, WB Saunders.

56. Koziol DE, Henderson DK: Risk analysis and occupational exposure to HIV and HBV, *Curr Opin Infect Dis* 6:506-510, 1993.

57. Kubiatowicz DO: *Important safety information (business letter communication)*, St Paul, May 4, 1990, Medical Device Division, 3M Health Care.

58. Lange JMA et al: Failure of zidovudine prophylaxis after accidental exposure to HIV-1, *N Engl J Med* 322:1375-1377, 1990.

59. Lemonick MD: The killers all around, *Time*, pp 183-185, September 12, 1994.

60. Looke DFM, Grove DI: Failed prophylactic zidovudine after needle-stick injury (letter), *Lancet* 335:1280, 1990.

61. Lynch P et al: Rethinking the role of isolation precautions in the prevention of nosocomial infections, *Ann Intern Med* 107:243-248, 1987.

62. Mahy BWJ, Centers for Disease Control and Prevention: *Overview of infectious diseases in the workplace*. Lecture at Baylor University Medical Center, Dallas, February 25, 1994.

63. Muldoon RL, Stanley ED, Jackson GG: Use and withdrawal of amantadine chemoprophylaxis during epidemic influenza A, *Am Rev Respir Dis* 133:487-491, 1976.

64. National Institute for Occupational Safety and Health: TB study funding announcement, *Federal Register* 58:148, 1993.

65. Noble RC: Infectiousness of pulmonary tuberculosis after starting chemotherapy: review of the available data on an unresolved question, *Am J Infect Control* 9:6-10, 1981.

66. Owens DK, Nease RF: Occupational exposure to human immunodeficiency virus and hepatitis B virus: a comparative analysis of risk, *Am J Med* 92:503-512, 1992.

67. Patterson JV, Hierholzer WJ Jr: The hospital epidemiologist. In Bennett JV, Brachman PS, editors: *Hospital infections*, ed 3, Boston, 1992, Little Brown.

68. Polder JA, Tablan OC, Williams WW: Personnel health services. In Bennett JV, Brachman PS, editors: *Hospital infections*, ed 3, Boston, 1992, Little Brown.

69. Rhame FS: The inanimate environment. In Bennett JV: *Hospitals infections*, ed 3, Boston, 1992, Little Brown.

70. Szuness W et al: Hepatitis B vaccine: demonstration of efficacy in a controlled clinical trial in a high risk population in the United States, *N Engl J Med* 303:833-841, 1980.

71. Thomas CL, editor: *Taber's cyclopedic medical dictionary*, ed 1, Philadelphia, 1973, FA Davis.

72. Williams WW, Centers for Disease Control: CDC guidelines for infection control in hospital personnel, *Infect Control* 4(Suppl):326-349, 1983.

CHAPTER

19

Assessment

Shirlee E. Maihoff

Outline

Key terms

Affective
Anemia
Anorexia
Anxiety
Cachexia
Cognitive
Depression
Empathy

Kwashiorkor
Leukopenia
Marasmus
Myelosuppression
Quality of life
Rehabilitation
Thrombocytopenia

ASSESSMENT DEFINED

The assessment of cancer patients and of systems in which they function provides the basis of effective cancer care.[34] The diagnosis of cancer can precipitate significant changes in the lives of the patient and family. These changes can be physiological, psychological, and spiritual. To understand the effect of the cancer diagnosis on a patient, significant other, or family, the diagnosis must be considered a process rather than an event. That process is dynamic and continuous and changes over time.

Information obtained through a continuous, systematic assessment allows the health care provider to (1) determine the nature of a problem, (2) select an intervention for that problem, and (3) evaluate the effectiveness of the intervention. The assessment should be continued as long as interventions are needed and wanted by the patient to facilitate an optimal quality of life. Assessment can be accomplished most effectively through a multidisciplinary approach and requires the efforts of the entire oncology team, including surgical oncologists, medical oncologists, radiation oncologists, oncology nurses, radiation therapists, social workers, dietitians, and pastoral counselors.

The importance of assessment in oncology

The assessment of cancer patients serves as the cornerstone for the structure of care. However, patient assessment is much more than obtaining a patient history. Patients come worried and often in pain. They feel extremely vulnerable and in need of help and understanding. Patients are often desperate to put their cancer problems behind them, receive treatment, and get on with their lives. They come hoping that health care providers will listen carefully and know the correct things to do to help them. Most patients want not only physical and psychological comfort, but also another person to firmly stand alongside them with genuine empathy at this vulnerable time. They want someone to resonate with their distress. All this intense emotion is presented after initial contact with the patient. Most people use their coping skills, but few fully reveal the extent of their feelings. Most adults convey varying degrees of ability to remain in control in an environment that appears strange at best and terrifying at worst.

Establishing a therapeutic relationship

Health professionals must recognize that the patient feels at a distinct disadvantage and must respect, reassure, and support even those who convey an incredible sense of confidence and comfort. At an initial encounter with a patient, acceptance, interest, and genuineness are imperative to establishing a therapeutic and healing relationship, which is critical to the healing process. Verbal and nonverbal communication between the patient and therapist is the basis of an effective therapeutic relationship. The box on the left lists helpful behaviors in working with patients, and the box on the right lists verbal and nonverbal behaviors that are not helpful.

To be effective in assessment, therapists must use communication skills that involve hearing verbal messages, perceiving nonverbal messages, and responding verbally and nonverbally to both kinds of messages.

Some anthropologists believe that more than two thirds of any communication is transmitted nonverbally. Therefore gestures, facial expressions, posture, personal appearance, and cultural characteristics must be interpreted to understand the patient. Nonverbal behavior provides clues to but not conclusive proofs of underlying feelings. However, research has proved that nonverbal cues (Table 19-1) tend to be more reliable than verbal cues.

Simple phrases to respond to negative nonverbal cues include, "You seem to be upset" and "You appear to be unhappy." The box on p. 310 provides an exercise for recognizing nonverbal cues.

Verbal messages are clearer than nonverbal messages. Verbal messages are composed of **cognitive** and **affective** content. Cognitive content comprises the actual facts and words of the message. Affective content may be verbal or nonverbal and comprises feelings, attitudes, and behaviors. The difference in hearing only the obvious cognitive content of a verbal message and hearing the cognitive *and* underlying affective messages is the difference between being an ineffective or effective listener. Affective messages express feelings and emotions. These messages are much more difficult to communicate, hear, and perceive than cognitive messages. Feelings can be grouped into four

---

Helpful Behaviors

Verbal

- Is nonjudgmental
- Uses understandable words
- Reflects and clarifies patient's statements
- Responds to real messages such as doubt and fear
- Summarizes or synthesizes the words of the patient
- Uses verbal reinforcers such as "I see" and "Yes"
- Appropriately gives information
- Uses humor at times to reduce tension

Nonverbal

- Maintains good eye contact
- Touches appropriately
- Nods head occasionally
- Has animated facial expressions
- Smiles occasionally
- Uses occasional hand gestures
- Has moderately calm rate of speech
- Has moderate tone of voice

Nonhelpful Behaviors

Verbal

- Preaches
- Blames
- Placates
- Directs and demands
- Gives advice
- Has patronizing attitude
- Strays from topic
- Talks about self too much
- Overanalyzes or overinterprets
- Intellectualizes
- Uses words patient does not understand
- Probes and questions extensively, especially "why" questions

Nonverbal

- Has poor eye contact
- Frowns
- Has expressionless face
- Has tight mouth
- Yawns
- Shakes pointed finger
- Has unpleasant tone of voice

Table 19-1	Nonverbal cues in a communicative relationship
Cue	**Example**
Eye contact*	Steady or shifty and avoiding
Eyes	Open, teary, closed, and excessively blinking
Body position	Relaxed, leaning (toward or away), and tense
Mouth	Loose, smiling, tight, and lip biting
Facial expression	Animated, painful, bland, and distant
Arms	Unfolded and folded
Body posture	Relaxed, slouching, and rigid
Voice	Slow, whispering, high-pitched, fast, and cracking
General appearance	Clean, neat, well-groomed, and sloppy

*Eye contact may vary in appropriateness based on cultural differences (e.g., Chinese persons do not consider eye contact appropriate with strangers).

Exercise for Nonverbal Cues

What do the following gestures mean to you? When you have completed this exercise, compare your answers with those of your classmates. Do you have different perceptions?

1. A patient refuses to talk and avoids eye contact with you.
2. A patient looks directly into your eyes and stretches her hands out with the palms up.
3. The patient with whom you are talking holds one arm behind her back and clenches her hand tightly while using the other hand to make a fist at her side.
4. A patient walks into the examination room for a radiation therapy consultation with the doctor, sits erect, and clasps his folded arms across his chest before saying a word.
5. A patient sits in the waiting room, slouches in his chair, says nothing, and has tears streaming down his cheeks.

---

major categories: anger, sadness, fear, and happiness. One feeling commonly masks and covers up another. For example, anger may mask fear because fear is at the root of much anger. A cancer patient who appears to be extremely angry may be quite afraid but not able to honestly show fear. The box that is located on p. 311 concerning cognitive and affective responses demonstrates the difference between the two levels of responding to patients.

Identifying underlying feelings in verbal messages is difficult at first and related to a person's comfortableness and proficiency in recognizing and expressing personal feelings. The health care professional must listen to patients' messages and identify their feelings rather than project personal feelings onto patients. This ability requires practice and awareness. Different people identify different underlying feelings for the same statement. Careful attention must be given to nonverbal and verbal cues when listening for the true feelings of patients.

Reflective listening involves responding with empathy. **Empathy** is defined as identifying with the feelings, thoughts, or experiences of another person. To arrive at the way the other person feels, the health care provider may ask inwardly, "If I were in this person's position, how would I feel?" A critical part of empathy is sharing feelings about the person's verbal communication. For example, empathic responses include, "Yes, I understand that . . . . I would feel angry too" and "Yes, I'm glad that . . . . It would make me feel good too."

People rarely communicate in a direct manner concerning the thoughts and feelings that they are having. Reflective listening is a way for a person to listen and communicate effectively. The consequences of good reflective listening are as follows:

- The person becomes aware of small problems and prevents them from developing into major problems.
- The person is perceived by others as concerned, warm, understanding, and fair.
- The person has more knowledge about others, which helps in relating to them in a real way.

Reflective listening is not the only form of verbal response that radiation therapists can use. Reflective listening is essential to developing verbal responses appropriate for the issues involved. Following are ten of the most commonly used and helpful verbal responses:

Minimal verbal response. *Minimal responses* are the verbal counterpart to the occasional head nodding. These are verbal clues such as "Yes," "Uh huh," and "I see" and indicate that the health care provider is listening to and understanding the patient.

Reflecting. *Reflecting* refers to health care providers communicating their understanding of the patient's concerns and perspectives. Health care workers can reflect the specific content or implied feelings of their nonverbal observations or communication they feel has been omitted or emphasized. The following are examples of reflecting: "You're feeling uncomfortable about finishing your treatments," "Sounds as if you're really angry at this disease," and "You really resent being treated like you're sick."

Paraphrasing. A *paraphrase* is a verbal statement that is interchangeable with a patient's statement. The words may be synonyms of words the patient has used. Paraphrasing acknowledges to patients that they are really being heard. The following is an example:

Patient: "I had a really bad night last night."
Therapist: "Things didn't go well for you last night."

Probing. *Probing* is an open-ended statement used to obtain more information. It is most effective when using

Excercise for Cognitive and Affective Responses

1. Patient: My skin is getting really red. I think you're burning me up.
   Cognitive Response: Are you putting that lotion on your skin?
   Affective Response: I hear your discomfort. It sounds like you're uncomfortable with your skin change. These are normal and temporary, and we're watching it every day.

2. Patient: My throat is getting sore. How much more sore is it going to get? I don't want one of those feeding tubes.
   Cognitive Response: Are you drinking acidic stuff, smoking, using your magic mouthwash?
   Affective Response: Sounds like the idea of a feeding tube is really frightening. That's not what happens with sore throats. The worst scenario is if it gets too sore, you'll have a couple days off!

3. Patient: It's only the second day of treatment and I have diarrhea!
   Cognitive Response: Well, what have you eaten?
   Affective Response: It's really kind of early for any diarrhea. What else do you think might be causing the diarrhea? Let's see the doctor and ask what she thinks.

4. Patient: I'm still in so much pain! When does this radiation start to work?
   Cognitive Response: Are you taking your pain medication?
   Affective Response: I'm sorry you're hurting, but everybody is different and sometimes it takes longer to get pain relief.

5. Patient: I sure am having trouble going to sleep. Is that normal?
   Cognitive Response: Well, how long is it taking you to go to sleep?
   Affective Response: Tell me what kinds of things are going through your mind while you're going to sleep.

6. Patient: I have a question and it's probably stupid, but I'm going to ask it anyway.
   Cognitive Response: No questions are stupid.
   Affective Response: I always appreciate patients who ask questions. It helps me know the things that are important to you.

statements such as "I'm wondering about . . .," "Tell me more about that," and "Could you be saying. . ." These statements facilitate much more open conversation than asking how, what, when, where, or who questions.

Clarifying. *Clarifying* is used to obtain more information about vague, ambiguous, or conflicting statements. Examples include the following: "I'm confused about . . .," "I'm having trouble understanding . . .," "Is it that . . .," and "Sounds to me like you're saying . . . ."

Interpreting. *Interpreting* occurs when the therapist adds something to the patient's statement or tries to help the patient understand underlying feelings. Health care providers may share their interpretation, the meaning, or the facts, thus providing the patient with an opportunity to confirm, deny, or offer an alternative interpretation. The patient may respond by saying, "Yes, that's it" or "No, not that but . . . ."

Checking out. *Checking out* occurs when therapists are genuinely confused about their perceptions of the patient's verbal or nonverbal behavior or have a hunch that should be examined. Examples are, "Does it seem as if . . ." and "I have a hunch that this feeling is familiar to you, are you saying . . . ." Therapists ask the patient to confirm or correct their perception or understanding of the patient's words.

Informing. *Informing* occurs when the therapist shares objective and factual information. An example is, "Your white blood cell count is extremely low, so it would be safer for you to avoid large crowds where the chances are higher of being exposed to bacteria and viruses."

Confronting. *Confronting* involves therapists making the client aware that their observations are not consistent with the patient's words. This response needs to be done with respect for the patient and extreme tact so that a defensive response is not elicited. An example of this is, "You say you're angry and depressed, yet you're smiling."

Summarizing. By *summarizing* the therapist condenses and puts in order the information communicated. This is extremely helpful when a patient rambles and has difficulty conveying the sequence of events. An example is, "I hear you saying . . . "

The box at the top of p. 312 is to help the individual to learn to recognize and identify the types of major verbal responses just discussed. The other box on p. 312 helps the individual to listen for feelings.

THE MULTIDISCIPLINARY APPROACH TO THE ASSESSMENT OF CANCER PATIENTS
General health assessment

One method of health assessment is the self-report. In a self-report, individuals disclose their perception of what is being measured. The box on p. 313 demonstrates a self-assessment tool that is useful in decreasing documentation time by the oncology professional while eliciting comprehensive information.

An alternative assessment method is for the oncology practitioner to do an interview. This often is done by the oncology nurse or radiation oncologist, but a radiation therapist may also conduct the interview. The history includes

Exercise for Recognizing and Identifying the Types of Major Verbal Responses

Read the following patient and therapist statements, and identify the therapist's response in each case as one of the 10 major verbal responses: minimal verbal response, paraphrasing, probing, reflecting, clarifying, checking out, interpreting, confronting, informing, or summarizing.*

1. Patient: I can't decide what to do. Nothing seems right.
   Caregiver: You're feeling pretty frustrated, and you want me to tell you what to do.
2. Patient: In our family the children don't do any of the work around the house.
   Caregiver: The children in your family don't do any housework.
3. Patient: My wife made me late for treatment today.
   Caregiver: Tell me more about that.
4. Patient: Do you think this is a good cancer center?
   Caregiver: The XYZ Association has ranked this cancer center number one in the state.
5. Patient: I guess that about covers it.
   Caregiver: Let's see if we can review what we've talked about today . . . . Does this seem right to you?
6. Patient: That's why I'm here. Dr. Jones said you were a good one to talk to.
   Caregiver: Let's see now. You want me to help you decide whether or not you should file for disability. Is that right?
7. Patient: Nobody in this world cares about anyone else.
   Caregiver: It's scary to feel that nobody at all cares about you.
8. Patient: Anyway, I'm unable to do it because it's too expensive. Besides, they won't help me anyway.
   Caregiver: Let me get this straight. You feel the tests will cost too much, and the results won't be worth the cost. Is that it?
9. Patient: I don't want to talk about it.
   Caregiver: You've told me that being open and honest about your illness is important to you, but you aren't willing to do that just now.
10. Patient: I have to go to the grocery store before picking up the children on the way home from my treatment.
    Caregiver: Oh, I see . . .

*See Appendix B for the answers to this exercise.

Exercise for Listening for Feelings

For each of the following statements, write what you think the person is really feeling. Ask yourself, "What are the underlying feelings here?"*

1. The doctor told me to come over here and have all these tests. I'll sit over here and wait until you're ready for me.
2. Have you heard anything about the new social worker? I'm supposed to see her at 3 PM.
3. Coming for treatment just doesn't seem to be helping me.
4. Are you going to see me again this week, Doctor?
5. Only 2 more weeks and I'm finished with my treatments.

*Discuss your answers with a small group in your class. Then look at all the possible answers in Appendix B.

the collection of data about the past and present health of each patient. A historical and physical evaluation should come from a referring physician, but a verification and current assessment should also be done.

Physical assessment

Table 19-2 lists physical aspects a therapist is responsible to assess daily and interventions for treatment. Some assessments are relative to the area being treated with radiation therapy. Specific areas in the physical realm in which assessment of the cancer patient is paramount include nutrition, pain, and biochemical balance (blood counts).

Nutritional assessment

Nutritional assessment involves the multidisciplinary oncology team. Oncology nurses are in an ideal position for the initial assessment of cancer patients and referrals to the nutrition specialist, or dietitian. In addition, therapists' awareness and knowledge in this area enable them to monitor patients under treatment and make appropriate referrals when needed.

Maintaining a good nutritional status is one of the most difficult challenges in treating cancer patients. Nutritional assessment is the critical first step in developing a comprehensive approach to the nutritional management of individuals with cancer. A complete list of components involved in nutritional assessment is outlined in the box that is located on p. 315.

After malnutrition is diagnosed, a plan of intervention is developed and implemented based on the information obtained in the nutritional assessment.

Weight loss is often the first physical change that alerts individuals with cancer to seek medical treatment. It is also frequently the first sign of malnutrition.

Specifically, the percent weight change is the most accurate measure of nutritional status. The percent weight change indicates the extent of tissue loss as a result of inadequate nutrition. For this reason, monitoring weight change weekly is imperative for patients who are undergoing radition therapy. A calculation of a percent weight change is found in Table 19-3.

Functional Health Pattern Patient Self-Assessment*

Health perception and health management

- Who provides your health and dental care?
- How often do you see your doctor and dentist?
- List the medication(s) you take. How much? How often?
- How much alcohol do you drink in a week?
- Do you smoke cigarettes and cigars? If so, how much?
- What allergies do you have? What happens when you have an allergic reaction?
- What other medical problems do you have?

Nutritional metabolic pattern

- Are you on any special diet?
- What did you eat yesterday (over the last 24 hours)?
- How much fluid do you drink each day?
- List the vitamins you take each day.
- Have you noticed any changes in your appetite? If yes, describe.
- Have you noticed any changes in your weight? If yes, describe.
- What foods do you avoid?
- Who cooks your meals?
- Do you wear dentures or partial plates?
- How do you take care of your skin? (What creams, lotions, or powders are you using?)
- Do you take baths or showers? How often?

Elimination pattern

- How often do you move your bowels?
- Do you have problems with diarrhea, constipation, or loss of control?
- What foods and medications do you use to regulate your bowels (laxatives, prunes, bran, and others)?
- How many times a day do you urinate?
- Have you had any changes such as loss of control, burning, frequency, or difficulty urinating?

Activity and exercise pattern

- Do you feel tired during the day? Is this new?
- What changes have you noticed in your energy level?
- What exercises do you do? How often?
- What do you do for relaxation and fun?
- Do you need help with ambulating, bathing, toileting, dressing, grooming, feeding, cooking, food shopping, housecleaning, or food preparation?

Sleep and rest pattern

- What time do you go to bed?
- What time do you get up?
- Do you have any problems sleeping?
- How do you feel when you wake up?
- Do you take any medications to help you sleep?

Cognitive and perceptual pattern

- Are you having problems hearing?
- Have you noticed any recent changes in your hearing?
- Do you use any hearing aids?
- Have you noticed any changes in your vision?
- How often do you have your eyes examined?
- Do you wear glasses or contact lenses?
- Are you experiencing any pain? If yes, where is the pain located? Describe it.
- What do you do to manage your pain?
- How does the pain affect your lifestyle?
- What is your occupation?

Roles and relationships pattern

- What is your marital status?
- Do you have children and grandchildren?
- With whom do you live?
- What changes in you family roles or relationships have you noticed since your illness?
- How do you anticipate that the radiation treatment will affect your daily routine?
- What is the best time for your radiation treatment?

Self-perception and conceptual pattern

- How would you describe yourself?
- What are your strengths and weaknesses?

Sexual and reproductive pattern

- Are you sexually active?
- Do you use any form of birth control?
- Have you had any changes in sexual relations?

Coping and stress-management pattern

- How do you handle major problems and stresses in your life?
- How are you coping with your life and diagnosis?
- What do you do to relax?
- What are your concerns regarding your treatment?

Value and belief pattern

- What is important in your life?
- Describe your spiritual needs.
- What part does religion play in your lifestyle?

Life and lifestyle patterns

- Describe your usual day.
- What means of transportation do you have?

Modified from Hirshfield-Bartek J, Dow KH, Creaton E: Decreasing documentation time using a patient self-assessment tool, *Oncol Nurs Forum* 17:251-255, 1990. Courtesy Beth Israel Hospital, Boston, Massachusetts.

*In the actual form, space is provided for patients' responses.

Table 19-2	Components of daily physical assessment

Side effects	Interventions
Skin reactions Erythema (3000-4000) cGy Dry and moist desquamation (4500-6000 cGy)	Instruct the patient to do the following: • Assess and monitor skin integrity and changes. • Use a moisturizing lotion after showering, and avoid port marks. • Avoid creams that contain alcohol. • Avoid exposing the treated area to heat, cold, wind, soaps, deodorant, and razor shaving. If skin erythema occurs, do the following: • Use moisturizing lotion according to the physician's orders. • Protect skin from further irritation, and wear loose cotton clothes. If skin breakdown occurs, do the following: • If dry desquamation has occurred, continue to use moisturizing lotion. • If the skin is tender, use cortisone cream as directed. • For moist desquamation, use Burrow's compresses and silver sulfadiazine creams per the physician's prescription. (The physician may consider temporarily stopping further treatment.) Try to aerate areas of skin breakdown, especially in skin folds.
Fatigue	Assess the energy level. Determine periods of increased fatigue. Assist patients to pace activities and listen to their bodies. Ensure adequate nutritional intake.
Sleep	Assess normal sleep patterns and changes. Evaluate the cause of problems.
Mouth changes (3000-4000 cGy)	Inspect the oral cavity. Assess the presence of stomatitis, xerostomia, mucositis, and taste changes. Instruct the patient about a soft, bland diet.
Diarrhea (2000-5000 cGy)	Assess the bowel function. Instruct the patient on a low-residue diet for use as diarrhea occurs. Use antidiarrheal medications as prescribed. Instruct the patient on perianal care.
Cystitis (>3000 cGy)	Assess the bladder function. Monitor for urinary retention or hematuria. Use antispasmodic medications as prescribed. Monitor for bladder infections.
Nausea and vomiting (1000-3000 cGy)	Anticipate nausea and vomiting in high-risk patients, and prevent nausea and vomiting by using antiemetics prophylactically before treatment and as needed continuously. Provide fluids to prevent dehydration. Refer or instruct the patient on a low-fat and low-sugar diet. Use nonpharmacological measures such as relaxation and guided imagery.
Pharyngitis and esophagitis (2000 cGy)	Assess pain during swallowing (dysphagia). Modify the diet to soft, nonspicy, and nonacidic foods. Use topical anesthetics and analgesics as prescribed (lidocaine mixed with Mylanta or Maalox [1:3]).
Alopecia (2000 cGy)	Protect the scalp from heat, cold, and wind. Suggest an appropriate head covering. Do the following to minimize scalp irritation: • Avoid frequent shampooing. • Avoid using blow dryers, hairsprays, gels, or other hair preparations. • Apply moisturizing lotion to the scalp. Explore issues related to body image (e.g., getting a wig or hairpiece at the start of treatment).
Pain	Assess the location and intensity. Instruct the patient on the importance of taking medications regularly.
Skin pallor	Monitor low hemoglobin, white blood cell, and platelet levels with weekly complete blood counts (CBCs).
Weight loss	Monitor once per week, and chart the results. Determine eating problems.

cGy, Centigray.

Components of the Nutritional Assessment

Medical history

- Duration and type of malignancy
- Frequency, type, and severity of complications (e.g., infections and draining lesions)
- Type and duration of therapy
- Specific chemotherapeutic agents used
- Radiation sites
- Antibiotics used
- Other drugs used
- Surgical procedures performed (site, type, and date)
- Side effects of therapy (diarrhea, anorexia, nausea, and vomiting)
- Concomitant medical conditions (diabetes, heart disease, liver failure, kidney failure, and infection)

Physical examination

- General appearance
- Condition of hair
- Condition of skin
- Condition of teeth
- Condition of mouth, gums, and throat
- Edema
- Performance status
- Identification of nutritionally related problems (fistula, pain, stomatitis, xerostomia, infection, constipation diarrhea, nausea, vomiting, and obstruction)

Dietary history

- 24-hour recall of foods eaten, including snacks
- Composition of food taken in 24 hours (calories and protein, caffeine, and liquor)
- Income
- Time of day meals and snacks eaten
- Past or current diet modifications
- Self-feeding ability
- Special cancer diet
- Vitamins, minerals, or other supplements
- Modifications of diet or eating habits as a result of treatment or illness
- Foods withheld or given on the basis of personal or religious grounds (e.g., kosher, vegetarian)
- Food preferences
- Food allergies or intolerances

Socioeconomic history

- Number of persons living in the home (ages and relationships)
- Kitchen facilities
- Income
- Food purchased
- Food prepared
- Amount spent on food per month
- Outside provision of meals

Anthropometric data

- Height
- Weight
- Actual weight as percentage of ideal
- Weight change as percentage of usual
- Triceps skinfold measurement
- Actual triceps skinfold as percentage of standard
- Midarm circumference
- Midarm muscle circumference
- Actual midarm muscle circumference as percentage of standard

Biochemical data

- Hematocrit
- Hemoglobin
- Serum albumin
- Serum transferrin
- Creatinine
- Creatinine height index
- Total lymphocyte count
- Delayed hypersensitivity response-skin testing
- Nitrogen balance
- Blood urea nitrogen
- Sodium, potassium, carbon dioxide, chloride
- Glucose

Modified from Groenwald SL et al: *Nutritional disturbances: cancer nursing principles and practice,* ed 3, Boston, 1993, Jones & Bartlett.

Nutritional consequences of cancer

Anorexia (loss of appetite resulting in weight loss) is a major contributor in the cause of cancer cachexia. **Cachexia** is a state of general ill health and malnutrition with early satiety; electrolyte and water imbalances; and progressive loss of body weight, fat, and muscle. Cachexia affects half to two thirds of patients with cancer.

Anorexia and taste alterations are two of the major causes of protein-calorie malnutrition in patients with cancer. The three forms of protein-calorie malnutrition are marasmus, kwashiorkor, and marasmus-kwashiorkor mix.

Marasmus, or *calorie* malnutrition, can be observed in patients who are slender or slightly underweight. It is characterized by weight loss of 7% to 10% and fat and muscle depletion. **Kwashiorkor,** or *protein* malnutrition, has an adequate intake of carbohydrates and fats but an inadequate intake of protein. Kwashiorkor in patients is often initially overlooked because they appear well nourished. This condition is characterized by retarded growth and development, muscle wasting, depigmentation of the hair and skin, edema, and depression of the cellular immune response. Marasmus-kwashiorkor mix, or protein and calorie malnutrition, is the

Table 19-3	Evaluation of weight change*	
Time	**Significant weight loss**	**Severe weight loss**
1 wk	1%-2%	> 2%
1 mo	5%	> 5%
3 mo	7.5%	> 7.5%
6 mo	10%	> 10%

From Blackburn GL et al: Nutritional and metabolic assessment of the hospitalized patient, *J Parent Ent Nutr* 1:17, 1977.
*Values charged are for percent weight change.

$$\text{Percent weight change} = \frac{\text{Usual weight} - \text{Actual weight}}{\text{Usual weight}} \times 100$$

most life-threatening form of malnutrition because it involves the depletion of fat and muscle stores and visceral protein stores. This condition is most commonly found in seriously ill, hospitalized patients who have had inadequate nutritional care throughout their illness. Marasmus-kwashiorkor mix is characterized by weight loss of 10% or greater in a 6-month period, decreased fat and muscle stores, depleted visceral protein stores, and depression of the cellular immune responses.

Pain assessment

Pain, one of the most feared consequences of cancer, is a complex process that has biological, social, and spiritual dimensions. All pain is real, regardless of its cause, and most pain is a combination of physiological and psychogenic factors. This phenomenon is connected to the essence of human existence and often precipitates questions about the meaning of life itself. Pain holds a great deal of power with the cancer patient experiencing it.

A multidimensional conceptualization of cancer pain as defined by Ahles, Blanchard, and Ruckdeschel[1] aids in understanding the scope of cancer pain. They propose five dimensions to consider in assessing and managing the experience of cancer pain: (1) physiological (organic etiology of pain), (2) sensory (intensity, location, and quality), (3) affective (depression and anxiety), (4) cognitive (the manner in which pain influences a person's thought processes and the way people view themselves or the meaning of pain), and (5) behavioral (pain-related behaviors such as medication intake and activity level).

McGuire[18] proposes a sixth dimension: sociocultural. This dimension involves the effects of cultural, social, and demographic factors that are related to the experience of pain.

Physiological dimension. Foley[10] described three types of pain (each with a different etiology) observed in cancer patients: (1) pain associated with direct tumor involvement, (2) pain associated with cancer therapy, and (3) pain unrelated to the tumor or its treatment.

Two important characteristics of pain are related to the etiology of pain: the duration and pattern of pain. *Duration* refers to whether pain is acute or chronic. *Acute pain* generally is a sudden onset with an identifiable cause lasting 3 to 6 months and responds to treatment with analgesic drug therapy and treatment of its precipitating cause. *Chronic pain* is the persistence of pain for more than 3 months with a less well-defined onset. Its cause may not be known. The second characteristic related to the etiology of pain (the pattern of pain) has three separate patterns: (1) brief, momentary, or transient; (2) rhythmic, periodic, or intermittent; and (3) continuous, steady, or constant. Melzack[20] first described these patterns in the McGill Pain Questionnaire (MPQ).

Sensory dimension. The second dimension (sensory) as set forth by Ahles, Blanchard, and Ruckdeschel[1] consists of pain location, intensity, and quality. The first component of establishing the location of pain is extremely important. One of the methods that can be used is to ask the patient to point with one finger to the site of the pain. Another method is to use a picture of the body and ask the patient to mark on the picture the location of the pain.

The second component is the intensity of the pain (i.e., the strength of its feeling). Intensity is the most commonly assessed aspect of pain. The goal is to translate the patient's description of intensity into numbers or words to provide an objective description. Visual analogue scales (VASs) and categorical scales are commonly used to quantify the intensity of pain. A VAS rates 0 (no pain) to 10 (severe pain). A categorical scale also has a numerical system with 0 (no pain), 1 (mild), 2 (discomforting), 3 (distressing), 4 (horrible), and 5 (excruciating). Descriptions of the pain may be helpful in determining its origin and implementing effective measures for its control. For example, burning, hot pain may indicate the involvement of nerve tissue. This type of pain does not do well with narcotic analgesics.

The third component of the sensory dimension is the quality of pain (i.e., the way it actually feels). In the MPQ, some of the most common terms used to describe the quality of pain are as follows: aching, hot-burning, sharp, tender, throbbing, cramping, stabbing, heavy, shooting and gnawing, splitting, tiring-exhausting, sickening, and fearful.

Affective dimension. The third dimension (affective) as defined by Ahles, Blanchard, and Ruckdeschel[1] consists of depression, anxiety, and other psychological factors or personality traits associated with pain. Anxiety and depression are critical factors that affect a patient's response to pain and ability to tolerate and cope with pain because anxiety often increases pain. Assessing which measure can be taken to decrease the pain is essential.

Cognitive dimension. The fourth dimension (cognitive) involves the way pain influences thought processes or the way persons view themselves. A patient can be asked, "Are

Table 19-4	Karnofsky Performance Status

Score (%)	Status
100	Normal—no complaints and no evidence of disease
90	Ability to carry on normal activity—minor signs or symptoms of disease
80	Normal activity with effort—some signs or symptoms of disease
70	Self-care—inability to carry on normal activity or do active work
60	Occasional assistance required but ability to care for most needs
50	Considerable assistance and frequent medical care required
40	Disability—special care and assistance required
30	Severe disability—hospitalization indicated, although death not imminent
20	Extreme sickness—hospitalization and active supportive treatment necessary
10	Moribund status—fatal processes progressing rapidly
0	Death

Modified from Yates JW, Chalmer B, McKegney FP: Evaluation of patients with advanced cancer using the Karnofsky Performance Status, *CA Cancer J Clin* 45:2220-2224, 1980.

Evaluating the Cancer Patient's Pain

- Believe the patient's complaint of pain.
- Take a careful history of the patient's pain complaint.
- Evaluate the patient's psychological state.
- Perform a careful medical and neurological examination.
- Order and review appropriate diagnostic studies.
- Treat the pain to facilitate the appropriate work-up.
- Reassess the patient's response to therapy.
- Individualize the diagnostic and therapeutic approaches.
- Discuss advance directives with the patient and family.

there any thoughts or images that may make your pain worse?" Some patients experience pain based on faulty logic. The following are examples of problem thinking by patients: "Nothing can be done to control the pain," "Pain is inevitable and should be tolerated," and "Doctors do not want to be bothered with complaints of pain." If undetected, these thoughts impair the assessment and management of pain.

Behavioral dimension. The fifth dimension (behavioral) includes a variety of observable behaviors related to pain. The assessment of pain behavior can include verbal and nonverbal responses such as moans, grimaces, and complaints. Estimates of physical activity are also important aspects of pain behavior. Factors such as physical exercise, time spent in bed, and ability to do chores have been used to measure pain behavior. An excellent tool for this is the Karnofsky Performance Status[35] (Table 19-4).

The use of analgesics and drugs should also be considered in the assessment of pain behavior. The type and amount of drug and the way the dose is scheduled is important. Patients are often afraid of narcotic pain medications and take them only after they are in pain. Therapists should encourage regular dosage and explain the importance of a stable blood-serum level, which is needed to interrupt the pain cycle. The duration of the effect of the drug and any mood change on administration should be noted.

Sociocultural dimension. The last dimension (proposed by McGuire[18] and added to Ahles, Blanchard, and Ruckdeschel's five dimensions[1]) consists of a variety of eth-

nic, cultural, demographical, spiritual, and related factors that influence a person's perception of and response to pain. Cultural and religious practices have a strong influence on the pain experience. Overt actions are accepted in some cultures, whereas other cultures consider such actions weak. A general value held by many Americans is that a good patient does not complain when in pain; a complainer has lost self-control. Unfortunately, health care professionals sometimes directly reinforce these beliefs.

Age, gender, and race may provide different pain experiences. Research shows that females and older individuals have increased verbal expressions of pain.

In considering the six dimensions of cancer pain, a holistic and multidisciplinary approach to assessment and management is essential. As stated, many factors contribute to the pain experience.

The multidimensional concept of cancer pain necessitates the involvement of various health care disciplines in assessment and management. Input is needed from many health caregivers, including oncologists, primary physicians, nurses, radiation therapists, social workers, pharmacists, psychologists, anesthesiologists, and occupational therapists.

Pain assessment has several purposes. First, it establishes a baseline for treatment and interventions. Second, it helps focus which interventions are best for the patient. Third, it enables the evaluation of chosen interventions. Pain assessment should be systematic, organized, and ongoing. In general, certain principles should be followed in evaluating the cancer patient who experiences pain (see the box above).

Tools to assess pain must be simple, short, and relevant for the patient. Pain-assessment tools can be classified according to the number of pain dimensions they assess. Multidimensional tools focus on two or more dimensions of the pain experience. Probably the most well-known and best example is the MPQ.[20]

The MPQ has the ability to assess in the sensory, cognitive, affective, and behavioral dimensions. Specifically, the MPQ elicits information about the location of pain; the intensity and periodicity of the pain; symptoms; effects on sleep,

INITIAL PAIN ASSESSMENT TOOL

Patient's Name _____

Diagnosis _____

Date _____

Age _____ Room _____

Physician _____

Therapist/Nurse _____

Location The patient or therapist marks the drawing.

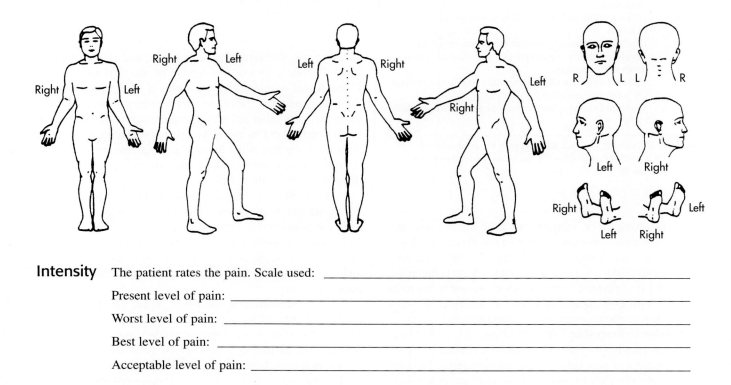

Intensity The patient rates the pain. Scale used: _____

Present level of pain: _____

Worst level of pain: _____

Best level of pain: _____

Acceptable level of pain: _____

activity, and eating; and patterns of the analgesic used. Two long forms and a short form are used.

A similar multidimensional tool is the Brief Pain Inventory (BPI).[5] The BPI was developed primarily for clinical use with patients in pain who were too ill to be subjected to long and exhausting assessment techniques. The BPI assesses the following dimensions: the history and site of pain; the intensity of pain at its worst, as its usual level, and at its present level; medications and treatments used to relieve the pain; the relief obtained; and the effect of pain on mood, interpersonal relations, walking, sleeping, working, and enjoyment of life. The BPI is a self-administered tool.

A third tool is the Memorial Pain Assessment Card (MPAC).[9] The MPAC consists of three visual analog scales. It is a short, easy-to-administer tool that measures pain inten-

sity, pain relief, and mood by choosing from a list of adjectives describing each. It can distinguish pain from psychological distress and can be used to study the subtle interaction of these factors.

A sample questionnaire for an initial pain assessment is shown above and on p. 319.

Radiation therapists are vital in the ongoing assessment of a patient's pain. Therapists see patients every day and can evaluate the level of pain and the way the patient is responding. Being aware of personal beliefs and biases about pain, learning how to listen and communicate, and asking key questions are imperative skills for holistic health caregivers.

Accurate assessment of pain is the first step toward understanding the experience as the patient perceives it. Good assessment promotes an essential therapeutic relationship

INITIAL PAIN ASSESSMENT TOOL—cont'd

Patient's Name _____

Diagnosis _____

Quality Use the patient's own words (e.g.," prick," "ache," "burn," "throb," "pull," "sharp")

_____

Onset, Duration, Variation, and Rhythms _____

Manner of Expressing Pain _____

What Relieves the Pain? _____

What Causes or Increases the Pain? _____

Effects of Pain (Note the decreased function and decreased quality of life)

Accompanying symptoms (e.g., nausea): _____

Sleep: _____

Appetite: _____

Physical activity: _____

Relationship with others (e.g., irritability): _____

Emotions (e.g., angry, suicidal, and crying): _____

Concentration: _____

Other: _____

Other Comments _____

Plan _____

Modified from McCaffery M, Beebe A: *Pain: clinical manual for nursing practice,* St Louis, 1989, Mosby.

between patient and caregiver. Assessment is the foundation in the process of finding an effective intervention for the devastating experience of pain for the cancer patient.

Blood

Hematological changes in cancer patients are critical for ongoing assessments because hematopoietic tissue exhibits a rapid rate of cellular proliferation. Hematopoietic tissue is especially vulnerable to cancer treatments (chemotherapy and radiation therapy). A **myelosuppression,** a reduction in bone marrow function, often results. The changes that may occur can result in anemia, leukopenia, and thrombocytopenia.

Anemia is a decrease in the peripheral red blood cell count. Without sufficient red blood cells, the circulatory system's oxygen-carrying capacity is impaired. This is due to a decrease in the hemoglobin level in the red blood cell, which serves as the carrier of oxygen from the lungs to tissues. Patients usually experience pale skin, muscle weakness, and fatigue (probably the most pervasive symptom). Normal blood values are found in Table 19-5.

Leukopenia is a decrease in the white blood cell count, thus increasing the risk of infection for the cancer patient. Because of chemotherapy or the disease process itself, patients may already have compromised immune systems. Therefore monitoring the white blood cell count during treatments is essential. (Normal values can be found in Table 19-5.) Because of patients' inability to fight disease, they need to reduce their exposure risks. Patients should be told to have minimal contact with others, especially if someone is sick. Health care workers also need to keep a distance if sick and at work.

Thrombocytopenia is a reduction in the number of circulating platelets. This decrease may be caused by a failure of the bone marrow to produce megakaryocyte cells, the precursors of platelets. This can be a result of various factors, such as chemotherapy, radiation therapy, the disease, or stress. The most significant factor that determines the risk of bone marrow depression related to radiation therapy is the volume of productive bone marrow in the radiation field. Therefore with large fields, monitoring counts is extremely important. Normal values for platelets can be found in Table 19-5.

Psychosocial assessment

Quality of life. A growing attention to the quality of life of cancer patients reflects the changing attitude of society and health care personnel. The value of cancer treatments is judged not only on survival, but also on the quality of that survival. The term **quality of life** has emerged in recent years to summarize the broad-based assessment of the combined affect of disease and treatment and the tradeoff between the two.

Cancer and its treatment, perhaps more than any other medical condition, becomes a major determinant of a patient's quality of life. The suggestion has been made in the literature that the emotional repercussions of cancer far exceed those of any other disease, and the emotional suffering cancer generates may actually exceed the physical suffering it causes. Therefore good quality-of-life information can make a major contribution in improving the management of cancer patients.

A more general definition of *quality of life* is a person's subjective sense of well-being derived from personal experience of life as a whole. The areas of life, or domains, most important to individuals resultantly have the most influence on their quality of life.

General agreement exists that the domains of quality of life for assessment should include physical, psychological, and social factors. In the physical domain the quality of life is affected by loss of function, symptoms, and limited activity as a result of the disease process and physical effects of treatments. In the psychological domain, five major emotional themes have been identified: (1) fear and anxiety generated by the diagnosis and compounded by inadequate communication with caregivers, (2) loss of personal control associated with the need to be dependent on those administering treatment, (3) uncertainty about the outcome of treatments, (4) the physician's persistent enthusiasm for cure, and (5) the debilitating effect of standard cancer treatments. In addition, loss of self-esteem and feelings of anxiety, depression, resentment, anger, discouragement, helplessness, hopelessness, isolation, and rejection are common.

Assessment. Many measures are available to assess quality of life, or health-related quality of life. This is, however, a double-edged sword. Those doing the assessing have choices and can choose tools based on specific characteristics of a particular disease site. However, this divides poten-

Table 19-5	Normal blood values*	
Level	**Percentage (range)**	
Hematocrit (Hct)		
Men	45 (38-54)	
Women	40 (36-47)	
Hemoglobin (Hgb)†		
Men	14-18 g/dl	
Women	12-16 g/dl	
Children	12-14 g/dl	

Blood counts	**Per cubic millimeter**	**Percentage**
Erythrocytes (RBCs)		
Men	5 (4.5-6) × 10	100
Women	4.5 (4.3-5.5) × 10	100
Reticulocytes		0-1
Total leukocytes (WBCs)	5000-10,000	100
Polymorphonuclear leukocytes‡	2500-6000	40-60
Bands	0-500	0-5
Lymphocytes	1000-4000	20-40
Eosinophils	50-300	1-3
Basophils	0-100	0-1
Monocytes	200-800	4-8
Platelets	200,000-500,000 (severely low < 20,000)	100

* Values may vary slightly according to the laboratory methods used.
† Severely low < 7.5 g/dl.
‡ Granulocytes, segmented neutrophils, and polymorphonuclear cells.
RBCs, Red blood cells.
WBCs, White blood cells.

tial data and makes comparisons of studies and research much more difficult. Following are some of the assessment tools* available to examine quality of life:

Quality of Life Index. The Quality of Life Index (QLI)[25] focuses on the present (within the last week) quality of a person's life. It clusters 14 items in 3 groups: general physical condition, normal human quality, and general attitudes as they relate to general quality of life. The patient responds by placing an X on a linear slide. The QLI can be found below.

Normal refers to the normal status before illness. The QLI is easy to use and practical. It has reliability and validity in its statistical components.

Functional Living Index—Cancer. The Functional Living Index—Cancer (FLIC)[29] is a 22-item scale on which patients indicate the affect of cancer on day-to-day living issues that assess the functional quality of life. It uses a seven-point Likert-type scale. This scale is often used in measuring attitudes and in the following ranges: strongly agree, agree, slightly agree, undecided, slightly disagree, disagree, and strongly disagree. This tool has been used extensively in oncology with predominantly positive results.

Functional Assessment of Cancer Therapy Scales. The Functional Assessment of Cancer Therapy (FACT) Scale[4] has 28 items and specifies subscales that reflect symptoms or problems associated with different diseases (head and neck, breast, bladder, colorectal, and lung cancers). The results yield information on the patient's well-being, social and family well-being, relationship with the physician, emotional well-being, and specific disease concerns. A form of this tool, called the *FACT–G,* can be found on pp. 322 and 323. This tool can also distinguish stages, metastatic from nonmetastatic diseases, and inpatients from outpatients.

*These tools are several of the cancer-specific, health-related, quality-of-life measures and approaches that are yielding good results.

QUALITY OF LIFE INDEX

With respect to your general physical condition, please place an X on the line at the point that best shows what is happening to you at the present time (within the past week):

General Physical Condition

1. How much *pain* are you feeling?	None	_____	Excruciating
2. How much *nausea* do you experience?	None	_____	Constant nausea
3. How frequently do you *vomit?*	Not at all	_____	Constant vomiting or retching
4. How much *strength* do you feel?	None	_____	Normal for me
5. How much *appetite do* you have?	None	_____	Normal for me

Important Human Activities

6. Are you able to *work* at your usual tasks (e.g., housework, office work, and gardening)?	Not at all	_____	Normal for me
7. Are you able to *eat*?	Not at all	_____	Normal for me
8. Are you able to obtain *sexual* satisfaction?	Not at all	_____	Normal for me
9. Are you able to *sleep* well?	Not at all	_____	Normal for me

General Quality of Life

10. How good is your quality of life (general QL)?	Extremely poor	_____	Excellent
11. Are you having *fun* (e.g., hobbies, recreation, and social activities)?	Not at all	_____	Normal for me
12. Is your life *satisfying*?	Not at all	_____	Normal for me
13. Do you feel *useful*?	Not at all	_____	Normal for me
14. Do you *worry about the cost* of medical care?	Not at all	_____	A great deal

Modified from Padilla GV et al: Quality of Life Index for patients with cancer, *Res Nurs Health* 6:117-126, 1983.

THE FACT–G SCALE

Fact–G (version 2)

Patient's Name _____

Diagnosis _____

Following is a list of statements that other people with your illness have said are important. By circling one number per line, please indicate how true each statement has been for you during the past 7 days.

	Not at all	A little bit	Some- what	Quite a bit	Very much

Physical Well-Being

	Not at all	A little bit	Some- what	Quite a bit	Very much
1. I have a lack of energy.	0	1	2	3	4
2. I have nausea.	0	1	2	3	4
3. I have trouble meeting the needs of my family.	0	1	2	3	4
4. I have pain.	0	1	2	3	4
5. I am bothered by side effects of treatment.	0	1	2	3	4
6. In general, I feel sick.	0	1	2	3	4
7. I am forced to spend time in bed.	0	1	2	3	4

8. How much does your physical well-being affect your quality of life?

Not at all 0 1 2 3 4 5 6 7 8 9 10 Very much

Social and Family Well-Being

	Not at all	A little bit	Some- what	Quite a bit	Very much
9. I feel distant from my friends.	0	1	2	3	4
10. I get emotional support from my family.	0	1	2	3	4
11. I get support from my friends and neighbors.	0	1	2	3	4
12. My family has accepted my illness.	0	1	2	3	4
13. Family communication about my illness is poor.	0	1	2	3	4

(If you answer "0," have a spouse/partner, or are sexually active, please answer questions 14 and 15. Otherwise, go to question 16.)

14. I feel close to my partner (or main support).	0	1	2	3	4
15. I am satisfied with my sex life.	0	1	2	3	4

16. How much does your social and family well-being affect your quality of life?

Not at all 0 1 2 3 4 5 6 7 8 9 10 Very much

Relationship With the Doctor

	Not at all	A little bit	Some- what	Quite a bit	Very much
17. I have confidence in my doctor(s).	0	1	2	3	4
18. My doctor is available to answer my questions.	0	1	2	3	4

19. How much does your relationship with the doctor affect your quality of life?

Not at all 0 1 2 3 4 5 6 7 8 9 10 Very much

THE FACT–G SCALE—cont'd

Fact–G (version 2)

Patient's Name _____

Diagnosis _____

	Not at all	A little bit	Some-what	Quite a bit	Very much
Emotional Well-Being					
20. I feel sad.	0	1	2	3	4
21. I am proud of the way I am coping with my illness.	0	1	2	3	4
22. I am losing hope in the fight against my disease	0	1	2	3	4
23. I feel nervous.	0	1	2	3	4
24. I worry about dying.	0	1	2	3	4

25. How much does your emotional well-being affect your quality of life?

        Not at all   0   1   2   3   4   5   6   7   8   9   10   Very much

	Not at all	A little bit	Some-what	Quite a bit	Very much
Functional Well-Being					
26. I am able to work (include work at home).	0	1	2	3	4
27. My work is fulfilling (include work at home).	0	1	2	3	4
28. I am able to enjoy life in the moment.	0	1	2	3	4
29. I have accepted my illness.	0	1	2	3	4
30. I am sleeping well.	0	1	2	3	4
31. I am enjoying my usual leisure pursuits.	0	1	2	3	4
32. I am content with the quality of my life right now.	0	1	2	3	4

33. How much does your functional well-being affect your quality of life?

        Not at all   0   1   2   3   4   5   6   7   8   9   10   Very much

Modified from Cella DF et al: The Functional Assessment of Cancer Therapy Scale: development and validation of the general measure, *J Clin Oncol* 11(3):570-579, 1993.

Coping strategies and responses—the patient. Over the past several decades a great deal of interest has been focused on assessing an individual's psychosocial adjustments to illness. The areas that comprise the realm of psychosocial issues are numerous. The North American Nursing Diagnosis Association (NANDA) has determined the content of psychosocial care (see the box below). Each of the diagnoses in the box must be assessed with adequate tools to substantiate data for the diagnosis and a clinically sound plan for care.

The affective responses that occur most frequently among cancer patients are anxiety and depression. The discussion about tools for assessment focuses on these two major areas.

A working definition for **anxiety** is an individual responding to a perceived threat affectively at an emotional level with an increased level of arousal associated with vague,

unpleasant, and uneasy feelings. The instrument used most often to measure anxiety in cancer patients is the State-Trait Anxiety Inventory (STAI).[31] The STAI is composed of two scales: the A-trait and A-state. On the A-state are 20 items with a 4-point scale with the following possible responses: not at all, somewhat, moderately so, and very much. Responses are summed to measure the way the subject feels at a particular moment. Scores demonstrate the level of transitory anxiety characterized by feelings of apprehension, tension, and autonomic nervous system–induced symptoms which are worry, nervousness and apprehension. The A-trait inventory is designed to measure a general level of arousal and predict anxiety proneness. Construct validity and reliability are established for this tool.

Irwin et al.[14] conducted a study of 181 patients receiving external beam radiation and found that all patients (males and females) exhibited higher anxiety scores than nonpatient norms before treatment. In this sample, higher anxiety scores were reported among females over males before treatment began, 1 week after treatment was completed, and 2 months after the completion of therapy. In general, patients showed significantly higher anxiety during rather than after treatment.

Every patient brings a history of coping strategies to the cancer experience. Patients use whatever has worked for them in the past in managing their anxiety. The box below lists effective and noneffective coping strategies.

Nursing Diagnoses Related to Psychosocial Care

- Adjustment, impaired
- Anxiety
- Body-image disturbance
- Caregiver role strain
- Coping, defensive
- Coping, family: potential for growth
- Coping, ineffective family: compromised
- Coping, ineffective family: disabling
- Coping, ineffective individual
- Decisional conflict (specify)
- Denial, ineffective and/or depression
- Family processes, altered
- Fear
- Social isolation
- Grieving, anticipatory
- Grieving, dysfunctional
- Risk for caregiver strain
- Impaired verbal communication (decreased attention and concentration)
- Impaired problem solving
- Ineffective management of therapeutic regimen: individual or family
- Knowledge deficit (specify)
- Noncompliance (specify)
- Parenting, altered, risk for
- Powerlessness related to illness and hospitalization
- Relocation stress syndrome
- Self-esteem disturbance
- Self-esteem, chronic low
- Self-esteem, situational low
- Sleep pattern disturbance related to anxiety and/or depression
- Social interaction, impaired
- Spiritual distress (distress of the human spirit)
- Violence, risk for: self-directed or directed at others

Modified from Gordon M: *Manual of nursing diagnosis.* New York, 1996, Mosby.

Effective and Noneffective Coping Strategies

Effective strategies
- Information seeking
- Participation in religious activities
- Distraction
- Expression of emotion and feeling
- Positive thinking
- Conservation of energy
- Maintenance of independence
- Maintenance of control
- Goal setting

Noneffective strategies
- Denial of emotion
- Minimization of symptoms
- Social isolation
- Passive acceptance
- Sleeping
- Substance abuse
- Avoidance of decision making
- Blame of others
- Excessive dependency

Modified from Miller JF: *Coping with chronic illness: overcoming powerlessness,* Philadelphia, 1983, Davis.

Depression is the second most common affective response in cancer patients. **Depression** is defined as the perceived loss of self-esteem resulting in a cluster of affective behavioral (change in appetite, sleep disturbances, lack of energy, withdrawal, and dependency) and cognitive (decreased ability to concentrate, indecisiveness, and suicidal ideas) responses. Depression plays a major role in the quality of life for cancer patients and their families. However, empirical and clinical reports indicate that depression is an underdiagnosed and probably undertreated response among persons with cancer.

Knowing the way to recognize depression is a critical skill for all oncology health caregivers. I have had experience with a patient with undiagnosed depression who, after receiving a radiation therapy treatment, returned home and committed suicide. The physicians, nurses, and therapists thought the patient who was experiencing severe sequelae in the head and neck radiation treatments was just a "quiet person." In retrospect the signs of depression were present, and no referral was made to a professional. The criteria for recognizing a depressed condition are the following (usually four of these are present nearly every day for at least 2 weeks):

1. Poor appetite or significant weight loss, or increased appetite or significant weight gain
2. Insomnia or hypersomnia (e.g., difficulty with falling asleep, awakening 30 to 90 minutes before time to arise, awakening in the middle of the night with difficulty going back to sleep, increased time of sleep, frequent naps)
3. Psychomotor agitation or retardation (noticeable to others, not just subjective feelings)
4. Loss of interest or pleasure in usual activities or decrease in sexual drive
5. Loss of energy (fatigue)
6. Feelings of worthlessness, self-reproach, or excessive or inappropriate guilt
7. Complaints or evidence of diminished ability to think or concentrate, such as slowed thinking or indecisiveness
8. Recurrent thoughts of death, suicidal ideation, wishes to be dead, or suicide attempt

The radiation therapist who sees and talks to the patient daily is in an excellent position to recognize signs of depression. Questions asked about a patient's eating or sleeping habits or energy level are essential. Therapists must listen and discern carefully the answers to these questions. The danger of routine is to ask how patients are doing and not hear what they are saying, whether through their words or nonverbal cues. Practicing and developing skills discussed in the first part of this chapter is critical for taking care of the whole patient.

Physiological changes such as sleep disturbance, change in weight, appetite disturbance, and decreased energy are experienced frequently by cancer patients as a result of their disease or treatment. In addition, a level of depression is certainly appropriate because cancer represents to patients a potential loss of not only life, but also body parts, image, function, roles, and relationships. The oncology team must assess whether the level of the depression is a change from previous functioning; the way this change occurs; and whether depression is persistent, occurs most of the day, occurs more days than not, and is present for at least a period of 2 weeks.

A variety of instruments are available to assess depression. These tools were designed for psychiatrically ill patients. Therefore the data are limited somewhat with respect to oncology populations.

The first tool is the Beck Depression Inventory (BDI).[3] This is a 21-item self-report scale used to assess symptoms of depression. Each item is composed of a set of statements graduating in severity of symptoms and measured on a scale of 0 to 3 with the higher score representing a more severe symptom. Subjects choose the statement in the tool that best describes their present feelings. The responses are tallied, and a level of depression is assessed.

The second tool is the Hamilton Rating Scale for Depression (HRS-D).[11] It is a 17-item self-report scale used to assess cognitive, behavioral, and physiological signs and symptoms of typical depression. The scores on each item are totaled in order to give a level of assessment of the depression.

Another tool is the Psychosocial Adjustment to Illness Scale (PAIS).[23] This tool is explicitly designed to assess a patient's psychosocial adjustment to medical illness in general. The PAIS is composed of 45 questions divided into the following six domains of psychosocial adjustment: health care orientation, vocational environment, domestic environment, sexual relationships, social environment, and psychological distress. Each of the domains is scored separately and summed. Morrow, Chiarell, and Derogatis' study reveals that the PAIS indicates an acceptable degree of reliability and initial confidence of validity.

Focusing on systematic and continuous assessment for signs and symptoms of psychosocial responses can improve the quality and quantity of survival for patients who have cancer.

Coping strategies and responses—the family. The dynamics of a diagnosis of cancer reach beyond the patient and extend to the entire family. Responses will vary with respect to economic and psychosocial resources, across developmental stages of the family, and with differing demands of the illness.

Life for families of cancer patients becomes complex. Family members must often learn new roles, self-care skills, and ways of relating to and communicating with each other, friends, and the health care team. To support family members, an assessment of their functioning to reveal problem areas may be necessary.

Instruments for assessing the family include the Family Functioning Index (FFI),[27] the Family APGAR* questionnaire,[30] and the Family Inventory of Resources for Management (FIRM).[17] The FFI is a 15-item self-report instrument designed to assess the dynamics of family interaction in families that contain children. Questions are designed to assess marital satisfaction, frequency of disagreement, communication, problem solving, and feelings of closeness and happiness.

The Family APGAR questionnaire[30] is a screening tool designed to assess the family from the view of the patient. The questionnaire consists of five questions on a 3-point scale. This tool does not assume institutional, structural, or cultural boundaries of a traditional family; therefore it has a wide application to the many configurations of the modern family.

The FIRM is a 69-item self-report questionnaire designed to assess the ability of the family to deal with stressors. This self-report is a 4-point Likert scale evaluating four factors: family strengths (esteem and communication), mastery and health, extended family social support, and financial well-being.

Rehabilitation. In cancer cases the focus is most often on the disease rather than its functional consequences. Cancer and its therapy can produce significant long-term and permanent functional losses, even in cases in which the goal is a cure. Each person with a disability needs opportunities for improving or at least maintaining functional ability, regardless of the cause of the disability. Often, little thought is given to aggressive rehabilitation of the cancer patient compared with patients having other conditions such as cardiac disease, a stroke, or a spinal cord injury. This occurs even though the 5-year survival rate for patients with cancer is currently about 50%. Rehabilitation in cancer is certainly relevant because the number of cancer survivors is growing.

Rehabilitation has been defined as the "dynamic process directed toward the goal of enabling persons to function at their maximum level within the limitations of their disease or disability in terms of their physical, mental, emotional, social and economic potential."[7]

In the early work by Mayer[16] the concept was set forth that cancer rehabilitation should encompass the theme of quality of survival—not just a person's life span, but also that individual's ability to live in the constraints of the disease. In their article, "Can life be the same after cancer treatment?" Veroness and Martino[33] stated that rehabilitation is the bridge leading the patient from diversity to normality. Mellette[19] expanded on the idea by suggesting that *prevention,* the initial avoidance of dysfunction, is the key word in discussing rehabilitation.

The National Cancer Rehabilitation Planning Conference, sponsored by the National Cancer Institute, identified four cancer-rehabilitation objectives[7]:

1. Psychological support after the diagnosis of cancer
2. Optimal physical functioning after the treatment of cancer
3. Early vocational counseling when indicated
4. Optimal social functioning as the ultimate goal of all cancer-control treatment

Probably one of the first major descriptions of a cancer-rehabilitation perspective is that of Dietz[6] in his book *Rehabilitation Oncology.* Dietz considers rehabilitation applicable to all patients who can learn and respond. He stressed readaptation as the synonym for rehabilitation because of widespread reluctance to view rehabilitation as relevant to the cancer patient. He further defined the term as accommodation or adjustment to personal needs for physical, psychological, financial, and vocational survival. He defined the initial goals of rehabilitation as the elimination, reduction, or alleviation of disability, and he defined the ultimate goal as the reestablishment of patients as functional individuals in their environments. Rehabilitation should begin at the earliest possible time, and it should continue throughout the entire convalescence until maximal benefit can be achieved.

Romassas et al.[28] developed a method to be used for assessing the rehabilitation needs of oncology patients. They devised an oncology clinic patient checklist designed to include rehabilitation concepts in the patient-assessment process. The patient was asked information regarding the following areas: fatigue; pain; nutrition; speech and language; respiration; bowel and bladder management; transportation; mobility; self-care and home care; vocational and educational interests and activities; and emotional, family, and interpersonal relationships.

As in other assessments, the evaluation for rehabilitative purposes is a dynamic event. It should continue as new issues arise or past issues recur and is best accomplished by a multidisciplinary team meeting the specific needs of each patient.

Cultural assessment

Cultural assessment refers to the systematic appraisal of the cultural beliefs, values, and practices of individuals and communities. Cultural beliefs and individual differences determine health behaviors in families and cultural groups. Many of the problems with health are the result of behavior and lifestyle.

Accepting and respecting patients for who they are is an important attribute of oncology caregivers. Being culturally sensitive is essential in caring for the whole patient. The box located at the top of p. 327 lists ways to develop cultural sensitivity.

---

*Adaptability, Partnership, Growth, Affection, and Resolve.

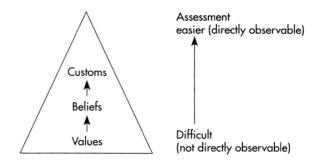

Fig. 19-1 A model of cultural strata. (Modified from Bellack J, Edlund B, editors: *Nursing assessment and diagnosis,* Boston, 1992, Jones & Bartlett.)

Cultural assessment has several key variables. Fig. 19-1 demonstrates a model of cultural strata useful in examining these variables. In this model, values are the foundation of beliefs that includes attitudes and behaviors. Values, which are most difficult to assess, are established early in childhood through an unconscious process of socialization.

Beliefs that include knowledge, opinions, and faith about life are built on an individual's values. Based on their knowledge, opinions, and faith, cultures view the origin, treatments, and responses to illness differently. Treatment of the whole cancer patient involves evaluating and understanding the patient's values and beliefs. This is especially important when these values and beliefs are different from or in direct conflict with those of the health caregiver and may impair the care of the patient.

Customs that are the result of values and beliefs are the most observable and assessable. These customs include dietary habits, religious practices, communication patterns, family structure, and health practices.

An extremely simple and short assessment model is proposed by Kleinman, Eisenberg, and Good.[15] They suggest the following questions*:

- What do you think caused your problems?
- Why do you think your sickness started when it did?
- What does your sickness do to you? How does it work?
- How severe is your sickness? Will it have a long or short duration?

*If time permits a more thorough cultural assessment, a longer tool can be used (see the box on p. 328).

- What kind of treatment do you think you should receive?
- What are the most important results you hope to receive from this treatment?
- What are the chief problems your sickness has caused you?
- What do you fear most about your sickness?

Cultural assessment enables the health care provider to develop a solid therapeutic relationship, which is a genuine collaborative effort between the patient and health care provider. This requires the person assessing to use good reflective listening skills and pay careful attention to all the cues. In addition, these cues need to be interpreted in the context of the patient's values, beliefs, and culture to be truly meaningful and helpful in treating and respecting the uniqueness of each cancer patient.

Spiritual assessment. In a holistic approach to care for cancer patients, dimensions of the total person need to be recognized and assessed. This includes the patient's spiritual concerns. In a presentation given at the White House Conference for Aging, Moberg[22] defined the *spiritual dimension* as pertaining to "man's inner resources especially his ultimate concern, the basic value around which all other values are focused, the central philosophy of life, which guides a person's conduct, the supernatural and non-material dimensions of human nature." The spiritual dimension encompasses a person's need to find satisfactory answers to questions that revolve around the meaning of life, illness, and death.

To help explore this dimension, Stoll[32] developed guidelines for the spiritual assessment of patients. She suggested the importance of understanding four areas related to this search for meaning and spirituality in patients' lives: (1) patients' concepts of God or deity, (2) their source of hope and strength, (3) the significance of their religious practices, and (4) the relationship between their spiritual beliefs and state of health.

Cultural Assessment Guide

Health beliefs and practices

- How does the client define *health* and *illness*?
- Are particular methods such as hygiene and self-care practices used to help maintain health?
- Are particular methods being used by the client for the treatment of illness?
- What is the attitude toward preventive health measures such as immunizations?
- Do health topics exist to which the client may be particularly sensitive or that are considered taboo?
- What are the attitudes toward mental illness, pain, handicapping conditions, chronic disease, death, and dying?
- Is a person in the family responsible for various health-related decisions, such as places to go, persons to see, and advice to follow?

Religious influences and special rituals

- Does the client adhere to a particular religion?
- Does the client look to a significant person for guidance and support?
- Do any special religious practices or beliefs affect health care when the client is ill or dying?
- What events, rituals, and ceremonies (birth, baptism, puberty, marriage, and death) are considered important in the life cycle?

Language and communication

- What language is spoken in the home?
- How well does the client understand English (spoken or written)?
- Do special signs of demonstrating respect or disrespect exist?
- Is touch involved in communication?
- Are there culturally appropriate ways to enter and leave situations (including greetings, farewells, and convenient times to make a home visit)?

Parenting styles and the role of family

- Who makes decisions in the family?
- What is the composition of the family? How many generations are considered a single family? Which relatives comprise the family?
- When the marriage custom is practiced, what is the attitude about separation and divorce?
- What is the role of and attitude toward children in the family?
- When do children need to be disciplined or punished? How is this done? In what way are physical punishment used (if any)?
- Do parents demonstrate physical affection toward their children and each other?
- What major events are important to the family? How are these events celebrated?
- Do special beliefs and practices surround conception, pregnancy, childbirth, lactation, and child rearing?

Dietary practices

- What does the family like to eat? Does everyone in the family have similar tastes in food?
- Who is responsible for food preparation?
- Are any foods forbidden by the culture? Are some foods a cultural requirement in observance of a rite or ceremony?
- How is food prepared and consumed?
- Do specific beliefs or preferences exist concerning food, such as those believed to cause or cure an illness?

From Stulc DM: The family as bearer of culture. In Cookfair JN: *Nursing process and practice in the community*, St Louis, 1990. Mosby.

Stoll notes that spiritual topics are emotionally laden and should be handled in the assessment process accordingly. They should probably be introduced late in an interview, perhaps as a continuation of psychosocial assessment. As with all questions asked patients, the basis for inquiry should be explained.

Spiritual support may bring comfort, peace, and for some, the reason for suffering. To facilitate the essential spiritual aspects of caring, oncology health care providers should do the following:

1. Assist patients to experience their own spirituality.
2. Listen carefully to the patient's expression of belief.
3. If possible, provide an appropriate environment and quiet time for reflection and contemplation.
4. Assist the patient in finding resources for spiritual fulfillment.

The willingness to allow a patient or family to be themselves by being present and supporting them is an essential part of working in oncology. In the spiritual realm, presence implies an unconditional acceptance of persons. To be present with a cancer patient or the family is to listen in the broadest sense to hear the communication clearly. Compassionate presence does not require many words. Sometimes it requires none.

Numerous tools are available for assessing spirituality. They include the Spiritual Well-Being Scale, the Religious Well-Being Scale,[26] the Existential Well-Being Scale,[8] Moberg's Indexes of Spiritual Well-Being,[22] and Hess' Spiritual Needs Survey.[13] Studies indicate a combination of these tools best yields the multifaceted nature of spirituality.

Hope. Hope is the key concept and an essential ingredient in the religious and spiritual aspects of care and a major component in the healing process. Spiritual persons inspire hope more by who they are than by their actions. Giving support with realistic hope is a powerful gift oncology caregivers can offer their patients. For some patients, hope is a major determinant between life and death.

A physician often becomes a symbol of hope. Through the physician's continued interest the patient does not despair. The fear of being abandoned by this person of hope can clearly alter the patient's behavior. Patients may protect their relationships with their physicians by not questioning them, limiting their complaints to them, and treating them as they wish to perceive them, as miracles workers. When this occurs the role of another member of the multidisciplinary team becomes paramount. Establishing a therapeutic relationship and applying good communication skills is essential in caring for this patient.

The literature and published research articles on hope number approximately 20. Of those articles, 10 involve patients with cancer. This suggests that cancer may have a greater effect on hope than other chronic illnesses. Key measurement instruments include the Nowotny Hope Scale,[24] Herth Hope Scale,[12] and Miller Hope Scale.[21]

The Nowotny Hope Scale is a 29-item scale designed to measure hope on six dimensions: confidence in outcomes, relationship to others, possibility of a future, spiritual beliefs, active involvement, and internal origin. This tool is a 4-point Likert-type scale that yields reliable and validated outcomes.

The Herth Hope Scale is a 32-item self-report scale to which patients respond, "does not apply to me" or "applies to me" to each item. A total hope score is attained by adding all the responses on each item. Reliability and validity estimates are determined. Herth's descriptive study investigated the relationship between hope and coping in 120 adult cancer patients receiving chemotherapy in a variety of care settings. A significant relationship was found between the level of hope and level of coping. In addition, patients with a strong religious faith had significantly higher mean scores on the Hearth Hope Scale than subjects with weak, unsure faith.

The Miller Hope Scale is a 40-item scale using a 5-point Likert format. The possible range of scores is 40 to 200, with a high score indicating high hope. Exemplary items include the statement, "I look forward to an enjoyable future." A low score item is, "I feel trapped, pinned down." The strength of this tool is strong reliability and validity.

Hope is a multidimensional construct that is more than goal attainment and has not been easily quantified. Hope is fundamental to meaning and transcendence for humans. For these reasons, including hope in holistic patient assessment is important.

SPECIAL CASES IN ASSESSMENT

Special attention must be given to meet the diverse needs of patients at different stages in life because cancer is a group of diseases that affects individuals across the life span.

Children

To provide holistic care to a child with cancer, assessing the needs and concerns of the child's primary caretakers (usually the parents) is essential. Parents experiencing a life-threatening diagnosis for their child is an extremely stressful event.

The assessment of children with cancer is a multidimensional task. Areas of functioning that should be considered are depression, withdrawal, anxiety, delinquency, achievement, family relations, and development.

The developmental level of children is directly related to the way they perceive, interpret, and respond to the diagnosis of cancer. A substantial amount of literature in nursing, medicine, psychiatry, psychology, and social work exists detailing the psychological effect of childhood cancer. The shock of diagnosis, discomfort and inconvenience of treatment, and burden of living with a life-threatening disease are sources of distress and disruption for the child with cancer, patients, siblings, and extended family members.

Those who provide health care to children with cancer have a key role in helping the child and family cope with situations. The study by Armstrong et al.[2] suggests that the overwhelming majority of children with cancer are normally adjusted. This is due in part to the caregivers' concern and help with coping.

Adolescents

Developmental theory suggests that adolescence is a crucial stage in the process of building self-esteem, forming perceptions about body image, establishing autonomy, and developing social functions. The adolescent with cancer experiences a disruption of these vital processes. As a result, assessment for the adolescent must consider and address these unique areas. The adolescent with cancer may face a loss of self-esteem because of the unfamiliar patient role. This role can cause the adolescent to feel inferior and dependent, thus inhibiting the developmental task of establishing independence.

Relationships with others and self-perception can change as the adolescent goes through treatment and is hospitalized. The unpredictability and uncertainty of cancer can limit the adolescent's sense of control and autonomy. Changes in body image, disruption of activities, and prescribed therapies can have a profound effect on the adolescent's self-image. Rapid changes in physical appearance as a result of treatments, disfigurement caused by the disease or amputation, or reduction in weight can confuse and impair the adolescent's self-perception.

These are complex processes that must be assessed and incorporated into the plan of care for the adolescent. The health care team needs to promote growth and developmental maturity while recognizing the burden that cancer places on the adolescent in meeting developmental tasks.

Older persons

As individuals enter the later stages of life, the risk of developing cancer increases. Specific attention to the sociological issues for older persons are crucial for appropriate assessment and treatment of cancer.

An important problem to assess in older persons is the amount of sensory and cognitive impairment that may be present. Assessing the ability of older patients to hear, see, or understand is paramount in their care. Recognizing any change from normal behaviors, usual routines, and social interactions is extremely important. Loss of physical health, limited economic resources, changes in family structure, and losses of social status greatly affect the quality of life for older persons. Obtaining a complete medical history that includes medications, the family health experience and history, the functional status, and current concerns is crucial to sound health care. The box on this page lists some suggestions for interviewing an older patient.

Ongoing communication is the key to assessing and working effectively with the older patient. The best way to promote ongoing communication is to communicate well from the start and to take time to establish a therapeutic and healing relationship.

Suggestions for Interviewing an Older Patient

- If feasible, gather preliminary data before the appointment. Request previous medical records, or have the patient or family complete a questionnaire at home or by phone.
- Try to avoid making patients tell their story more than once.
- In the review of systems, ask about difficulty sleeping, incontinence, falling, depression, dizziness, or loss of energy.
- Pace the interview. An older patient may need extra time to formulate answers.
- If the patient has difficulty with open-ended questions, use yes-or-no or simple-choice questions.
- Encourage patients and their caregivers to bring a list of their main concerns and questions to help ensure that the issues important to them are discussed.
- Ask patients to bring with them all the medications they are taking (prescription and over-the-counter).
- Ask about the patient's functional status, such as eating, bathing, dressing, cooking, and shopping. Sudden changes in these areas are valuable diagnostic clues.
- Determine whether the patient is a caregiver. Many older women care for spouses, older parents, or grandchildren. Patients' willingness to report symptoms depends on whether they think they can afford to get sick.

Modified from Gastel B: *Working with your older patient: a clinician's handbook,* Bethesda, Md, 1994, National Institute on Aging, National Institute on Health.

Review Questions

Essay

1. What is assessment?
2. What is included in the cognitive content of a message? Give an example.
3. What is included in the affective content of a message? Give an example.
4. What is involved in an empathic response?
5. What are the 10 most common verbal responses in affective communication?
6. What is the assessment responsibility of radiation therapists for daily treatment in the following areas?
   - Skin reactions
   - Fatigue
   - Diarrhea
   - Cystitis
   - Alopecia
   - Pain
   - Sleep
   - Mouth changes
   - Pharyngitis and esophagitis
   - Nausea and vomiting
   - Skin pallor
   - Weight loss
7. What is frequently the first sign of malnutrition?
8. What is cachexia?
9. What are two important characteristics related to the etiology of pain?
10. What is leukopenia?
11. What are the major symptoms of depression?
12. List five ways to be culturally sensitive.

Questions to Ponder

1. Why is doing an assessment in oncology important?
2. What is the basis of an effective therapeutic (communication) relationship?
3. Why is observing nonverbal communication so important?
4. What are the three purposes of pain assessment?
5. Why is rehabilitation of the cancer patient important?
6. What are four areas related to the search for meaning and spirituality in patients' lives?
7. Describe five helpful methods in interviewing an older patient.

REFERENCES

1. Ahles TA, Blanchard EB, Ruckdeschel JC: The multidimensional nature of cancer-related pain, *Pain* 17:277-288, 1983.
2. Armstrong GD et al: Multidimensional assessment of psychological problem in children with cancer, *Res Nurs Health* 5:205-211, 1982.
3. Beck AT, Beamesderfer A: Assessment of depression: the Depression Inventory. In Pichot P, Olivier-Martin R, editors: *Psychological measurements in psychopharmacology: modern problems in pharmopsychiatry,* vol 7, Basel, 1974, Karger.
4. Cella DF et al: The Functional Assessment of Cancer Therapy Scale: development and validation of the general measure, *J Clin Oncol* 11(3):570-579, 1993.
5. Daut RW, Cleeland CS, Flannery RC: Development of the Wisconsin Brief Pain Questionnaire to assess pain in cancer and other disease, *Pain* 17:197-210, 1983.
6. Dietz JH: *Rehabilitation oncology,* New York, 1981, John Wiley & Sons.
7. Dudas S, Carlson CE: Cancer rehabilitation, *Oncol Nurs Forum* 15(2):183-188, 1988.
8. Ellison CW: Spiritual well-being: conceptualization and measurement, *J Psy Theology* 11(4):330-340, 1983.
9. Fishman B et al: The Memorial Pain Assessment Card: a valid instrument for the evaluation of cancer pain, *Cancer* 60:1151-1158, 1987.
10. Foley KN: Pain syndromes in patients with cancer. In Bonica JJ, Ventafridda V, editors: *Advances in pain research and therapy,* vol 2, New York, 1979, Raven Press.
11. Hamilton M: A rating scale for depression, *J Neurol Neurosurg Psychiatry* 23:56-62, 1960.
12. Herth KA: The relationship between level of hope and level of coping response and other variables in patients with cancer, *Oncol Nurs Forum* 16:67-72, 1989.
13. Hess JS: Spiritual Needs Survey. In Fish S, Shelly JA, editors: *Spiritual care: the nurse's role,* Downers Grove, Ill, 1983, Intervarsity Press.
14. Irwin PH et al: Sex differences in psychological distress during definitive radiation therapy for cancer, *J Psychosoc Oncol* 4:63-75, 1986.
15. Kleinman A, Eisenberg L, Good B: Culture, illness and care: clinical lessons from anthropologic and cross-cultural research, *Am Intern Med* 88:251-258, 1978.
16. Mayer NH: Concepts in cancer rehabilitation, *Semin Oncol* 2:393-398, 1975.
17. McCubbin HI, Comew J: FIRM: Family Inventory of Resources for Management. In McCubbin HI, Thompson AI, editors: *Family assessment inventories for research and practice,* Madison, Wis, 1987, University of Wisconsin-Madison.
18. McGuire DB: Cancer-related pain: a multidimensional approach, *Dissert Abst Int* 48(3):Sec B:705, 1987.
19. Mellette SJ: Rehabilitation issues for cancer survivors:psychosocial challenges, *J Psychosoc Oncol* 7:93-109, 1989.
20. Melzack R: The McGill Pain Questionnaire: major properties and scoring methods, *Pain* 1:277-299, 1975.
21. Miller JF: Development of an instrument to measure hope, *Nurs Res* 37(1):6-9, 1988.
22. Moberg D. Spiritual well-being: background and issues, Washington DC, 1971, White House Conference on Aging.
23. Morrow GR, Chiarell RJ, Derogatis LR: A new scale for assessing patient's psychosocial adjustment to medical illness, *Psy Med* 8:605-610, 1978.
24. Nowotny ML: Assessment of hope in patients with cancer: development of an instrument, *Oncol Nurs Forum* 16:57-61, 1989.
25. Padilla GV et al: Quality of Life Index for patients with cancer, *Res Nurs Health* 6:117-126, 1983.
26. Paloutzian R, Ellison CW, Lonelines S: Spiritual well-being and quality of life. In Piplair A, Perlman D, editors: *Loneliness sourcebook of current theory research and therapy,* New York, 1982, Wiley Interscience.
27. Pless IB, Satterwhite BB: A measure of family functioning and its application, *Soc Sci Med* 7:613-620, 1973.
28. Romassas ED et al: A method for assessing the rehabilitation needs of oncology outpatients, *Oncol Nurs Forum* 10(3):17-21, 1983.
29. Schipper H et al: Measuring the quality of life of cancer patients: the Functional Living Index–Cancer: development and validation, *J Clin Oncol* 2(5):472-483, 1984.
30. Smilkstein F: The family APGAR: a proposal for a family function test and its use by physicians, *J Fam Pract* 6:1231-1239, 1978.
31. Spielberger C, Gorusch R, Lushene R: *Manual for the State-Trait Anxiety Inventory,* Palo Alto, Calif, 1970, Consulting Psychologists Press.
32. Stoll RI: Guidelines for spiritual assessment, *Am J Nurs* 79:1574-1577, September 1979.
33. Veroness V, Martino G: Can life be the same after cancer treatment? *Tumori* 64:345-351, 1978.
34. Yasko JM: A model for the assessment of the client with cancer. In Yasko JM, editor: *Guidelines for cancer care symptom management,* Reston, Va, 1983, Reston Publishing.
35. Yates JW, Chalmer B, McKegney FP: Evaluation of patients with advanced cancer using the Karnofsky Performance Status, *CA Cancer J Clin* 45:2220-2224, 1980.

BIBLIOGRAPHY

The American Psychiatric Association: *DSM III–R (diagnostic and statistical manual of mental disorders*, ed 3, Washington, DC, 1987, The Association.

Blackburn GL et al: Nutritional and metabolic assessment of the hospitalized patient, *J Parent Ent Nutr* 1:17, 1977.

Gastel B: *Working with your older patient: a clinician's handbook,* Bethesda, Maryland, 1994, National Institute on Aging, National Institute on Health.

Gordon M: *Manual of nursing diagnosis,* New York, 1987, McGraw-Hill.

Groenwald SL et al: *Nutritional disturbances: cancer nursing principles and practice,* ed 3, Boston, 1993, Jones & Bartlett.

Hirshfield-Bartek J, Dow KH, Creaton E: Decreasing documentation time using a patient self-assessment tool, *Oncol Nurs Forum* 17:251-255, 1990.

McCaffery M, Beebe A: *Pain: clinical manual for nursing practice,* St Louis, 1989, Mosby.

Miller JF: *Coping with chronic illness: overcoming powerlessness,* Philadelphia, 1983, Davis.

Stulc DM: The family as bearer of culture. In Cookfair JN, editor: *Nursing process and practice in the community,* St Louis, 1990, Mosby.

Stulc P: The family as bearer of culture. In Cookfair JN, editor: *Nursing process and practice in the community,* St Louis, 1990, Mosby.

Trip-Reimer T: Cultural assessment. In Bellack J, Edlund B, editors: *Nursing assessment and diagnosis,* Boston, 1992, Jones & Bartlett.

20

Pharmacology and Drug Administration

Lynda N. Reynolds

Outline

Key terms

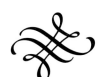

Although the administration of drugs is not the primary role of the radiation therapist, it is a crucial part of overall patient care.[2] The therapist may personally administer medications specific to radiation therapy, such as contrast media, anesthetics, or intravenous (IV) fluids. The therapist must also know all the drugs a patient is taking and for what purpose.

The radiation therapist interacts closely with patients in radiation oncology and may be the first to notice adverse reactions or unusual symptoms as these reactions or symptoms appear. Competent patient care requires that the therapist have a general knowledge of pharmacology and specific details of each patient's medication history. With a basic understanding of medications and their common side effects, the therapist will be able to distinguish an expected side effect from an adverse reaction that requires medical intervention.

DRUG LEGISLATION

The Federal Food, Drug, and Cosmetic Act of 1938 and the Controlled Substance Act of 1971 govern the labeling, availability, and dispensation of all drugs in the United States.[10] Radiation therapists must remain abreast of information about the drugs in use in their profession. Safer and more effective drugs, such as nonionic contrast media, are continually being developed. Legislation requires extensive testing of all new drugs before they can be used on patients; however, the value and drawbacks of medications are proved through their actual daily use. The therapist administering these drugs plays an important role in providing feedback to the pharmacology community.

DRUG NOMENCLATURE

Pharmacology is the science of drugs, which includes the sources, chemistry, and actions of drugs. The list of drugs available for medical use changes constantly as new formulas are developed. Each drug has at least four separate names—its chemical name (chemical formula), **generic name** (coined by the original manufacturer), official name (usually the same as the generic name), and brand or trade name (the drug's name in official publications).[9,10,14] Several manufacturers may produce the same generic drug but call that drug by different brand names. Radiation therapists and all health professionals need to easily access this drug name information. The best resources available are the *Physicians' Desk Reference (PDR)*, *United States Pharmacopeia (USP)*, and specific drug packaging.

PHARMACOLOGICAL PRINCIPLES

The way in which drugs affect the body is called **pharmacodynamics.** Each drug has a unique molecular structure enabling it to interact with a specific enzyme or a corresponding cell type. The drug attaches itself to a target site in the body called the *receptor site* in the same way that two puzzle pieces interlock. The combined effect alters the behavior of the targeted cells or enzyme and causes physiological changes in the patient.

The way that drugs travel through the body to their receptor sites is called **pharmacokinetics.** A drug must be administered so that the body can absorb it, distribute it to the necessary sites, metabolize it, and excrete the excess. Many individual factors cause these steps to vary within each patient; the effectiveness of and reaction to a drug may differ greatly from one patient to another.

Absorption

Every drug must be absorbed into the bloodstream to be effective. The dosage and speed of absorption depend on factors such as the route of entry, the pH of the recipient environment, the solubility of the formula, and the drug's interaction with body chemicals while in transit.[10,14]

Distribution

A drug travels through the circulatory system to its receptor site(s) and then connects with the molecular structure for which it was designed. The drug may need to bind with a certain protein or cross specific membranes to produce the desired response. Many drugs cross the placental villi and affect the fetus. Fewer drugs can cross the blood-brain barrier. Some medications may be stored in the tissues for later use.

Metabolism

The liver detoxifies nearly all foreign substances entering the body, including drugs, and changes them into inactive, water-soluble compounds that can be excreted by the kidneys.[10] The breakdown of drugs into waste matter may also involve chemical processes and enzyme reactions in the blood and other organs such as the gallbladder, lungs, and intestines. If drugs accumulate or react synergistically with other substances in the body or the organs are damaged, metabolism and excretion of the drugs may be difficult.[14]

Excretion

Most drugs leave the body through the kidneys. The lungs sometimes expel those drugs that break down into gases. The sweat glands, tear ducts, salivary glands, intestines, and mammary glands can also eliminate small quantities of drugs. The rate of excretion depends on the body's systems and, especially with many medications used in radiation therapy, the drug's half-life and concentration in the tissues.

VARIABLES AFFECTING PATIENT RESPONSE

The caregiver must consider the numerous factors that determine patient response to drugs. The following section discusses several of these factors.

Patient-related variables

Age. Young children and older adults generally require smaller than average doses, although for different reasons. In children and infants the organs are still developing. Determining dosages by using body weight is safer than using age, but this calculation remains imprecise because of the child's immature metabolism.[13] Children may be hypersensitive to medications, so administration of minimal doses and close monitoring of their responses is the usual process. Getting the prescribed dose into children can be challenging, because they frequently cannot swallow pills, spit out liquid preparations, reject suppositories, and fight injections.

Older adults require smaller (or sometimes larger) doses because age decreases the efficiency of their organs. Their circulation slows, enzymes are depleted, sensitivities develop, absorption becomes impaired, and the liver and kidneys can no longer detoxify efficiently.[9,10,13,14] In addition, elderly patients frequently take multiple medications that may interact negatively. Elderly patients should be monitored to ensure that the dosage of the medications they are taking is appropriate.

Weight and physical condition. Average doses are based on the median 150-lb, healthy adult. The dose needs to be adjusted for heavier or lighter patients, and body mass must be taken into account because obesity or excessive thinness affects circulation and organ efficiency. A damaged liver or kidneys, an electrolyte imbalance, poor circulation, nutritional deficiency, infection, and other physiological disorders should be considered to determine the optimum dosage.[10]

Gender. Women have a lower average body weight than men and metabolize drugs differently. Women's hormone profiles and the amount and distribution of their body fat differ greatly from those of men and influence the dosage of medications needed. The difference in fluid balance between the genders is another important factor for figuring dosage. The added complication of pregnancy is critical because many drugs affect the fetus.

Personal and emotional requirements. Patients react differently to drugs. Caffeine is a common example; some people can drink coffee all day and have no trouble sleeping, whereas others cannot tolerate caffeine. As a result, patients have unique needs and must be evaluated individually. Patients with negative attitudes or anxiety require higher levels of sedation than calm patients with positive outlooks. Although some patients prefer to take minimum doses of medication, others see drugs as cure-alls.[13] Health care professionals must relate to patients as individuals and be alert to each patient's emotional response to the drugs administered.

Drug-related variables: nontherapeutic reactions

An important difference exists between unpleasant but expected side effects and adverse drug responses or complications. Side effects are expected reactions to medication; complications are *unexpected* reactions to medications that range from mild to severe.[10] In radiation therapy the treatment, diagnostic contrast media used, and various medications taken before and after treatment combine to produce toxicities and discomfort for the patient.

Allergic reactions. Allergic reactions result from an immunological reaction to a drug to which the patient has already been sensitized. In an allergic reaction the drug acts as an antigen, and the body develops antibodies to that drug. The result may range from a light rash to life-threatening **anaphylactic shock.** Once an allergy develops, subsequent exposures to that drug cause increasingly severe symptoms. Penicillin is a common allergenic drug.

Tolerance. Tolerance occurs if the body adapts to a particular drug and requires ever greater doses to achieve the desired effect. For example, the body develops a tolerance for narcotics extremely quickly. If overused, antibiotics become increasingly less effective by killing not only the bad bacteria but also the good. Antibiotics may also leave the patient susceptible to further infection. Bacteria that survive antibiotic use can mutate within the patient into strains that are resistant to the antibiotic during subsequent use.[14] The patient may need to switch to a different drug if the first one loses its effectiveness.

Cumulative effect. A cumulative effect develops if the body is unable to detoxify and excrete a drug quickly enough or if too large a dose is taken.[13] Unless the dosage is adjusted, the drug accumulates in the tissues and can become toxic. In some cases the cumulative effect is desirable, such as with medications prescribed to prevent depression.

Idiosyncratic effects. Idiosyncratic effects are the inexplicable and unpredictable symptoms caused by a genetic defect within the patient.[13] These symptoms are completely different from the expected symptoms and may occur the first time a drug is given.

Dependence. Drug dependency can result from extensive exposure to drugs for pain relief. The majority of persons who become drug dependent do so because of physiological or psychological problems.

Drug interactions. Drug interactions occurring between two or more drugs or a combination of food and drugs can create or produce positive or negative effects in patients. This interaction of drugs may result in synergism, which increases a drug's effects; interaction can also result in antagonism, which decreases a drug's effects. For example, alcohol and sedatives taken together produce a toxic reaction, whereas an antiemetic given with anesthesia can be therapeutic. Older adults commonly take many different medications, and the interactions of these drugs can cause the bodies of these people to go into toxic shock. The person administering medications should *never* mix drugs without consulting a drug compatibility chart or checking with a pharmacist.

The therapist should also be familiar with the term **iatrogenic disease**. This disease results from long-term use of a drug that damages organs or causes other disorders over time.

In these nontherapeutic responses the drugs used to treat disease may also cause disease. The therapist should remain aware of complications caused by drug administration.

PROFESSIONAL DRUG ASSESSMENT AND MANAGEMENT
Assessing the patient's medication history

The patient is the managing partner in the business of self-medication. Although the health care professional may educate and evaluate the patient regarding drug use, the patient is ultimately responsible for self-medication. If the patient is forgetful, confused, depressed, or taking several medications simultaneously or has inadequate diet and exercise habits, it may be difficult to differentiate between poor compliance and additional medical needs. For example, impaired liver or kidney function may indicate toxicity from drug overuse, lack of improvement from a prior disease, poor distribution from sluggish circulation, an allergic reaction, damaged organs from alcohol or drug abuse, or a negative response from drug interaction. The assessment is further complicated because the person recording the medical history must rely on the patient's verbal description and inadequate recollection.

Despite these difficulties the therapist must assess the patient's drug use during the patient evaluation by documenting every drug the patient is taking (including alcohol) and looking especially for overuse and underuse of prescribed drugs.[4,5,9,10,14,16,17] Misuse of drugs can influence the outcome of radiologic diagnosis or treatment. An accurate medication history is essential to proper diagnosis and treatment (see the section on "legal aspects").

Applying the Five Rights of Drug Safety

The Five Rights of Drug Safety are as follows: (1) to identify the *right* patient, (2) to select the *right* medication, (3) to give the *right* dose, (4) to give the medication at the *right* time, and (5) to give the medication by the *right* route.[5,7,9,10,13,14,17]

Checking the patient's name on the door or looking at the chart in the slot is not enough; the therapist should check the identification bracelet *and* ask patients to give their name if possible. If the patient's name is called and the patient nods or smiles, this does not mean that the name has been called correctly. The patient may have nodded or smiled in acknowledgment. A patient may be too young to understand, may not have a hearing aid in place, may not speak English as a primary language, or may be drowsy and have misheard. Checking the patient's identification bracelet is *essential*.

The therapist does not bear the primary responsibility for choosing the correct dose; however, as with all caregivers, the therapist must continually watch for errors. Even if the physician or nurse (in the case of standing orders) has prescribed the drug, the therapist involved should *always* check the dosage.[9,10,13,14,17] Extremely old or young patients have special requirements, as do people of different weights, genders, physical conditions, allergic statuses, and emotional conditions. The dosage should *always* be doublechecked.

Although a physician (not a therapist) must prescribe the medications, the therapist may confirm that the physician has ordered the proper drug for the patient and that the drug ordered is also the drug being administered. The patient usually knows if a medication order seems different. This can be a "red flag" for a therapist to check for a change in the medication or an error. Every patient deserves to receive the correct medication every time. Therefore the written order should always be checked against the patient's chart and the drug label.

Some drugs can be administered in more than one way; other drugs should only be given by a particular route. If a drug is administered incorrectly, the consequences may range from injury to death. In the radiologic sciences profession a drug given by the wrong route can also skew a procedure's results. **Contrast media,** in particular, needs to be delivered to the proper location by the correct route in order to enhance the images that facilitate the diagnosis or treatment. The route of entry should *always* be doublechecked.

Giving a drug at the wrong time can have serious consequences. Such consequences can include poor absorption, fluctuation of blood or serum levels, enhanced side effects, or less than optimal diagnostic capability in the case of contrast media. A drug that has been ordered before surgery or before a diagnostic procedure must be administered punctually because the procedure is scheduled for a particular time and depends on the drug's effect. Although medicating an entire ward of patients at one time is a challenge, patients deserve to receive medications *on time*.

Implementing proper emergency procedures

If a drug emergency occurs, the therapist or another health care professional must follow proper emergency procedures. Each hospital has its own emergency codes and procedures. At the onset of an emergency the therapist's first duty is to summon help by "calling a code." The therapist should know the location of emergency supplies within the area and the way to administer oxygen and perform cardiopulmonary resuscitation (CPR).

Types of emergencies that the radiation therapist is most likely to see are shock, anaphylaxis, cardiac or respiratory failure, pulmonary embolism, and fainting. Recognizing symptoms and delivering the appropriate treatment are required skills for therapists.[2] If a reaction develops while a contrast medium is being administered, the therapist must stop the treatment immediately and call the oncologist. The patient must *never* be left alone.

The ability to handle medical emergencies comes from hands-on experience. The amount of material regarding hands-on-training is too broad to be dealt with adequately here; however, all radiation therapists should seek extensive education in this area.

DRUG CATEGORIES RELEVANT TO RADIATION THERAPY

Oncology patients have specific symptoms or indications for certain types of drugs. In radiation therapy, for example, patients may require certain drugs, such as antidiarrheals and antiemetics, to relieve the symptoms of the therapy and other drugs, such as contrast media, to facilitate the pretherapy diagnosis.

Pharmacologists classify drugs in the following ways: according to the effects of the drug on particular receptor sites, such as bronchodilators or cardiovascular drugs; in terms of the symptoms that the drug relieves, such as aspirin for reducing fever; by chemical group, such as antihistamines and anticoagulants; or by the effects of the drug on body systems, such as tranquilizers and antidepressants.[1,5,15,17] These categories not only overlap, but often a single drug can be used in order to treat multiple conditions, whereas several different drugs can be used to treat a single condition. The following categories of drugs contain the common medications that are administered to oncology patients for conditions that may precede or relate to the radiation therapy treatment.

Analgesics relieve pain. Narcotic analgesics for moderate-to-severe pain are made from opium, such as morphine, codeine, and Demerol. These narcotic analgesics are not only addictive, but they can cause adverse side effects. Nonnarcotic analgesics, such as Tylenol, Darvon, and aspirin are not addictive but are also not strong enough to relieve severe pain.

Anesthetics suppress the sensation of feeling by acting on the central nervous system. General anesthetics, such as Pentothal, depress the entire central nervous system, thereby rendering the patient unconscious so that major surgery can be performed. Local anesthetics, such as Novocain, act only on the nerves in a small area. Xylocaine, as a viscous solution, is used to treat inflamed mucous membranes in the mouth and pharynx.

Antianxiety drugs are mild tranquilizers that help calm anxious patients and relieve muscle spasms. Equanil, Valium, and Librium are antianxiety drugs that may be used concurrently with radiation therapy treatments.

Antibiotics suppress the growth of bacteria. Examples include *erythromycin,* which is usually prescribed for respiratory tract infections, and penicillin and tetracycline, which are broad-spectrum antibiotics effective against a variety of bacterial infections.

Anticoagulants prevent blood from clotting too quickly in cases of thrombosis or if an IV line needs to be kept open. The most commonly used drugs in this category are Coumadin, which is administered orally, and heparin, which is always administered parenterally.

Anticonvulsants inhibit or control seizures. The most commonly used drugs in this category are Klonopin, which is used orally to prevent petit mal seizures, and Dilantin, which is administered orally or parenterally to treat grand mal seizures.

Antidepressants act as serotonin uptakes in the brain. The most commonly used drugs that are categorized as antidepressants are Prozac and Zoloft. Other antidepressants, such as Elavil, act on the serotonin and norepinephrine. Antidepressants generally take a month or longer to work. In addition, they can be addictive, and they frequently react negatively with other drugs.

Antidiarrheal drugs control the gastrointestinal distress that frequently results from bacterial infections, the administration of other medications, or radiation therapy treatments. Two examples of antidiarrheal drugs are Lomotil and Imodium.

Antiemetics prevent nausea and vomiting, especially if they are given before symptoms develop. These are frequently used to alleviate side effects of chemotherapy and radiation therapy. Commonly used antiemetics include Compazine, Phenergan, and Tigan.

Antihistamines are usually used to treat allergies but can also be found in cold remedies and motion sickness tablets. Because many drugs trigger allergic reactions in susceptible patients, antihistamines are frequently administered to patients before surgery. Benadryl, Phenergan, and Chlor-Trimeton are common antihistamines.

Antihypertensives lower the blood pressure. Catapres, Lopresor, and Serpasil are all antihypertensives. Hypertension can become a factor in most medical procedures, thereby making this drug category relevant to all health care disciplines.

Antiinflammatory drugs reduce inflammation. Although they do not work as quickly as corticosteroids they may have fewer side effects. Commonly used antiinflammatory drugs include Motrin, Feldene and Naprosyn.

Antineoplastic drugs are chemotherapeutic agents used by oncologists to treat tumors. Chemotherapy, a treatment modality that uses antineoplastic drugs, can be extremely aggressive and cause adverse side effects. Chapter 8 discusses antineoplastic drugs in greater detail.

Antiseptics, although not actually drugs because they are not taken internally, are used externally to sterilize equipment and intravenous sites and to prevent infection. Alcohol and Betadine are commonly used antiseptics.

Contrast media enhance the visibility of internal tissues for diagnostic imaging. Oncologists depend on these agents in order to pinpoint target areas for radiation therapy treatments.[1,5,8,15]

Corticosteroids reduce inflammation and are sometimes used to treat adrenal deficiency. Common examples of corticosteroids are Decadron and Solu-Cortef.

Diuretics remove fluid from the cells. They are used to treat edema and are often used with antihypertensives to lower blood pressure. Fluids and electrolytes must be watched closely for imbalance whenever diuretics are used. Commonly used diuretics include Diamox, Diuril, and Lasix.

Hormones are used to augment endocrine secretion. Estrogen (Premarin) is given to females; methyltestosterone (Metandren) is given to males. This category of drugs can also be used to treat neoplastic conditions in the opposite sex. Insulin is a hormone commonly used to treat diabetes. Synthroid is a hormone commonly used to treat thyroid disorders.

Narcotics are federally controlled substances that relax the central nervous system and relieve pain. Some examples include codeine, Demerol, and morphine.

Radioactive isotopes that are used in nuclear medicine as diagnostic imaging agents include technetium 99m and iodine 131. Radioactive isotopes that are used in radiation therapy for therapeutic purposes include phosphorus 32 and strontium 89.

Sedatives can calm anxious patients and relax the central nervous system, thereby inducing sleep or unconsciousness. Barbiturates, such as seconal and Nembutal, can be addictive. Examples of nonbarbiturate sedatives include Ativan, Benadryl, and Versed. Chloral hydrate is the sedative most often used to sedate children.

Skin agents are used to keep the skin soft and supple while reducing the pain and itching caused by erythema. Some examples include hydrocortisone 1%, Aquaphor, and Eucerin.[6]

Tranquilizers relieve anxiety. Two examples are Librium and Valium.

CONTRAST MEDIA

Some departments do not administer contrast agents. However, with such emerging technology as computed tomography simulation, contrast media is becoming increasingly important.

Contrast agents allow the oncologist to enhance the visibility of soft tissue and other areas with low natural contrast. Each diagnostic imaging examination has unique requirements, and every oncology department has its own protocols for the imaging procedures that are performed. The following are fundamental principles that every therapist needs to understand whenever dealing with radiographic contrast media.

Types of contrast agents

The two basic categories of contrast agents are negative (radiolucent) and positive (radiopaque).[1,5,15] Radiolucent agents have low atomic numbers and, as a result, are easily penetrated by x-rays. The spaces containing these compounds (usually in the form of gases) appear dark on the radiographs. Air and carbon dioxide are the most common negative contrast media. Air alone can sometimes provide sufficient contrast for radiography of the larynx or other parts of the upper respiratory system.

Radiopaque agents have high atomic numbers and absorb x-ray photons, so the spaces filled with these agents appear opaque on the film. For some procedures, negative and positive contrast media are given together to demonstrate certain internal structures. For example, diagnostic tests of the stomach and large intestine usually use barium sulfate combined with air or carbon dioxide as the contrast media.

Heavy metal salt

Barium sulfate, a heavy metal salt, is the most commonly used contrast agent for gastrointestinal tract examinations.[1,5,15] This contrast agent is delivered orally or rectally in an aqueous (water-based solution) suspension. Barium

sulfate coats the lining of the alimentary organs, and because it is radiopaque the contrast is extremely high. Hazards and inconveniences with the use of barium sulfate are that it requires additives to facilitate ingestion and prevent clumping and it must be concentrated to coat the organs. However, if it is too thick, barium sulfate will not flow easily and is difficult to swallow. Barium sulfate can irritate the colon and cause cramping and can stimulate the body to absorb too much fluid, thus leading to hypervolemia or pulmonary edema. Barium sulfate can cause peritonitis if used in patients with a perforation of the colon or vaginal rupture, and constipation. If preexisting conditions contraindicate the use of barium sulfate, oncologists will prescribe water-soluble iodides instead.

Organic iodides

As with barium sulfate, iodine atoms have been proved to be one of the best contrast elements for imaging. Iodine atoms attach to water-soluble carrier molecules or oil-based ethyl esters and dispatch to certain areas of the body. These atoms then displace water in the cells and absorb x-ray photons in those regions.

Most of the conventional, older compounds are highly toxic ionic iodine agents. These compounds are ionic because their molecules split into two particles (i.e., one negatively charged particle and the other positively charged) whenever they come in contact with body fluids. This splitting results in twice as many iodine particles going into solution in the plasma. The chemical structure of these particles pulls water from the cells, and because so many of the offending particles exist, the fluid balance of the body may be severely affected. The **ionic contrast media** are said to have **high osmolality**, a high number of particles in solution.[1] The large amount of iodine provides greater contrast but also increases toxicity and viscosity. The most common ionic iodides used are meglumine iodine salts and various sodium iodine salts.

The charged ions are irritants and can cause allergic reactions. **Nonionic contrast media** have been developed for this reason. Nonionic contrast media has **low osmolality**, the iodides remain intact instead of splitting, and therefore they agitate the cells less. No charged ions are introduced into the body. These agents are equally effective but cost much more than ionic agents, so some oncology departments reserve them for allergy-prone patients. Two common nonionic contrast agents are iopamidol and iohexol.

Some contrast agents have characteristics of ionic and nonionic agents (called *ionic dimers*); they have low osmolality because the molecules are larger and do not have an osmotic (water-moving) effect, but they split and are therefore still ionic.[1,15] An example of this type of contrast agent is sodium meglumine ioxaglate.

Iodinated contrast media are generally viscous, especially at room temperature. This causes discomfort to the patient, although the discomfort can be eased somewhat by heating the solution to body temperature before injection. Some iodinated contrast media are so viscous that they are best injected by a power injector.

The three aforementioned iodides are all aqueous. Iodinated contrast media can also be oil based. Oil-based agents do not dissolve in water and therefore stay in the body longer. They are unstable and decompose if exposed to light or heat. They are also difficult to disseminate. Propyliodine, used for bronchography, is an oil-based compound.

ABSORPTION AND DISTRIBUTION OF CONTRAST MEDIA

Each type of radiographic imaging requires specific contrast media and sometimes a sophisticated route of delivery. Intravenously injected media display a rapid, systemic absorption level. Direct injection of contrast media allows optimal imaging of the organ or joint before the media are absorbed into the bloodstream and excreted. If the intestinal tract is being imaged, ionic contrast media cause increased fluid in the intestines and improve intestinal contractions (peristalsis), thereby producing a better image.

Radiographic imaging of the gallbladder may be performed after the patient swallows contrast media tablets. These tablets travel through the stomach and small intestine, continue through the blood to the liver, are absorbed into the bile, and are finally sent into storage in the gallbladder. This procedure normally takes 12 hours and may require 24 hours with an additional dose of tablets. The contrast media may be inhibited by dysfunction of any of the organs involved. In many situations, ultrasound imaging of the gallbladder first obviates the need for diagnostic x-ray images and contrast media and then yields instant results.

Certain procedures, such as urography (pyelography), involve a timed sequence of radiographs taken as the contrast agent progresses through the urinary system.[1,5,15] When myelography is performed with water-soluble media, the body absorbs the media rapidly, and images must be made immediately after an injection.

The most efficient and least toxic use of contrast media requires the patient to comply with preparation instructions such as fasting and enemas, which ensure diagnostic-quality images by using the least amount of contrast media. This requires an accurate patient history to avoid unnecessary adverse reactions, as well as the optimum dose being given by the correct route so that the distribution and metabolism of the contrast media illuminate the desired area. Table 20-1 shows some of the common procedures performed with contrast media.

Metabolic elimination of contrast media

Radiology is invasive whenever large volumes of foreign materials must be introduced into the body to facilitate imaging. Contrast media are not drugs in the curative sense; they are nontherapeutic, toxic substances.

Aqueous contrast agents generally absorb quickly into the bloodstream and are excreted through the kidneys. Because of their osmotic action, ionic media significantly change the body's metabolism. In some instances, ionic media dehydrate the cells; in other situations the vascular system becomes overhydrated. The metabolism of ionic agents should be monitored carefully. IV fluids, which may be essential for dehydrated cells, can cause damage if the vascular system is overhydrated.[5]

Excretion of contrast media usually occurs through the kidneys. Extravasation, or accidental leakage into the surrounding tissues, may require the media to be suctioned surgically. Bronchial media can usually be expelled by coughing; large volumes of aqueous media found in the bladder or kidneys may be drained by a catheter.

Patient reactions to contrast media

Water displaced by the osmotic action of iodine particles in the plasma is forced into cells or drawn to specific areas. The excess fluid can saturate and distend the blood vessels, inundate the vascular system and cause hypovolemia, or cause shock by withdrawing too much water from the vessels. The osmostic action of ionic molecules can also cause dramatic fluctuations in kidney function. These fluctuations in function can be counteracted by giving IV fluids. Ionic iodine compounds can provoke allergic reactions ranging from **urticaria** (hives) to anaphylactic shock in susceptible patients.

Nonionic media or water-soluble ionics are toxic to the kidneys. Patients with renal disease, diabetes, allergies, asthma, sickle cell anemia, thyroid disease, pregnancy, old age, hypertension, or coronary disease may suffer life-threatening reactions to contrast agents and should be carefully evaluated. Children and older adults are often unable to tolerate the dehydration caused by ionic contrast media.

If a patient is going to react to contrast media, the reaction usually happens very quickly (i.e., within a few minutes of administration of the compound). The therapist must be alert and able to recognize the danger signs of anaphylactic shock, pulmonary edema, asthma attack, or cardiac arrest, and the therapist must be ready to take immediate remedial action. Nonthreatening reactions such as mild nausea, diarrhea, urticaria, dry mouth, headache, anxiety, chills, and itching can be handled by supportive communication and general patient care.

ROUTES OF DRUG ADMINISTRATION

General information regarding the numerous routes of administration and the effects of each can be found in clinical textbooks.[1,4,5,7,9,10,13-15,17] The following four administration routes are particularly important for radiation therapy and radiologic imaging: oral, mucous membrane, topical, and parenteral.

Radiation therapy patients receive specific medications before and after the radiation treatments. Medications

Table 20-1	Common diagnostic imaging procedures that use constrast media	
Procedure	**Route of administration**	**Contrast agent**
Angiography (cardiac, renal, cerebral, and thoracic)	Intraarterial	Diatrizoate meglumine 60% Diatrizoate sodium 50% Iopamidol 61.2% Iohexol
Arthrography	Direct injection	Diatrizoate meglumine 60% Sodium meglumine ioxaglate Air
Bronchography	Intratracheal catheter	Propyliodone oil
Cholangiography	IV	Iodipamide meglumine 10.3% Diatrizoate sodium 50%
Cholecystography	Oral	Ipodate sodium (500 mg) Iopanic acid (500 mg)
Computed tomography	IV injection or infusion	Ioversol 68% Diatrizoate meglumine 60% Iohexol
Cystography	Urinary catheter	Iothalamate meglumine 17% Iothalamate sodium 17% Diatrizoate meglumine 17%
Discography	Direct injection	Diatrizoate meglumine 60% Diatrizoate sodium 60%
Esophography	Oral	Barium sulfate 30% - 50%
Hysterosalpingography	Cervical injection	Iothalamate meglumine 60%
Lymphography	Direct injection	Ethiodized oil
MRI	IV injection	Gadolinium
Myelography	Intrathecal (lumbar puncture)	Iohexol
Pyelography	Instillation via catheter	Diatrizoate meglumine 20% Diatrizoate sodium 20% Methiodal sodium 20%
Sialography	Catheter	Iothalamate meglumine 60%
Splenoportography	Percutaneous injection Catheter	Diatrizoate meglumine 60% Diatrizoate sodium 50% Sodium meglumine ioxaglate
Upper and lower GI	Oral/rectal	Barium sulfate
Urography and nephrography	IV injection	Diatrizoate meglumine 60% Iodamide meglumine 24% Sodium meglumine ioxaglate Iohexol
Venography	IV injection	Ioxaglate meglumine Ioxaglate sodium Diatrizoate meglumine 60%

IV, Intravenous; *MRI,* magnetic resonance imaging; *GI,* gastrointestinal.

administered before radiation treatments are for sedation and diagnostic purposes; medications given after radiation treatments are palliative (i.e., for relief of distressing symptoms). Therapists must clearly understand the way to administer medications, whether their knowledge is firsthand or as a supporting role. The remainder of this chapter discusses specific ways to administer drugs and the resultant patient care.

Oral administration

The oral route of administration is safe, simple, and convenient for the patient and caregiver. Drugs taken by mouth absorb slowly into the bloodstream and are less potent but longer lasting than drugs given by injection.[1,5,7,9,10,13-15] The risk of infection is also less from oral administration than from any other route. Some patients are unable to take oral preparations because of vomiting or nausea, unconsciousness, intubation, required fasting before tests or surgery, difficulty swallowing, or refusal to cooperate. The latter two occurrences are especially common with children.

In radiation therapy, some types of contrast media used for pretreatment diagnosis *must* be administered orally.[1,5,13] Palliative medications administered after the therapy are frequently given by mouth. Whenever oral medications are given, the caregiver should do the following:

1. Wash the hands.
2. Read the label and medication order before and after preparing the dose.
3. Identify the patient.
4. Check for allergies.
5. Assess the patient by recording vital signs.
6. Prepare the medicine accurately without touching it.
7. Confirm the order with the physician.
8. Give water or other more palatable liquid, such as ice chips, orange juice, or a strong-tasting chaser, if indicated.
9. Elevate the patient's head.
10. Observe and ensure that the medicine is swallowed.
11. Discard medication paraphernalia.
12. Rewash the hands.
13. Record the medication administration in the patient's chart.

Some physicians encourage self-administration of drugs. However, the therapist should be aware that depressed patients in particular may hide and store drugs for later suicide attempts.

Mucous membrane administration

Some drugs cannot be given orally because gastric secretions inactivate the medications or because the drugs have a bad taste or odor, damage teeth, or cause gastric distress. If a drug has one of these potential side effects, it can be given via mucous membranes by suppository in the rectum, urethra, or vagina.

Some medications can be inhaled in a medicated mist, directly applied by swabbing or gargling, or administered by irrigating the target tissue by flushing the tissue with sterile or medicated fluid. Some medications can be instilled by drops into a body cavity. For example, in pyelography the drops are instilled into the ureters via catheters. Medications can also be dissolved under the tongue by sublingual administration. All these methods have a systemic effect, although some affect the system more rapidly than others. Regardless of the route used, the person administering the drug must never compromise sterility by touching the drug directly.

Topical administration

Topical drugs are frequently needed after the skin is disturbed by radiation therapy.[6] Topical applications are used for antiseptics preceding injections, ointments, lotions, as well as for transdermal patches such as patches dispensing scopolamine, estrogen, or nicotine, which must deliver medicine slowly and at a constant level. If the caregiver is administering topical drugs, gloves should be worn to avoid introducing infection and absorption of the medication.

Parenteral administration

Parenteral administration means that the medication bypasses the gastrointestinal tract. Taken literally, this includes the topical and some mucous membrane routes, but the word *parenteral* colloquially means "by injection."

A drug administered parenterally is absorbed rapidly and efficiently; none of the drug is destroyed by digestive enzymes, so the dosage is usually smaller.[13-15,17] Medications are administered parenterally in the following situations: (1) the drug would irritate the alimentary tract too much to be taken orally; (2) a rapid effect is needed, such as during an emergency; (3) drugs need to be dispensed intravenously over time; and (4) the patient is unconscious or otherwise unable to take oral medications (e.g., if the patient is fasting, nil per os [NPO] or nothing by mouth, is given before surgery or tests).

Parenteral administration carries with it the danger of infection from piercing the skin and an increased risk of unrecoverable error because of rapid absorption. Injections also cause genuine fear in some patients. Injection sites can also become damaged from long-term parenteral therapy.

Parenteral administration is categorized by the depth of the injection and location of the injection site (Fig. 20-1). The following are the four most common parenteral routes[15]:

1. **Intradermal**—a shallow injection between the layers of the skin
2. **Subcutaneous**—a 45- or 90-degree injection into the subcutaneous tissue just below the skin
3. **Intramuscular**—a 90-degree injection into the muscle used for larger amounts or a quicker systemic effect
4. **Intravenous**—an injection directly into the bloodstream that provides an immediate effect

The therapist will inevitably be a member of a health care team that administers drugs by less common parenteral routes as well. Other routes pertaining to radiation oncology include the following: (1) intrathecal administration, in which medications are injected directly into the spinal canal, such as contrast media or chemotherapeutic agents; (2) intratracheal administration, in which medications are administered directly into the trachea; (3) intracranial administration, in which medications are administered directly into the brain; and (4) catheterization, which includes urinary catheterization.[6] The administration of drugs by these routes is performed by the physician or anesthesiologist with the therapist acting as a support person.

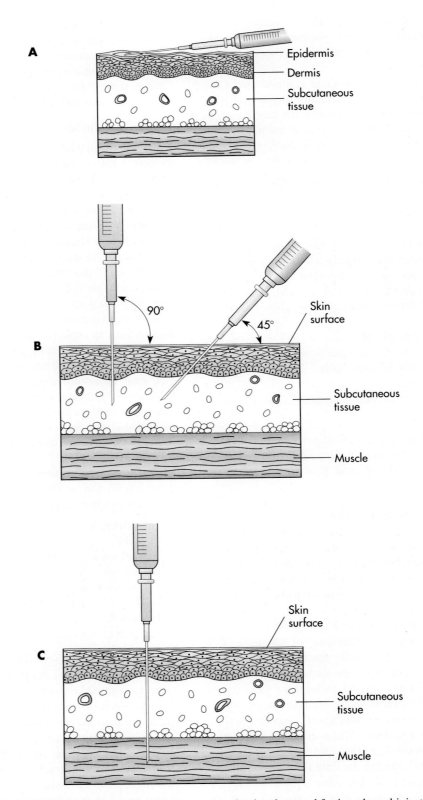

Fig. 20-1 A, The syringe is positioned almost parallel to the skin with the bevel pointed upward for intradermal injections. The medication is deposited right under the skin, forming a small, raised area. **B,** The syringe is positioned at a 45- or 90-degree angle to the skin for subcutaneous injections. The medication is deposited in the subcutaneous tissue just below the skin. **C,** The syringe is positioned at a 90-degree angle for intramuscular injections. The medication is deposited in the muscular area just below the subcutaneous tissue.

IV ADMINISTRATION

Of the four parenteral routes, the IV route is the one most often used by therapists. IV injections, or **venipuncture,** are within the scope of practice for radiation therapists in most states.[2] This technique is best learned by hands-on experience.

From the patient's viewpoint, the therapist should have error-free preparation, appropriate equipment, flawless venipuncture technique, and a caring bedside manner. Even if all these requirements are met, venipuncture is still hazardous. The therapist administering drugs through an IV route must never leave the patient alone during the procedure but must continuously monitor the patient.

Different methods of IV administration serve different purposes. The safest method is continuous infusion, in which the medication is mixed with a large volume of IV solution and given gradually over time. The drug can be piggybacked onto the main IV line by means of a special valve so that the medication can be administered intermittently at prescribed levels.[9,10,13-15] The caregiver lowers the volume of IV fluid administered while the drug is infused; this usually takes less than an hour. Then the volume is restored to the primary level.

If a patient needs intermittent medication but not a continuous fluid IV, the caregiver can use a heparin lock. With the use of a heparin lock, a catheter is inserted into the vein and anchored to the patient's arm. The drug can be infused through this port. The tube is then sealed off whenever it is not in use. The advantage of a heparin lock is that the vein is only punctured once.

A third method of IV injection is a bolus, or push, of a concentrated dose of medication injected by a syringe directly into the vein or through the IV port. This method requires diligent observation of the patient because the effect is rapid and can be irreversible.

Administering bolus injections

Certain medications, including contrast media, must be administered at full strength. If the patient has an IV line in place, the therapist must temporarily stop the IV flow while the bolus is injected to avoid mixing the solutions. However, the IV line should remain in place because radiopaque materials are highly toxic, and when reactions happen quickly, the patient IV line allows the patient to receive immediate remedial treatment.

After the same preliminaries (i.e., checking the medication, identifying the patient, washing the hands) are completed, the bolus of medicine can be injected. The injection port of the catheter should be wiped with alcohol or the heparin lock should be flushed with sterile saline, and then the drug may be slowly injected into the port. If the medication enters the vein too quickly, the body may go into speed shock, a severe, life-threatening reaction caused by the toxicity of the drug. The correct rate for injecting the drug should be specified on the package or in the medication order. The catheter should then be rewiped with alcohol or the heparin lock should be flushed and refilled with heparin solution. Only then can the IV flow be restored.

If the medication is to be given as a one-time injection, the drug is prepared in the syringe and attached to the needle; then the medication is injected at the time of venipuncture. This type of medication comes packaged in ampules or vials, each of which has its own specific requirements for use. An ampule contains a single dose of medicine; the tip is snapped off, and the drug is drawn into a syringe through a filter needle. A vial has a rubber stopper, and the needle is inserted through that stopper to draw out the medicine (Fig. 20-2). Usually multidose vials are not used because of possible contamination, but if the vial contains more than one dose, a new needle should be used and the opening of the vial must be wiped with alcohol before every use.

If the medication is not directly delivered by a vein, an IV port (Fig. 20-3, *A* and *B*) may be used. After the port is in place, the therapist or another caregiver can connect the appropriate equipment to the catheter or cannula. Chemotherapy is often administered through a different type of vascular access port such as the Hickman, Groshong, Port-A-Cath, and Infusaid (Fig. 20-3, *C*).[13]

Two major types of IV injections pertain to radiation therapists: drugs requiring dilution and drugs requiring delivery by IV bolus. Most contrast media, if not given orally, are injected by bolus. Drugs that are diluted or solutions for the maintenance of fluid levels are administered slowly by IV drip.

IV infusion and venipuncture equipment

Before the actual venipuncture or injection takes place, the health care professional must gather all the necessary equipment. Interruption of the procedure to find missing equipment is extremely unprofessional and erodes the patient's confidence in the caregiver. The IV equipment can be prepared with the tubing capped and ready to attach before performing the venipuncture or after the IV port is in place. The timing of the preparation depends on institutional policy or the physician's orders.

In the case of an IV drip, such equipment includes IV tubing with a clamp on it, the vacoliter or plastic drip bag, a stand on which to hang the bag of solution, an IV filter, and a meter to measure the flow rate. The most common place for sterility to be compromised is in the two ends of the tubing; neither the end going into the sterile solution nor the end connecting with the IV catheter should *ever* be touched, even with gloves.[1,5,7,9,11,14,17] If either end is inadvertently touched, it must be sterilized before use or discarded and replaced.

IV equipment varies according to the drug and dosage. The equipment tray should include a tourniquet, antiseptic swabs, gloves, a syringe, a needle, cotton balls, the correct drug, and adhesive bandages. Any catheters, tubing, drip bot-

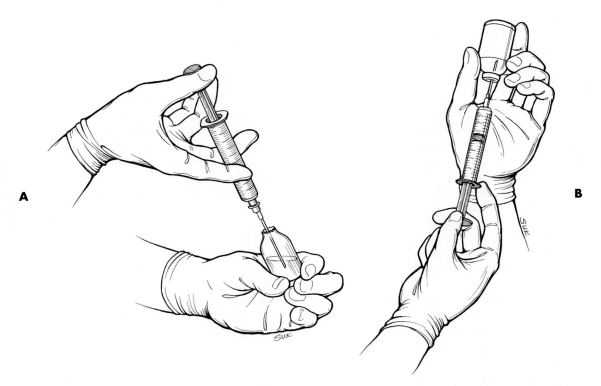

Fig. 20-2 **A,** This drawing shows the way to remove the medication from an ampule. The medication is removed by pulling back on the plunger of the syringe. The therapist should be careful not to contaminate the needle when inserting and removing the needle from the ampule. **B,** This drawing shows the removal of medication from a vial. The rubber stopper must be cleaned with alcohol before the needle is inserted into the vial. The same amount of air must be injected into vial as will be withdrawn to equalize the pressure in the vial.

tles, poles, and monitors required should also be in place before the procedure begins.

The type of medication and physical characteristics of the patient determine which instrument should be used for IV injection. For a one-time injection of 30 ml or less, a regular needle (i.e., 18 to 20 gauge, depending on the viscosity of the drug and size of the patient's veins) and a syringe should suffice. An infusion that takes place over a longer time requires a butterfly set, which is a special steel needle attached to two plastic "wings" taped to the skin. This butterfly set anchors the needle in the vein.

Whenever the infusion requires a large volume of fluid or needs to be administered over an extremely long period of time, a plastic catheter can be inserted into the vein. Because the tubing is flexible and soft, it allows the patient to move around and is less irritating than a rigid, metal needle. Two kinds of venous catheters exist; one is a narrow tube inserted through a hollow needle, and the other has the needle through the tube. The through-the-needle catheter is generally longer and thinner and can be inserted deeper into the vein. This type of catheter is commonly used for antineo-

plastic drugs. After the catheter is in place and taped down, the needle is removed.

Dosage, dose calculation, and dose response

Medication charts list standard measurements (i.e., metric or apothecary), their abbreviations, and recommended doses for most common medicines. Table 20-2 lists common abbreviations used for prescribing medications.[5,10,17] Health care personnel must invariably calculate individual doses for their patients if the standard packaging differs from the amount ordered. To calculate the quantity ordered, the therapist or nurse must multiply or divide the dose required by the packaged amount to make sure the two are in the same unit of measurement. The math should *always* be double-checked.

Doses for children should be calculated according to the child's weight or body surface area. The latter is more accurate because it also takes into account the child's height and body density.[10,13] Although the specifics of dose calculation are beyond the scope of this chapter, a good nursing or pediatrics text will explain the way to compute the correct dose.

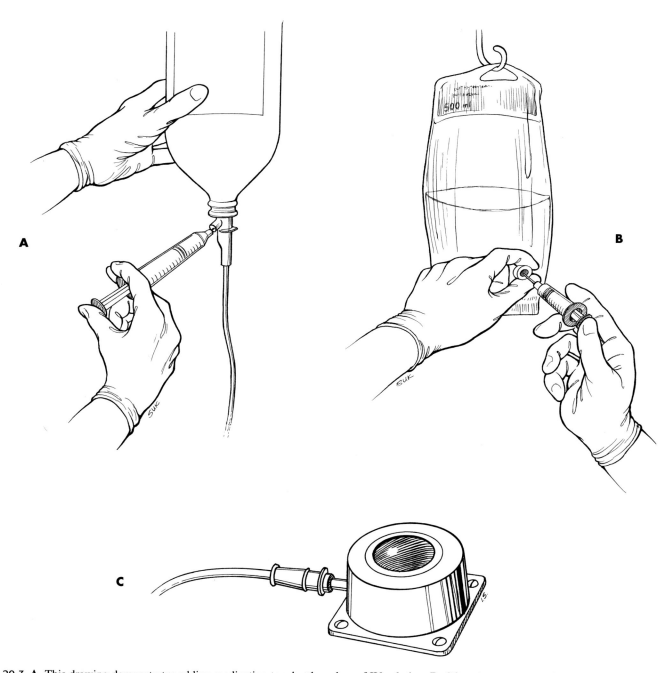

Fig. 20-3 A, This drawing demonstrates adding medication to a bottle or bag of IV solution. **B,** Often there are ports closer to the needle insertion site where a bolus of medication can be injected. **C,** Chemotherapy is often administered through a vascular access port.

Table 20-2	Common abbreviations used for prescribing medications
Abbreviation	**Meaning**
a.c.	Before meals
bid	Twice a day
h	Hour
h.s.	At bedtime
IM	Intramuscular
IV	Intravenous
ml	Milliliter
p.c.	After meals
PO	By mouth
p.r.n.	As necessary
q	Every
q3h, q4h, and so on	Every 3 hours, every 4 hours, and so on
qd	Every day
qh	Hourly
qid	Four times each day
qod	Every other day
stat	At once
SC/Subq	Subcutaneous
tid	Three times a day

Whenever drugs are administered by IV, the dosages must be calculated according to the total volume of fluid the patient receives (except in the case of a bolus injection). This calculation must be carefully monitored because flow and absorption rates can fluctuate. Also, the drug must be given in the correct dilution, at the appropriate rate, and in the correct amount. Controlling the dosage in single injections or piggyback deliveries is easier than in long-term IV treatment.

Many factors can affect the delivery rate of an IV injection. The flow can be interrupted by a kink in the tubing, a clot in the needle or catheter, the needle tip pressing against the vein wall, or a problem at the site of entry. The drip rate may depend on the patient's absorption rate, which always varies greatly from one person to another. Sudden fluctuations in flow rates happen frequently because of mechanical problems with the equipment or because the patient dislodges the catheter. All these factors influence the accuracy of delivery whenever drugs are infused intravenously.

Initiation of IV therapy

Patient education. Before any IV drugs are administered, therapists should identify themselves to the patient, assess the patient's condition, and explain the procedure. Assessment involves taking an allergic history or reading the patient's chart if a history has already been taken, taking the blood pressure for a baseline reading, determining whether the patient has had any medication that affects blood clotting, and asking the patient (not the nurse) whether the patient has been fasting.[1,7,8,10,14,15,17]

The therapist must educate the patient by explaining the procedure. The physician is responsible for explaining the reason the procedure is needed; the therapist can ease any anxiety the patient may have by describing the process and answering questions. Iodinated contrast media can produce adverse reactions within minutes after being administered, so the therapist must explain the symptoms and the way that the patient should handle these symptoms *before* administering the drug.

Infusion of medication. The procedure[1,5,7,9,11,13,14,17] for starting a drip infusion after venipuncture has been performed and an IV line is in place is as follows:

1. Wash the hands.
2. Assess the patient. Ask the patient about allergies to drugs.
3. Triple-check the physician's orders against the solution label.
4. Check the bag or vacoliter for an expiration date, signs of contamination (such as discoloration, cloudiness, or sediment), and cracks or leaks.
5. Put on gloves. Use safety glasses if required by the institution.
6. Remove the metal cap and rubber diaphragm from the bottle or bag without touching the rubber stopper.
7. Close the clamp on the tubing, attach the in-line filter, and insert the spike of the drip chamber into the rubber stopper without touching the sterile end.
8. Invert the fluid container and hang it on an IV pole 18 to 24 inches above the vein.
9. Release the clamp, remove the cap covering the lower end of tubing, and allow the fluid to flow through the tube to get rid of air bubbles. (If air is left in the tubing, it will be forced into the vein.) Close the clamp.
10. Recap the lower end of the tubing until venipuncture is complete.
11. Discard paraphernalia according to institutional policy.
12. Remove the gloves and rewash the hands.
13. Record the drug administration in the patient's chart.

Site selection for venipuncture

The site chosen for venipuncture depends on the drug to be administered and the length of time the IV line will be in place (Fig. 20-4, *A*). The large antecubital vein is convenient for drawing blood or for injecting a single dose or viscous solution, but this vein is inappropriate for a long-term IV therapy because it hinders the patient's mobility. The best choices for long-term infusion include sites above the anterior wrist (lower cephalic, accessory cephalic, and basilic veins) or veins on the posterior hand (basilic, metacarpal, and cephalic veins) (Fig. 20-4, *B*).[10] If the patient is right-handed, putting the IV line into the left arm allows the patient to use the dominant arm.

Certain contraindications at a specific venipuncture site mean that a different site should be chosen. These contraindications include scar tissue or hematoma that necessitates injection above this site, infection or skin lesions that could introduce infection into the bloodstream, burns, col-

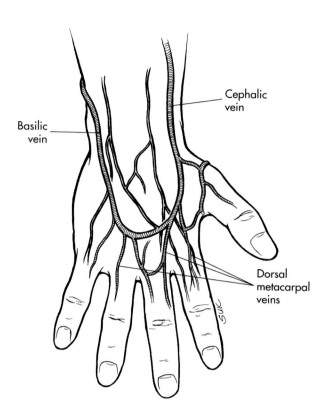

A

Accessory
cephalic
vein

Cephalic
vein

Radial
vein

Antecubital
vein

Medial
cubital
vein

Basilic
vein

Antebrachial
vein

B

Basilic
vein

Cephalic
vein

Dorsal
metacarpal
veins

Fig. 20-4 **A,** Venipuncture sites of the forearm. **B,** Venipuncture sites of the wrist and hand.

lapsed veins, or veins too small for the chosen gauge of the needle. Special techniques apply if a patient has rolling veins, has **phlebitis,** is on dialysis, or is extremely obese. If the patient is taking blood thinners, extra compression is needed.

Venipuncture technique

The venipuncture may be performed after the preliminaries, such as patient identification, collection of supplies, and patient assessment, are completed. The procedure[11] is as follows:

1. Position the patient. The patient should be sitting or lying down, and the arm should be placed in a relaxed position. The arm may need to be anchored to an arm board if the patient is extremely active.

2. Wash the hands and put on gloves. All **universal precautions** should be followed because of potential contact with body fluids. These precautions include wearing gloves, a mask, and protective eyewear; properly handling needles; and disposing of used equipment into containers for biohazardous material.

3. Apply the tourniquet tightly in a way that it can be removed with one hand. The tourniquet should be about 2 to 4 inches above the puncture site.

4. Choose a vein. It may be necessary to tap or stroke the vein or to have the patient make a fist to enhance distention of the vein (Fig. 20-5).

5. Apply an antiseptic by using a circular motion to cleanse the venipuncture site. If local anesthetic is being used, inject it intradermally at this time.

6. Anchor the vessel by placing the thumb about 1 inch below the puncture site and pulling the skin taut. This will prevent the vein from "rolling."

7. Insert the needle parallel to the vein, bevel side up, at a 30-degree angle, and then flatten the needle to a 10- to 15-degree angle. If the angle is too shallow, the needle will skim between the skin and vein; if the angle is too deep, the needle will penetrate the posterior wall of the vein and cause bleeding into the tissues. When blood flows back into the syringe or hub of the cannula, the needle is in the vein. Allowing the blood to fill the hub before attaching tubing ensures that air bubbles are not trapped in the line.

8. Remove the needle from the catheter. Attach the IV tubing or syringe. Release the tourniquet and push the catheter deeper into the vein and up to the hub, if possible.

9. Place an antiseptic swab or patch over the puncture site, and fix the catheter in place with adhesive tape.

10. Attach the IV tube, release the clamp, and start the infusion. Monitor the flow until the desired rate is established.

11. Discard paraphernalia according to institutional policy.

12. Remove the gloves and rewash the hands.

13. Record the medication procedure in the patient's chart.

Hazards of IV fluids

Perhaps the biggest challenge of administering drugs intravenously is to get the drug into the vein without introducing foreign microorganisms that can cause infection. No one should ever touch the fluid ports, needle, ends of tubing, or any other part of the equipment through which germs could pass into the bloodstream. Diligent observation of the venipuncture site allows the caregiver to recognize symptoms of sepsis at its earliest stage.

IV infusion carries unique hazards with it. Any swelling around the injection site accompanied by cool, pale skin and possibly hard patches or localized pain is a sign of **infiltration.** This can occur if the catheter or IV needle has pulled out of the vein and the fluid has seeped into the adjacent subcutaneous tissue. Infiltration can also occur if the IV bottle is hung too high, the hydrostatic pressure is so great that the vein cannot absorb the fluid quickly enough, and the fluid

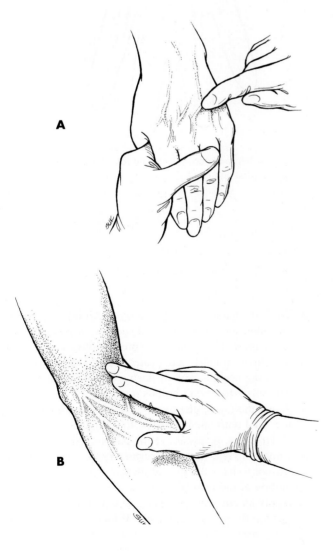

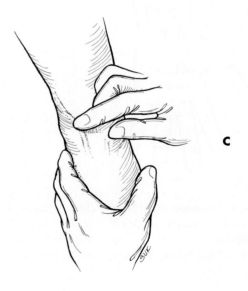

Fig. 20-5 Techniques to distend veins include tapping the vein (**A**), gently stroking the vein (**B**), and having the patient make a fist (**C**).

saturates the surrounding tissue. If the therapist mistakenly misses the vein and injects contrast media into the tissues surrounding the vein, the result is a similar condition called **extravasation,** which is not only painful but can cause severe tissue damage.[9,10,13,14,17]

Other hazards to IV infusion include an allergic reaction to the drug, an air embolism caused by failing to eliminate air bubbles in the equipment, a metabolic or an electrolyte imbalance, edema caused by the dressing being too tight at the site or too much fluid, speed shock from too rapid a delivery, drug incompatibility, thrombus (blood clots), and phlebitis. Phlebitis can be avoided if the needle is a small enough gauge that the blood can flow around it. Nevertheless, any time veins are invaded or the bloodstream is opened to the air, inflammation and blood clots are potential hazards. A keep vein open (KVO) drip keeps the blood from clotting at the site; likewise, the heparin in a heparin lock prevents the injection site and bloodstream from developing clots.

Sudden increases in fluid volume introduced by IV equipment can accidentally occur. If the patient is extremely frail or has a head trauma, a sudden overload can be fatal. Any time fluid is infused too quickly, the excess can collect in the lungs, thereby causing pulmonary edema. Rapid infusion can also result in an overdose of the medication. Too little fluid may result in dehydration or an insufficient dose of the required medication. These are only a few of the reasons that monitoring IV lines closely is crucial.

Discontinuation of IV therapy

Because the potential for contamination is so high in IV therapy, the infusion set should be changed every 24 to 48 hours. If IV therapy must be continued for a longer period of time, changing to a new venipuncture site may be necessary, depending on the condition of the original site. Most of the drugs that therapists administer are infused over a short period of time, through a single site.

To remove the IV line, the therapist needs to gather the following supplies: sterile gauze pads (or bandages), gloves, tape, and a tourniquet. After the patient has been properly identified, these steps[1,10] should be followed to discontinue IV therapy:

1. Wash the hands.
2. Clamp off the IV tubing and remove the tape holding the catheter in place.
3. Put on gloves.
4. Remove the needle or catheter along the angle at which it was inserted.
5. Press a gauze pad immediately over the puncture site until the bleeding stops. Before taping the gauze or applying a bandage, inspect the site to make sure no artifacts, such as broken catheters or bits of dressing, are left in the wound. If they are, tie the tourniquet above the wound, and call the physician.
6. After the wound is clean, apply a bandage.
7. Dispose of the IV materials properly.
8. Rewash the hands.
9. Record the appropriate information in the patient's chart.

LEGAL ASPECTS

First and foremost, the scope of practice for radiation therapists includes the delivery of radiation to treat disease. It also requires patient care, including comfort, dignity, education, monitoring, and documentation.[2] Increasingly, the practice of venipuncture and the administration of IV medications and contrast media are also included.

The therapist may not legally diagnose, interpret radiographs, reveal test results to patients or family members, prescribe drugs, admit or discharge patients, or order tests. Those duties belong to the physician. The therapist, like every health care professional, is legally required to report incidents or errors and is allowed to act without liability in an emergency if no other care is available (the Good Samaritan laws).

The therapist is legally liable for administering competent treatments and accurately communicating with the patient. The two most common complaints leading to malpractice suits in radiology and oncology are false-negative or false-positive diagnoses of fractures or cancers and the misadministration of contrast media.[3] The oncologist does not bear these risks alone. The radiation therapist is part of the team and on the front line of patient care.

Although radiation oncology team members cannot be held accountable for poor health results, they are liable if they act negligently or cause injury. Because the profession can be so hazardous, it is in everyone's best interest that efforts be taken to communicate *all* risks before any treatment takes place. Every precaution must be taken in the actual treatment of each patient.

Different states have different laws regulating the radiation therapist's scope of practice. Currently, 27 states allow therapists to perform venipuncture. In these states, legal obligations that apply to radiation therapists and are associated with administering drugs and monitoring IV agents exist. Other laws, such as those governing restraint of a patient for diagnostic imaging and dispensing of drugs, may also apply.

Documentation of administration

The medical record is a legal document and is evidence for the caregiver and patient in the event of confusion or litigation.[3,8] Therefore it is in the therapist's best interest to make sure the information in the chart is thorough and accurate. For example, if the patient verbally informs the therapist of a sensitivity to iodine and the therapist fails to pass on the information or record it in the chart, the therapist could be held liable for adverse reactions. A previously documented sensitivity should be apparent in the patient's permanent record, and in this situation the therapist is responsible for noticing and making sure the physician is also aware of the sensitivity.[8]

The patient's chart or medical record is often the primary means of communication among the members of a health care team. Each patient is often treated by several different professionals, all of whom need to know the entire medical history to do their jobs effectively.

Accurate documentation protects the patient from errors in treatment; likewise, accurate documentation protects the caregivers from making procedural, ethical, or legal errors. Every medication, every treatment procedure, every diagnostic test, and even verbal communication should be documented in the patient's permanent medical record.

Although each medical institution is allowed to develop its own system of record keeping, certain standard contents are required by the various accrediting bodies in the medical profession; these include the following:

1. Patient identification and demographic information
2. Medical history, including family history, allergies, and previous illnesses
3. Nature of the current complaint and a report of examinations and treatments.
4. Orders for and results of any tests or procedures
5. Record of all medications, whether self-administered, prescribed, or professionally administered. The information should include but is not limited to time, route, dosage, site of administration, and caregiver's signature
6. Physician's notes, instructions, and conclusions
7. Informed consent form[12]

Documentation of any complications or adverse reactions to a medication is especially critical to the medical record of any patient.[1,3,5,8,10,13] A sensitivity to any medication must be prominently displayed in the patient's record. Remedial action taken to counteract the complication must also be recorded.

The therapist bears the responsibility for understanding the way to read the chart accurately and enter information in the record. A written error should not be erased or "whited-out" but should have a single line drawn through it and initialed (so that the original is legible). The information should be rewritten, dated, and initialed.

Medical records are confidential and may not be released without the patient's consent. Orders of any kind *must* be signed by the attending health care professional.

Informed consent

Radiation therapy and diagnostic imaging require **informed consent** from the patient. In addition to the general consent form the patient signs when entering a health care facility, each radiation therapy procedure requires a separate form in the patient's record.[15]

Especially in cases of radiation administration and ionic contrast media in which the potential risk is so high, a grey area about what constitutes "informed" consent exists. If a patient agrees in writing to receive ionic contrast media but suffers a reaction, the oncologist could be held liable if that oncologist failed to inform the patient that nonionic agents were available. The issue of cost (e.g., nonionic media costs considerably more than ionic media) should not determine how much the physician tells the patient. Open communication about risk and cost are part of the patient's legal rights.

Informed consent expectations and documentation varies by state and institution. Informed consent forms generally include the name of the authorized physician; a description of the procedure and associated medications; an assurance that the purpose, benefit, risk, and any alternative options have been imparted and understood; an area where patients can write in their words what the procedure entails; and a disclaimer, which does not always hold up in court, releasing the caregiver and facility from liability, if complications develop or the treatment fails.

SUMMARY

The technique of venipuncture and assisting in the administration of IV drugs and contrast media are crucial skills required for the practice of radiation therapy. The descriptions in this chapter do not qualify a radiation therapist to perform those actions but are intended only as an overview. The therapist must study the principles of pharmacology and must have hands-on experience before performing these techniques on patients. The therapist who is knowledgeable in all pertinent aspects of drug administration contributes an invaluable service to the success of the radiation therapy team.

Review Questions

Listing

1. List the Five Rights of Drug Safety.

   _____

   _____

   _____

   _____

   _____

Multiple Choice

2. Which of the following is *not* a patient-related variable affecting response to medications?
   a. Weight
   b. Physical condition
   c. Tolerance
   d. Emotional requirements
   e. Age
3. What is the way drugs affect the body?
   a. Pharmacokinetics
   b. Metabolism
   c. Pharmacodynamics
   d. Drug effectiveness
4. Which of the following is *not* a parenteral route of administration for medications?
   a. Subcutaneous
   b. Instillation
   c. Intravenous
   d. Intramuscular
5. The type of drug given to cancer patients to relieve nausea and vomiting is which of the following:
   a. Antacid
   b. Emetic
   c. Cathartic
   d. Antiemetic
6. A combination of two drugs can sometimes cause an effect greater than the sum of the effects of each drug alone. This effect is known as which of the following?
   a. Cumulative effect
   b. Idiosyncratic effect
   c. Synergistic effect
   d. Antagonistic effect

7. The abbreviation *qod* stands for which of the following?
   a. Once daily
   b. Once every other day
   c. Daily
   d. None of the above

Matching

8. Match the following drug categories with its expected action.

   a. _____ Decadron   I. Antiseptic
   b. _____ Hydro-   II. Antidiarrheal
           cortisone 1%   III. Sedative
   c. _____ Dilantin   IV. Skin agent
   d. _____ Betadine   V. Corticosteroid
   e. _____ Xylocaine   VI. Radioactive
   f. _____ Heparin   isotope
   g. _____ Imodium   VII. Diuretic
                                VIII. Analgesic
                                IX. Anticoagulant
                                X. Anesthetic
                                XI. Anticonvulsant

Essay

9. Define *extravasation*.
10. Describe the difference between a side effect from a drug and a complication from a drug.

Questions to Ponder

1. You are charting a dose of medication administered in the oncology department. You recorded the wrong route of administration. You "whiteout" the error and rewrite the appropriate route to correct the record. Is this an acceptable method to correct the record? If not, what is the correct method?

2. Why is following universal precautions during drug administration important?
3. Discuss the importance of parenteral drug administration.
4. Compare the gender differences in the absorption of medications.
5. Analyze the differences between ionic and nonionic contrast media.

REFERENCES

1. Adler AM, Carlton R, editors: *Introduction to radiography and patient care,* Philadelphia, 1994, WB Saunders.
2. American Society of Radiologic Technologists: *Radiation therapist's scope of practice,* Albuquerque, 1993, The Society.
3. Brice J: Imaging and the law: simple tactics minimize exposure to malpractice, *Diagnostic Imaging* 14(3):43-46, 1992.
4. Cosgriff JH, Anderson DL: *The practice of emergency care,* ed 2, Philadelphia, 1984, JB Lippincott.
5. Ehrlich RA, McCloskey ED: *Patient care in radiography,* ed 4, St Louis, 1993, Mosby.
6. Holleb A, Fink DJ, Murphy GP: *Clinical oncology: a multidisciplinary approach for physicians and students,* Atlanta, 1991, The American Cancer Society.
7. Kemp BB, Pillitteri A, Brown P: *Fundamentals of nursing: a framework for practice,* ed 2, Glenview, Ill, 1989, Scott, Foresman.
8. Lucchese DR, Eikman EA: The medical-legal implications of contrast agent use, *Applied Radiology* 18(12):36-37, 1989.
9. Narrow BW, Buschle KB: *Fundamentals of nursing practice,* ed 2, New York, 1987, John Wiley & Sons.
10. Potter PA, Perry AG: *Basic nursing: theory and practice,* St Louis, 1987, Mosby.
11. Roberts GH, Carson J: Venipuncture tips for radiologic technologists, *Radiol Technol* 65(2):107-115, 1993.
12. Schwartz HW: *Current concepts in radiology management,* Sudbury, Mass, 1992, American Healthcare Radiology Administrators.
13. Smith SF, Duell DJ: *Clinical nursing skills: nursing process model basic to advanced skills:* ed 3, Norwalk, Conn, 1992, Appleton & Lange.
14. Taylor C, Lillis C, LeMone P: *Fundamentals of nursing,* Philadelphia, 1989, JB Lippincott.
15. Torres LS: *Basic medical techniques and patient care for radiologic technologists,* ed 4, Philadelphia, 1993, JB Lippincott.
16. Wieck L, King EM, Dyer M: *Illustrated manual of nursing techniques,* ed 3, Philadelphia, 1986, JB Lippincott.
17. Wolff LV et al: *Fundamentals of nursing,* ed 7, Philadelphia, 1983, JB Lippincott.

A

Glossary

ablation The surgical excision or amputation of any part of the body.

accreditation A process of voluntary external peer review, in which a nongovernmental agency grants public recognition to an institution or specialized program of study that meets current qualifications and educational standards. This recognition is determined through initial and subsequent periodic evaluation.

adjuvant A form of therapy used with another therapy.

advocate A supporter who can act as a professor and friend. The advocate assists patients by ensuring that their needs are fulfilled and their rights enforced.

affective Content that may be verbal or nonverbal and comprises feelings, attitudes, and behaviors.

agreement state A state that enters into an agreement with the Nuclear Regulatory Commission to assume the responsibility of enforcing regulations for ionizing radiation.

allergic reaction A reaction resulting from an immunological reaction to a drug to which the patient has already been sensitized.

alopecia A partial or complete lack of hair.

anaphylactic shock A severe reaction (marked by respiratory arrest and vascular shock) to a sensitizing substance such as insect stings, contrast media, and penicillin.

anemia A decrease in the peripheral red cell count.

anesthetic An agent that produces complete or partial loss of sensation with or without loss of consciousness.

anorexia Loss of appetite resulting in weight loss.

antibody A protein substance manufactured by the immune system's plasma cells in a defensive response to the presence of a specific antigen.

antigen A substance or pathogen that is viewed as foreign by a person's immune system and induces the formation of antibodies.

asepsis A condition free from germs.

asymptomatic The absence of symptoms. A patient who does not have or experience symptoms is asymptomatic.

attributable risk Risk that can be linked to a specific disease.

autoclave A device used for sterilization by steam under pressure.

autonomy The quality or state of being self-governing; self-directing freedom, especially moral independence.

barium sulfate Heavy metal salt; the most commonly used contrast agent for examinations of the gastrointestinal tract.

baseline study An initial study performed so that future studies can be compared with the original values.

battery The touching of a person without permission.

beam modifiers Devices that change the shape of the treatment field or distribution of the radiation at depth.

becquerel (Bq) A Standard International (SI) unit of radioactivity that equals 1 disintegration per second.

beneficence The doing or producing of good; acts of kindness and charity.

betatron A megavoltage unit that can provide x-ray and electron therapy beams from less than 6 to more than 40 MeV.

bimodal Occurring with two peaks of incidence. With Hodgkin's disease the disease occurs with greater frequency during the young adult years and then again in the fifth or sixth decade of life.

biopsy The surgical removal of a small tissue sample from a solid tumor to determine the pathology for the diagnosis of disease.

bolus Material whose interaction with radiation (attenuation coefficient) is similar to tissue.

brachytherapy Radiation treatment of disease accomplished by inserting radioactive sources directly into the tumor site.

Bragg peak A sharp increase in the dose distribution curve of a charged particle at a particular depth.

cachexia A state of general ill health and malnutrition with early satiety, electrolyte and water imbalances, and progressive loss of body weight, fat, and muscle.

carfusion A dyelike liquid usually containing silver nitrate and phenol in a fuchsin base; magenta liquid that can be painted onto patients by using thin sticks or swabs.

carrier A person who carries a specific pathogen but is free of signs or symptoms of the disease and yet capable of spreading the disease.

case manager A member of the health care team who is assigned to manage the continuum of care for the patient.

cell cycle The sequence of recurring biochemical and morphological events observed in a population of reproducing cells.

cellular differentiation The degree to which a cell resembles its cell of origin in morphology and function.

certification A process by which a governmental or nongovernmental agency or association grants authority to an individual who has met predetermined qualifications to use a specific title.

cesium A radioactive isotope with a half-life of 30 years that is commonly used as a low-dose brachytherapy source.

chemotherapy The use of chemical agents to induce specific effects on disease.

chromosomes The gene-bearing protein structures in the nucleus of animal cells.

civil law The law that governs relationships between individuals.

cobalt 60 A radioactive isotope with a half-life of 5.26 years that is used as a source for external-beam radiation therapy.

cognitive Pertaining to an individual's basic reasoning processes.

collegial model A cooperative method of pursuing health care for the provider and patient. It involves sharing, trust, and consideration of common goals.

collimation The definition of radiation beam size and dimensions.

colonization The presence of an agent that is infectious but does not initiate an immune response.

colostomy The surgical construction of an artificial excretory opening from the colon on the surface of the abdominal wall.

communication The ability to transfer concrete and abstract information from one person to another person or a group of people while keeping the same meaning. Communication can be verbal, nonverbal, or a combination of the two techniques.

compensator A beam modifier that changes radiation output relative to loss of attenuation over a changing patient contour.

consequentialism The evaluation of an activity by weighing the good against the bad or the way a person can provide the greatest good for the greatest number.

contact therapy unit A machine that operates at potentials of 40 to 50 kV and uses an extremely short source-skin distance.

contractual model A model that maintains a business relationship between the provider and patient; a sharing of information and responsibility.

contrast media High-density substances used radiographically to visualize internal anatomy for diagnostic imaging.

convalescence The period of recovery after an illness.

covenant model A model that deals with an understanding between the patient and health care provider and is based on traditional values and goals.

critical structures Normal tissue whose radiation tolerance limits the deliverable dose.

critical thinking The freedom to use the cognitive process to allow the union of theory and practical experiences to be mastered; the use of learned information to heighten edification through the use of cognitive, affective, and psychomotor domains.

cumulative effect An effect that develops if the body is unable to detoxify and excrete a drug quickly enough or if too large a dose is taken.

curie (Ci) A historical unit of radioactivity that equals 3.7×10^{10} Bq.

curriculum The body of courses and formally established learning experiences presenting the knowledge, principles, values, and skills that are the intended consequences of a program's formal education.

cyclotron A charged particle accelerator used mainly for nuclear research and more recently for generating proton and neutron beams.

cytoplasm All the cellular protoplasm except the nucleus and its contents. It consists of a watery fluid (cytosol) in which numerous organelles are suspended.

cytoxic The ability to kill cancer cells.

D_o A graphic representation of the cell's radiosensitivity.

D_q The quasithreshold dose or a measure of the cell's ability to accumulate and repair sublethal damage.

daily treatment record A document recording the actual treatment delivery.

definitive A course of radiation therapy in which the objective is to cure by eradication of the disease.

deontology The use of formal rules of right and wrong for reasoning and problem solving.

deoxyribonucleic acid (DNA) A large, double-stranded nucleic acid molecule that carries the genetic material of the cell on the chromosomes. This genetic information is composed of a sequence of nitrogen bases and molecular subunits.

depression The perceived loss of self-esteem resulting in a cluster of affective behavioral (e.g., change in appetite, sleep disturbances, lack of energy, withdrawal, and dependency) and cognitive (e.g., decreased ability to concentrate, indecisiveness, and suicidal ideas) responses.

doctrine of foreseeability A principle of law that holds a person liable for all consequences of any negligent acts to another individual to whom a duty is owed and should have been reasonably foreseen under the circumstances.

doctrine of personal liability The doctrine stating that all persons are liable for their own negligent conduct.

doctrine of res ipsa loquitur ("the thing speaks for itself") A doctrine, which is an accepted substitute for the medical expert, requiring the defendant to explain an incident and convince the court that no negligence was involved.

doctrine of respondent superior A legal doctrine that holds an employer liable for negligent acts of employees occuring while they are carrying out their orders or otherwise serving their interests.

domain A group of job activities related on the basis of required skills and knowledge.

dose maximum (D_{max}) The point or depth at which maximum absorbed dose occurs.

droplet nuclei The residual remains of airborne pathogens after the evaporation of moisture.

drug interactions The mutual or reciprocal action or influence between drugs and/or food that can create positive or negative effects in the body.

elapsed days The total time over which treatment is delivered (protracted).

electron shields (cutouts) Collimate and shape electron treatment fields.

electronic portal imaging devices (EPID) A system producing near real-time portal images on a computer screen for evaluation.

electrons Negatively charged subatomic particles that can be accelerated by a variety of machines or are emitted from decaying isotopes and used for external beam treatment and brachytherapy.

empathy Identifying with the feelings, thoughts, or experiences of another person.

en bloc A French term meaning "in one block." In surgical cancer care, it means "in one specimen."

endoplasmic reticulum A continuous membrane in the cellular cytoplasm containing the ribosomes.

engineering model A model that identifies the caregiver as a scientist dealing only in facts and does not consider the human aspect of the patient.

epidemiology The division of medical science concerned with the study of defining the distribution and determinants causing disease and injury in human populations.

ethics The discipline dealing with what is good and bad, with a concern for moral duty and obligations; a set of moral principles or values; a theory or system of moral values; the principles of conduct governing an individual or professional group .

etiology The study of the causes of disease.

excisional biopsy The removal of the entire tumor by cutting it out so that a diagnosis can be made.

exenteration (pelvic) The radical removal of most or all pelvic organs.

extrapolation number (n) Part of a graphic representation of a cell-survival curve, determined by extrapolating the linear portion of the curve back until it intersects the y-axis.

extravasation Accidental leakage into the surrounding tissues; a discharge or escape (e.g., of blood) from a vessel into the tissues.

feathering The migration of a gap between treatment fields through the treatment course.

field size The dimensions of a treatment field at the isocenter (usually represented by width × length).

fomite Any inanimate object (vehicle) involved in the transmission of disease.

fractionation Radiation therapy treatments given in daily fractions (segments) over an extended period of time, sometimes up to 6 to 8 weeks.

free radical An atom or atom group in a highly reactive transient state that is carrying an unpaired electron with no charge.

gamma rays Electromagnetic radiation emitted from decaying isotopes and used for external-beam treatment and brachytherapy.

genome The complete complement of hereditary factors as found on a haploid distribution of chromosomes.

germ theory The hypothesis that microorganisms cause disease.

Golgi apparatus A cytoplasmic organelle consisting of flattened membranes that modify, store, and route products of the endoplasmic reticulum.

grenz ray Low-energy x-rays in the range of 10 to 15 kV.

half-life The time necessary for a radioactive substance to decay to half, or 50% of its original activity.

half-value layer The thickness of absorbing material necessary to reduce the x-ray intensity to half its original value.

hinge angle The measure of the angle between central rays of two intersecting treatment beams.

hospice A program that provides care for patients who have limited life expectancy. The care is provided in the patient's home or a hospital setting.

hypothesis A prediction of the relationship between certain variables.

iatrogenic Disease or illness created as a result of the treatment or diagnosis of another condition.

idiosyncratic response (effects) The inexplicable and unpredictable symptoms caused by a genetic defect in the patient.

immobilization device A device that reproduces the treatment position while restricting movement (i.e., casts, masks, or bite blocks).

immunoglobulin The system of closely related, though not identical, proteins capable of acting as antibodies. Humans have five main types.

immunotherapy Therapy producing or increasing immunity.

incidence The occurrence of a particular disease over a period of time in relationship to the entire population.

incident Any happening not consistent with the routine operation of the hospital or routine care of a particular patient.

incisional biopsy The act of cutting into tissue to remove part of the tumor so that a diagnosis can be made.

incubation The time interval between exposure to infection and the appearance of the first sign or symptom characteristic of the disease.

infiltration A swelling around the injection site accompanied by cool, pale skin and possibly hard patches or localized pain.

informed consent An assurance that the purpose, benefit, risk, and any alternative options have been explained and understood and a disclaimer (which will not always hold up in court) releasing the caregiver and facility from liability if complications develop or the treatment fail.

interdisciplinary All the disciplines cooperating in the management of the disease process, as in the cancer-management team.

interlocks Safety switches blocking or terminating radiation production.

interstitial radiation therapy The insertion of radioactive sources into the tissue to treat the disease.

intracavitary radiation therapy The insertion of radioactive sources into naturally occurring body cavities to treat the disease.

intradermal A shallow injection between the layers of the skin.

intramuscular A 90-degree injection into the muscle. It is used for large amounts or quick systemic effect.

intravenous An injection directly into the bloodstream providing an immediate effect.

invasion of privacy Revealing confidential information or improperly and unnecessarily exposing a patient's body.

ionic contrast media Media having high osmolality or a high number of particles in isolation. The large amount of iodine provides greater contrast but also increases toxicity and viscosity. Meglumine iodine salts and various sodium iodine salts are the most common ionic iodides used.

ionizing radiation The ejection of an electron from an atom, thus resulting in a charged particle or ion.

iridium A radioactive isotope with a half life of 74 days. It is used in wire form for interstitial brachytherapy.

irradiated volume The volume of tissue receiving a significant dose (e.g., > 50%) of the specified target dose.

isocenter The point of intersection of the three axes of rotation (gantry, collimator, and base of couch) of the treatment unit.

isodose curve The plotted percentage depth dose at various points in the beam along the central axis and elsewhere.

isodose lines Lines connecting points of equivalent relative radiation dose.

justice The quality of being just, impartial, or fair; treatment that is fair or adequate.

Karnofsky score A standardized numerical rating scale that describes the performance status of the patient. A patient is assigned a numerical value from 0 to 100 depending on daily functionality.

kilovoltage units Equipment carrying out external-beam treatment by using x-rays generated at voltages up to 500 kVp.

kilovolts peak (kVp) Unit of measurement for x-ray voltages. (1 kV equals 1000 V of electrical potential.)

kwashiorkor Protein malnutrition that includes an adequate intake of carbohydrates and fats but an inadequate intake of protein.

LD$_{50/30}$ The lethal effect of acute whole-body exposure, in which 50% of the total population exposed is effected in 30 days.

law of Bergonié and Tribondeau The law stating that ionizing radiation is more effective against cells that are (1) actively mitotic, (2) undifferentiated, and (3) having a long mitotic future.

legal concepts The sum of artificial rules and regulations by which society is governed in any formal and legally binding manner.

legal ethics The study of the law mandating certain acts and forbidding others under penalty of criminal sanction.

leukopenia A decrease in the peripheral white blood count, thus increasing the risk of infection for the cancer patient.

libel Written defamation of character.

licensure A process by which an agency or government grants permission to an individual to work in a specific occupation after finding the individual has attained the minimal degree of competency to ensure the health and safety of the public.

life experiences Information gathered through a normal day's activity and useful for enhancing an existing cognitive knowledge base. Life experiences can be used to promote knowledge and elevate functionality.

linear accelerator A radiation therapy treatment unit that accelerates electrons and produces x-rays or electrons for treatment.

linear energy transfer (LET) The rate at which energy is deposited by charged particles (incident or secondary) as they travel through matter.

localization The geometrical definition of the tumor and anatomical structures using anatomical or surface marks for reference.

lysosome A membranous sac containing hydrolytic enzymes and found in the cellular cytoplasm. It functions in intracellular digestion.

marasmus Calorie malnutrition that is observed in patients who are slender or slightly underweight and characterized by weight loss of 7% to 10% and fat and muscle depletion.

medical record All components used to document chronologically the care and treatment rendered to a patient.

megavoltage equipment Units using x-ray beams of energy 1 MeV or greater.

melanoma A dark pigmented malignant tumor arising from the skin.

metastasis The transmission of a disease from an original site to one or more sites elsewhere in the body.

milliamperes (mA) Units of measurement for x-ray currents in which the ampere (A) is a measure of electrical current.

mitochondria A cytoplasmic organelle serving as the site of cellular respirations and energy production.

mitosis Indirect cell division involving the nucleus and cell body.

monoclonal antibody An antibody derived from hybridoma cells that can be used to identify tumor antigens.

moral ethics The study of right and wrong as it relates to conscience, God, a higher being, or a person's logical rationalization.

multidisciplinary The use of several disciplines at the same time.

mutation Change; transformation.

myelosuppression A reduction in bone marrow function.

negligence The neglect or omission of reasonable care or caution.

neutrons Neutral subatomic particles used for the treatment of some cancers.

nonionic contrast media Media having low osmolality. The iodides remain intact instead of splitting; therefore they agitate the cells less. These agents are equally effective but cost much more than ionic agents.

nonmaleficence Not doing wrong or harm to an individual.

nosocomial Infection acquired in a hospital.

nuclear membrane The membranous envelope enclosing the nucleus and separating it from the cytoplasm.

nucleoli A rounded internuclear organelle serving as the site of construction of the ribosomes.

nucleoside A compound composed of a nitrogenous base and a five-carbon sugar. With the addition of a phosphate group, a nucleoside becomes a nucleotide.

nucleotide A compound composed of a nitrogenous base, five-carbon sugar, and phosphate group. Nucleotides are the basic building blocks of the nucleic acids RNA and DNA.

nucleus A conspicuous cytoplasmic organelle containing most of the genetic material (a small amount is located in the mitochondria) and nucleolus.

Occupational Safety and Health Administration (OSHA) An administrative regulatory agency requiring employers to ensure the safety of workers.

oncogene Genetic material with the potential to cause cancer.

organelle One of many membrane-bound particles suspended in the cytoplasm of cells and having specialized functional characteristics.

orthovoltage therapy (deep therapy) Treatments using x-rays produced at potentials ranging from 150 to 500 kV.

osmolality A property of a solution that depends on the concentration of the solute per unit of solvent.

oxygen-enhancement ratio (OER) The comparison of the response of cells to radiation in the presence and absence of oxygen:

$$OER = \frac{\text{Radiation dose under hypoxic /anoxic conditions}}{\text{Radiation dose under oxic conditions to produce the same biological effect}}$$

palliation The objective of radiation therapy when the disease has reached the stage that a cure is no longer possible.

paraneoplastic syndrome A syndrome that arises from the metabolic consequences of cancer on tissues far from the cancer site.

parenteral Medication bypassing the gastrointestinal tract. Taken literally, this would include the topical and some mucous membrane routes, but the word has come colloquially to mean "by injection."

pathogenicity The ability of an infectious agent to cause disease.

penumbra An area or region at the beam's edge where the radiation intensity falls to 0.

peroxisome An intracellular enzyme-containing body that participates in the metabolic oxidation of various substrates.

pharmacodynamics The way drugs affect the body.

pharmacokinetics The way drugs travel through the body to their receptor sites.

pharmocology The science of drugs and their sources, chemistry, and actions.

phlebitis Inflammation of a vein.

polypeptide A chain of many amino acids linked by peptide bonds. Polypeptides are the subunits of proteins.

portal verification The documentation of treatment portals through radiographic images or electronic portal imaging devices.

priestly model A model that provides the caregiver with a godlike, paternalist attitude by making decisions *for* the patient and not *with* the patient.

prognosis The estimation of life expectancy.

proliferation The rapid and repeated reproduction of a new part (e.g., through cell division).

prospective A study in which the theory of the cause of a condition or disease is tested by examining those who have a particular characteristic or trait. The population to be examined is selected in the beginning of the study.

protein A complex biological compound composed of amino acids. Linked together in a genetically determined, three-dimensional sequence, 20 different amino acids are commonly found in proteins.

protocols Treatment regimens based on clinical or scientific hypotheses and designed to compare the results of different methods of treatment for the same disease.

protraction The time over which total dose is to be delivered.

psychosocial Psychological support of the patient during the course of disease, with the recognition that social aspects of the treatment and disease prognosis may require special care.

quality of life A person's subjective sense of well-being derived from current experience of life as a whole.

quality-assurance (QA) program A series of activities and documentation performed with the goal of optimizing patient care.

radiation therapy domain The confines of the radiation therapy department and the socialization that takes place inside. It is a limited physical environment in which a wide sampling of ethnicity gathers daily and creates a miniature society in which many social interactions occur among clusters of patients and between patients and staff members.

radioactive decay The process of an unstable nuclei emitting radiation.

radiographic cassette A holder for radiographic film used in portal imaging or simulation.

radiolysis The initial event in the radiolysis (splitting) of water involves the ionization of a water molecule, thus producing a water ion.

radiopaque marker A material with a high atomic number used to document structures radiographically.

radioprotectors Certain chemicals and drugs that diminish the response of cells to radiation.

radiosensitizers Certain chemicals and drugs that enhance the response of cells to radiation.

random error Variation in individual treatment setup.

randomization A method by which patients are blindly assigned to participate in specific portions of a protocol called an *arm.* The use of randomization ensures an equitable distribution of patients in each arm without prejudices that can later be blamed for unfair patient selection and can be detrimental to the outcome of the trial.

randomize To make random for scientific experimentation.

recombinant DNA technology (genetic engineering) Techniques that facilitate the manipulation and duplication of pieces of DNA.

Reed-Sternberg cells Cells characterized by large, abnormal, multinucleated cells.

rehabilitation The dynamic process with the goal of enabling persons to function at their maximal level within the limitations of their disease or disability in terms of physical, mental, emotional, social, and economic potential.

relative biological effectiveness (RBE)

$$RBE = \frac{\text{Dose from 250 keV x-ray}}{\text{Dose from test radiation to produce the same biological effect}}$$

reproductive failure A decrease in the reproductive integrity or the ability of a cell to undergo an infinite number of divisions after radiation.

retrospective A study of a group of individuals all having the same disease and common characteristics that might have caused the disease.

ribosome An organelle constructed in the nucleolus and concerned with protein synthesis in the cytoplasm.

risk management The process of avoiding or controlling the risk of financial loss to the staff members and hospital or medical center.

sarcoma A malignancy arising from other than epithelial tissues of the body.

scientific revival The intellectual resurgence of the sixteenth century.

scope of practice The body of courses and formally established learning experiences presenting the knowledge, principles, values, and skills that are the intended consequences of formal education; the defining document to guide radiation therapists through the day-to-day responsibilities of the profession.

separation The measurement of the thickness of a patient along the central axis or at any other specified point in the irradiated volume.

shielding block Field-shaping material that reduces beam transmission to less than 5% of the original intensity.

simulation A process carried out by the radiation therapist under the supervision of the radiation oncologist. It is the mock-up procedure of a patient treatment with radiographic documentation of the treatment portals.

simulators Radiographic x-ray units that mimic all the movements and parameters of the treatment units. They are used for imaging the target volume during treatment planning.

skin squames Superficial skin cells that serve as vehicles for airborne pathogens.

slander Oral defamation of character.

source head The housing for shielding that contains the device for positioning the cobalt 60 source.

stratified Segregate populations according to certain specific characteristics.

subcutaneous injection A 45- or 90-degree injection into the subcutaneous tissue just below the skin.

superficial therapy Treatment with x-rays produced at potentials ranging from 50 to 150 kV.

Surveillance, Epidemiology, and End Results (SEER) program A program initiated in 1973 to collect data in an effort to determine the epidemiology and etiology of cancer.

systemic error Variation in the translation of the treatment setup from the simulator to the treatment unit.

target volume An area of a known and presumed tumor.

TD$_{5/5}$ The tolerance of normal tissue where a tissue dose is associated with a 5% complication rate within 5 years.

TD$_{50/5}$ The tolerance of normal tissue where a tissue dose is associated with a 50% complication rate within 5 years.

thrombocytopenia A reduction in the number of circulating platelets.

titers A measurement of the number of specific antibodies in a person's body or blood specimen.

tolerance The body's adaptation to a particular drug and requirement of ever greater doses to achieve the desired effect.

tort law The type of law that governs rights between individuals in noncriminal actions. This law deals with violations of civil as opposed to criminal law.

transcription The process resulting in the transfer of genetic information from a molecule of DNA to a molecule of RNA.

translation The process resulting in the construction of a polypeptide in accordance with genetic information contained in a molecule of RNA.

transmission filters Filters that allow the transmission of a predetermined percentage of the treatment beam.

travel time The length of time for a cobalt 60 source to advance and retract.

treatment console The operating center where timers and system-monitoring indicators are displayed.

treatment field (portal) The volume exposed to radiation from a single radiation beam.

treatment volume Generally larger than the target volume, the treatment volume encompasses the additional margins around the target volume to allow for limitations of the treatment technique.

tuberculin skin test (Mantoux test) An intradermal injection of purified protein derivative (PPD) or tuberculin used to test for exposure to tuberculosis.

tumor registry A tracking mechanism for cancer incidence, characteristics, management, and results in cancer-treatment facilities for patients diagnosed with cancer.

tumoricidal dose A dose high enough to eradicate the tumor.

tumor-suppressor gene A gene whose presence and proper function produces normal cellular growth and division. The absence or inactivation of such a gene leads to uncontrolled growth or neoplasia.

universal precautions The method of infection control in which any human blood or body fluid is treated as if it were known to be infectious.

urticaria Hives.

vacuole A membrane-bound cavity in the cytoplasm of a cell having a variety of storage, secretory, and metabolic functions.

Van de Graaff generator An electrostatic accelerator designed to accelerate charged particles. In radiation therapy procedures the unit produces high-energy x-rays typically at 2 MeV.

vector An animal, usually an arthropod, that carries and transmits a pathogen capable of causing disease.

venipuncture Puncture of a vein.

verification simulation A final check that each of the planned treatment beams covers the tumor or target volume and does not irradiate normal tissue structures.

virtue ethics The use of practical wisdom for emotional and intellectual problem solving.

virulence The relative power of a pathogen to cause disease. Severity expressed in terms of *morbidity* and *mortality*.

wedge A beam modifier that changes the angle of the isodose curves. The angle is defined relative to the horizontal plane at depth.

wipe test A test done to evaluate the contamination or leakage of a sealed radioactive source.

x-rays Electromagnetic radiation that is produced when a fast electron stream hits a target. The energy of the resultant x-ray beam increases with the voltage that accelerates the electrons.

Answers to Review Questions

CHAPTER 1

1. Cellular differentiation
2. Antioncogenes
3. Sarcomas
4. Carcinomas
5. Tumor staging
6. a. Anatomical site
   b. Cell of origin
   c. Biological behavior
7. a. Age
   b. Culture
   c. Support system
   d. Education
   e. Family background
8. a. Surgery
   b. Radiation therapy
   c. Chemotherapy
   d. Immunotherapy

CHAPTER 2

1. c
2. b
3. d
4. a
5. c
6. c
7. c
8. b
9. d
10. a

CHAPTER 3

1. a
2. d
3. c
4. b
5. d
6. d
7. c
8. c
9. True
10. True

CHAPTER 4

1. b
2. d
3. a
4. d
5. a
6. c
7. c
8. b

CHAPTER 5

1. a
2. c
3. d
4. b
5. b

CHAPTER 6

1. a. IV
   b. I
   c. III
   d. II
   e. IV
2. a. III
   b. I
   c. III
   d. II
   e. II
   f. I
3. d
4. a
5. d
6. a. False
   b. False
   c. True
   d. True
   e. False
   f. False
   g. True
   h. True
   i. False
   j. False
7. Adenine, guanine, thymine, and cytosine; adenine, guanine, uracil, and cytosine
8. A five-carbon sugar, a nitrogenous base, and a phosphate group; a five-carbon sugar and a nitrogenous base.
9. Exfoliative cytology, needle aspiration, and open biopsy

CHAPTER 7

1. Teamwork
2. Tumor
3. Regional
4. a
5. b

CHAPTER 8

1. c
2. c
3. d
4. a
5. a
6. e
7. S phase
8. Daunorubicin and doxorubicin
9. Combination

CHAPTER 9

1. b
2. c
3. d
4. a
5. c

CHAPTER 10

1. c
2. b
3. a
4. c
5. a

CHAPTER 11

1. d
2. c
3. c
4. a
5. c
6. d
7. c
8. d
9. d
10. b

CHAPTER 12

1. e
2. b
3. b
4. b
5. b
6. b
7. d

CHAPTER 13

1. c
2. b
3. c
4. b
5. a
6. b

CHAPTER 14

1. b
2. b
3. b
4. a
5. b
6. a

CHAPTER 15

1. Adequate dosage could not reach deep-seated tumors, and normal tissues were not spared.
2. Inferior
3. Aluminum filter
4. Cyclotron
5. Magnetic field
6. d
7. b
8. c
9. a
10. e
11. d
12. a
13. c
14. b

CHAPTER 16

1. d
2. b
3. b
4. a
5. c
6. a
7. b
8. b
9. d
10. a

CHAPTER 17

1. Formal classroom education or life experiences
2. 1964
3. ARRT, JRCERT, and ASRT
4. Didactic and clinical
5. Do-not-resuscitate order, living will, and health care proxy
6. Verbal or nonverbal
7. Advocate
8. Community education
9. A direct link to a specific cancer and effective clinical or pathological examinations
10. 1992

CHAPTER 18

1. Epidemiology
2. Carrier
3. OSHA
4. TB and hepatitis C
5. Acid fast bacilli
6. Incubation, clinical illness, and convalescense
7. Ethlene oxide
8. The presence or absence of moisture and the distance they can travel
9. Notify the employer who is then obligated to provide hypoallegenic gloves or other suitable solution
10. Household bleach; to clean up blood or other body fluids
11. Testing positive for a disease at a later date after first testing negative immediately after exposure

CHAPTER 19

1. Assessment is a dynamic and continuous process that involves listening and hearing the concerns of patients at the physical, psychological, emotional, and spiritual levels. It should include the determination of the problem, the selection of an intervention, and the evaluation of effectiveness.
2. Cognitive content includes the actual facts and words of the message.
   Example: "I only slept 2 hours last night."
3. Affective content involves the feelings, attitudes, and behaviors behind the words. It can be verbal or nonverbal.
   Example: "While you were awake, what kinds of things were going through your mind?"
4. *Empathy* is defined as identifying with the feelings, thoughts, or experiences of another person.
5. The ten most common verbal responses in reflective listening are minimal verbal response, reflecting, paraphrasing, probing, clarifying, interpreting, checking out, informing, confronting, and summarizing.
6. The daily assessment responsibilities of radiation therapists are as follows (complete answers on a chart titled "Components of Daily Physical Assessment"):
   Skin reactions—Monitor and give lotion instructions.
   Fatigue—Assess, probe reasons, and counsel.
   Sleep—Assess and evaluate patterns.
   Mouth changes—Inspect and instruct regarding diet.
   Pharyngitis and esophagitis—Evaluate pain, diet, and medication.
   Diarrhea—Assess bowel function, instruct regarding a low-residue diet, and check medications.
   Cystitis—Assess bladder function, infections, and medication.
   Nausea and vomiting—Assess antiemetic use and diet, and use visual imagery if needed.
   Alopecia—Instruct regarding the care of the scalp, and address body-image issues if needed.
   Pain—Assess the location and intensity of the pain, and evaluate the administration of medications.
   Skin pallor—Monitor CBC counts.
   Weight loss—Weigh weekly, monitor daily eating, and offer helpful suggestions.
7. Weight loss is often the first physical change indicating the possibility of cancer.
8. *Cachexia* is a state of general ill health and malnutrition with early satiety, electrolyte and water imbalances, and progressive loss of body weight, fat, and muscle.
9. The duration and pattern of pain are the two most important characteristics of the etiology of pain.
10. *Leukopenia* is a decrease in the white blood cell count, which increases the risk of infection.
11. The major symptoms of depression are changes in appetitie, sleep disturbances, lack of energy, withdrawal, reduced ability to concentrate, indecisiveness, and suicidal ideas.
12. • Recognize that cultural diversity exists.
    • Respect persons as uniqe individuals.
    • Evaluate your own cultural beliefs.
    • Be willing to modify health care delivery to honor the client's beliefs.
    • Do not expect every person in a culture to behave in exactly the same way.

Answers to Exercise for Recognizing and Identifying the Types of Major Verbal Responses
1. Reflecting
2. Paraphrasing
3. Probing
4. Informing
5. Summarizing
6. Checking out
7. Interpreting
8. Clarifying
9. Confronting
10. Minimal verbal response

Answers to Exercise for Listening for Feelings
1. Fear of illness or pleasure of attention from physician
2. Anxiety about the new social worker or excitement about meeting her
3. Discouragement or fear of not responding to treatment
4. Fear of rejection or loneliness
5. Anticipation of being finished or fear of losing the support that "doing something" gives

CHAPTER 20

1. Right patient, right drug, right dose, right time, and right route
2. c
3. c
4. b
5. d
6. c
7. b
8. a. V
   b. IV
   c. XI
   d. I
   e. X
   f. IX
   g. II
9. The discharge or escape of blood or fluid into tissues
10. Side effects are physiological responses to a medication other than the desired response. Most drugs produce some side effects in some patients. Complications are unexpected reactions to medications and can range from mild to severe.

Index

362